CHITOSAN-BASED HYDROGELS

*Functions
and
Applications*

CHITOSAN-BASED HYDROGELS

Functions
and
Applications

Edited by
Kangde Yao • Junjie Li
Fanglian Yao • Yuji Yin

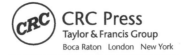

CRC Press
Taylor & Francis Group
Boca Raton London New York

CRC Press is an imprint of the
Taylor & Francis Group, an **informa** business

CRC Press
Taylor & Francis Group
6000 Broken Sound Parkway NW, Suite 300
Boca Raton, FL 33487-2742

First issued in paperback 2017

© 2012 by Taylor & Francis Group, LLC
CRC Press is an imprint of Taylor & Francis Group, an Informa business

No claim to original U.S. Government works
Version Date: 20110602

ISBN 13: 978-1-138-07684-6 (pbk)
ISBN 13: 978-1-4398-2114-5 (hbk)

Visit the Taylor & Francis Web site at
http://www.taylorandfrancis.com

and the CRC Press Web site at
http://www.crcpress.com

Contents

Preface

Chitosan is a deacetylated derivative of chitin, which is an abundant marine resource that can be obtained from the shells of shrimps or crabs. Chemically, it is a linear polysaccharide composed of randomly distributed β-(1–4)-linked D-glucosamine (deacetylated unit) and N-acetyl-D-glucosamine (acetylated unit). It is a unique natural base polysaccharide whose structural units are similar to those of glycosaminoglycans of the extracellular matrix (ECM). As a result, chitosan has the advantage of being multiply bioactive, which can be taken advantage of in constructing biomaterials of different applications. At the same time, a large number of active hydroxyl and amino groups are available within chitosan molecules. In order to produce various chitosan derivatives, these groups can be set as target sites for chemical modification. Chitosan molecules undergo different types of degradation reactions that result in different degradation products with different molecular weights, some of which will take part in the synthesis of ECM. To optimize the physical, mechanical, and biological properties of these materials, different kinds of chitosan networks are designed and produced, resulting in chitosan-based biomaterials. These biomaterials are used to make a variety of medicines, drug controlled-release carrier, tissue-engineering scaffolds, and immobilized enzymes. With the development of stem-cell technology, chitosan-based biomaterials are also used as scaffolds for stem cells, which will regulate the proliferation and differentiation of cells. Today, more and more papers and patents on chitosan-based materials are emerging. However, very few of these materials can be merchandised, which means that more work needs to be done to fill the gap between research and production. Recognizing this situation, the authors try to summarize progress in the research and development of chitosan-based biomaterials, which they think will not only inspire those who contribute to the research and development of chitosan-based biomaterials, but will also provide the basis for future research.

Kangde Yao and Junjie Li

Contributors

Liandong Deng
School of Chemical Engineering and
    Technology
Tianjin University
Tianjin, People's Republic of China

Xigang Leng
Institute of Biomedical Engineering
Chinese Academy of Medical
    Sciences and Peking Union
    Medical College
Tianjin, People's Republic of China

Junjie Li
Tissue Engineering Research Center
Academy of Military Medical
    Sciences
Beijing, People's Republic of China

and

School of Chemical Engineering and
    Technology
Tianjin University
Tianjin, People's Republic of China

Jian Shen
College of Chemistry and Environment
    Science
Nanjing Normal University
Nanjing, People's Republic of China

Dayong Teng
China National Offshore Oil Corp
    (CNOOC)
Tianjin Chemical Research and Design
    Institute
Tianjin, People's Republic of China

Changyong Wang
Tissue Engineering Research Center
Academy of Military Medical
    Sciences
Beijing, People's Republic of China

Kang Wang
School of Chemical Engineering and
    Technology
Tianjin University
Tianjin, People's Republic of China

Yuliang Xiao
College of Pharmaceutical Sciences
Taishan Medical University
Taian, People's Republic of China

Fanglian Yao
School of Chemical Engineering and
    Technology
Tianjin University
Tianjin, People's Republic of China

Kangde Yao
Research Institute of Polymeric
    Materials
Tianjin University
Tianjin, People's Republic of China

Yuji Yin
School of Material Science and Engineering
Tianjin University
Tianjin, People's Republic of China

Jin Zhao
School of Material Science and
    Engineering
Tianjin University
Tianjin, People's Republic of China

Lianyin Zheng
Institute of Biological Engineering
Zhejiang University
Hangzhou, People's Republic of China

Aiping Zhu
College of Chemistry and Chemical
    Engineering
Yangzhou University
Yang Zhou, People's Republic of China

Dunwan Zhu
Institute of Biomedical Engineering
Chinese Academy of Medical Sciences
    and Peking Union Medical College
Tianjin, People's Republic of China

Jiangfeng Zhu
Qingdao Institute of Bioenergy and
    Bioprocess Technology
Chinese Academy of Sciences
Qingdao, People's Republic of China

1

From Chitin to Chitosan

Dayong Teng

CONTENTS

1.1 Chitin

1.1.1 Discovery and Origin

Chitosan usually exists in nature as chitin, which is a natural macromolecular compound, namely, a polysaccharide formed by connecting N-acetyl-2-amino-2-deoxy-D-glucoses through β-(1,4) glycoside bonds. The structural formula of chitosan is shown in Figure 1.1. Chitosan is formed when some acetyls are removed from chitin. Usually, products with over 60% deacetylation degree (DD) or that can be dissolved in dilute acid are called chitosan.

In 1811, H. Braconnot, a French professor of natural science history, repeatedly treated mushroom with a warm dilute alkali solution and finally harvested white fibroid residues [1]. He believed that they were celluloses from mushroom and named the residues fungine. In 1823, another French scientist, A. Order, separated the same substance from the elytra of beetles. He named the compound chitin because he thought that the compound was a new cellulose. In 1843, J. L. Lassaigne found that chitin contains nitrogen, which proved that chitin is not a cellulose, but a new compound with fiber quality. In 1878 glucosamine and acetic acid in chitin were identified by G. Ledderhose through hydrolysis, and in 1894 E. Gilson further proved that chitin contains glucosamine. Later research showed that chitin is formed by polymerizing N-acetylglucosamine.

In 1859, a Frenchman, C. Rouget, boiled chitin in a concentrated alkali solution for a while and found that the product can dissolve in organic acid after washing it [2]. In 1894, F. Hoppe-Seiler confirmed that the product is deacetylated chitin and therefore named it chitosan.

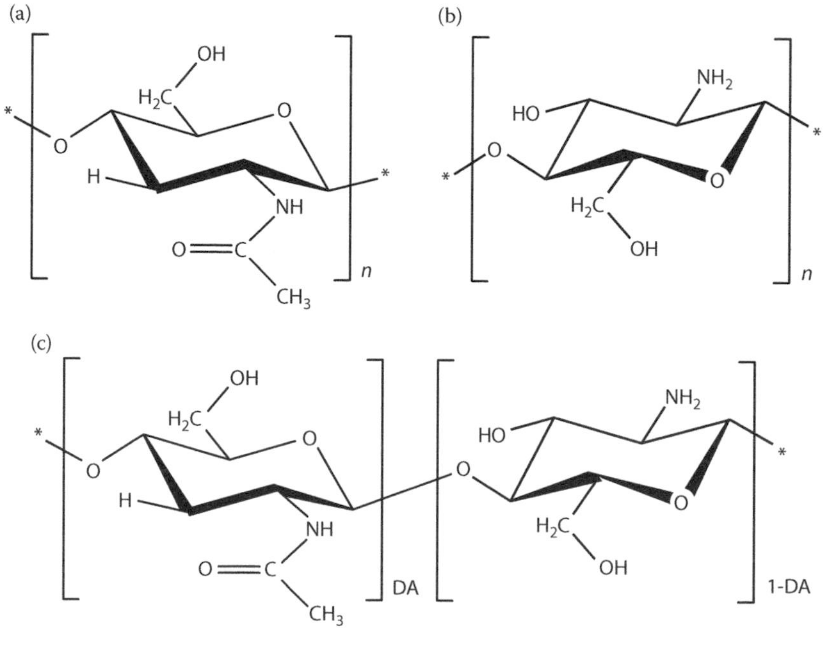

FIGURE 1.1
Chemical structure of (a) chitin and (b) chitosan repeat units. (c) Structure of partially acetylated chitosan, a copolymer characterized by its average degree of acetylation DA.

1.1.2 Existence

As a natural organic compound, cellulose content is the largest on Earth, followed by chitin content. Cellulose is produced from plants and chitin is produced from animals. It is estimated that approximately 10 billion tons of chitin can be biosynthesized in nature each year. Chitin is also a natural nitrogen-containing organic compound with the largest content on Earth, except for protein. Sources of chitin are the following.

1. Arthropods: the primary source is crustacea such as shrimp and crab whose chitin contents are 58–85%, and the secondary source is insects (e.g., locust, butterfly, mosquito, fly, and silkworm chrysalis) whose chitin contents are 20–60%, and myriapods and arachnids.

2. Molluscs include amphineura, gasteropods, scaphopoda, lamellibranch, and cephalopods whose chitin contents are 3–26%.

3. Annelids include archiannelida, chaetopoda, and hirudinea, some of which contain little chitin whereas others contain 20–38% chitin.

4. Protozoans, namely unicellular animals, include mastigophora, sarcodina, sporozoa, and ciliatea, which contain a little chitin.

5. Coelenterates include hydrozoa, scyphozoa, and actinozoa, some of which contain little chitin while others contain 3–30% chitin.

6. Seaweed: the primary source is green algae, which contains just a little chitin.

7. Fungi include ascomycetes, basidiomycetes, and phycomycetes whose chitin contents are from trace to 45% chitin. Only a few fungi do not contain chitin.

8. Others include rigid parts of animal joints, hoofs, and feet and joints of muscles and bones.

All the chitins found in nature exist as complex compounds rather than as separated or alone. In the shells of insects and the exoskeletons of molluscs, chitins combine with proteins to harden the cuticles of insects by cross-linking with polyhydric phenol. In fungi, chitins combine with other polysaccharides such as cellulose [3].

Chitins can be divided into α-, β-, and γ-chitins due to hydrogen bonds. α-Chitin comprises two antiparallel polysaccharide chains. β-Chitin comprises two parallel polysaccharide chains. γ-Chitin comprises three parallel polysaccharide chains, two of which are in the same direction. α-Chitin is the most stable one; thus it has the largest content, and the other two types can transform into α-chitin if conditions permit. Different configurations lead to different functions. α-Chitin can be found in parts with high hardness (e.g., the cuticle of arthropods) and usually combines with shell protein or inorganic compounds. γ-Chitin and β-chitin exist in soft and firm parts. All the three chitins can be found in inkfish: α-chitin forming a thin esophageal epithelium in the stomach, β-chitin forming the skeleton, and γ-chitin forming a thick esophageal epithelium in the stomach [4].

1.1.3 General Situation of Research and Production

Between 1811 (when chitin was first identified) and 1910, there were only 20 research papers on chitin and chitosan in the literature. In the 1930s, the very first patent for industrial preparation of chitosan and a patent for the preparation of chitosan film and chitosan fiber were issued in the United States, which had promoted research on chitin and chitosan. But chitin and chitosan did not attract research attention until the 1970s. In 1977, scientists began to be attracted by this resource due to the first monograph of Professor Muzzarelli from Cambridge University and the First International Conference on Chitin and Chitosan [5]. The *First International Conference on Chitin and Chitosan* was held in Boston from April 11, 1977 to April 13, 1977, and scientists from the United States, the former Soviet Union, Japan, Norway, Canada, South Africa, Belgium, Britain, Nigeria, India, Italy, and Chile attended this conference. During the conference 47 reports were submitted, which focused on distribution of chitin and chitosan in nature, the separation method, properties, and applications in different fields, especially application of chitin and chitosan in wastewater treatment. This conference was a milestone in the research, development, and applications of chitin and chitosan.

Thereafter, many countries started to provide investments, resources, and labor power for research and industrial applications of chitin and chitosan. During this period, Japan had made great achievements in research and applications [6]. Many of their findings were advanced. Moreover, other countries and regions such as China, Korea, Singapore, and Thailand also had some valuable findings in research. From then on, China began to play an increasingly important role in research in Asia and the world.

In October 1996, the Chinese Chemical Society held the first *China Chemical and Application Symposium on Chitin* in Dalian, opening Chinese chitin/chitosan academic exchanges. In November 1997, the *Chitin Resources Research and Development Seminar* was held in Qingdao. In October 1999, the Chinese Chemical Society held the second *China Chemical and Application Symposium on Chitin* in Wuhan, and during the meeting, the Chinese Chemical Chitin Seminar was formally established. In 2001, the third *China Chemical and Application Symposium on Chitin* was held in Zhejiang Yuhuan County; it was a milestone in chitin/chitosan research. Then, in 2004, the fourth *China Chemical and Application Symposium on Chitin* was held in Guangxi Beihai. In 2006, the fifth *China Chemical and Application Symposium on Chitin* held in Nanjing had a profound influence, and in order to confirm the need for developing and promoting application research, the meeting was renamed the fifth *Chinese Chemical Society Chitin Chemical Biology and Application Technology Symposium*. From the contents of the papers presented at the conference, fundamental research and innovation achievements significantly increased, and the number of young researchers increased significantly, indicating a vigorous development period for Chinese chitin/chitosan research. In June 2006, the Chinese Chemical Society professional committee on chitin, the Chinese Society of Biotechnology professional committee on sugar biotechnology, and the Chinese Society of Oceanography professional committee on marine bioengineering sponsored a chitin and its derivatives conference in Qingdao, and more than 30 experts leading research on chitin/chitosan made a congress report. From the report, research on medicine and biological materials has become a focus, indicating that chitin/chitosan have a wide range of potential applications in nanobiomaterials, bioactive materials, and environmental-friendly functional materials.

Since 1977 when the first *International Conference on Chitin and Chitosan* was held in Boston, another 10 conferences on the same topic have been held. The eighth, ninth, and tenth conferences held in Japan, Canada, and France, respectively, were greatly enhanced in scale, number of attendees, and topics, reflecting that scientists highly value chitin and chitosan. Several monographs on chitin and chitosan were also published abroad [7–9].

Over the last 10 years, chemical modification methods of chitin/chitosan have improved a lot owing to the development of environment-friendly functional materials and subjects merging. The modifications not only helped research on the structure–activity relationship, but also contributed to the development of special functional polymer materials. Chitin and chitosan relevant research and product development are in full swing now.

An upsurge of interest in chitin/chitosan and their derivatives has swept the globe, and thus many countries are putting more efforts into relevant research and development. Since 2000, the number of research papers on chitin/chitosan has been increasing linearly. These usually concentrate on the application of chitin/chitosan and their composites in biomedical fields such as tissue engineering, gene vectors, and drug carriers, which indicates that chitin/chitosan and their derivatives are important in the research and application of biomaterial in the twenty-first century.

Now, in industrial preparation, chitin is formed by removing calcium carbonates and proteins from waste shrimp shells and crab shells from aquatic product factories by steeping them in acid and alkali solutions. This technique has many inherent shortcomings; for instance, the raw materials are hard to collect, preserve, and transport owing to limitations of location and season; resources of raw material are very different; the quality of products can hardly be controlled; and large amounts of calcium carbonate in the shells make extraction of chitin difficult, which increases cost and generates plenty of wastewater [10]. Therefore, new chitin resources have drawn a lot of attention: for example, various insects that are abundant in nature such as pine moth [11], myiasis [12], silkworm chrysalis [13], and cicada slough [14].

1.2 Deacetylation

Chitosan can be harvested by removing acetyls from chitin, but to eliminate all acetyls is not easy. Chitosan can be made by a chemical method or an enzyme method. Chitosans available in the market are formed by removing acetyls from chitin through strong base hydrolysis. The equation is shown in Figure 1.2.

1.2.1 Chemical Method

The chemical method for preparing chitosan includes the alkali fusion method, the concentrated alkali solution method, the alkali catalysis method, and the hydrazine hydrate method. The main performance indexes of chitosan are DD and relative molecular weight or viscosity. To date, quite a few researchers have studied chitosan preparation and have made significant achievements [15,16]. Research findings on the extraction process of chitosan from shrimp and crab shells are shown in Figure 1.3.

The alkali fusion method is used in the early period, comprising the following steps: fusing chitin and solid potassium hydroxide directly in a nickel crucible, melting them at

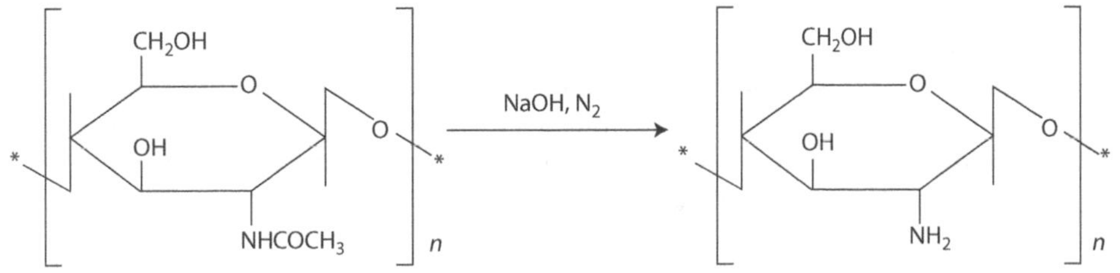

FIGURE 1.2
Preparation of chitosan by base hydrolysis of chitin.

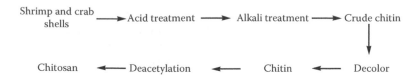

FIGURE 1.3
Preparation process of chitosan.

180°C for 30 min under nitrogen protection, transferring the mixture into ethanol solvent to form gelatinous depositions, washing the depositions with water to neutral pH in order to form rough chitosan, dissolving the rough product in 5% formic acid, neutralizing the solution by using diluted NaOH to form deposits, filtering the mixture, washing the deposits to neutral, and forming refined chitosan by repeating the said steps. The product undergoes serious main chain degradation and hence the relative molecular weight is small; also, the method is complicated. As a result, it was abandoned. The concentrated alkali solution method is the most popular one, in which raw materials react with 40–50% NaOH solution at 100–130°C for 0.5–6 h and chitosans with different DDs are generated. The concentration of alkali solution, reaction temperature, reaction time, and shape of solid chitin are closely related to DD.

The concentration of alkali solution, reaction temperature, and reaction time are the main factors affecting chitosan performance (viscosity and DD). Orthogonal experiments show that all three factors can influence the performance to varying degrees, and the most important one is NaOH concentration [17]. Considering the main quality standards of chitosan, which are viscosity and DD, the preparation method includes the following steps: mixing milled chitin with 45–50% NaOH in a weight/volume ratio of 1:10, reacting the mixture at about 90°C for 8–10 h, controlling the temperature carefully and stirring the mixture continuously during the reaction, washing the product with water to neutral, and drying the product to form white chitosan powder. To accelerate deacetylation, discontinuous water washing can be used.

In homogeneous phase, when DD is about 50%, chitosan will have good water solubility. However, when the reaction occurs in heterogeneous phase, the product is water insoluble despite 50% DD [18]. Analysis of chemical structure proves that acetamino and amino irregularly distribute in chains of the water-soluble chitosan with 50% DD, breaking molecular orderliness; that is why the product is water soluble. The water-soluble chitosan has high solubility and is alkali soluble, so that the modification reaction can be carried out in alkali conditions, expanding the range of chitosan research and application [19]. Although deacetylation in homogeneous phase can generate water-soluble chitosan, the reaction must occur in concentrated alkali solution and a large amount of solvent is needed for desalting in the late stage; therefore, this method is not applicable for industrial use.

The concentrated alkali solution method requires largely excess NaOH, which is a waste product. Organic solvent can strongly permeate chitin and help alkali enter the chitin as a diluting medium; thus organic solvent will reduce the amount of alkali while chitosan with high DD can still be formed. A batch process can form chitosan with high DD and high quality. When the reaction temperature is 60°C, acetone will produce higher DD and relative molecular weight than ethanol. However, the product is yellowish and difficult to wash when the solvent is acetone. When the reaction temperature is 80°C, water is worse than ethanol as reaction medium because it causes low DD, unsatisfactory color, and makes the product hard to wash. Therefore, ethanol is the best medium for deacetylation. Ethanol with a certain polarity and penetrability can efficiently penetrate into chitosan to increase reaction efficiency. When the reaction occurs at 80°C with ethanol as the medium for 3 h, DD can reach 90% if the weight ratio of chitosan to NaOH to ethanol is 1:3:16, while DD is 80% in the traditional method [20].

Microwave radiation heating greatly reduces alkali treatment time compared with the traditional heating technique for preparing chitosan, and makes chitosan have high DD and solubility. In 1979, Peniston tried to prepare chitosan by treating chitin with microwave radiation in the normal alkali solution method for the first time [21]. Chitosan with 85% DD can be formed by the normal alkali solution method by reacting in 50% NaOH solution at 100°C for 10 h. When microwave is used, only 80°C and 18 min are enough for chitosan with over 80% DD. The semi-dry microwave method can also be applied for chitosan preparation, comprising the following steps: uniformly mixing a concentrated alkali solution with chitin, which is milled into a certain granularity in advance to form a paste, deacetylating in a microwave oven, washing the product using hot water to neutral, steeping the product in methanol, and drying the product in vacuum to form white or yellow grains [22].

The microwave radiation greatly shortens deacetylation time and lowers energy consumption. But radiation also seriously breaks the chitin chain, making the product low in relative molecular weight. Hence the method is particularly suitable for making chitosan with high DD and low relative molecular weight. Microwave treatment increases the reactivity of chitin and the reaction rate of deacetylation; hence the reaction time is shortened and the alkali amount is reduced. It is a good way of saving material and lowering energy consumption, so that the product cost of chitosan is saved. The industrial microwave reactor will definitely bring remarkable benefits if it is developed.

The alkali solution catalysis method is suitable for chitosan with high DD and high relative molecular weight. This method uses thiophenol and dimethylsulfoxide in addition to NaOH. The thiophenol is transformed into sodium thiophenol with deoxidizing and catalytic functions in NaOH solution. Therefore, the reaction is accelerated and chain breakage is prevented. The reaction medium is an alcohol–water solution of NaOH. The phase transfer catalyst is cheap and harmless polyethylene glycol with good human compatibility (no need to remove the catalyst after reaction). The reaction condition is moderate and with high DD, which can be obtained when concentration of NaOH is 35%, reaction temperature is 90°C, reaction time is 3 h, and concentration of the phase transfer catalyst is 5%. This technique can remove protein and prevent the degradation of chitin when alkali concentration is low. It lowers acid and alkali consumption and shortens the production period [23]. But it can only be used for preparing small amounts of samples in the laboratory.

1.2.2 Enzyme Method

Chitin deacetylase can hydrolyze acetyls of chitin, and so it may replace the hot concentrated alkali method for producing high-quality chitosan. Chitin deacetylase was first found in *Mucor rouxii* of zygomycetes in 1974 [24]. Electrophoretically pure chitin deacetylase from *Mucor rouxii* with specific activity 13.33 U/mg can be formed by immune affinity chromatography, and the yield is 29.1% [25]. Chitin deacetylases from different sources differ with respect to relative molecular weight, isoelectric point, optimum pH, inhibitor, and distribution, leading to different physiological functions. The reaction mechanism of the chitin deacetylase from *Mucor rouxii* is multipoint attack mode; specifically, the enzyme systematically hydrolyzes acetyls from the nonreducing end of the binding site after it binds to a substrate chain, and then leaves the substrate and binds to another one. There is no binding tendency between the enzyme and molecular sequence of the substrate [26]. Strains that produce a large amount of extracellular deacetylase with high activity are very valuable in the production of chitin deacetylase and the production of chitosan by the catalytic method.

The chitin deacetylase method could replace the hot concentrated alkali method because it prevents serious environmental pollution, lowers energy consumption, and solves the problem that product treated with hot concentrated alkali has uneven DD and low relative molecular weight. The product formed by the enzyme method can be used for producing new functional materials. Nevertheless, there are still some problems such as low yields of deacetylase-producing strains and low enzyme activity. Moreover, natural chitins are crystals, not a good substrate for deacetylase. Hence, many preparations still need to be carried out before the chitin deacetylase method can be used in the industrial production of chitosan.

The microorganism culture method is another hotspot of chitosan research, which removes acetyls by catalyzing the substrate with enzymes produced by microorganisms. From the 1980s, Japan and the United States began to study chitosan production by microbial fermentation [27–29], followed by China from the early 1990s. Currently, the research concentrates on breeding of the strain and optimization of the culture medium. The chitosan formed by this method is similar to the chitosan from shelled animals in terms of DD and relative molecular weight, while its metal ion adsorption capacity is much higher. So the product is particularly suitable for treating heavy-metal-ion-containing wastewater. The antibacterial ability of the food preservative made of the product is 1–2 times that of the food preservative made of chitosan from shelled animals. It can be seen that the microorganism culture method has good prospects.

1.3 Control of Quality

1.3.1 Deacetylation Degree

The DD of chitosan, namely the content of free amino in chitosan chains, is a technical index of great importance. The DD of chitosan directly relates to solubility in diluted acid, viscosity, ion exchange ability, flocculability, reaction capacity with amino, and other aspects.

DD can be defined as the ratio of residues without acetyls to all residues of chitosan. Quite a few methods can be used for measuring DD, such as alkalimetry (acid–base titration [30–33], electrolytic titration [34–35], and hydrobromide titration [36]), infrared spectroscopy [37–41], refractive index [42], colloid titration [43,44], thermal analysis [45], gas chromatography [46], ultimate analysis [46], ultraviolet (UV) spectrometry [44,45], and trinitrophenol spectrophotometry [37]. The most common method is acid–base titration, followed by infrared spectroscopy and electrolytic titration.

Acid–base titration is the simplest method with good repetitiveness for measuring the content of free amino in chitosan, and does not require special instruments. This method is particularly suitable for monitoring weight during production. The mechanism is that the alkali free amino in chitosan can be protonated by acid quantification to form a chitosan colloid solution, then the dissociative hydrogen ions can be titrated by alkali, and acid combined by free amino can be figured out by the difference of acid for dissolving chitosan and alkali for titrating.

Precautions in acid–base titration are as follows: (1) To prevent the error caused by hydrochloric acid degrading the main chain of chitosan, the sample should be dissolved at room temperature and not at high temperature. (2) The higher the DD, the larger the solubility of the sample, and vice versa. Hence some samples need to be treated overnight. (3) The deacetylation is uneven, usually resulting in incomplete dissolution. If data from three measurements are very different, the sample should be measured again. (4) The sample must be neutral, or the result may be incorrect. The sample that is not neutral should be washed to neutral or the data should be corrected. (5) The influence of oxygen in the atmosphere can be ignored, and hence nitrogen protection is not necessary. (6) Obvious agglutination lowering the measured values should be prevented. (7) The color of the colloid solution with large viscosity changes slowly when the titration end point is near, and hence the operator should pay attention to the rate of titration.

DD can be measured by the absorption peak of characteristic groups in the infrared spectrum of chitosan [47]. In this method, it is not necessary to dissolve chitosan by solvent or solution, which means that the infrared spectrum can be directly obtained by using dry powder. By using a series of samples with known DDs, a standard curve can be plotted by using the absorption peak ratio of special bands such as amide I or amide II to a certain band. The DD of the tested sample can be determined by using the curve. Compared with acid–base titration, the error is larger in this method. But the infrared spectrum is more convenient and samples used in the method can be recycled. Dryness is significant to the repeatability of experimental data. Generally, the amide I peak is hardly affected by water while the amide II peak is not; hence the sample must be dried carefully. Furthermore, the sample must be ground into very fine powder, or the absorption peak will not be sharp enough, making the determination of peak height inaccurate.

Electrolytic titration has the same mechanism as acid–base titration, but is different from the end point determination method, which means that electrolytic titration uses a potential curve while acid–base titration uses a single indicator or indicator mixture [34].

Electrolytic titration comprises the following steps: dissolving chitosan in a standard hydrochloric acid solution in a small beaker, measuring the standard NaOH titration process by a potentiometric titrimeter, recording pH when 0.25–0.5 mL of NaOH is used, recording pH more frequently when the end point is near, plotting a pH–V curve by using pH as the vertical coordinate and the volume of NaOH as the horizontal ordinate, finding the volume of NaOH corresponding to the equivalent point, and calculating DD by the given formula.

There are still some disadvantages: (1) Chitosan that separates out before and after the end point may cover the electrode film, influencing the measurement of pH. (2) It is different to find out the equivalent point on the titration curve, which is usually shaped as S, causing personal error in the determination of the end point.

1.3.2 Molecular Weight

Relative molecular weights of chitin and chitosan can be measured by gel permeation chromatography [48], steam osmotic pressure method, membrane osmometry, end group method [49], viscosity measurement, light scattering method, and coupled light scattering–gel permeation chromatography. Gel permeation chromatography is applied for measuring weight-average relative molecular weight and number-average relative molecular weight. The light scattering method is applied for measuring weight-average relative molecular weight. The viscosity measurement is applied for measuring viscosity-average relative molecular weight.

The greatest advantage of high-performance liquid chromatography (HPLC) in relative molecular weight measurement is that it can absolutely measure the relative molecular weight and determine relative molecular weight distribution. Special instrument and guide samples for relative molecular weights have been developed; thus, HPLC is now a common method for measuring relative molecular weight and relative molecular weight distribution. The light scattering method is another common method, especially the coupled light scattering–gel permeation chromatography method used for absolutely measuring relative molecular weight. The end group method does not need a special device and is easy to operate; hence it is widely used. However, error in the end group method is somewhat large.

Viscosity can be measured by many methods with different physical significance. During production of chitosan, viscosity is usually measured by a rotational viscometer. The result is apparent viscosity, which means quantification of the chitosan viscosity property in using, but the molecular weight cannot be figured out through this value. Inherent viscosity can be measured by a Ubbelohde viscometer, which is the most common method for measuring the viscosity of chitosan. Inherent viscosity is apparent viscosity when the concentration of high polymer is infinitely low. High-performance capillary electrophoresis is featured with high resolution, high sensitivity, and fast separation rate, and is widely used for measuring the molecular weight of low-molecular-weight chitosan (chitosan oligosaccharide). The chain of chitosan oligosaccharides is modified by negative charges, chromophores, and fluorophores. Chitosan oligosaccharides can be separated by electrophoresis due to molecular size, because each oligosaccharide in a complex of different oligosaccharides has just one charge. The separated oligosaccharides can be identified by laser-induced fluorescence detection, and then polymerization degrees of the oligosaccharides can be determined according to peak time. The percentage of oligosaccharides of different polymerization degrees in the hydrolysate can be determined by peak areas.

1.3.3 Structure Identification

Structure identification and characterization can be carried out by paper chromatography, thin-layer chromatography (TLC), infrared absorption spectroscopy, UV absorption spectroscopy, mass spectrometry, nuclear magnetic resonance, ultimate analysis, x-ray diffraction, and free amino content (or DD) [50]. Low-molecular-weight chitosans of different polymerization degrees can be separated by a silica gel thin layer with developing solvent made of ethyl acetate, ethanol, water, and ammonia water in the ratio 5:9:1:1.5. Chromatography reproducibility of TLC and the linear relation between number of residues and Rf are good [51,52].

The configurations of glycoside bonds and the substitution state of hydroxyls and amino can be determined by the infrared spectrum. The infrared spectrum shows similar structure characterizations of high-molecular-weight chitosans and low-molecular-weight chitosans when they are pressed with KBr and scanned at 400–4000 cm^{-1}. Characteristic absorption bands such as the O–H stretching vibration absorption band at 3450 cm^{-1}, the C–H stretching vibration absorption band at 2867 cm^{-1}, and the amide absorption bands at 1665 and 1550 cm^{-1} appear in the spectrum. The low-molecular-weight chitosan shows a strong –OH absorption band at 3450 cm^{-1} due to increased hydroxyl [53].

Main peaks such as the N–H stretching vibration at about 3400 cm^{-1} and the N–H bending vibration at about 1600 cm^{-1} do not move before and after chitosan is degraded, but strengths change due to decreased molecular weight. This further confirms that the concerted reaction goes by cracking β-(1,4) glycoside bonds of chitosan, and the polysaccharide ring does not change in structure after degradation.

UV spectrometry is used for analyzing the structure of chitin. Normal polysaccharides do not have chromophores or conjugated groups. However, chitin is different; it has an acetyl on C_2 of each residue as chromophore, so that it absorbs UV.

^{1}H nuclear magnetic resonance is used for identifying the configuration of the glycoside bond in polysaccharide. Most chemical shifts δ of polysaccharide are within 4.0–5.5 ppm. Protonic signals of C_2–C_6 within 4.0–4.8 ppm are hard to analyze; only the protonic signal of C_1 within 4.8–5.5 ppm is easy to analyze. The chemical shift scope in ^{13}C nuclear magnetic resonance up to 200 ppm is much wider; thus signals can be separated, making the location determination of carbon atoms and the identification of the configuration and conformation of a molecule available. The relative height of the peak in resonance is proportional to the number of carbon atoms; hence, the percentages of different residues can be calculated according to the relative heights of peaks of different anomeric carbons. It can be concluded that ^{13}C nuclear magnetic resonance is more useful than ^{1}H nuclear magnetic resonance [50].

1.3.4 Ash Content

Ash content is an important index for the preparation of food-grade and pharmaceutical-grade chitosans and can be measured by the normal method: carbonizing chitosan in a crucible by an electric stove and igniting it by a high-temperature electric stove until weight is constant. The ash index is the ratio of the weight after igniting to the original weight. The ash content of common chitosan products is as follows: industrial grade ≤1.0, food grade ≤0.5, and medical grade ≤0.2.

1.3.5 Nitrogen Content

Both chitin and chitosan are polysaccharides containing aminos. The theoretical nitrogen content of chitin with all N-acetyls, aminos, and acetaminos and without crystal water is 6.9%. The theoretical nitrogen content of chitosan that has 100% DD and is not deaminated is 8.7%. Nondeamidation is emphasized because wet fresh shrimp and crab shells will automatically deaminate due to microbes after exposure to air for 1 week, just like protein. Therefore, DD of the sample not undergoing deamidation can be found in Table 1.1 after measuring nitrogen content, and the known DD of the sample can be found as well.

Nitrogen content can be determined by the Kjedahl method, like protein. This method comprises the following steps: damaging organic compounds in the sample by sulfuric acid and transforming nitrogen-containing compounds into ammonium sulfate, adding strong alkali to the mixture, distilling to remove ammonia, absorbing ammonia by boric acid, and titrating the solution by using acid to measure nitrogen content. The sample must be totally dried until no free water or crystal water exists, and cannot contain nitrogen-containing compounds such as nitrate or nitrite.

TABLE 1.1

Relationship between Nitrogen Content and DD

Nitrogen content	6.9	7.0	7.1	7.2	7.3	7.4	7.5	7.6	7.7	7.8
DD	0	6	11	17	22	28	33	39	44	50
Nitrogen content	7.9	8.0	8.1	8.2	8.3	8.4	8.5	8.6	8.7	
DD	56	61	67	72	78	83	89	94	100	

1.3.6 Water Content

"Water" here shall be defined as free water (adsorbed water) and part of the crystal water of chitin or chitosan. All crystal water cannot be removed by drying under normal pressure.

Water content is measured by the following steps: accurately weighing 1–2 g of chitosan sample, drying it at 105°C for 4 h until the weight is constant, and calculating weight loss in order to determine water content according to the following formula, where W is the weight of chitosan and Wt denotes the weight of chitosan after drying.

$$\text{Water content} = (W - Wt)/W \times 100\%$$

1.4 Physical Properties

1.4.1 Structure Characteristic

Despite the alteration due to deacetylation, chitosan from crab tendon possesses a crystal structure showing an orthorhombic unit cell with dimensions $a = 0.828$, $b = 0.862$, and $c = 1.043$ nm (fiber axis). The unit cell comprises four glucosamine units; two chains pass through the unit cell with an antiparallel packing arrangement. The main hydrogen bonds are O3⋯O5 (intramolecular) and N2⋯O6 (intermolecular) [54]. The crystal structures of salts and derivatives have also been determined, for instance, for chitosan ascorbate and salicylate, among others. The structural unit is presented in Figure 1.4 [55].

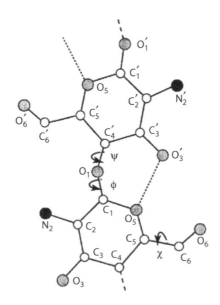

FIGURE 1.4

Chemical structure of a disaccharide segment of chitosan, showing position numbering. Two angles, psi and ø, defining the chain conformation and the angle chi defining the O6 orientation are shown. Dashed lines denote the O3–O5 hydrogen bonds. Hydrogen bonds connecting various positions of adjacent chains are omitted.

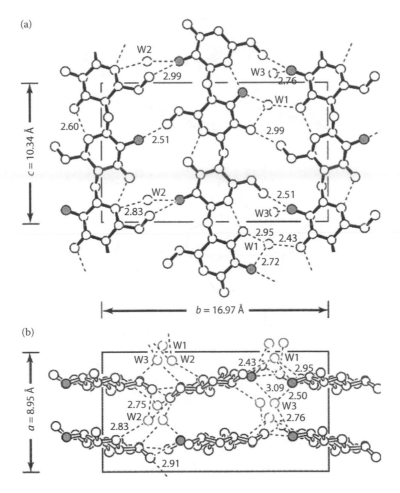

FIGURE 1.5
Packing arrangement of hydrated (tendon) chitosan projected along the *a*-axis (a) and along the *c*-axis (b). Filled circles denote nitrogen atoms. All hydrogen atoms are omitted, and hydrogen bonds are shown as dashed lines. The letter "w" is the oxygen atom of the water molecule.

As shown in Figure 1.5 [56], each chitosan chain takes an extended twofold helix: in other words, a zigzag structure. Chitosan chains on the *c*-axis are up chain, whereas those in the unit cell are down chain. That is, in this crystal, chitosan chains are packed in an antiparallel manner. Along the *b*-axis, the up chain and the down chain are bonded by hydrogen bonds to make a sheet structure, and these sheets are stacked along the *a*-axis (Figure 1.5b). Water molecules are present between these sheets and stabilize this crystal structure. Because water molecules are included in this crystal, the tendon polymorph is a hydrated crystal. This polymorph is the most abundant in chitosan samples; that is, commercially available chitosan samples have this crystal although their crystallinity is different.

When tendon chitosan was immersed in water and heated at around 200°C, the resultant chitosan specimen gave another crystal. This crystal was called the annealed polymorph. This change in chitosan crystal is an irreversible process. Figure 1.6 shows the molecular and crystal structure of annealed chitosan [57–59]. The chitosan chain along the *c*-axis is

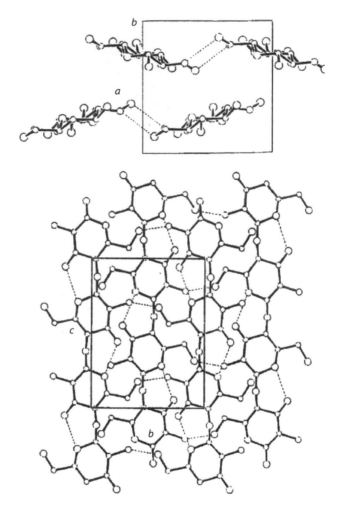

FIGURE 1.6
Projections of the crystal structure of chitosan in the anhydrous (annealed) polymorph on the *ab* (top) and *bc* (bottom) planes. All hydrogen atoms are omitted, and hydrogen bonds are shown as dashed lines.

up chain, and the neighbor is down chain, that is, they are also packed in an antiparallel fashion. However, there is no water molecule in this crystal, indicating that this is an anhydrous crystal. Different from the previous tendon polymorph, neighbor chains having parallel direction are bonded by direct hydrogen bonds to make a sheet, and neighbor sheets having antiparallel direction are stacked along the *a*-axis. Each chitosan chain takes an extended twofold helix, zigzag structure, similar to the tendon polymorph. Thus, only the zigzag structure has been found in chitosan crystals so far. This structure is also similar to those of chitin and cellulose.

1.4.2 Infrared Spectroscopy and Nuclear Magnetic Resonance

FTIR spectra of α- and β-chitin samples are shown in Figure 1.7. The C=O stretching region of the amide moiety, between 1600 and 1500 cm^{-1}, is quite interesting because it yields dif-

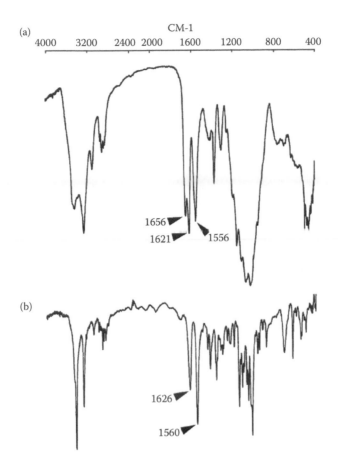

FIGURE 1.7
FTIR spectra of chitin for (a) single crystals of α-chitin and (b) deproteinized dried β-chitin from the tube of *Tevnia jerichonana*.

ferent signatures for α-chitin and β-chitin. For α-chitin, the amide I band is split at 1656 and 1621 cm^{-1}, whereas it is unique, at 1626 cm^{-1}, for β-chitin. In contrast, the amide II band is unique in both chitin allomorphs: at 1556 cm^{-1} for α-chitin and at 1560 cm^{-1} for β-chitin. The occurrence of two amide I bands for α-chitin has been the subject of debate. The band at 1656 cm^{-1}, which occurs at similar wavelengths in polyamides and proteins, is commonly assigned to stretching of the C=O group hydrogen bonded to N–H of the neighboring intrasheet chain. Regarding the 1621 cm^{-1} band, which is not present in polyamides and proteins, its occurrence may indicate a specific hydrogen bond of C=O with the hydroxymethyl group of the next chitin residue of the same chain [60]. This hypothesis is reinforced by the presence of only one band in this region for *N*-acetyl D-glucosamine [61]. Also, in α-chitin, the band at 1621 cm^{-1} is modified in deuterated water, whereas the band at 1656 cm^{-1} remains nearly unaffected [62]. Other possibilities may also be considered, as the band at 1621 cm^{-1} could be either a combination band or an enol form of the amide moiety [61].

Spectra of chitosan are shown in Figure 1.8. The spectra differences between chitosan and chitin are amide band, –NH$_2$ band, and hydrogen. For chitosan, the amide I band is

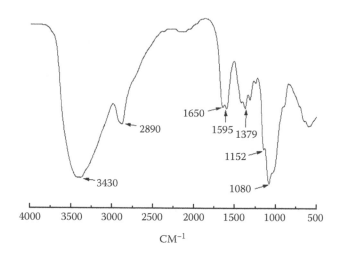

FIGURE 1.8
FTIR spectra of chitosan.

unique, at 1650 cm⁻¹, indicating that the *N*-acetyl amino still exists in chitosan and its absorption intensity is weaker than that of chitin. The band at 1595 cm⁻¹ is assigned to –NH₂ and does not exist in chitin. The other bands of chitosan are similar to those of chitin: 3430 cm⁻¹ for O–H stretching, 2890 cm⁻¹ for C–H stretching, 1379 cm⁻¹ for symmetric distortion vibration bands of –CH₃, 1152 cm⁻¹ for C–O–C stretching, and 1080 cm⁻¹ for C–O stretching.

Figure 1.9 [63] gives the ¹HNMR spectrum obtained for chitosan dissolved in D₂O containing DCl (pD approximately 4). The signal at 1.95 ppm allows determination of the acetyl content by reference to the H-1 signal at 4.79 ppm for the D-glucosamine residue and at 4.50 ppm for the H-1 of the *N*-acetyl-D-glucosamine unit at 85°C.

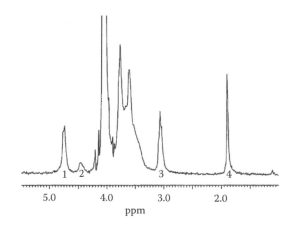

FIGURE 1.9
¹HNMR spectrum of chitosan in D₂O, pH 4, *T* = 85°C, conc. 5 g/L: (1) H-1 of glucosamine units, (2) H-1 of *N*-acetylglucosamine, (3) H-2, and (4) protons of the acetyl group of *N*-acetylglucosamine.

1.5 Chemical Properties

1.5.1 O-Acylation and N-Acylation

Chitin and chitosan may react with various derivatives of organic acids such as anhydride and acyl chloride to obtain aliphatic or aromatic acryls of different molecular weights. Such a reaction is most studied among all the chitosan relevant reactions.

Residues of the chitosan include hydroxyls and aminos; hence acylation may occur at hydroxyls to form ester or at aminos to form amide. A hydrogen atom on a nitrogen atom of an acetamino of chitin is still active despite the fact that the acetamino is changed to amido. This hydrogen atom can react if conditions permit. Hydroxyls on residues of chitin and chitosan include C6 hydroxyls and C3 hydroxyls, which are secondary hydroxyls. C6 hydroxyl as primary hydroxyl can freely spin in space due to small steric hindrance whereas C3 cannot due to large steric hindrance. For this reason, C6 is more active in reaction than C3. On the other hand, aminos on the residues are more active than the primary hydroxyls. However, activity is not the only factor influencing acylation; reaction site is also determined by reaction solvent, structure of acylating agent, catalyst, and reaction temperature. Moreover, acylation hardly forms a single product, which means that N-acylation and O-acylation occur at the same time or C6 acylation and C3 acylation occur at the same time. If C3, C6, and C2-NH are all acylated, the product is fully acylated chitosan, which is actually fully acylated chitin.

Strong intramolecular and intermolecular hydrogen bonds of chitin make the structure especially tight, and thus acylation is difficult. Usually, the acylating agent is anhydride and the reaction medium is the corresponding acid. Catalyst is a must and the reactant must be cooled during reacting. Commonly used catalysts include hydrogen chloride, methanesulfonic acid, perchloric acid, and so on. Main chain degradation is slight if the catalyst is methanesulfonic acid or perchloric acid. Chitosan contains several aminos, making acylation easier than chitin, and therefore a catalyst is not necessary. The reaction medium is methanol or ethanol.

The preparation method of fully acrylated chitin comprises the following steps: dispersing 1 g of chitosan powder that is dried sufficiently in 150 mL of methanol, adding excess acetic anhydride (2–3 mol larger than glucosamino of chitosan), stirring the mixture at room temperature for 16 h, filtering it, washing the filter cake with methanol twice, steeping the filter cake in 50 mL of 0.5 mol/L ethanol–KOH solution for 16 h, filtering the mixture, washing the filter cake with methanol sufficiently, dehydrating the mixture with ether, and drying the product naturally in air. The yield is almost stable.

This preparation method is of significance because it is difficult to form fully acylated chitin by using chitin, and chitin may degrade, causing molecular weight decline. These problems can be solved by using chitosan as the raw material. Fully acylated chitin fiber or film has excellent strength but is complex to make. Instead, acylation of chitosan will form fully acylated chitin of good performance and with lower cost.

The above method is suitable for making other acylates by using different carboxylic anhydrides. Fatty acid anhydride with more than six carbon atoms should be heated in reflux for over 16 h instead of reacting at room temperature.

As amino is more active than C6 hydroxyl, which makes acylation primarily occur at amino, the O-acylated chitosan is hard to form. Hence, aminos of chitosan are protected in advance (e.g., by benzaldehyde) before acylation and unprotected after acylation, and the acylation condition is moderate. Grant et al. [64,65] formed fully acylated chitosan by butyryl through the following steps: mixing 2.1 g of chitosan powder with 11 mL of methanesulfonic acid, stirring the mixture at 0°C for 30 min until the solution is homogeneous, dripping 125 mmol of butyric anhydride into the liquid, stirring at 0–5°C for 2 h, placing the mixture at –20°C overnight, pouring the mixture into 300 mL of acetone the next day for depositing, filtering, and extracting deposits by acetone for 18 h, and drying the deposits. On replacing butyric anhydride with 20 mmol of benzoyl chloride, the product is fully benzoylated chitosan.

N-acylation of chitosan is useful. The same steps as the preparation method of fully acylated chitin with less acetic anhydride will form N-acylated chitosan, namely, chitin. Corresponding acylates can be formed when acetic anhydride is replaced with propionic anhydride, butyric anhydride, or caproic anhydride. Amido acid derivatives of chitosan can be formed if the acylating agent is diacid anhydride (succinic anhydride, maleic anhydride, or phthalic anhydride). The derivatives are soluble in water, dilute acid, dilute alkali, or some organic solvents and have good hygroscopicity and water-retaining property [66,67].

1.5.2 Esterification Using Inorganic Oxygen Acids

Hydroxyls of chitin and chitosan, especially C6 hydroxyls, can be esterified by using inorganic oxygen acids or their anhydrides. Such reactions are similar to cellulose reactions. Aminos of chitosan can be esterified as well.

Sulfates of chitin and chitosan are the focus of esterification using inorganic oxygen acids. Studies on this subject have not subsided since 1953 because these esters are like heparin in structure and also have anticoagulation function. However, heparin is hard to extract and produce and is expensive, and may increase plasma fatty acid concentration. A cheap substitute for heparin with better anticoagulation function and no side effects can be formed by designing chitosan sulfate of a certain structure and molecular weight.

The esterifying agents for chitin and chitosan are concentrated sulfuric acid, a mixture of sulfur dioxide and sulfur trioxide, chlorosulfonic acid, and so on. Reactions are usually heterogeneous reactions. Chitosan 6-O-sulfate is prepared by the following steps [68]: cooling 40 mL of 95% H_2SO_4 and 20 mL of 98% HCl-SO_3 at 0–4°C, adding 1 g of chitosan to the solution, slowly heating the mixture to room temperature during stirring, stirring for 1 h, pouring the mixture into 250 mL of cold ether, filtering the mixture, washing the filter cake with cold ether, dissolving the deposit in water, neutralizing the solution with 0.5 mol/L $NaHCO_3$, dialyzing it with water, filtering and drying the product by freezing; or forming a formic acid solution of chitosan, keeping the pH at 2–7, slowly dripping 1 mol/L $CuSO_4$ solution into the solution until chitosan–Cu chelate appears, stirring for 16 h, filtering, grinding wet deposits, washing them with dry DMF, mixing them with 30 mL of anhydrous DMF, cooling the mixture to 0–2°C, dripping anhydrous DMF solution of pyridine-sulfur trioxide that is six times the chelate in mol, heating to 25°C, stirring for 16 h, ending the reaction by using saturated $NaHCO_3$, filtering, dialyzing the filter cake with water and drying the product by freezing. Chitosan 6-O-sulfate can also be formed by a mixture of 95% H_2SO_4 and 98% $HClO_4$.

Chitosan 6-O-sulfate is a polyampholyte and is soluble in water. It has stable conformation in solution because sulfate groups form strong hydrogen bonds with aminos, C3 hydroxyls, and the oxygen bridge of pyranose (Figure 1.10).

Chitosan 6-O-sulfate and chitosan 3-O-sulfate can be formed by changing chitosan into formate, acetate, perchlorate, nitrate, hydrochloride, or hydrobromide, dissolving it in DMF, adding cold chlorosulfonic acid to the solution, and stirring. Besides esterification,

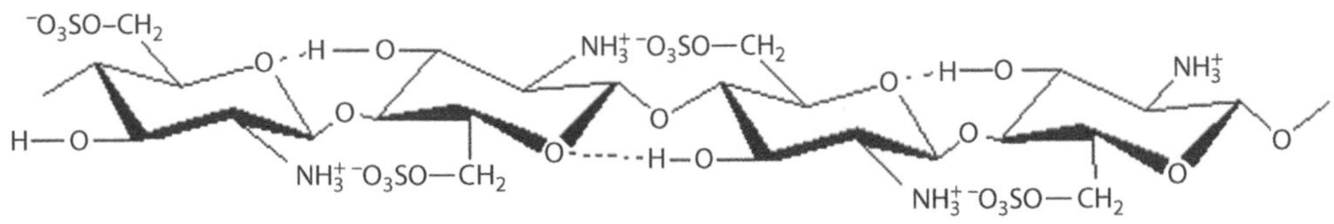

FIGURE 1.10
Conformation of chitosan 6-O-sulfate in solution.

sulfuric groups will be formed on aminos when a DMF solution of chitosan reacts with chlorosulfonic acid at 80°C.

O-sulfate and N-sulfuric groups will be formed when chitosan reacts with excess SO_3-DMF in homogeneous phase. The product is amorphous and has better anticoagulant activity than heparin.

Like cellulose, chitin can be transformed into xanthate by carbon disulfide after being treated with alkali. See Figure 1.11.

Sodium chitosan N-xanthate, which is a brilliant yellow powder, can be formed by adding chitosan in a water solution of carbon disulfide and sodium hydroxide, reacting at 60°C for 6 h, and pouring the mixture into acetone. The powder is water soluble and has strong heavy-metal-chelating capacity. The chelate composites are insoluble in water and can be removed by filtering. So xanthate is an effective heavy-metal remover. Chitosan fibers can be made by spraying a water solution of the xanthate. The equation is shown in Figure 1.12.

Phosphates of chitin and chitosan can be formed by treating them with phosphorus pentoxide in methanesulfonic acid. Chitin phosphate has water solubility increasing with degree of substitution. In case the aminos are unprotected, the chitin is water soluble at a low degree of substitution and water insoluble at a high degree of substitution due to the formation of phosphate. Prolonging the reaction time will increase the degree of substitution, but in the meantime the main chain will degrade.

1.5.3 Etherification

Ethers, such as methyl ether, ethyl ether, benzyl ether, hydroxylethyl ether, hydroxylpropyl ether, cyanoethyl ether, and carboxylmethyl ether, can be formed by hydroxyls of chitin and chitosan and hydrocarbylation agents. Such reactions have attracted more attention in recent years, and subsequently a few new materials have been developed.

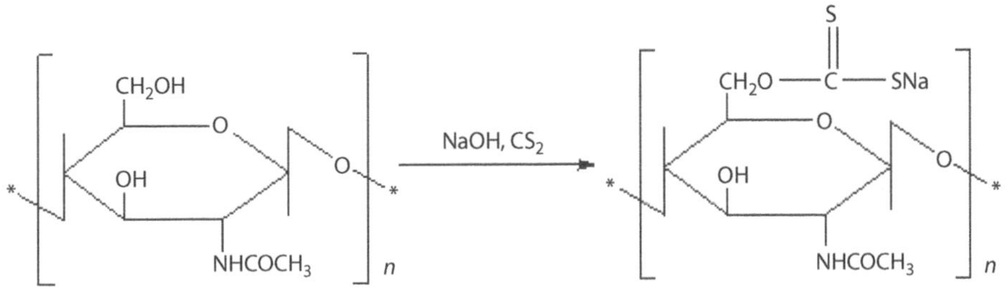

FIGURE 1.11
Transformation of chitin to xanthate.

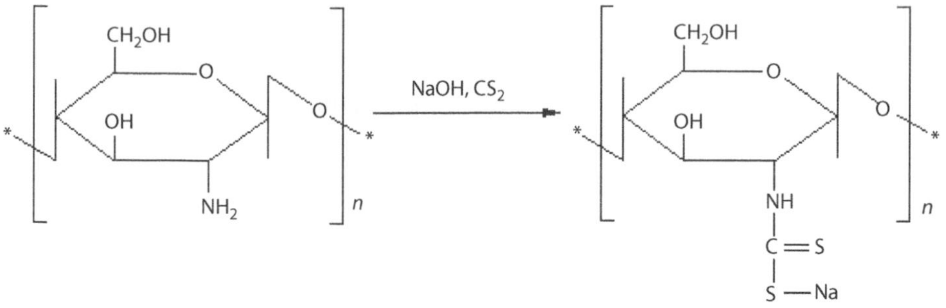

FIGURE 1.12
Transformation of chitosan to xanthate.

Etherification of chitin includes the following steps: making frozen basified chitin by using chitin and concentrated alkali, directly dispersing it in alkyl halide, slowly stirring at 12–14°C for 24 h, neutralizing by using dilute acetic acid, filtering and drying deposits in air, washing them with ethanol, water, and ethanol in sequence, dehydrating with acetone, and drying the product. The alkyl halide is 10 times the residues in mol. The substitution degree is unrelated to the amount of alkyl halide. Generally, substitution degrees are low. Some believe that it is because of temperature, whereas others think it is because of the tight structure of chitin. Actually, the main cause is the low activity of alkyl halides. The substitution degree can be increased only by increasing the reactivity. Primary reactions of alkyl halides and chitosan are N-alkylation followed by O-alkylation (etherified chitosan).

Chitosan and dimethyl sulfate form methyl ether in alkali medium by the following steps [69]: dissolving 38 g of chitosan in 1000 mL of 1 mol/L HCl, slowly adding 500 g of granular NaOH in the solution, stirring until the mixture becomes a paste, adding 500 mL of water in the paste, stirring, adding 200 mL of cold dimethyl sulfate to the paste in 1 h, stirring for 8 h, carefully adding 40 g of NaOH and 40 mL of dimethyl sulfate to the mixture in baths, stirring for 48 h, neutralizing with concentrated hydrochloric acid, dialyzing by using water for 4 h, concentrating the liquid to the smallest volume, and drying by freezing to form 36 g of chitosan methyl ether whose substitution degree is 29%. Most substituted groups are hydroxyls, which are turned into ether. A few aminos are also substituted to form *N*-methyl chitosan.

Site control of etherification is theoretically significant. Chitin is a macromolecule with complex structure, high crystalline degree, and large molecular weight. C6 hydroxyls and C3 hydroxyls are alike despite their different levels of activity. In particular, neither of them can react in homogeneous phase. So it is extremely complicated to increase the substitution degree, not to mention control of the reaction site. Just a few etherified chitins or acylated chitins with substitution degrees of 2 (two hydroxyls are completely substituted) have been reported so far. Jiang [70] was successful in directly changing chitin into fully benzylated chitin by liquid–solid phase transfer catalysis, and conveniently prepared 6-*O*-benzyl chitin and 3,6-*O*-di-benzyl chitin by controlling the amount of NaOH.

Both chitin and chitosan are available for cyanoethylation with acrylonitrile in the alkali condition, which forms *O*-cyanomethyl ether and causes many side reactions. One side reaction is hydrolysis of the cyano of cyanomethyl ether by alkali, forming *O*-propionamido chitin and sodium *O*-carboxylethyl chitin. The cyanoethyl etherification

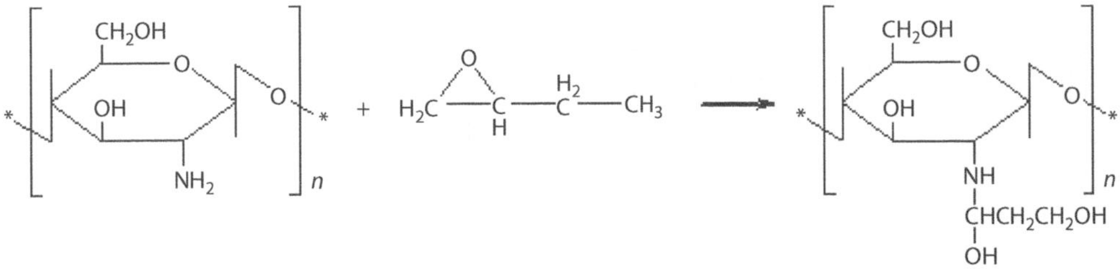

FIGURE 1.13
Addition reaction of chitosan and glycidol.

of chitosan forms 6-O-cyanoethyl chitosan at 20°C without influencing aminos. When the reaction temperature reaches 70°C, 30% aminos will be substituted by cyanoethyl.

1.5.4 N-Alkylation

Aminos of chitosan are primary aminos with lone-pair electrons and strong nucleo-philicity. They are involved in many reactions. N-alkylation is also of great importance in addition to N-acylation. Each acetamino of chitin is stable because there is only one hydrogen atom on the nitrogen atom. However, the substitution reaction is still available in the strong condition.

In the reaction of chitosan and alkyl halide, N-alkylation begins first [71]. The addition reaction of chitosan and epoxides forms *N*-alkylates and introduces two hydrophilic hydroxyls at a time. As shown in Figure 1.13, the N-substituted product formed by glycidol and chitosan is water soluble.

When chitosan reacts in a water solution of excess glycidol, two H atoms on the amino of chitosan will be substituted to form *N,N*-dihydroxyl *n*-butyl chitosan, which is water soluble.

In neutral medium, chitosan easily reacts with aromatic aldehyde or ketone or aliphatic aldehyde to form Schiff base. Such a reaction is useful in research and applications of chitosan. On the one hand, it protects aminos by protective groups that can be easily removed after the reaction, so that hydroxyls can react freely. On the other hand, Schiff bases formed by special aldehydes can be used for synthesizing useful *N*-derivatives via sodium borohydride reduction.

Chitosan Schiff bases are prepared by the following steps [72]: dispersing 1 g of chitosan powder into methanol, adding 3 mol of aldehyde to the mixture, extracting it by methanol via a Soxhlet extractor for 4 h, washing with ether, removing residual aldehyde, and drying by air. Neither aliphatic aldehyde nor aromatic aldehyde can completely change all aminos of chitosan into Schiff base.

The chitosan Schiff bases can be decomposed by acids to recycle chitosan; for example, chitosan-salicylaldehyde Schiff base can be decomposed by 5% acetic acid.

Chitosan and formaldehyde hydrate form *N*-hydroxylmethyl chitosan by condensing, as shown in Figure 1.14 [73].

The H remaining on the N can further react with one molecule of formaldehyde to form *N*-dihydroxylmethyl derivative, as shown in Figure 1.15.

The N-monosubstituted product turns into a Schiff base of formaldehyde and chitosan after one molecule of water is removed.

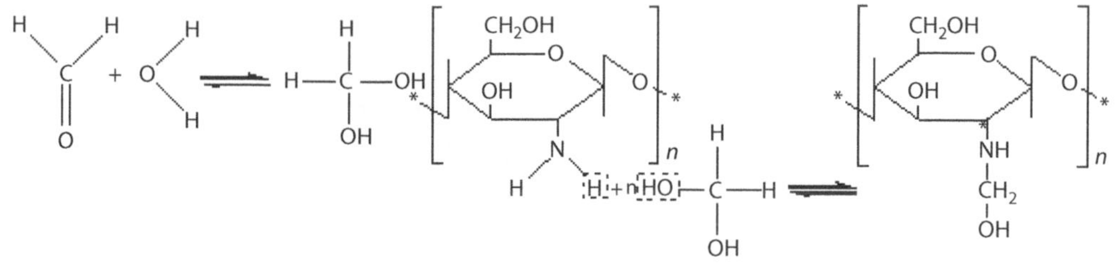

FIGURE 1.14
Reaction of chitosan and formaldehyde hydrate.

The Schiff base of formaldehyde and chitosan can be reduced by $NaBH_3CN$ to form *N*-methyl chitosan [74]. The method comprises the following steps [75]: suspending 20 g of chitosan powder with 2 L of water, adding 20 mL of glacial acetic acid to the suspension, stirring to dissolve glacial acetic acid, adding formaldehyde of the calculated amount in two batches, stirring for 30 min, adjusting the pH to 4.5 by using NaOH solution, dissolving 5 g of $NaBH_4$ in 50 mL of water, adding the solution to the reactant in 1 h during stirring, reacting for 1 h until the pH is 5.5, adjusting the pH to 10 by using alkali until *N*-methyl chitosan deposits, filtering, washing deposits with water to neutral, and extracting them with ethanol and ether via a Soxhlet extractor to remove the remaining formaldehyde and inorganic compounds.

A similar method can be used to prepare *N*-dimethyl chitosan: adding 50 mL of glacial acetic acid to 2 L of water, adding 50 g of 100–200 mesh chitosan to the solution, stirring the mixture to dissolve solid and form a solution of pH 3.2, adding 500 mL of 35% formaldehyde solution, stirring strongly to immediately form *N*-methylene chitosan gel, keeping it still for 12 h, adding 13 g of $NaBH_4$ in 8 h, reacting at 15–20°C until the pH is 4.0, which shows that the reaction is complete, adjusting the pH to 9.0 by using NaOH solution, washing the gel with water, and using acetone for depositing, filtering, and extracting deposits by using ether in a Soxhlet extractor to obtain a white powder that is insoluble in acetic acid or hydrochloric acid.

A small amount of formaldehyde cross-links chitosan, increasing the viscosity and even changing the solution into a gel. The specific steps are as follows: swelling chitosan by 95% ethanol for 2 h, adding excess salicylaldehyde to the mixture, stirring in reflux for 8 h, filtering to harvest the yellow product, extracting it by using ethanol in a Soxhlet extractor for 24 h to get salicylaldehyde chitosan Schiff base, and reducing it by $NaBH_4$ in methanol

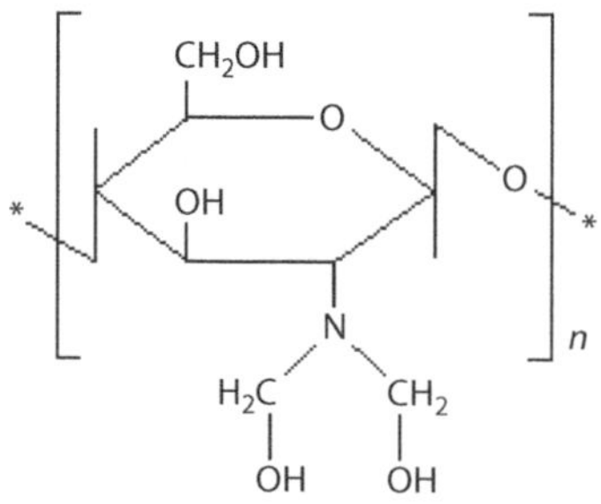

FIGURE 1.15
N-dihydroxylmethyl derivative of chitosan.

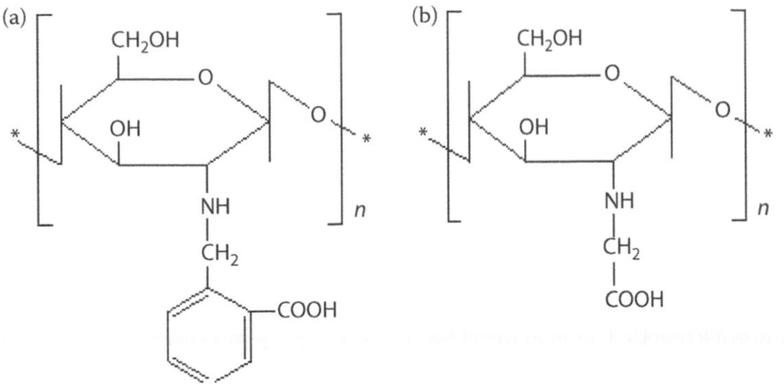

FIGURE 1.16
(a) *N*-carboxylbenzyl chitosan and (b) *N*-carboxylmethyl chitosan.

to form *N*-hydroxylbenzyl chitosan [76]. The product specifically chelates Cu and Hg. The product is *N*-carboxylbenzyl chitosan when salicylaldehyde is replaced by phthalaldehydic acid, and the product is *N*-carboxylmethyl when chitosan reacts with glyoxylic acid [77,78]. The said compounds become insoluble metal chelates after combining with transition metal ions in water solution, which are easy to separate from water. The compounds are soluble in acid and alkali solutions and their structures are shown in Figure 1.16. Glyoxal, glutaraldehyde, and dialdehyde starch are usually used as the cross-linking agents for chitosan. If the reaction is controlled properly, the expected Schiff base can be formed. Only one aldehyde group of dialdehyde is used for reacting, which means that the rest are available for other reactions.

Aminos exist on chains of the chitosan. Muzzarelli and Tanfani [75] claim that *N*-trimethyl chitosan quaternary ammonium salt iodide can be formed from methyl iodide and chitosan as shown in Figure 1.17.

The specific steps are as follows: drying 5 g of *N*-dimethyl chitosan at 80°C overnight, adding it to a mixture including 100 mL of anhydrous acetonitrile and 2.5 mL of methyl iodide, stirring at 35°C continuously in the anhydrous condition for 30 h, and extracting the product by using ether in a Soxhlet extractor to remove the remaining methyl iodide. Finally, 6.1 g of the final water-insoluble product is formed.

Considering one residue, the quaternary ammonium salt has a quaternary ammonium group on C2 of the pyranoid ring of the anhydroglucose unit. All carbon atoms of the anhydroglucose unit are asymmetric carbon atoms except for C6. The asymmetric carbon atom may give quaternary ammonium salt special biological activities, for example, selective bactericidal effect. A phase transfer catalyst with asymmetric carbon atoms may have some special effects on phase transfer catalysis in asymmetric organic synthesis.

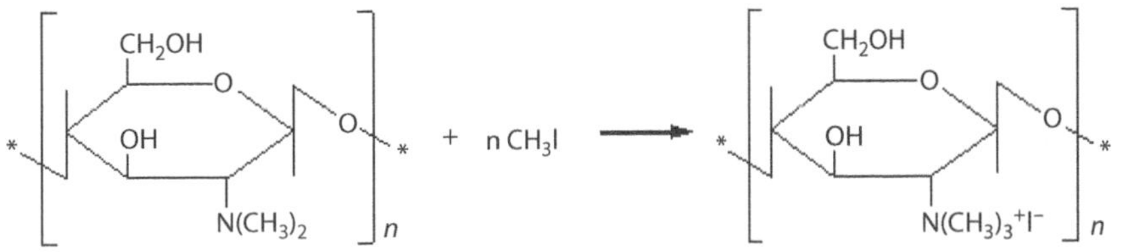

FIGURE 1.17
N-trimethyl chitosan quaternary ammonium salt iodide.

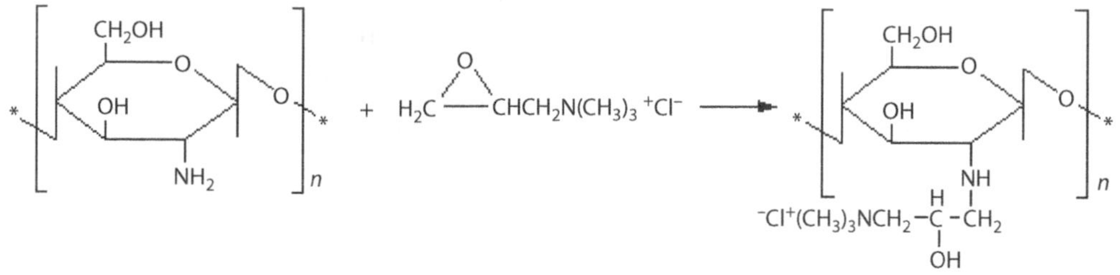

FIGURE 1.18
Chitosan hydroxypropyltrimethyl ammonium chloride.

There is another structure for chitosan quaternary ammonium salt: instead of directly binding the quaternary ammonium group with C2, a low-molecular-weight quaternary ammonium is bound to amino. For instance, as shown in Figure 1.18, chitosan hydroxy-propyltrimethyl ammonium chloride is formed by mixing a water solution of glycidyl trimethyl ammonium chloride and chitosan in the mol ratio 3:1 in isopropanol at 90°C for 8 h, followed by filtering, washing, and drying the product.

Chitosan amino has two H atoms and so the theoretical substitution degree can reach 200%. In the said reaction, it is 127.71% and the product has good water solubility. In fact, the N-acylation part has referred to such a quaternary ammonium salt. This method can be applied for preparing a series of chitosan quaternary ammonium salts of the same structure.

1.5.5 Oxidation

Chitin and chitosan can be oxidized by oxidants whose mechanisms are complicated. Different oxidants require different pH values and form different products by different mechanisms. They may oxidize C6 hydroxyl into an aldehyde group or carboxyl, oxidize C3 hydroxyl into carbonyl (ketone synthesis), and eliminate partly aminos or acetaminos, even damage the pyranoid ring and glucosidic bond. Common situations are described below.

Periodic acid degradation is frequently used in polysaccharide structure research. Periodic acid selectively cracks dihydroxyl or trihydroxyl. Chitin does not have such a structure, and so it cannot be oxidized by periodic acid. The amino on C2 of chitosan has similar properties to hydroxyl and so each residue consumes one molecule of periodic acid and releases 0.6–0.7 mol/L ammonia in oxidization when the pH is 4.1.

Hydrolysis of chitosan by dilute hydrochloric acid can be accelerated using a little sodium nitrite due to oxidative deamination. Chitosan oligosaccharides of different molecular weights can be obtained by controlling the amount of sodium nitrite. For example, chitosan oligosaccharide of average polymerization degree 13 can be formed by dissolving 2 g of chitosan in 100 mL of 6% acetic acid, reacting with 85.5 mg of sodium nitrite at 20°C for 30 min and adjusting the pH to 7.4 with NaOH solution.

Primary hydroxyls of chitin and chitosan can be oxidized to form chitin oxide and chitosan oxide, which are polysaccharide acids. Sodium salts formed by acids are water soluble. The most significant finding is that chitosan is turned into a compound similar to heparin in structure after its aminos are sulfated and primary hydroxyls are oxidized [79]. Such a compound is an alternative to heparin and is prepared as follows: dissolving 10 g of chitosan acetate powder in 50 mL of water, adding 200 mL of acetic acid to the solution, distilling to form syrup, repeating the steps until the product cannot be dissolved by acetic acid, adding acetic acid to the syrup to 1 L, slowly adding 12 mL of 60% perchloric acid solution forcefully, and stirring until needle-like deposits, namely chitosan perchlorides, are formed.

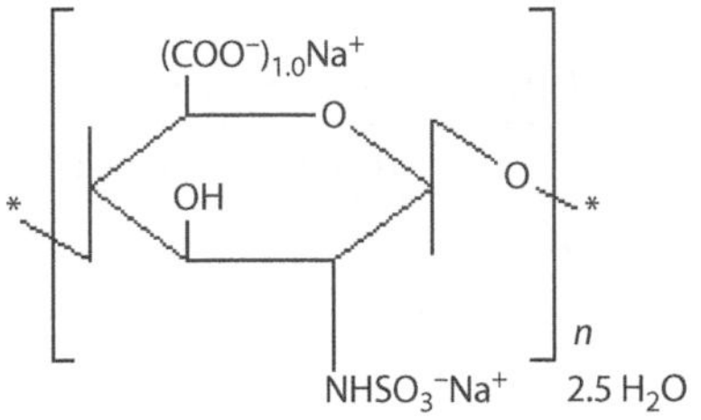

FIGURE 1.19
Chitosan heparin analogues.

The heparin alternative can be formed by the following steps: dissolving 3 g of CrO_3 in 3 mL of water and 30 mL of acetic acid, adding the solution to a suspension of chitosan perchloride during fast stirring, reacting at 25°C for 30 min, adding CrO_3 solution of equal amounts in the reactant, stirring for 30 min, adding 2 g of CrO_3, stirring for 1 h, decomposing excess CrO_3 by using 25 mL of methanol after reaction, stirring for 15 min, keeping it still, removing the supernatant carefully, filtering, washing deposits with methanol until the methanol is colorless and acid free, washing deposits with ether, drying them in vacuum to form 9.7 g of chitosan perchloride whose primary hydroxyls are oxidized into carboxyls, dissolving the product in pyridine, treating the solution with chlorosulfonic acid, and neutralizing by using 1 mol/L NaOH solution to transform the perchloride on aminos into sulfate and make carboxyls react with Na. The product is quite like heparin in infrared spectrometry (Figure 1.19).

1.5.6 Chelation

Each residue of chitin and chitosan has an acetyl or an amino on C2 and a hydroxyl on C3. They are flat bonds so that they can chelate metal ions with certain ion radii at certain pH values. Chitosan is able to chelate more metal ions.

Muzzarelli [80] points out that chitosan combines metal ions by ion exchange, absorption, and chelation. Chitosan will not change in structure but in property due to chelation. Usually, its color changes after chelation, such as red chelate formed by chitosan and titanium ion, orange chelate formed by chitosan and metavanadate, green chelate formed by chitosan and trivalent chromium, orange chelate formed by chitosan and hexavalent chromium, yellowish-brown chelate formed by chitosan and ferrous, yellowish-green chelate formed by chitosan and ferric, pink chelate formed by chitosan and cobalt ion, green chelate formed by chitosan and nickel ion, and blue chelate formed by chitosan and copper ion.

Chitosan cannot chelate alkali metals or alkaline earth metals; therefore, chitosan may separate transition metal ions from a solution of alkali metal or alkaline earth metal by chelating as shown in Table 1.2. The most convincing example is as follows: after treating

TABLE 1.2

Coexistence of Alkaline Metal Ions and Transition Metal Ions

Ions	Accumulation Rate (%)				
	1 h	2 h	8 h	18 h	24 h
Cr^{3+}		33	71	91	94
Cr^{3+} + 10% NaCl	35	42	74	93	95

TABLE 1.3

Coexistence of Different Transition Metal Ions

Ions	Accumulation Rate (%)					
	1 h	4 h	8 h	16 h	20 h	24 h
Cu^{2+}	31.8	70	79	93.5	98.6	98.8
$Cu^{2+} Cr(VI)$	8	58	71	86.7	95.4	96.2
$Cr(VI)$	18	40	60	74	85	90.3
$Cr(VI) Cu^{2+}$	14	34	43	65.2	65.4	72.1

100 mL of 0.4 mol/L $(NH_4)_2SO_4$, which contains nanogram grade zinc ions marked by isotope, by chitosan powder column and testing isotope, the result shows that all the zinc ions marked by isotope remain at the upper part of the column and only ammonium sulfate is left the eluate, which means that all the zinc ions are chelated by chitosan. The chitosan can also separate trace copper ions from ammonium sulfate solution.

In solution containing two or more transition metal ions, chitosan chelates ions with more suitable radii first. For example, since nickel ions are more suitable for chitosan than ferrous ions, they can be separated from the solution by chitosan chromatography, which retains nickel ions in the column and almost all the ferrous ions are left in the eluate. Table 1.3 shows interactions between Cu ions and a few Cr(VI) ions in solution and the opposite. Such interactions exist between Cu ions and chromate, and other transition metal ions (for instance, ferrous ions) strongly affect Cu ions (Table 1.4).

Different oxide valences determine different chelation capacities (Table 1.5). For example, ferrous ions are easy to remove from the chitin column whereas ferric ions are not.

The combination of chitosan and transition metal ions will be influenced by anions. Chlorine ions inhibit the amount of combined metal ions whereas sulfates increase it. Due to soluble chitosan acetate, the solution contains acetates that change the surface property of chitosan. Sulfonic acid can chelate metal ions itself, and so it also inhibits the combination of chitosan and metal ions.

A number of papers on the chelation mechanism of chitosan and copper have been published. Experiments prove that four residues chelate one copper molecule [81], as shown in Figure 1.20.

Chitosan combines with an Fe molecule and three molecules of water based on two glucose residues [82].

Guan et al. [83] believe that the coordination number of a coordination polymer formed by metal and organic macromolecule cannot be simply determined by elementary analysis; instead, the coordination number of the central ion should be determined by the vibration effect of the photoelectron spectrograph or measured by the conductimetric method.

TABLE 1.4

Influence of Ferrous Ion on Cupric Ions

Ions	Accumulation Rate (%)				
	1 h	4 h	8 h	16 h	20 h
Cu^{2+}	31.8	70	79	93.5	98.6
Fe^{2+}	30	32	34	36	37
Fe^{2+}, Cu^{2+}	14	15	16	18	18

TABLE 1.5

Accumulation Rate of the Same Metal Ions and Different Valences

Ions	Accumulation Rate (%)				
	1 h	2 h	4 h	6 h	12 h
Fe^{3+}	88	92	95	96	96
Fe^{2+}	30	32		34	36

According to conductivity, infrared spectrometry, electron spin resonance spectrometry, and photoelectron spectrography, they assume that one Ni^{2+} ion combines with O of C3 hydroxyl and N of aminos of three glucosamines to form a chitosan-Ni(II) coordination polymer with six coordinate bonds. According to infrared spectrometry, electron spin resonance spectrometry, and photoelectron spectrography, they assume that one La^{3+} ion combines with O of C3 hydroxyl and N of aminos of five glucosamines to form a chitosan-Ni(II) coordination polymer with 10 coordinate bonds.

Moreover, chitosan is especially significant for absorption of transuranic elements, actinide elements, and lanthanides. The technique for extracting uranium isotopes from seawater by chitosan film or fiber has good prospects.

1.5.7 Graft Copolymerization

There are many active groups on chitin and chitosan available for graft copolymerization, which changes the functions of chitin and chitosan to meet some special needs. Research on graft copolymerization began in 1979, but did not make significant progress until the 1990s.

Graft copolymerization can be carried out by the chemical method, the radiation method, and the mechanical method, although only the chemical method and the radiation method have been reported so far. Based on the reaction mechanism, the methods include free-radical-induced graft copolymerization and ion-induced graft copolymerization.

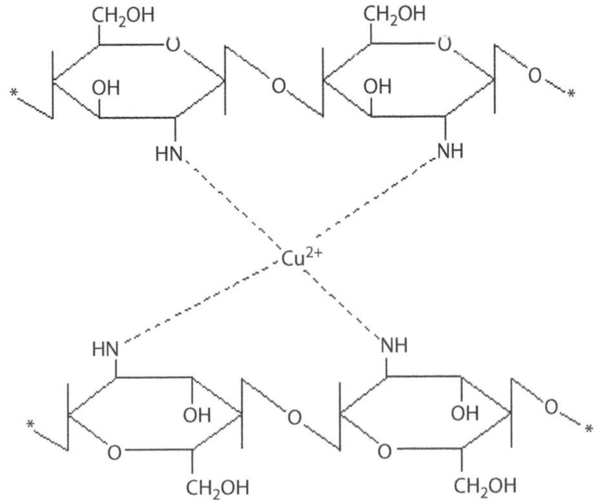

FIGURE 1.20
Chelation mechanism of chitosan and copper.

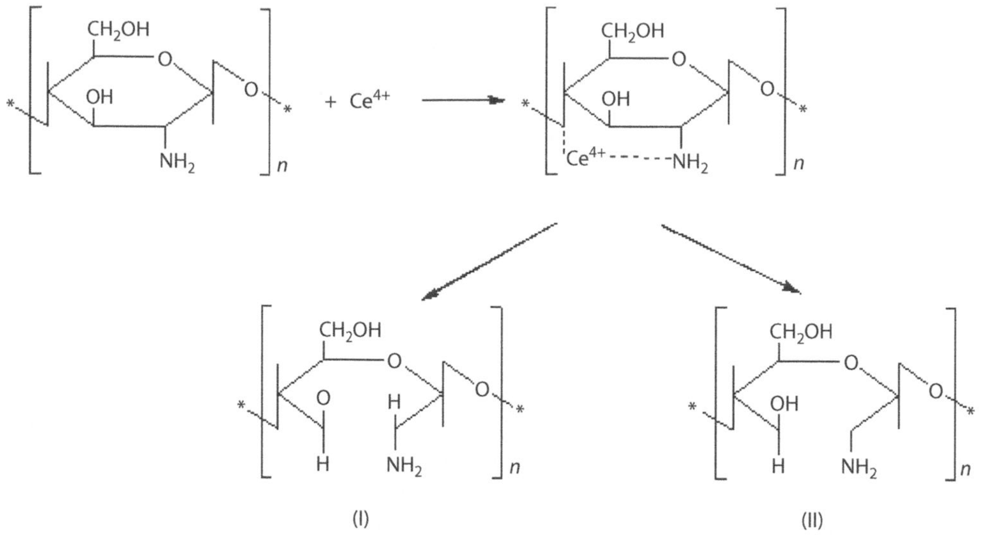

FIGURE 1.21
Oxidation–reduction initiating reaction mechanism by cerium ions.

A key factor of free-radical-induced graft copolymerization is the generation of free radicals. There are four initiators for generating free radicals in free-radical-induced graft copolymerization of chitin and chitosan.

The oxidation–reduction initiator is frequently used in graft polymerization. Cerium ion is a common initiator for promoting allyl monomers such as acrylic acid, acrylate, acrylamide, methyl methylacrylate, and styrene to graft with residues of chitin or chitosan [84–88]. The reaction is carried out by adding cerium nitride or cerium ammonium sulfate to a mixture of chitin or chitosan, water, and allyl monomer, and heating them in heterogeneous phase. Grafting degree increases with monomer concentration, but does not necessarily lead to increased percentage grafting. The initiator is available over a certain concentration because chitin or chitosan is a reductive polysaccharide whose reducing end groups consume a certain amount of initiator; thus graft polymerization occurs only when the initiator is beyond that amount [89]. In 1993, Li et al. [86] put forward the complete mechanism of cerium ions as a graft polymerization initiator. The mechanism can be described as follows: Ce^{4+} ions react with C2–NH_2 and C3–OH of residue to form a complex, –CH=NH (I) and –CH (OH)(II) free radicals are formed by disproportionating, cerium ions oxidize II into carbonyl free radicals at temperatures higher than 40°C for initiating graft polymerization, the reaction continues and I is hydrolyzed into aldehyde and ammonium ions at temperatures higher than 90°C, and aldehyde is further oxidized into carbonyl free radicals for initiating polymerization. The reactions are described in Figure 1.21.

Persulfate used as the initiator forms an oxidation–reduction system with sodium bisulfite or ferrous sulfate [90–91]. The system is cheap and convenient to operate, and does not remain in the graft polymer. Wei et al. [92] believe that the reaction mechanism is as shown in Figure 1.22. The reactions are chain propagation and chain termination.

Except for the reactions mentioned above, the oxidization–reduction reaction of persulfate and aminos of the chitosan may also occur to form macromolecular free radicals. The H_2O_2–Fe system is another common oxidation–reduction initiator that initiates the reaction

$$S_2O_8^{2-} + HSO_3^- \longrightarrow SO_4^{2-} + *SO_4^- + *HSO_3$$

$$*SO_4^- + HSO_3^- \longrightarrow SO_4^{2-} + *HSO_3$$

$$*HSO_3 + \text{Chitosan} \longrightarrow \text{Chitosan} * + H_2SO_3$$

$$\text{Chitosan} * + M \longrightarrow \text{Chitosan} - M *$$

$$*HSO_3 + M \longrightarrow HSO_3 - M *$$

FIGURE 1.22
Oxidation–reduction initiating reaction mechanism by persulfate.

of chitosan and methyl methylacrylate in water solution [93]. The mechanism is probably as in Figure 1.23. The reaction is graft polymerization of chitosan with free radicals and monomers.

A research paper published in 1979 claimed that tributylborane can be used as an initiator for the graft polymerization of chitin [94]. The mechanism includes the following steps: first, water diffuses into the main chain of chitin to solvate chitin; second, solvated chitin forms a complex with tributylborane; and third, monomer diffuses into chitin and reacts with the complex to generate macromolecular free radicals for initiating graft polymerization. Tributylborane is not a universal initiator.

Azodiisobutyronitrile is a common initiator for free radical polymerization and can also be used for initiating graft polymerization of chitosan and an alkyl monomer [95]. In a heterogeneous reaction, acrylonitrile and methyl methylacrylate can only graft aminos of chitosan if the initiator is azodiisobutyronitrile, and the product is insoluble in dilute acid. Only if the monomer is ethenyl ethanoate, graft polymerization will occur at sites other than amino and the product is soluble in 2% acetic acid. In a homogeneous reaction, ethenyl ethanoate can only graft aminos, and the solubility of the product in dilute acid is limited.

Radiation is also used for initiating graft polymerization. To date, only γ-rays of ^{60}Co can be used for graft polymerization of chitin and chitosan.

Maximal percentage conversion and percentage grafting can be obtained when chitin and styrene are irradiated by γ-rays at 30°C in water. This proves that water can permeate into chitin for solvating, which damages the hydrogen bonds between chitin molecules and increases the diffusivity of styrene, so that the reaction becomes easier [96]. High percentage grafting of chitosan powder and styrene can be obtained when styrene is turned into a 50% water solution. Differently, chitosan film can be grafted without solvent,

$$H_2O_2 + Fe^{2+} \longrightarrow *OH + OH^- + Fe^{3+}$$

$$*OH + Fe^{2+} \longrightarrow OH^- + Fe^{3+}$$

$$*OH + H_2O_2 \longrightarrow H_2O + *OOH$$

$$*OOH + H_2O_2 \longrightarrow *OH + O_2 + H_2O$$

$$*OH + \text{Chitosan} \longrightarrow \text{Chitosan} * + H_2O$$

FIGURE 1.23
Oxidation–reduction initiating reaction mechanism by the H_2O_2–Fe system.

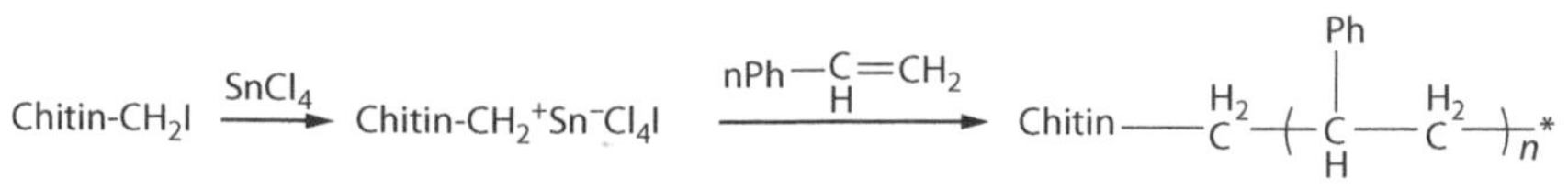

Chitin-CH$_2$I $\xrightarrow{\text{SnCl}_4}$ Chitin-CH$_2^+$Sn$^-$Cl$_4$I $\xrightarrow{n\text{Ph}-\underset{\text{H}}{\overset{}{\text{C}}}=\text{CH}_2}$ Chitin$-\underset{}{\overset{\text{H}_2}{\text{C}}}-\left(-\underset{\text{H}}{\overset{\text{Ph}}{\text{C}}}-\underset{}{\overset{\text{H}_2}{\text{C}}}-\right)_n^*$

FIGURE 1.24
Ion induced graft polymerization

but only trace homopolymers of styrene can be formed. Percentage grafting is remarkably increased when the solvent is 30% methanol–20% water. It is thus clear that the graft reaction changes with the physical structure of chitosan. In the same condition, ethenyl ethanoate cannot graft chitin or chitosan, acrylamide forms gel products that are hard to separate, and methyl methylacrylate reacts with chitosan with 94.2% grafting degree and 84% grafting efficiency. The largest grafting degree of chitosan and hydroxylethyl acrylate appears when the ratio of water to methanol is the best [97].

The UV method completes the reaction in a short time and is suitable for preparing a large amount of samples. Methyl methylacrylate grafts chitin or chitin oxide when they are irradiated by a low-pressure mercury lamp [98]. Chitin oxide is better for such a reaction. The possible cause is carbonyl. 10% DMF obviously increases grafting degree.

Moreover, grafting degrees of UV-irradiated chitin iodide at room temperature [99] and polymerization of chitin thiol and styrene in DMSO [100] are 97%.

Research on ion-induced graft polymerization is limited; however, one method was introduced with the following steps (Figure 1.24): dispersing chitin iodide in nitrobenzene, and adding Lewis acid SnCl$_4$ to the mixture for grafting styrene via cation graft polymerization [101].

Another method for *N*-carboxylic anhydride graft polymerization of chitosan and nonallyl monomer comprises the following steps [102]: dispersing chitosan powder in DMSO, adding *N*-carboxylic anhydride to the solution, stirring at room temperature for about 1 week to form gel swelled by water and DMSO, diluting with water, repeatedly centrifuging the mixture to remove polypeptide, and depositing from acetone to form a new graft polymer that is a polysaccharide peptide. The grafted groups are aminos and the polypeptide for grafting has about six amino acid residues.

1.5.8 Cross-Linking

Chitin and chitosan can cross-link by aldehydes or anhydrides with two functional groups. Such a reaction forms stable products that are insoluble and difficult to swell. The products can be used as carriers for chromatographic fractionation or immobilized enzymes. Chitosan needs to be cross-linked on various occasions.

Mostly, cross-linking occurs between molecules. However, intramolecular cross-linking exists as well. Primarily, the cross-linking reaction forms Schiff base by the amino of chitosan and aldehyde. The reaction between aldehyde and hydroxyl does not occur so frequently. Common cross-linking agents include glutaraldehyde, formaldehyde, and glyoxal, and reaction can occur in both water and heterogeneous medium at room temperature. The reaction rate is high and the pH range is wide.

Additionally, quite a few methods can introduce active groups during cross-linking. For example, when using epoxy chloropropane to cross-link chitosan powder in dilute alkali solution [103,104], hydroxyls are generated between crossbonds. Cyanuric chloride [105], toluene diisocyanate [106], and chloromethyl thiirane [107,108] are also available.

1.6 The Standard as Biomaterials

Chitosan is a degradable material with good biocompatibility in the medical field; thus it can be used for preparing sutures, artificial blood vessels, and artificial skin. It is effective in treating cancer, cardiovascular disease, and wounds and can be made into intelligent controlled release agents and slow release agents. With respect to health care, western academia considers chitosan as the sixth key element in addition to protein, fat, sugar, vitamin, and inorganic salt because it strengthens immunity, resists aging, prevents disease, and adjusts physiological function [109].

1.6.1 Standard of Chitosan as Biomaterials

In solution, the cationic nature of chitosan gives this polymer a mucoadhesive property. Chitosan salts can be used as a matrix or scaffold material as well as in nonparenteral delivery systems for challenging drugs. Chitosan salts have been shown to increase the transport of polar drugs across the nasal epithelial surface.

American Society for Testing and Materials (ASTM) F 2103-01 [110] is a standard guide for the characterization and testing of chitosan salts as starting materials intended for use in biomedical and tissue-engineered medical product applications. The purpose of this guide is to identify key parameters relevant for the functionality and characterization of chitosan salts for the development of new commercial applications of chitosan salts for the biomedical and pharmaceutical industries. Key parameters include the degree of deacetylation, molecular mass and viscosity in aqueous solution, dry matter content, ash content, insolubles, endotoxin content, protein content, heavy-metal content, and microbiological safety. This guide provides chemical and physical test methods of these key parameters, product development considerations, and safety and toxicology aspects of chitosan.

The People's Republic of China pharmaceutical industry standards (YY/T) 0606.7 [111] is a standard of tissue-engineered medical products—part 7: chitosan and this standard reference the ASTM standard mentioned above. This standard is applicable to chitosan as starting materials intended for use in tissue-engineered medical products and surgical implant applications. This standard provides terms and definitions of chitosan, requirements of chitosan products, test methods and inspection rules, packaging, transportation, and storage of products.

SC/T (The People's Republic of China Fisheries Industry Standard) 3403 [112] is a standard of chitin and chitosan. This standard provides detailed specifications and requirements of chitosan products (Table 1.6).

1.6.2 Status of Chitosan Products

Golden-Shell Biochemical Co. Ltd., founded in 1994, is the largest enterprise in the line of chitin and its ramifications in China. Major products include D-glucosamine HCl, D-glucosamine sulfate, *N*-acetyl-D-glucosamine, chitosan, high-density chitosan, chitosan-ase, oligosaccharide, and fish collagen powder. Moreover, they developed special molecular weight chitosan, water-soluble chitosan, paper-making chitosan, sugar-refining chitosan, pharmaceutical chitosan, cosmetic moisturizing chitosan, and so on. Table 1.7 shows the standard of common chitosan products.

TABLE 1.6

Specifications and Requirements of Chitosan Products

	Low	Medium	High	Ultrahigh
DD (%)	<75.0	75.0–89.0	90.0–95.0	>95.0
Viscosity (mPa/s)	<50	50–499	500–1000	>1000
Color and luster	Industrial grade Off-white to yellowish		Food grade Off-white to yellowish, glossy	
Appearance	Flaker or powder			
Smell	Allowing a small amount of natural odor			
Water content (%)	≤12.0		≤10.0	
Ash content (%)	≤2.0		≤0.5	
Insolubles (%)	—		≤1.0	
pH	6.5–8.5			
	Requirements			
Arsenic (mg/kg)	≤1.0			
Heavy metals (mg/kg)	≤10			
Total colony count (cpu/kg)	≤1000			
Pathogenic bacteria	—			

TABLE 1.7

The Standard of Common Chitosan Products

Items	Medical Grade	Food Grade	Industrial Grade
Appearance	Off-white powder	Off-white powder	Off-white to yellowish semitransparent flaker or powder
Deacetylation[a] degree	>90%, 95%	>85%, 90%, 95%	>70%, 80%, 85%
pH value	7.0–8.0	7.0–8.0	7.0–8.0
Loss on drying	<8.0%	<10.0%	<12.0%
Residue on ignition	<1.0%	<1.5%	<2.0%
Insoluble matter	<1.0%	<1.0%	<2.0%
Heavy metals (count as load)	≤10 ppm	≤10 ppm	
Arsenic	≤0.5 ppm	≤0.5 ppm	
Total plate count	≤1000 cfu/g	≤1000 cfu/g	
Viscosity[b]	50–800 mPa/s		
Particle size	40 mesh, 60 mesh, 80 mesh, 100 mesh		

Packing for medical and food grade: 20.0 kg, 25.0 kg/fiber drum (Φ = 38.0 cm × 48.0 cm or Φ = 42.0 cm × 60.0 cm), or according to demand.

[a] They can supply high-purity chitosan with DD > 95%.

[b] The viscosity is determined at 20°C with 1°C chitosan in 1°C acetic acid.

References

1. Braconnot, H. 1811. Sur La nature des champignons. *Ann Chi Phys* 79: 265–304.
2. Rouget, C. 1859. Des substances amylacees dans le tissue des animux, specialement les Articules (Chitine). *Compt Rend* 48: 792–795.
3. Ruiz-Herrera, J. 1978. *Proceedings of First International Conference on Chitin/Chitosan*. R. A. A. Muzzarelli and E. R. Pariser, eds. MIT Sea Grant Program Report MITSG 78-7 11.
4. Rudall, K. M. 1963. The chitin/protein complexes of insect cuticles. *Adv Insect Physiol* 1: 257–313.
5. Muzzarelli, R. A. A. 1977. *Chitin*. Oxford: Pergamon, pp. 255–265.
6. Kurita, K. 2001. Controlled functionalization of the polysaccharide chitin. *Prog Polym Sci* 26(9): 1921–1971.
7. Muzzarelli, R., Jeuniaux, C., and Gooday, G. W. 1986. *Chitin in Nature and Technology*. New York, NY: Plenum Press.
8. Roberts, G. A. F. 1992. *Chitin Chemistry*. London: Macmillan Press.
9. Goosen, M. F. A. 1997. *Applications of Chitin and Chitosan*. Lancaster, PA: Technomic Publishing.
10. Heyn, A. N. J. 1936. Further investigations on the mechanism of cell elongation and the properties of the cell wall in connection with elongation. *Protoplasma* 25(1): 372–396.
11. Liu, G. Q., Zhang, K. C., and Wang, X. L. 2003. Advances in insects as food resources in China. *The Fifth International Conference on Food Science & Technology Proceedings* (Vol. II). Beijing: Chinese Books Press, pp. 263–266.
12. Masuoka, K., Ishihara, M., and Asazuma, T. 2005. The interaction of chitosan with fibroblast growth factor-2 and its protection from inactivation. *Biomaterials* 26(16): 3277–3284.
13. Zhang, M., Haga, A., and Sekiguchi, H. 2000. Structure of insect chitin isolated from beetle larva cuticle and silkworm (*Bombyx mori*) pupa exuvia. *Int J Biol Macromol* 27(1): 99–105.
14. Meng, X. and Xu, M. 2000. The preparation and analysis of chitin from the Cigala shell. *Hebei Chem Eng Ind* 23(1): 28–29.
15. Bough, W. A., Salter, W. L., and Wu, A. C. 1978. Influence of manufacturing variables on the characteristics and effectiveness of chitosan products. I. Chemical composition, viscosity, and molecular weight distribution of chitosan products. *Biotechnol Bioeng* 20(12): 193–194.
16. Seiichi, M., Masaru, M., and Reikichi, I. 1983. Highly deacetylated chitosan and its properties. *J Appl Polym Sci* 28(6): 1909–1917.
17. Zeng, M. 1992. The research of chitosan preparation condition. *Fisheries Sci* 11(10): 9–13.
18. Sannan, T., Kutita, K., and Iwakur, Y. 1976. Studies on chitin II. Effect of deacetylation on solubility. *Macromol Chem* 177(12): 3589–3600.
19. Kurita, K., Yoshida, A., and Koyama, Y. 1988. Studies on chitin 13: New polysaccharids/polypeptide hybrid materials based on chitin and poly γ-methyl L-glutamate. *Macromolecules* 21(6): 1579–1583.
20. Wang, A. and Yu, X. 1998. Preparation of high deacetylated chitosan by dissolving-precipitated method. *Fine Chem* 15(6): 17–18.
21. Peniston, Q. P. 1979. Process for activating chitin by microwave treatment and improved activated chitin product. US Patent 4159932.
22. Guo, G. and Zhong, H. 1994. The preparation of chitosan by semi-dry method with microwave treatment. *Nat Prod Res Dev* 6(4): 103–106.
23. Sun, J., Li, Y., and Yu, Z. 2006. Preparation of chitosan using PEG as phase transfer catalyst. *J Huaihai Inst Technol: Nat Sci Edn* 15(2): 48–50.
24. Martinou, A., Kafetzopoulos, D., and Bouriotis, V. 1995. Chitin deacetylation by enzymatic means: Monitoring of deacetylation processes. *Carbohydr Res* 273(2): 235–242.
25. Chung, L. Y., Schmidt, R. J., and Hamlyn, P. F. 1994. Biocompatibility of potential wound management products: Fungal mycelia as a source of chitin/chitosan and their effect on the proliferation of human F1000 fibroblasts in culture. *J Biomed Mater Res* 28(4): 463–469.

26. Iason, T., Nathalie, Z., and Aggeliki, M. 1999. Mode of action of chitin deacetylase from *Mucor rouxii* on *N*-acetylchitooligosaccharides. *Eur J Biochem* 261: 698–705.

27. Hang, Y. D. 1990. Chitosan production from *Rhizopus oryzae* mycelia. *Biotechnol Lett* 12(12): 911–912.

28. Ravi Kumar, M. N. V. 2000. A review of chitin and chitosan applications. *React Funct Polym* 46(1): 1–27.

29. Kafetzopoulos, D., Martinou, A., and Bouriotis, V. 1992. Bioconversion of chitin to chitosan: Purification and characterization of chitin deacetylase from *Mucor rouxii*. *Proc Natl Acad Sci USA* 90(7): 2564–2568.

30. Broussignac, P. 1968. Chitosan: A natural polymer not well known by the industry. *Chim Ind Genie Chim* 99(9): 1241–1247.

31. Domszy, J. G. and Roberts, G. A. F. 1985. Evaluation of infrared spectroscopic techniques for analyzing chitosan. *Macromol Chem* 186(8): 1671–1677.

32. Chen, Z. and Guo, S. 1990. Improvement of alkali method determining amino in chitosan. *Chem Bull* (10): 42–43.

33. Wu, X., Zeng, Q., Zeng, F., and Zhang, L. 2004. A discussion on determination of the deacetylation degree of chitosan by alkali titration method. *Guangzhou Food Sci Technol* 20(4): 96–97.

34. Sannan, K. K. and Iwakura, Y. 1976. Studies on chitin, 2. Effect of deacetylation on solubility. *Macromol Chem* 177(12): 3589–3600.

35. Ke, H. and Chen, Q. 1990. Potentiometric titration chitosan by linear method. *Chem Bull* (10): 44–46.

36. Lin, R., Jiang, S., and Zhang, M. 1992. Determination of deacetylation degree. *Chem Bull* (3): 39–42.

37. Sannan, T., Kurita, K., Ogura, K., and Iwakaru, T. 1978. Studies on chitin: 7. I.R. spectroscopic determination of degree of deacetylation. *Polymer* 19(4): 458–459.

38. Rathke, T. and Hudson, S. 1993. Determination of the degree of *N*-deacetylation in chitin and chitosan as well as their monomer sugar ratios by near infrared spectroscopy. *J Polym Sci Part A: Polym Chem* 31(3): 749–753.

39. Miya, M., Iwamoto, K., Yoshikawa, S., and Mima, S. 1980. I.R. spectroscopic determination of CONH content in highly deacylated chitosan. *Int J Biol Macromol* 2(5): 323–324.

40. Muzzarelli, R. A. A. and Tanfani, F. 1980. The degree of acetylation of chitins by gas chromatography and infrared spectroscopy. *J Biochem Biophys Methods* 2(5): 299–306.

41. Neugebauer, W. A., Neugebauer, E., and Brzezinski, R. 1989. Determination of the degree of *N*-acetylation of chitin–chitosan with picric acid. *Carbohydr Res* 189: 363–367.

42. Wang, W., Qin, W., Li, S., and Bo, S. 1991. The molecular weight of chitin. *Chinese J Appl Chem* 8(6): 85–87.

43. Hiroshi, T. 1952. Method of colloid titration (a new titration between polymer ions). *J Polym Sci* 8(2): 243–253.

44. Wang, W., Li, S., and Qin, W. 1989. Colloid titration method to measure the amino concentration of chitosan. *China Surf Detergent Cosmetics* (2): 36–38.

45. Alonso, G., Penichi-Covas, C., and Nieto, J. M. 1983. Determination of the degree of acetylation of chitin and chitosan by thermal analysis. *J Thermal Anal* 28(1): 189–193.

46. Lal, G. S. and Hayes, E. R. 1984. Determination of the amine content of chitosan by pyrolysis–gas chromatography. *J Anal Appl Pyrol* 6(2): 183–193.

47. Moore, G. K. and Roberts, G. A. F. 1981. Reactions of chitosan: 3. Preparation and reactivity of Schiff's base derivatives of chitosan. *Int J Biol Macromol* 3(5): 337–341.

48. Domard, A. and Cartier, N. 1989. Glucosamine oligomers: 1. Preparation and characterization. *Int J Biol Macromol* 11(5): 297–302.

49. Imoto, T. and Yagshito, K. 1971. A simple activity measurement of lysozyme. *Agric Biol Chem* 35(7): 1154–1156.

50. Wu, J. 2001. Determination of mean relative molecular mass of chitosan–oligosaccharide by photometric analysis. *Chem World* 42(6): 293–295.

51. Capon, B. and Foster, R. L. 1970. The preparation of chitin oligosaccharides. *Chem Soc* 3(12): 1654–1655.
52. Jiang, T. 1996. *Chitin*. Beijing: China Environmental Science Press, pp. 149–152, 377–380.
53. Fang, Z., Liu, W., Wei, X., and Han, B. 2005. The separation of chito-oligosaccharides by HPLC with TLC. *Periodical Ocean Univ China* 35(1): 113–115.
54. Yui, T., Kobayashi, H., Kitamura, S., and Imada, K. 1994. Conformational analysis of chitobiose and chitosan. *Biopolymers* 34(2): 203–208.
55. Ravi Kumar, M. N. V., Muzzarelli, R. A. A., Muzzarelli, C., Sashiwa, H., and Domb, A. J. 2004. Chitosan chemistry and pharmaceutical perspectives. *Chem Rev* 104: 6017–6084.
56. Okuyama, K., Noguchi, K., Miyazawa, R., Yui, T., and Ogawa, K. 1997. Molecular and crystal structure of hydrated chitosan. *Macromolecules* 30(19): 5849–5855.
57. Yui, T., Imada, K., Okuyama, K., Obata, Y., Suzuki, K., and Ogawa, K. 1994. Molecular and crystal structure of the anhydrous form of chitosan. *Macromolecules* 27(26): 7601–7605.
58. Yui, T., Ogasawara, T., and Ogawa, K. 1995. Miniature crystal models of the anhydrous form of chitosan. *Macromolecules* 28(23): 7957–7958.
59. Okuyama, K., Noguchi, K., Hanafusa, Y., Osawa, K., and Ogawa, K. 1999. Structural study of anhydrous tendon chitosan obtained via chitosan/acetic acid complex. *Int J Biol Macromol* 26(4): 285–293.
60. Focher, B., Naggi, A., Torri, G., Cosani, A., and Terbojevich, M. 1992. Structural differences between chitin polymorphs and their precipitates from solutions—Evidence from CP-MAS ^{13}CNMR, FT-IR and FT-Raman spectroscopy. *Carbohydr Polym* 17: 97–102.
61. Pearson, F. G., Marchessault, R. H., and Liang, C. Y. 1960. Infrared spectra of crystalline polysaccharides. V. Chitin. *J Polym Sci* 13: 101–116.
62. Iwamoto, R., Miya, M., and Mima, S. 1982. Vibrational polarization spectra of a-type chitin. In: Hirano, S., Tokura, S., eds. *Chitin and Chitosan. Proceedings of the Second International Conference on Chitin and Chitosan*. Sapporo: The Japanese Society of Chitin and Chitosan, pp. 82–86.
63. Rinaudo, M. 2006. Chitin and chitosan: Properties and applications. *Prog Polym Sci* 31: 603–632.
64. Grant, S., Blair, H. S., and Mckay, G. 1988. Water-soluble derivatives of chitosan. *Polym Commun* 29(11): 342–344.
65. Grant, S., Blair, H. S., and Mckay, G. 1989. Structural studies on chitosan and other chitin derivatives. *Macromol Chem* 190(9): 2279–2286.
66. Uenoyama, H., Shimizu, K., and Oshima, T. 2007. Cosmetics with specified pH for common use among humans and pet animals. *Jpn Kokai Tokkyo Koho* 14pp.
67. Watabe, K., Sawada, M., and Tsunakawa, S. 1997. Cosmetic packs containing chitosan organic acid salts and pullulan. *Jpn Kokai Tokkyo Koho* 4pp.
68. Terbojevich, M., Carraro, C., Cosani, A., Focher, B., Naggi, M., and Torri, G. 1989. Solution studies of chitosan 6-*O*-sulfate. *Macromol Chem* 190(11): 2847–2855.
69. Wolfrom, M. L., Vercellotti, J. R., and Horton, D. 1964. Methylation studies on carboxyl-reduced heparin. 2-amino-2-deoxy-3,6-di-*O*-methyl-α-D-glucopyranose from the methylation of chitosan. *J Org Chem* 29(3): 547–550.
70. Jiang, T. 1984. Benzylated of *N*-acetyl glycosaminoglycan by phase transfer catalysis. *Chinese Sci Bull* 29(13): 792–795.
71. Wang, A. and Yu, X. 1998. Study on the preparation and properties of alkyl–chitosan derivatives. *J Funct Polym* 11(1): 83–86.
72. Moore, G. K. and Roberts, G. A. F. 1982. Reactions of chitosan: 4. Preparation of organosoluble derivatives of chitosan. *Int J Biol Macromol* 4(4): 246–249.
73. Synowiecki, J., Sikorski, Z. E., Naczk, M., and Piotrzkowska, H. 1982. Immobilization of enzymes on krill chitin activated by formaldehyde. *Biotechnol Bioeng* 24(8): 1871–1876.
74. Hall, L. D. and Yalpani, M. 1980. Synthesis of luminescent probe–sugar conjugates of either protected or unprotected sugar. *Carbohydr Res* 78(1): C4–C6.
75. Muzzarelli, R. A. A. and Tanfani, F. 1985. The *N*-permethylation of chitosan and the preparation of *N*-trimethyl chitosan iodide. *Carbohydr Polym* 5(4): 297–307.

76. Qu, R. and Ma, Q. 1995. Preparation of chitosan derivatives and their adsorption behaviour. *Chinese J Appl Chem* 12(2): 117–118.
77. Muzzarelli, R. A. A. and Tanfani, F. 1982. N-(carboxymethyl) chitosans and N-(o-carboxybenzyl) chitosans: Novel chelating polyampholytes. *Chitin chitosan, Proceedings of the Second International Conference.* Muzzarelli, R. A. A., eds. MIT Sea Grant Program, Cambridge, MA, 45–53.
78. Muzzarelli, R. A. A., Tanfani, F., Emanuelli, M., and Mariotti, S. 1982. *N*-(o-carboxybenzyl) chitosans: Novel chelating polyampholytes. *Carbohydr Polym* 2(2): 145–147.
79. Horton, D. and Just, E. K. 1973. Preparation from chitin of $(1 \rightarrow 4)$-2-amino-2-deoxy-β-D-glucopyranuronan and its 2-sulfoamino analog having blood-anticoagulant properties. *Carbohydr Res* 29(1): 173–179.
80. Muzzarelli, R. A. A. 1973. *Natural Chelating Polymers.* Oxford: Oergamon Press.
81. Yaku, F. and Koshijima, T. 1978. In *Proceedings of the First International Conference on Chitin/Chitosan.* Muzzarelli, R. A. A., and Pariser, E. R., eds. MIT Sea Grant Program, Cambridge, MA, 386pp.
82. Nieto, J. M., Peniche, C., and Bosque, J. D. 1992. Preparation and characterization of a chitosan-Fe (III) complex. *Carbohydr Polym* 18(3): 221–224.
83. Guan, H., Cheng, X., and Tong, Y. 1999. Coordination number of coordination polymer for chitosan with Ni^{2+} and chitosan with La^{3+}. *J Funct Polym* 12(4): 431–435.
84. Kurita, K., Kawata, M., and Kayama, M. Y. 1991. Graft copolymerization of vinyl monomers onto chitin with cerium (IV) ion. *J Appl Polym Sci* 42(11): 2885–2891.
85. Lagos, A., Yazdani-Pedram, M., and Reyes, J. 1992. Ceric ion-initiated grafting of poly(methyl acrylate) onto chitin. *J M S-Pure Appl Chem A* 29(11): 1007–1015.
86. Lee, Y. C., Kim, K. S., and Shin, J. S. 1989. Graft polymerization of methyl methacrylate onto chitin initiated by ceric salt. *Polymer (Korea)* 13(5): 442–446.
87. Ren, L., Miura, Y., and Nishi, N. 1993. Modification of chitin by ceric salt-initiated graft polymerisation—Preparation of poly(methyl methacrylate)-grafted chitin derivatives that swell in organic solvents. *Carbohydr Polym* 21(1): 23–27.
88. Ren, L. and Tokura, S. 1994. Structural aspects of poly (methyl methacrylate)-grafted β-chitin copolymers initiated by ceric salt. *Carbohydr Polym* 23(1): 19–25.
89. Yang, J., He, D., Wu, J., Yang, H., and Gao, Y. 1984. The study of the grafting polymerization of methyl methacrylate on chitin film initiated by ceric salt. *J Shandong Coll Oceanol* 14(4): 58–62.
90. Yazdani-Pedram, M., Lagos, A., and Campos, N. 1992. Comparison of redox initiators reactivities in the grafting of methyl methacrylate onto chitin. *Inter J Polym Mater* 18(1–2): 25–37.
91. Shantha, K. L., Bala, U., and Rao, K. P. 1995. Tailor-made chitosans for drug delivery. *Eur Polym J* 31(4): 377–382.
92. Wei, D., Luo, X., Deng, P., and Tao, J. 1995. Study on the emulsion graft copolymerization of butyl acrylate onto chitosan. *Acta Polym Sin* (4): 427–433.
93. Lagos, A. and Reyes, J. 1988. Grafting onto chitosan. I. Graft copolymerization of methyl methacrylate onto chitosan with Fenton's reagent ($Fe^{2+} - H_2O_2$) as a redox initiator. *J Polym Sci Part A: Polym Chem* 26(4): 985–991.
94. Kojima, K., Yoshikuni, M., and Suzuki, T. 1979. Tributylborane-initiated grafting of methyl methacrylate onto chitin. *J Appl Polym Sci* 24(7): 1587–1593.
95. Blar, H., Guthric, T., and Law, T. 1987. Chitosan and modified chitosan membranes I. Preparation and characterisation. *J Appl Polym Sci* 33(2): 641–656.
96. Shigeno, Y., Kondo, K., and Takemoto, K. 1980. Functional monomers and polymers. LXX. Adsorption of iodine onto chitosan. *J Appl Polym Sci* 25(5): 731–738.
97. Singh, D. K. and Ray, A. R. 1994. Graft copolymerization of 2-hydroxy ethylmethacrylate onto chitosan films and their blood compatibility. *J Appl Polym Sci* 53(8): 1115–1121.
98. Takahashi, A., Sugahara, Y., and Hirano, Y. 1989. Studies on graft copolymerization onto cellulose derivatives. XXIX. Photo-induced graft copolymerization of methyl methacrylate onto chitin and oxychitin. *J Polym Sci Part A: Polym Chem* 27(11): 3817–3828.

99. Kurita, K., Inoue, S., and Yamamura, K. 1992. Cationic and radical graft copolymerization of styrene onto iodochitin. *Macromolecules* 25(14): 3791–3794.

100. Kurita, K., Hashimota, S., and Yoshino, H. 1996. Preparation of chitin/polystyrene hybrid materials by efficient graft copolymerization based on mercaptochitin. *Macromolecules* 29(6): 1939–1942.

101. Kurita, K. and Inoue, S. 1989. *Chitin Source Book: A Guide to Research Literature*. Pariser, E. R., and Lombard, D., eds. New York, NY: John Wiley and Sons. 365.

102. Aiba, S., Minoura, N., and Fujiwara, Y. 1985. Graft copolymerization of amino acids onto partially deacetylated chitin. *Int J Biol Macromol* 7(2): 120–121.

103. Wang, G., Qian, S., Huang, G., Yan, L., and Mo, S. 2005. Preconcentration of trace Pt on cross-linked chitosan and its determination by graphite furnace atomic absorption spectrometry. *Chem J Int* 7(1): 3

104. Wang, M., Huang, G., Qian, S., Jiang, S., Wan, Y., and Chau, Y. K. 1997. A novel preconcentration technique using cross-linked chitosan for determination of mercury by CVAAS. *Fresenius' J Anal Chem* 358(7–8): 856–858.

105. Fouda, M., Zorjanovic, J., and Knitte, D. 2005. Biological, medical and pharmaceutical application of chitosans. *Zsigmondy Colloquium with the Annual Meeting of the Swiss Group of Colloid and Interface Science*. Bern, pp. 3–4.

106. Huang, R., Chen, G., Sun, M., Hu, Y., and Gao, C. 2006. Studies on nanofiltration membrane formed by diisocyanate cross-linking of quaternized chitosan on poly(acrylonitrile) (PAN) support. *J Mem Sci* 286(1–2): 237–244.

107. Xu, Y. and Ni, C. 1991. Synthesise and adsorption properties of chelating resins obtained by the reaction of chitosan with chloromethylthiirane. *Acta Polym Sin* (1): 57–63.

108. Hu, Y., Xu, Y., Feng, C., and Dong, S. 1992. Study on chelating resins. XIX. The syntheses and adsorption properties of chelatin resins based on chitosan. *Ion Exchange Adsorp* 8(3): 229–233.

109. Ledderhose, G. 1876. Ueber salzsaures glycosamin. *Chemische Berichte* 9(2): 1200–1201.

110. ASTM F2013-01 *Standard Guide for Characterization and Testing of Chitosan Salts as Starting Materials Intended for Use in Biomedical and Tissue-Engineered Medical Product Applications*.

111. YY/T (The People's Republic of China pharmaceutical industry standards) 0606.7 Tissue engineered medical products-part 7: Chitosan.

112. SC/T (The People's Republic of China Fisheries Industry Standard) 3403 Chitin and Chitosan.

2

Chitosan Derivatives

Junjie Li, Liandong Deng, and Fanglian Yao

CONTENTS

2.1 Introduction

Chitosan displays interesting properties such as biocompatibility and biodegradability, and its degradation products are nontoxic, nonimmunogenic, and noncarcinogenic. Therefore, chitosan has prospective applications in many fields such as biomedicine, waste water treatment, functional membranes, and flocculation. However, the commercial or practical use of chitin and chitosan (including monomers and oligomers) has been confined to the unmodified forms. For a breakthrough in utilization, chemical modification to introduce a variety of functional groups will be a key point. For this purpose, more fundamental studies on chemical modification will be required. Fortunately, chitosan is an amenable molecule. Without disturbing the degree of polymerization (DP) of chitosan, one can chemically modify this acquiescent polymer because it provides functional groups as primary amine and primary as well as secondary hydroxyl groups in its monomers.

2.2 *N*-Alkyl-Chitosans

The primary amino groups of chitosan undergo Schiff reaction with aldehydes and ketones to yield the corresponding aldimines and ketimines, which are converted to an *N*-alkyl derivative by reduction with sodium borohydride (NaBH$_4$) or sodium cyanoborohydride (NaBH$_3$CN) among other reducing agents (Figure 2.1). The choice of the reducing agent is

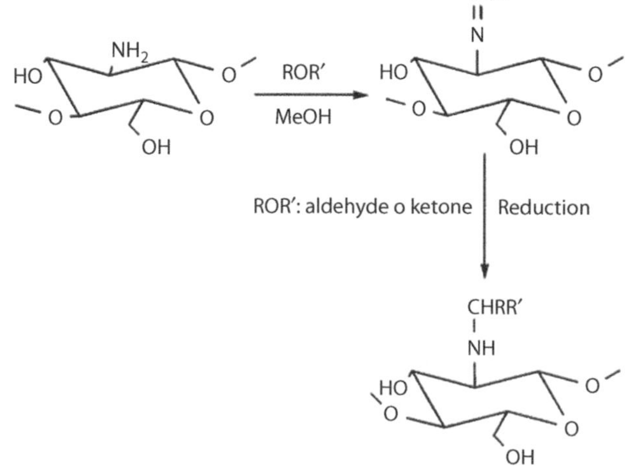

FIGURE 2.1
Synthesis of *N*-alkyl chitosans.

crucial to the success of the reaction because the reducing agent must reduce imines selectively. $NaBH_3CN$ is widely used in reductive alkylation systems because it is more reactive and selective than standard reducing agents. However, it is highly toxic and generates toxic by-products such as HCN or NaCN. Therefore, the use of this reducing agent is not acceptable in green synthesis [1,2].

The existence of hydrophobic interactions between alkyl chains improves the physicochemical properties of solutions of modified chitosans. Rinaudo et al. [3] have studied the bulk and interfacial properties of a series of alkylated chitosans having different alkyl chain lengths (C3, C6, C8, C10, and C12) and two degrees of substitution (DSs), 2% and 5%. The optimum alkyl chain length was C12 and the degree of grafting was 5% to obtain physical gelation based on the formation of hydrophobic domains. The cross-linking was essentially controlled by the salt concentration. Hydrophobic interactions produced highly non-Newtonian behavior with large thinning behavior; this behavior was suppressed in the presence of cyclodextrins (CDs) able to cap the hydrophobic alkyl chains. The interfacial properties of chitosan derivatives were tested for air/aqueous solution interfaces. Specifically, the role of their structure in the kinetics of film formation was examined, showing that an excess of external salt favors stabilization of the interfacial film. Derivatives with a higher DS and longer alkyl chains were more efficient and gave a higher elastic modulus compared to the model surfactant as a result of the chain properties.

Apart from rheological studies and the application of chitosan alkyl derivatives as rheological modifiers, especially in aqueous-based formulations in various industrial domains such as paints, oil recovery, cosmetics, and food, alkyl chitosan derivatives have been used in drug delivery systems, tissue engineering, and several technological applications. Klotzbach et al. [4,5] modified chitosan with butanal, hexanal, octanal, or decanal aldehydes to prepare a biocompatible and biodegradable hydrophobic chitosan membrane that can replace Nafion® for electrode coatings in both sensor and fuel cell applications. Several enzymes such as glucose oxidase, alcohol dehydrogenase, formate dehydrogenase, lactic dehydrogenase, glucose dehydrogenase, and formaldehyde dehydrogenase were successfully immobilized and voltammetric studies were carried out. This is the first evidence which shows that hydrophobically modified chitosan can be used at the anode of a biofuel cell.

N-Succinyl-N-octyl chitosan (SOCS), which can form micelles in aqueous media, has been prepared by modifying the amino group with hydrophobic long-chain alkyl functionality and a hydrophilic succinyl moiety [6]. Doxorubicin (DOX), a model antitumor drug, was successfully loaded into SOCS micelles and a sustained release pattern was observed. The *in vitro* antitumor activity studies indicated that DOX-loaded SOCS micelles were more cytotoxic than free DOX.

2.3 Quaternized Chitosan

Chitosan has been extensively evaluated for its mucoadhesive and absorption enhancement properties. The positive charge on the chitosan molecule gained by the acidic environment in which it is soluble seems to be important for absorption enhancement. However, chitosan is not soluble in medium except below pH 5.6. This limits its use as a permeation enhancer in body compartments where the pH is high. In this regard there is a need for chitosan derivatives with increased solubility, especially at neutral and basic pH values.

Quaternization of chitosan is an effort in this direction. *N,N,N*-Trimethyl chitosan chloride (TMC) with much higher aqueous solubility than chitosan in a much broader pH and concentration range overcomes this problem, as demonstrated by its use as an absorption enhancer for test drugs such as buserelin, octreotide acetate, 9-desglycinamide-8-arginine vasopressin, fluorescein-isothiocyanate dextran (FD4, MW4400), mannitol, and so on [7]. The trimethylation of chitosan also allows maintenance or improvement of the mucoadhesive properties of starting chitosans, depending on quaternization degree. In particular, mucoadhesive properties increase with increasing degree of quaternization (DQ).

Quaternization of chitosan was successfully carried out by using iodomethane, iodoethane, or dimethylsulfate or by grafting with a compound that contains the quaternary ammonium moiety itself.

2.3.1 Quaternization of Chitosan Using Iodomethane

Quaternization (methylation) of the primary amino groups of chitosan was carried out using iodomethane in an alkaline solution of *N*-methyl pyrrolidinone (NMP). Quaternization is based on the nucleophilic substitution of the primary amino group on the C-2 position of chitosan with iodomethane and sodium iodide used as a catalyst. Muzzarelli and Tanfani [8] first prepared *N,N,N*-trimethyl chitosan iodide (TMI) by reacting *N,N*-dimethylated chitosan (DMC), which had previously been prepared by treating chitosan with formaldehyde followed by reduction with NaBH$_4$, with iodomethane in acetonitrile at 35°C for 30 h. Chitosan with a high DQ of 60% was obtained, but it was not soluble in water. Domard et al. [9] prepared TMC by reacting chitosan, suspended in NMP, with iodomethane in the presence of sodium hydroxide and iodomethane at 36°C for 3 h (Figure 2.2). A DQ of 64% was obtained after repeated quaternization. The chloride counterion was changed to an iodide one using ion-exchange resin in order to enhance the stability of quaternized chitosan. It was noted that chitosan with DQ greater than 25% is soluble in water. It was found that not only the primary amino groups but also the hydroxyl groups of chitosan were quaternized [10]. Repeated quaternization through subsequent additional steps resulted in chitosan with DQ higher than 85%, but it produced a poorly water-soluble TMC due to a large amount of O-methylation [11].

Hamman and Kotzé [12] studied the effects of the type of base and the amount of quaternization on DQ and molecular weight of TMC. Increases in DQ ranged from 21% to 59% with an increase in the amount of quaternization. The intrinsic viscosity value showed that dimethylaminopyridine used as a base did not cause polymer degradation compared with sodium hydroxide. However, the disadvantage of dimethylaminopyridine is that it provided a low DQ ranging from 7% to 10%, even though the amount of quaternization was increased. In addition, DQ can be slightly increased from 10% to 34% if the two bases,

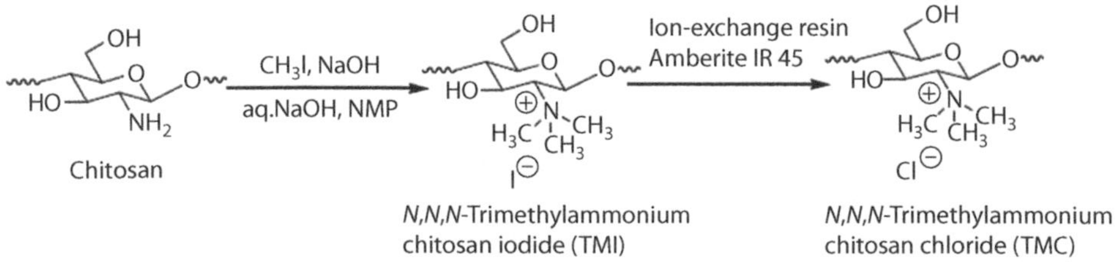

FIGURE 2.2
Synthesis of TMC.

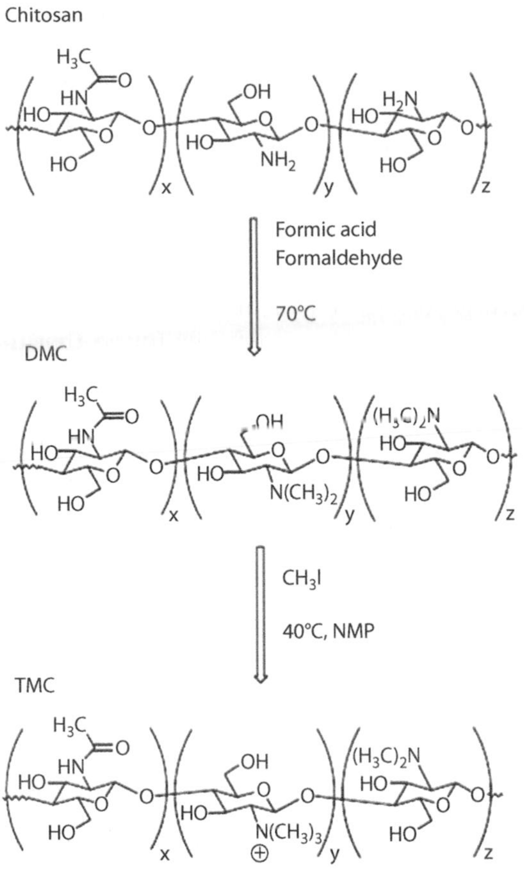

FIGURE 2.3
Two-step synthetic pathway for the preparation of TMC avoiding O-methylation.

dimethylaminopyridine and sodium hydroxide, are used together. Snyman et al. [13] synthesized TMC with various conditions based on the methods of Sieval et al. [11] and Hamman and Kotze [13]. They found that DQ was in the range of 22–59%, depending on the number of repeated reaction steps. DQ was increased by increasing the number of repeated reaction steps. Moreover, the decrease in intrinsic viscosity and molecular weight of the starting chitosan correlated with the increase in the number of repeated reaction steps. This was due to the effects of time, alkali, and temperature. Curiti et al. [14] found that the chemoselectivity of the N-methylation of chitosan was affected by the addition of excess sodium hydroxide and iodomethane. Therefore, O-methylation was favored when a larger excess of these reagents was used. Polnok et al. [15] investigated the effects of quaternization of the chitosan process and types of base. They found that a DQ higher than 75% was necessary to repeat the reaction steps. However, an increase in the number of reaction steps provided high O-methylation, which would decrease the aqueous solubility of TMC.

Runarsson et al. [16] synthesized TMC by changing the solvent system from NMP to an N,N-dimethylformamide/water mixture (50:50) and performed the reaction without the aid of a catalyst—for example, sodium iodide. This significantly reduced O-methylation since N,N-dimethylformamide/water seems to lower the reactivity of the hydroxyl group sufficiently in order to keep the O-methylation down. They found that DQ was in the range of 0–74% depending on the reaction conditions accompanying N-monomethylation, N,N-dimethylation, and O-methylation. Based on this solvent system, they also recently claimed to achieve a high DQ ranging from 81% to 88% by the "one-pot" synthesis procedure. They suggested a protection group strategy for more selective N-quaternization (sequence of N-phthaloylation, O-tritylation, N-deprotection, N-methylation, and O-deprotection) [17]. Recently, Verheul et al. [18] synthesized TMC without O-methylation using two steps (Figure 2.3). In the first step, a formic acid–formaldehyde methylation (Eschweiler–Clarke) was used to synthesize the N,N-dimethylated chitosan (DMC). Quaternization of DMC was performed by using iodomethane in NMP without the assistance of a catalyst for the last step. Moreover, they found that the molecular weight of TMC slightly increased with increasing DQ, implying that no chain scission occurred during synthesis.

2.3.2 Quaternization of Chitosan Using Glycidyl Trimethylammonium Chloride

Glycidyl trimethylammonium chloride (GTMAC) was selected as a quarternizing agent because it has a quaternary ammonium group itself. When a primary amino group at C-2 of chitosan reacted with GTMAC, the chain of the quaternary ammonium group obtained was longer than that of TMC. Loubaki et al. [19] synthesized and characterized GTMAC-modified chitosan by reacting chitosan with GTMAC (*cf.* Figure 2.4). The reaction was performed in water at 60°C for 15 h. The complete DQ was obtained by using the molar ratio of GTMAC:GlcN of chitosan as 6:1. They found that N-monoalkylation was obtained under this condition.

Daly and Manuszak-Guerrini [20] developed a method for the synthesis of N-(2-hydroxy) propyl-3-trimethylammonium chitosan chloride (HPTC) using commercially available Quat-188 salt, 3-chloro-2-hydroxypropyl trimethylammonium chloride, under the basic condition. This product was called chitosan Quat-188. Under this condition, Quat-188 readily generated the corresponding epoxide, which reacted in both the primary amino groups and hydroxyl groups of chitosan via a nucleophilic substitution pathway to introduce the quaternary ammonium substituent (*cf.* Figure 2.5). It is important to note that sodium hydroxide concentration affects the generation of the epoxide form of Quat-188. If a high sodium hydroxide concentration is used, it will not only activate the polysaccharide but will also hydrolyze Quat-188 and produce large amounts of the diol [21,22].

Recently, Sajomsang et al. [23] quaternized N-aryl chitosan derivatives, which contained different electron-donating and electron-withdrawing substituents, using Quat-188 (cf. Figure 2.6). Iodine was used as a catalyst and the pH of the reaction condition was maintained at 8 at room temperature for 48 h. To obtain complete quaternization, the reaction was heated up to 50°C for 24 h. Even when the reaction was performed at room temperature and the pH was adjusted to 8, O-alkylation could occur in this condition.

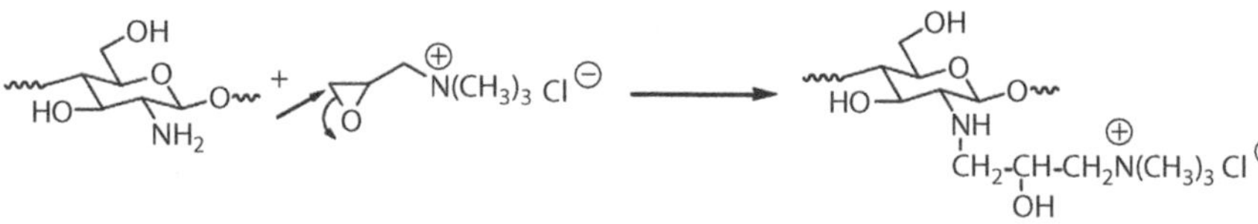

FIGURE 2.4
Reaction of chitosan with GTMAC.

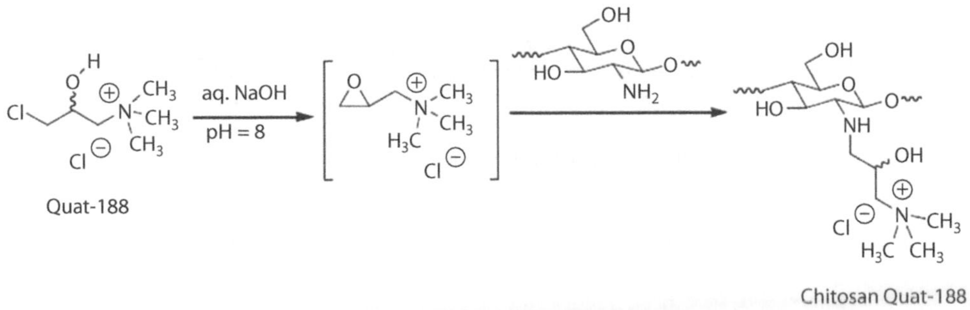

FIGURE 2.5
Reaction of chitosan with 3-chloro-2-hydroxypropyl trimethylammonium chloride (Quat-188).

2.3.3 Quaternization of Chitosan Using Other Quaternizing Agents

De Britto and Assis [24] synthesized TMC by using dimethylsulfate as the methylating agent. They suggested that dimethylsulfate is less expensive and less toxic than iodomethane. Moreover, it has a higher boiling point than iodomethane and no solvent is required for the reaction. The quaternization of chitosan was performed in mixtures of sodium hydroxide solution and sodium chloride and refluxed with a methylating agent at room temperature or at 70°C. They found that DQ was in the range of 15–52%, depending on reaction time and temperature. Moreover, undesirable O-methylation and polymeric degradation were also observed to have taken place in the reaction.

2.3.4 Quaternization of Chitosan Derivatives

Alkylation of TMC produces amphiphilic polymeric molecules because it possesses both charged groups and nonpolar linear hydrocarbon branches in the chitosan backbone. Kim

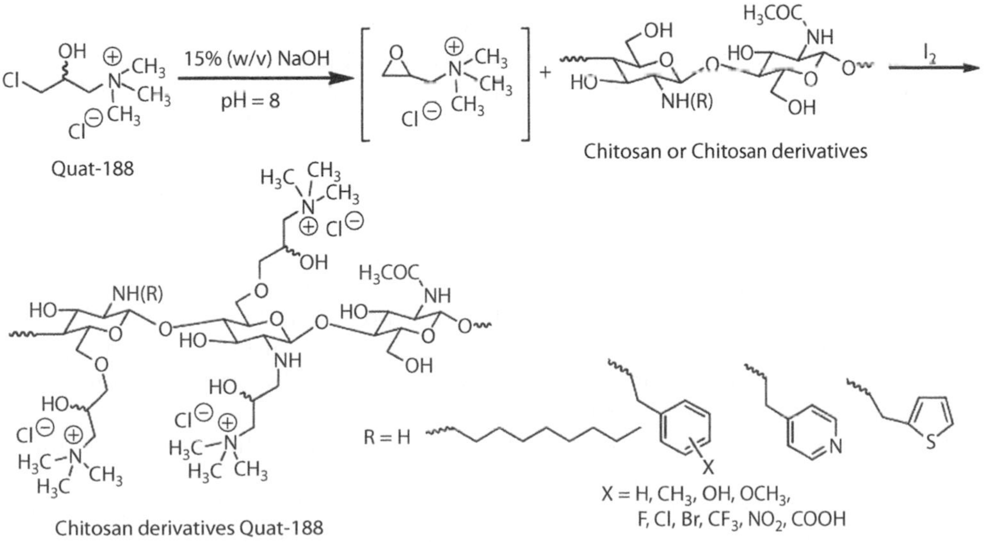

FIGURE 2.6
Synthesis of quaternized chitosan and quaternized *N*-aryl chitosan derivatives using Quat-188.

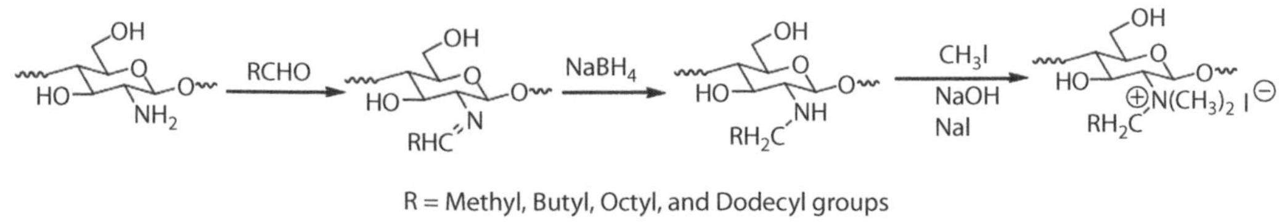

R = Methyl, Butyl, Octyl, and Dodecyl groups

FIGURE 2.7
Synthesis of quaternized *N*-alkyl chitosan derivatives using iodomethane as a quaternizing agent.

and Choi [25] and Kim et al. [26] prepared quaternized *N*-alkyl chitosan derivatives containing alkyl substituents of different chain lengths. The reaction was carried out in two steps: N-alkylation and quaternization. In the first step, chitosan reacted with formaldehyde, butyraldehyde, *n*-octylaldehyde, and *n*-dodecylaldehyde. Then the resulting Schiff bases were reduced with NaBH$_4$. In the last step, the *N*-alkyl chitosan derivatives were quaternized with iodomethane in the presence of sodium hydroxide as base and NMP (Figure 2.7). The trimethylated and triethylated 6-NH$_2$-6-deoxy chitosans were synthesized by Sadeghi et al. [27]. The 6-NH$_2$-6-deoxy chitosan was prepared in four steps: phthaloylation, tosylation, amination, and deprotection of the phthaloyl group. Then methylation and ethylation were carried out at both C-2 and C-6 of 6-NH$_2$-6-deoxy chitosan using iodomethane and iodoethane in the presence of sodium hydroxide and NMP, respectively. The DQs of trimethylated and triethylated 6-NH$_2$-6-deoxy chitosans were 65% and 51%, respectively.

Holappa et al. [28] synthesized chitosan *N*-betainates with various DSs. An efficient five-step synthetic route (N-phthaloylation, 6-O-triphenylmethylation, removal of the *N*-phthalimido moiety, addition of the *N*-betainate, and chitosan *N*-betainates) was developed for the full N-substitution of chitosan (Figure 2.8). Previously, N-acylation of chitosan with betaine was performed in aqueous acidic solutions, but it did not yield sufficient substitution degrees. To overcome this problem, an organo-soluble 6-O-triphenylmethyl chitosan intermediate was used as the starting material for N-acylation reactions to enable reactions in homogeneous reaction mixtures in organic solvents.

Furthermore, novel quaternary ammonium chitosan derivatives were synthesized by the same group [29]. *N*-Chloroacyl-6-O-triphenylmethylchitosan was used as the starting material for the synthesis of quaternary ammonium chitosan derivatives through reaction with four tertiary amines: pyridine, *N*-methylpyrrolidone, triethylamine, and tributylamine (*cf.* Figure 2.9).

The quaternary piperazine derivatives of chitosan were synthesized in two ways [30]. First, 1,4-dimethylpiperazine reacted with *N*-chloroacyl-6-O-triphenylmethylchitosan in the presence of potassium iodide and NMP under argon at 60°C for 72 h (Figure 2.10a). Second, 4-carboxymethyl-1,1-dimethylpiperazinium iodide or 1-carboxymethyl-1,4,4-trimethylpiperazi-1,4-dium diiodide reacted with 6-O-triphenylmethylchitosan using a coupling agent (Figure 2.10b). They found that the quaternary ammonium moiety can be selectively inserted into either one or both of the piperazine nitrogens, yielding structurally uniform chitosan derivative structures.

Sajomsang et al. [31,32] synthesized quaternary ammonium chitosan containing aromatic moieties, particularly aromatics bearing *N,N*-dimethylaminobenzyl and *N,N*-dimethylaminocinnamyl groups, based on the method of Curiti et al. [14]. In addition, quaternized *N*-(4-pyridylmethyl)chitosan was also synthesized. Quaternization occurred among *N,N*-dimethylaminobenzyl, *N,N*-dimethylcinnamylamino, and *N*-pyridylmethyl groups and the primary amino groups of chitosan (Figure 2.11). The total DQ of each

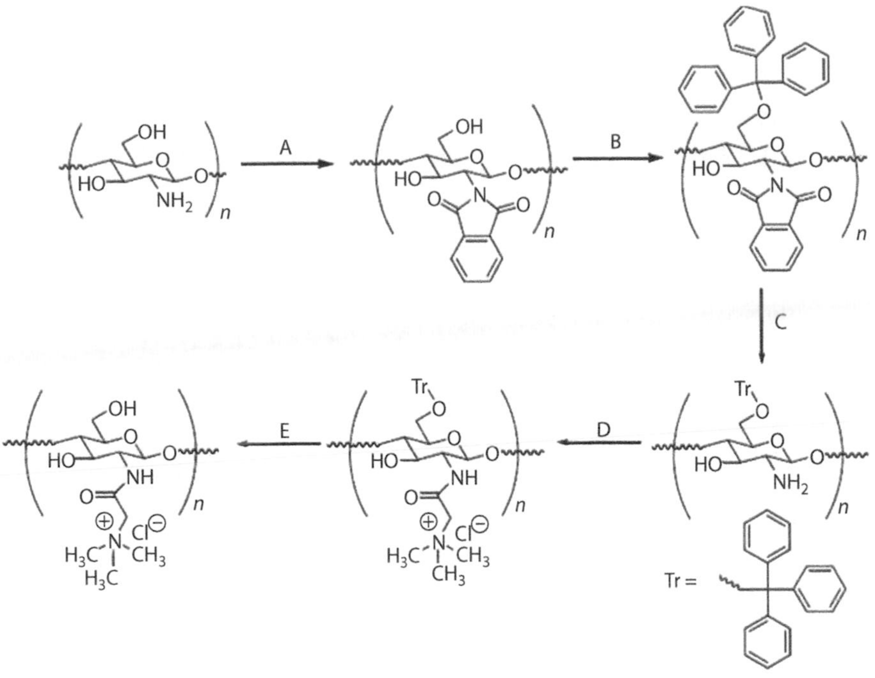

FIGURE 2.8
Synthetic route for the preparation of chitosan *N*-betainates: (A) phthalic anhydride, DMF/water, 120°C, (B) triphenylchloromethane, pyridine, 90°C, (C) hydrazine monohydrate, water, 120°C, (D) *N*-chlorobetainyl chloride (1, 2, and 4 equivalents), pyridine, room temperature, and (E) aq. HCl, room temperature.

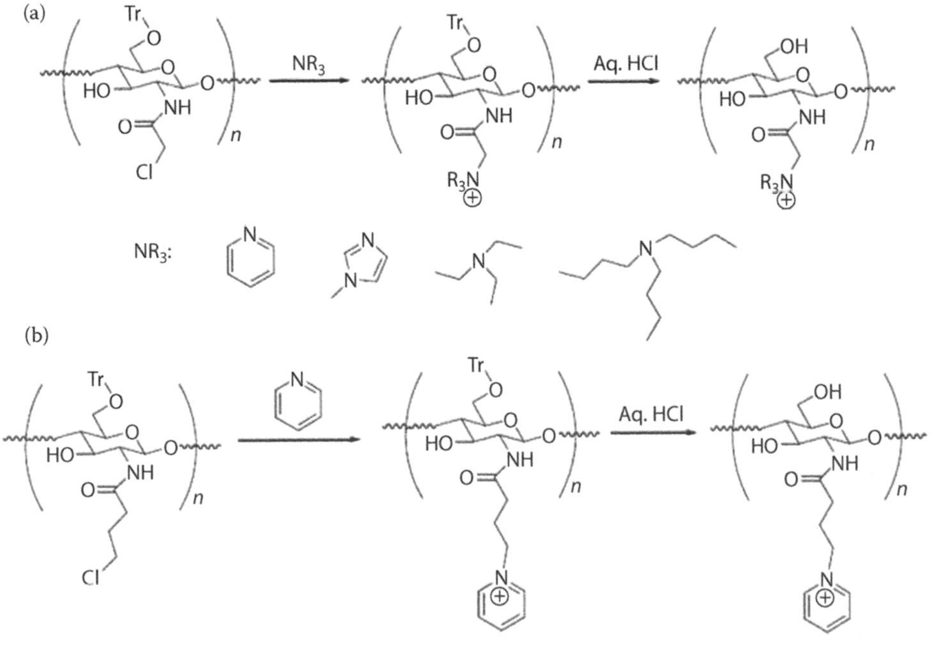

FIGURE 2.9
Synthetic route for the preparation of various quaternary ammonium chitosan derivatives via *N*-chloroacyl-6-triphenylchitosans (a and b).

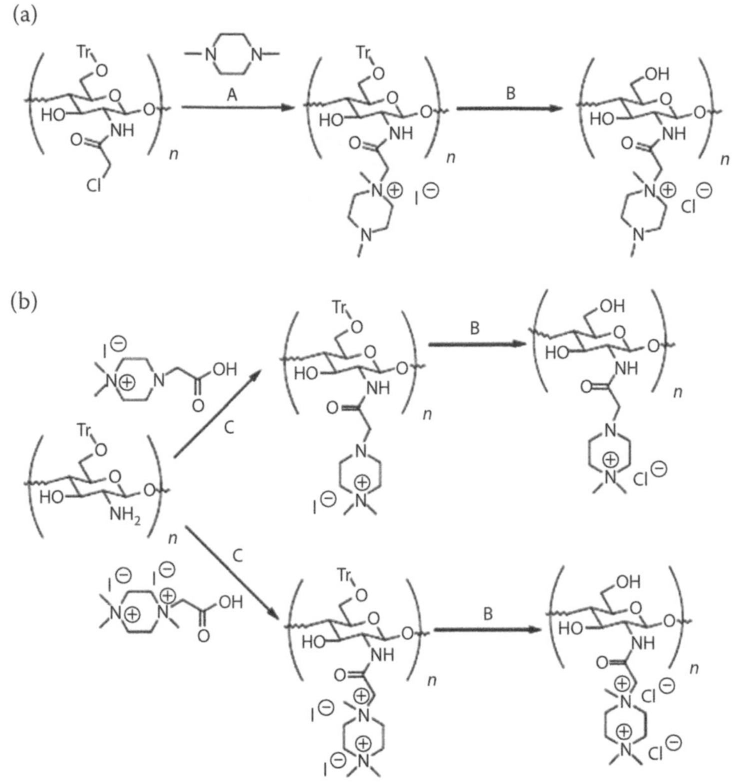

FIGURE 2.10
Synthetic route for the preparation of quaternary piperazine derivatives of chitosan: (A) KI, NMP, 60°C, (B) aq. HCl, room temperature, and (C) DCC, HOBt, NMP, room temperature.

chitosan derivative varied depending on the DS and the sodium hydroxide concentration used in quaternization.

2.4 Acyl Chitosan

Comparing N-alkylation with acylation, the latter is more versatile because it allows the introduction of hydrophobic moieties at amino, alcohol, or both residues. Moreover, the introduction of a hydrophobic moiety with an ester linkage allows the action of lipase-like enzymes, these derivatives being very interesting as biodegradable materials. *N*-Acyl chitosan derivatives with different purposes have been synthesized as shown in Table 2.1 [33].

2.4.1 *N*-Acyl Chitosan

N-Acyl derivatives of chitosan can be easily obtained from acyl chlorides and anhydrides (*cf.* Figure 2.12). In a general way, acylation reactions carry out frequently in mediums as aqueous acetic acid/methanol, pyridine, pyridine/chloroform, trichloroacetic acid/ dichloroethane, ethanol/methanol mixture, methanol/formamide, or DMA–LiCl [60]. Due

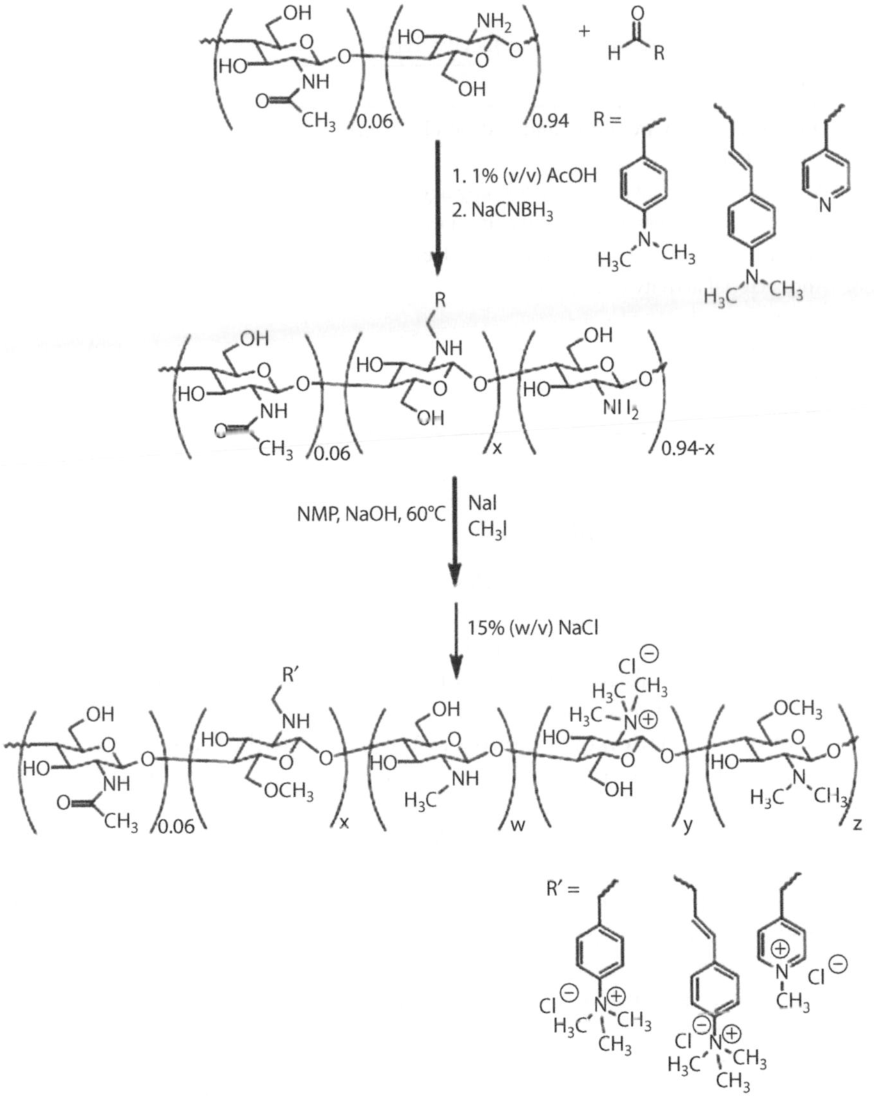

FIGURE 2.11
Synthesis of the quaternary ammonium chitosan containing aromatic moieties.

to fairly different reactivities of the two hydroxyl groups and the amino group on the repeating unit of chitosan, acylation can be controlled at the expected sites, that is, on amino [61–63], hydroxyls [64], or both groups [65–68]. The introduction of hydrophobic branches generally endows the polymers with new physicochemical properties such as the formation of polymeric assemblies, including gels [69], polymeric vesicles [70], Langmuir–Blodgett films [71,72], liquid crystals [73,74], membranes [75], and fibers [76,77]. Hydrophobic associating water-soluble polymers have emerged as a new class of industrially important macromolecules. Some of these are intended to mimic the endotoxins. The introduction of hydrophobic branches also endows the polymers with a better soluble range than chitosan itself.

TABLE 2.1

Applications of Acyl-Chitosan Derivatives

Application	References
Drug delivery (hydrophobic and hydrophilic drugs)	[34–46]
DNA delivery	[47–49]
Polymeric surfactants, foaming forming agents	[50]
Artificial viscosifiers (biomedical and pharmaceutical application)	[50]
Dispersant/coating of nanoparticles (biolabeling and biosensoring)	[51,52]
Antibacterial activity (biomedicine)	[47]
Smart materials	[53–56]
Tissue engineering	[38]
One-step purification of IgG	[57]
LB layers	[58,59]

2.4.1.1 Acyl Derivatives from Anhydrides

N-Succinyl-chitosan (NSCS), with a well-designed structure and the ability to self-assemble in regular nanosphere morphology, has been successfully synthesized [78]. The *in vitro* cell culture indicates that NSCS is nontoxic and has cell compatibility. The interactions between NSCS and bovine serum albumin (BSA) were studied [34]. It has been demonstrated that BSA binds to NSCS with a molar ratio of 30:1. This study demonstrates the potential of the NSCS matrix for encapsulation of proteins or other hydrophilic bioactive drugs.

Stearoyl, palmitoyl, and octanoyl chitosan derivatives with DSs from 0.9% to 29.6% have been prepared [79]. The N-fatty acylations were carried out by reacting carboxylic anhydride with chitosan in dimethylsulfoxide (DMSO). The chitosan derivative-based micelles were spherical in shape, their sizes being in the range of 140–278 nm. The properties of palmitoyl-chitosan micelles such as encapsulation capacity and controlled release ability of the hydrophobic model drug ibuprofen (Ib) were evaluated [36]. Experimental results indicated that the loading capacity of palmitoyl-chitosan was approximately 10%. The drug release strongly depended on pH and temperature; low pH and high-temperature accelerated drug release markedly.

Chitosan was selectively N-acylated with acetic, propionic, and hexanoic anhydrides under homogeneous conditions in order to prepare *N*-acetyl chitosan (NACS), *N*-propionyl chitosan (NPCS), and *N*-hexanoyl chitosan, respectively [47]. NACSs with different N-acetylation degrees were obtained by controlling the degree of N-acetylation. Intramolecular aggregation of NPCS and NACS was stronger with NPCS than with NACS. Hydrophobic interaction of N-acylated chitosan substituted with longer acyl chains was stronger. With moderate DS, intramolecular aggregation occurs predominantly.

2.4.1.2 Acyl Chitosan Derivatives from Acyl Chlorides

Oleoylchitosans (OCSs) have been synthesized by reacting chitosan with oleoyl chloride [37]. The hemolysis rates of OCS nanoparticles tested in different conditions were well within permissible limits (5%). OCS nanoparticles showed no cytotoxicity to mouse embryo fibroblasts. DOX was efficiently loaded into OCS nanoparticles (encapsulation efficiency: 52.6%). The drug was rapidly and completely released from the nanoparticles (DOX–OCS nanoparticles) at pH 3.8, whereas at pH 7.4 there was a sustained release after a burst release.

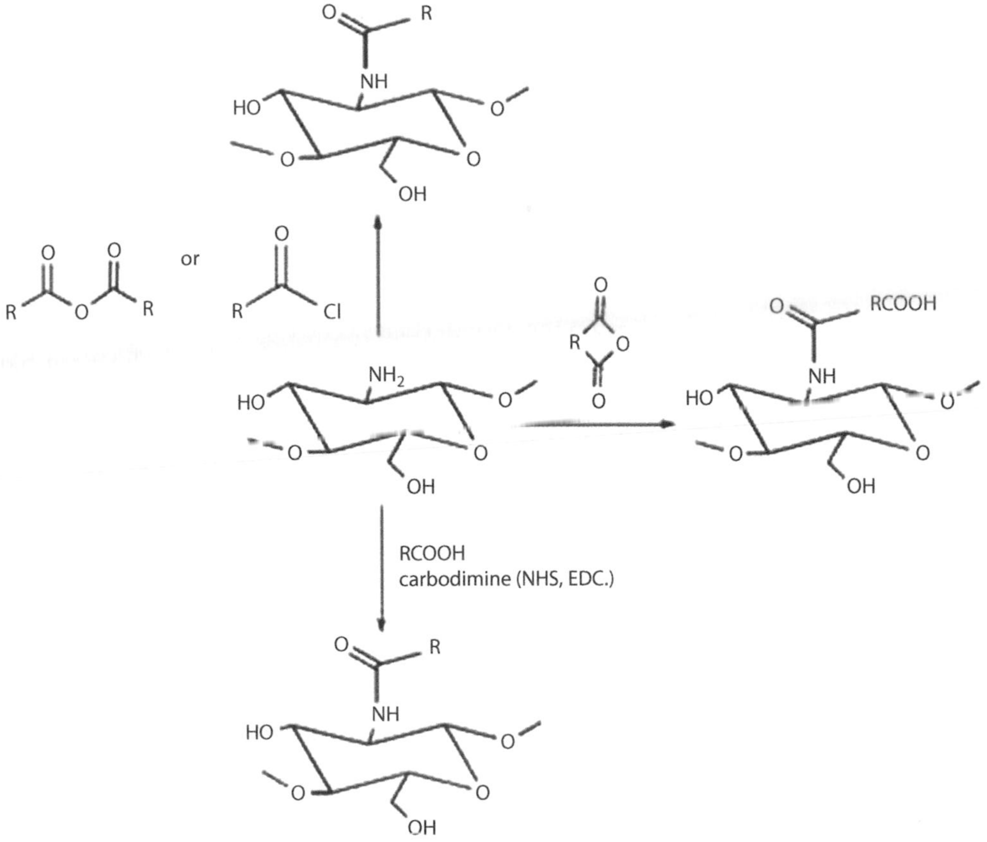

FIGURE 2.12
Synthesis of acyl-chitosans.

The inhibitory rates of DOX–OCH nanoparticle suspension to different human cancer cells (A549, Bel-7402, HeLa, and SGC-7901) significantly outperformed that of DOX solution.

2.4.1.3 Acyl Chitosan Derivatives from Coupling Reactions

An aniline pentamer chitosan derivative with electroactivity was prepared by a coupling reaction [38]. Due to its amphiphilic property, this derivative is able to self-assemble into spherical micelles, which makes the potential application of these polymers in drug delivery possible. The use of these polymers as scaffold materials in neuronal tissue engineering was evaluated; noncytotoxicity, degradability in the presence of enzymes, and biocompatibility were observed. Moreover, differentiation of PC-12 cells seeded on pure chitosan and on the three electroactive samples with 2.5%, 4.9%, and 9.5% AP, respectively, in the presence of exogenous nerve growth factor (NGF) was assessed for up to 5 days. The PC-12 cells on samples containing AP showed neurite extension, and some of them even formed intricate networks, while those on chitosan showed much fewer neurites.

Linoleic acid has been covalently conjugated to chitosan or chitosan derivatives via a 1-ethyl-3-(3-dimethylaminopropyl)carbodiimide-mediated (EDC-mediated) reaction to generate amphiphilic chitosan derivatives. Linoleic-chitosan nanoparticles have been used for the adsorption of trypsine (TR) [40]. Environmental factors (e.g., pH, concentration of

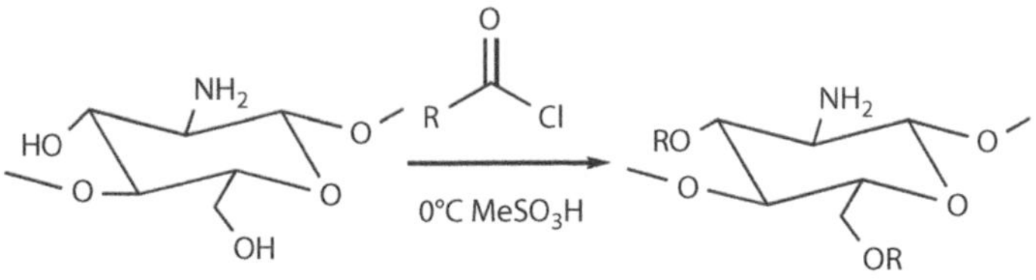

FIGURE 2.13
Synthesis of *O*-acyl-chitosans.

urea, or NaCl) can affect TR loading on the nanoparticles. The thermal stability of TR load-ing on nanoparticles was significantly improved compared to free TR. On the other hand, adriamycin (ADR) has been physically entrapped in self-aggregates based on linolenic-carboxylchitosan derivatives [41]. The drug loading (DL) experiments indicate that loading capacity and efficiency increase with increasing concentration of ADR. ADR is slowly released from chitosan self-aggregates for about 3 days.

Stearic acid has also been coupled to chitosan via activation with EDC for DNA and drug delivery applications [49]. Stearic acid–chitosan oligosaccharide micelles showed a critical micelle concentration (CMC) of 0.035 mg/mL (DS 25.4%). Due to their cationic prop-erties, the micelles could compact the plasmid DNA to form micelle–DNA complex nano-particles, which can efficiently protect the condensed DNA from enzymatic degradation by DNase I. You et al. [54–56] demonstrated that stearic acid–chitosan micelles show pH-sensitive properties, thus favoring intracellular delivery of encapsulated drug.

2.4.2 *O*-Acyl Chitosan

Since the amino group is more active than the two hydroxyl groups, protection is often necessary in order to prepare *N,O*-acyl chitosan with a refined substitution pattern. Nishimura et al. [80] reported the preparation of amphiphilic chitosans by using an *N*-phthaloyl chitosan as an intermediate. However, this method needs several steps for the protection and deprotection of the amine groups. Seo et al. [66] also reported a heteroge-neous method to prepare *N,O*-acyl chitosan by using *N*-acyl chitosan as a precursor. However, the resultant *N,O*-acyl chitosans had lower DSs and showed poor solubility in organic solvents. At the same time, a new method for selective O-acylation of chitosan in methanesulfonic acid (MSA) was proposed [64]. This method is based on the idea that the amine groups are protonated through the formation of a salt with MSA, which is disad-vantageous for a nucleophilic displacement reaction. As a result, the substitution occurs preferentially on the hydroxyl groups of chitosan. *O*-Acyl chitosans are prepared from acyl chlorides in the presence of MSA (MeSO$_3$H) (Figure 2.13).

Acryloyl chitosan (AcCS) has been synthesized by a homogeneous reaction of chitosan and acryloyl chloride using MSA as the solvent and catalyst [81,82]. Concentrated solutions of AcCS/acrylic acid were investigated by polarized optical microscopy, and cholesteric mesophase was found above the critical concentration of 45 wt%.

2.4.3 Controlled *N,O*-Acylation of Chitosan

The *O*-acyl chitosans synthesized via an MSA protection method generally dissolve in *N,N*-dimethylacetamide (DMAc). Therefore, further N-acylations could be conducted on the *O*-acyl chitosans in homogeneous systems using DMAc as the solvent (Figure 2.14).

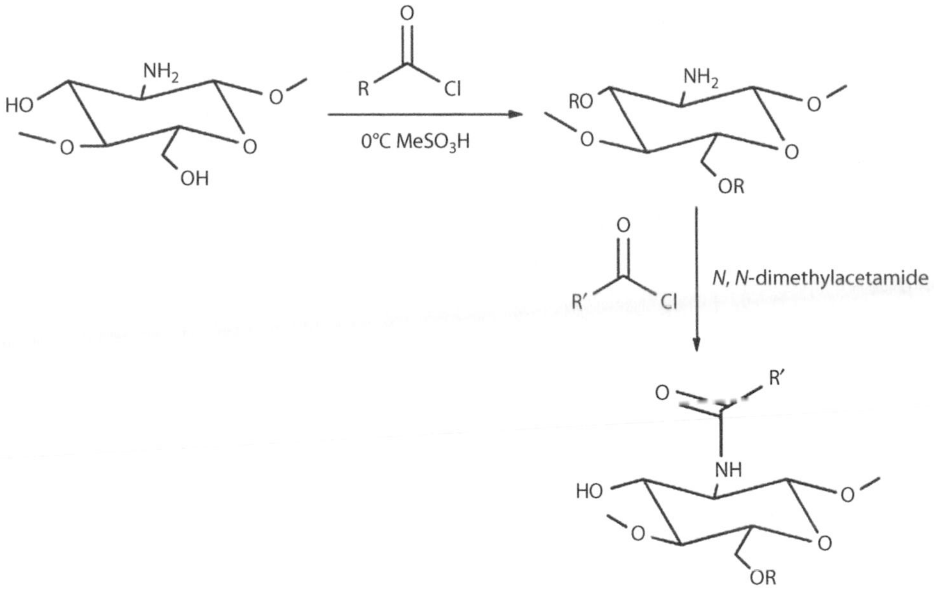

FIGURE 2.14
Controlled synthesis of *N,O*-acyl-chitosans in the presence of MSA.

O-Octanoyl, *N*-cinnamate chitosan, and *N*-*O*-hexanoyl chitosan derivatives have been synthesized using the aforementioned methodology [59,83]. *N,O* amphiphilic derivatives containing *N*-phthaloyl moieties can be easily prepared by a coupling reaction in the presence of dicyclohexylcarbodiimide [46]. For instance, *N*-phthaloylchitosan-g-polyvinylpyrrolidone (PHCS-g-PVP) has been synthesized by grafting PVP onto a chitosan derivative whose amino groups have previously reacted with phthalic anhydride. Polymeric micelles were prepared by the dialysis method and showed a CMC of 0.83 mg/L. Prednisone acetate was incorporated into the polymeric micelles with a loading capacity of around 45%. *In vitro* tests showed that the release of prednisone acetate from the micelles was continuous with no initial burst.

2.5 Carboxyalkyl Chitosans

O/N-Carboxymethyl chitosan is one of the most investigated derivatives of chitosan, obtained under controlled reaction conditions with sodium monochloroacetate. The process of carboxyalkylation introduces acidic groups on the polymer backbone. On introducing carboxyl groups into the amino groups of chitosan, amphoteric polyelectrolytes containing both cationic and anionic fixed charges are prepared. By varying the DS of the carboxyl-bearing group, we can obtain various charge densities on the molecular chain, which provide a convenient way of controlling pH-dependent behavior. This amphoteric polyelectrolyte has attracted considerable interest in a wide range of biomedical applications, such as wound dressings, artificial bone and skin, bacteriostatic agents, and blood anticoagulants, due to its unique chemical, physical, and biological properties, especially its excellent biocompatibility [84–88]. The presence of both carboxyl groups and amino

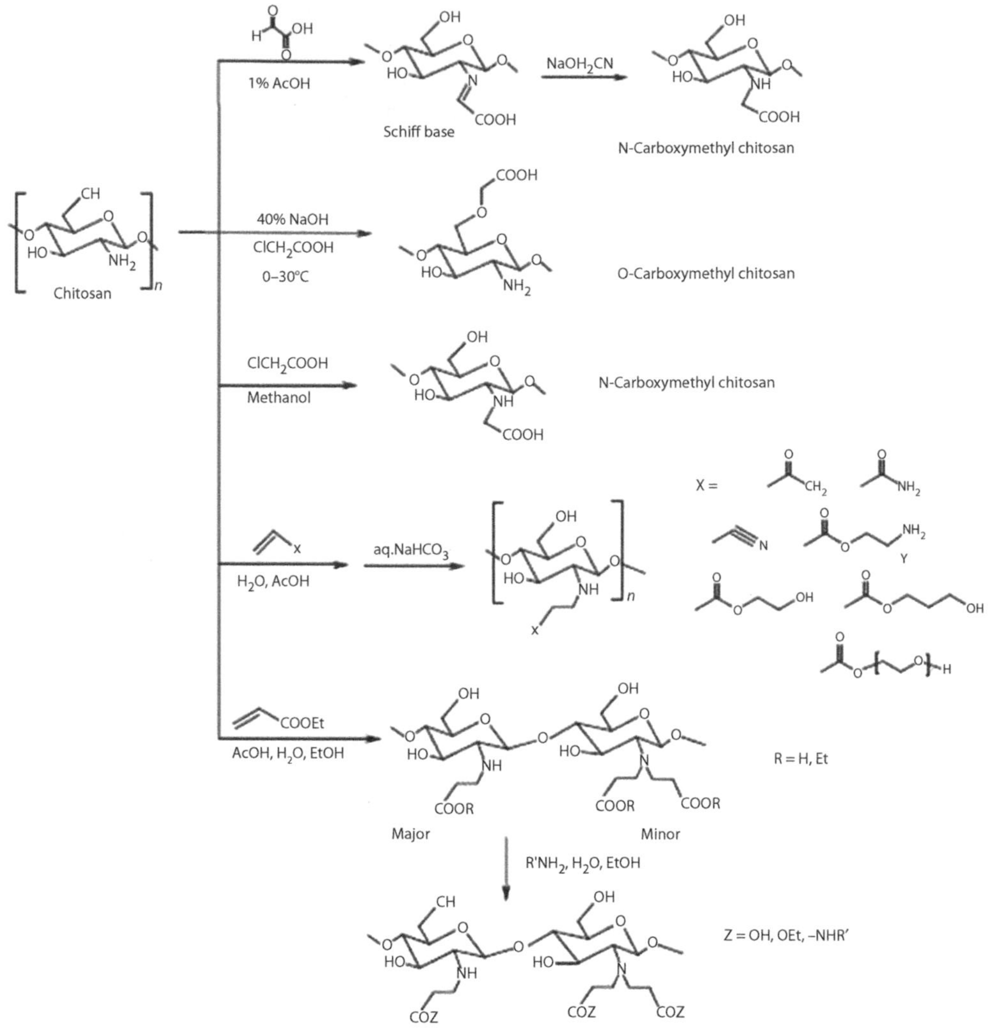

FIGURE 2.15
Carboxylation of chitosan. Depending on reaction conditions, O-carboxylated, N-carboxylated, or N,O-carboxylated chitosan can be obtained.

groups in Carboxymethyl chitosan macromolecules elicits special physicochemical and biophysical properties. It is interesting for pharmaceutical applications because of their novel properties, especially for controlled or sustained drug delivery systems [89].

N- and *O-*Carboxyalkylation takes place when chitosan reacts with monohalocarboxylic acids using different reaction conditions to control the selectivity of the reaction (Figure 2.15) [90]. Carboxyaldehydes have been used to selectively produce *N-*carboxyalkyl chitosan derivatives by reductive amination. Vinilic polymers (such as acrylic acid) have also been used to produce *N-*carboxyalkyl chitosan derivatives.

By using glyoxylic acid, water-soluble *N-*carboxymethyl chitosan is obtained: the product is a glucan-carrying pendant glycine group [91]. This reaction extends the range of pH (pH > 7) in which chitosan is water soluble, but a phase separation due to the balance between positive and negative charges on the polymer was observed at 2.5 < pH < 6.5.

With the proper selection of the reactant ratio, that is, with equimolar quantities of glyoxylic acid and amino groups, the product is in part N-monocarboxymethylated (0.3), N,N-dicarboxymethylated (0.3), and N-acetylated depending on the starting chitosan (0.08–0.15) [92]. N-Carboxymethyl chitosan is not only soluble in water, but has unique chemical, physical, and biological properties such as high viscosity, large hydrodynamic volume and film, and gel-forming capabilities, all of which make it an attractive option in connection with its use in food products and cosmetics [93]. Carboxymethyl chitosan is used in the development of different protein drug delivery systems as superporous hydrogels, pH-sensitive hydrogels, and cross-linked hydrogels [94–97]. N,N-Dicarboxymethyl chitosan has been shown to possess good chelating abilities and its chelate with calcium phosphate favored osteogenesis while promoting bone mineralization [85].

N-Phthaloyl-carboxymethyl chitosan (CMPhCS) has been successfully prepared by reacting N-phthaloylchitosan with chloroacetic acid in isopropyl alcohol [98]. CMPhCS existed as a flexible chain in the aqueous solution and aggregated gradually to form sphere aggregates in the mixture solution of H$_2$O-DMF. Micelles were self-assembled from N-phthaloyl-carboxymethylchitosan (CMPhCS) in a DMF-H$_2$O mixture solution, and they were used to evaluate drug deliveries of levofloxacine hydrochloride (Lfloxin). The results indicated that the CMC of CMPhCS in aqueous solution was 0.20 mg/mL. Moreover, Lfloxin and BSA could be controlled for release within 72 h in sodium phosphate buffer (pH 7.4) [99].

Sashiwa et al. applied the Michael reaction of various acryl reagents with chitosan [100]. With the application of water-soluble acryl reagents for this reaction, novel types of functional groups were introduced by a simple procedure. The reagents tried are hydroxyethyl acrylate, hydroxypropyl acrylate, acrylamide, acrylonitrile, and poly(ethylene glycol) (PEG)-acrylate. Reaction of chitosan with acrylonitrile gives cyanoethyl chitosan, whereas reaction of chitosan with ethyl acrylate in aqueous acidic medium gives an N-carboxyethyl ester intermediate that can be easily hydrolyzed to free acid or used as an intermediate to substitute with various hydrophilic amines, without requiring protecting groups [101].

2.6 Sulfated Chitosan

Chemical modification of the amino and hydroxyl groups of chitosan with sulfate can generate products for pharmaceutical applications. Sulfonation reactions of polysaccharides can give rise to a structural heterogeneity in polymer chains, but on the other hand some structures that emerge from random distribution can reveal good features for biological functions. Sulfated chitosans, which represent the nearest structural analogs of the natural blood anticoagulant heparin, show anticoagulant, antisclerotic, antitumor, and antiviral activities [102–106]. Chitosan derivatives having N- and/or O-sulfate groups either alone or in conjunction with other substituents have been widely examined as potential heparinoids. Vikhoreva et al. [107] synthesized chitosan sulfates by sulfation of low-molecular-weight chitosan (M_W 9000–35,000 Da). They used oleum as sulfating agent and dimethylformamide as medium, and demonstrated that chitosan sulfates with reduced molecular weight show a regular increase of anticoagulant activity, for example, heparins.

The sulfation of chitin was reported as far back as 1954 [108]. Over the following several decades, effort was extended to prepare N- and/or O-sulfated-chitins and chitosans using various reaction conditions and sulfating reagents (Table 2.2). Wolfrom and Shen-Han [109], Horton and Just [110], Nishimura et al. [111], Terbojevich et al. [112], Gamzazade et al.

TABLE 2.2

Sulfating Reagents and Reaction Positions of Chitosan or Its Derivatives

Chitosan or its Derivatives	Sulfating Reagents	Reaction Media	Sulfating Positions	References
Chitosan	Concentrated sulfuric acid	/	O-6, O-3, and N-2	[119]
Low-molecular-weight chitosan	Oleum	Dimethylformamide	O-6 and O-3	[120]
Chitosan	$Me_3N–SO_3$	Water/Na_2CO_3	O-6, O-3, and N-2	[121]
Chitosan		Water	N-2	[122]
Chitosan		Water	N-2	[123]
	SO_3-pyridine	Pyridine	O-3 and N-2	[124]
	SO_3-pyridine	Pyridine	O-3	[124]
R^2 = H, –$COCH_3$, octyl, lauryl. or –$CH_2CH_2O(CH_2CH_2O)$ mCH_3	$ClSO_3H$ or DMF-SO_3	DMF	O-6, O-3, and N-2	[125–128]
Chitosan	SO_3-pyridine	5% LiCl/DMAc	O-3 and O-6	[129]
Chitosan		8:1 (v/v) acetonitrile/water	N-2	[130,131]

[113], Drozd et al. [105], and Vongchan et al. [114] have all reported the preparation of N-sulfated Carboxymethyl chitosan, *O*-sulfated chitin, 6-O-sulfated chitosan and multi-substituted sulfated chitosan using $HClSO_3$. Hirano et al. [115,116] and Nishimura et al. [111] and Nishimura and Tokura [117] used a SO_3-DMF complex to prepare sulfated-chitin and sulfated-6-*O*-(carboxymethyl)chitin, while Terbojevich et al. [112] reported the selective 6-O-sulfation of chitosan with SO_3-pyridine complex. Holme and Perlin [118] and Gamzazade et al. [113] used the SO_3-Me3N complex and the SO_3-pyridine complex,

respectively, to prepare N-sulfated-chitosan. Compared to chlorosulfonic acid, the sulfur trioxide–organic solvent complexes are mild and less destructive.

We aimed to generate compounds having lowest toxicity for determining the pharmacological structure–function relationships among different backbone structures and differently arranged functional groups compared to those of heparin and heparan sulfate. Solely or in combination, N-sulfo, O-sulfo, N-acetyl, and N-carboxymethyl groups were introduced into chitosan with the highest possible regioselectivity and completeness and defined distribution along the polymer chain [132].

N-Sulfonation: N-Sulfonation of chitosan or 6-*O*-sulfochitosan in a homogeneous aqueous solution using the trimethylamine-SO$_3$ complex according to Holme and Perlin [118] resulted in almost complete N-acetyl-N-sulfochitosan without sulfation at C-3 and without a decrease in the original NAc content.

6-O-Sulfonation: Focher et al. [133] described a method for regioselective 6 O-sulfonation of chitosan. These workers used a copper complex for simultaneous intermediate protection of the amino groups at C-2 and the OH group in the 3-position of the saccharide backbone. Application of this method to chitosan (DD 0.86) was highly regioselective and complete without changes in NAc content and without reaction at C-3.

3,6-di-O-sulfonation: Because chitosan (DD 0.86) or carboxymethylated chitosan (0.86) is insoluble in DMF, the phthalimido group as the intermediate protecting group was introduced to solubilize the polymer. 3,6-O-disulfonation was carried out with the SO$_3$-pyridine complex, which when followed by deprotecting the amino group with hydrazine hydrate resulted in a highly sulfated chitosan derivative with a sulfate DS at C-3 of 0.97 and at C-6 of 0.79 [125].

3-O-Sulfonation: In heparin chemistry, there is a known sulfato transfer reaction for specific 3-O-sulfonation from glucosamine-N-sulfonate units, which is not applicable to chitosan. Therefore, Yao et al. [125] first completely sulfated both the 3- and 6-position of the glucosamine moiety, and then tried to use specific 6-O-desulfonation reactions from heparin chemistry to obtain 3-O-sulfonation chitosan [134].

Generally, the chemical derivatization reactions of chitin or chitosan were conducted under heterogeneous or semiheterogeneous conditions due to chitin's poor solubility in common organic solvents. Consequently, the attainment of a high degree of sulfation was difficult, with poor selectivity for the site of sulfation (C-6, C-3, or N-2 positions), inevitably resulting in multisubstituted derivatives unless tedious preprotection and deprotection steps were taken [111,124]. The uncertainty regarding degree of sulfation at the individual positions led to structure–activity relationship ambiguities. Finally, heterogeneous reactions are known for their poor reproducibility, limiting industrial production and practical applications. Zou and Khor [129] and Baumann and Faust [132] presents carefully prepared and characterized sulfated-chitins whose anticoagulant reactivity can be specifically related to the structure of the material. 6-O and 3,6-O-sulfated-chitins with degree of sulfation ranging from 0.53 to 1.91 were prepared under mild and homogeneous conditions, in a controllable manner, in a 5% LiCl/DMAc solvent system. Sulfation at room temperature yielded only monosubstituted 6-O-sulfated-chitins, whereas elevated temperatures gave 3,6-O-disulfated-chitins. Sulfation at the two positions resulted in different effects on the structural features of sulfated-chitins, the C-3 position being more subject to structural variation than the 6-O position. At low degree of sulfation, both the 6-O and 3,6-O-sulfated-chitins showed structural heterogeneity that eased as degree of sulfation increased, becoming more homogeneous and uniform.

Chitosan sulfates have been shown to possess anticoagulant and hemagglutination inhibition activities due to structural similarity to heparin [105, 106, 135–138]. By sulfation of chitosan, some of the amino groups are converted to anionic centers and the polymer attains better polyelectrolyte properties, which can be focused on developing potential drug carriers in the form of micelles or microcapsules [291,308]. N-Alkyl-O-sulfated chitosan has amphiphilicity since it carries long-chain alkyl groups having hydrophobic nature and sulfated groups having hydrophilic nature. This amphiphilic polymer has been shown to form micelles with physical entrapment of water-insoluble drugs such as taxol in significant concentrations [126,139]. The polyelectrolyte character is also revealed to be useful to form micrometer-sized hollow shells by means of a layer-by-layer technique, and permeation of the macromolecular fluorophore was observed [140]. Apart from these valuable biological properties, chitosan sulfates exhibit high sorption capacities as expected, and are of great advantage in metal ion recovery [123].

2.7 Phosphorylated Chitosan

The introduction of phosphonic acid or phosphonate groups onto chitin and chitosan by reaction of a phosphorylating agent onto the amino groups is known to increase the chelating properties [141–143] of chitin and chitosan and could modify its solubility. Several techniques (*cf.* Figure 2.16) for obtaining phosphate derivatives of chitin and chitosan have been proposed because of the interesting biological and chemical properties of such compounds.

The reaction of chitin with phosphorus pentoxide was found to give water-soluble phosphorylated chitin of high DS, constituting a strategy to overcome this major drawback of chitin and its derivatives. Phosphorylated chitin (P-chitin) and chitosan (P-chitosan) were prepared by heating chitin or chitosan with orthophosphoric acid and urea in DMF [144–146]. Urea is added to the reaction media to act as a reaction promoter. P-chitin and P-chitosan were also prepared by the reaction of chitin or chitosan with phosphorus pentoxide in MSA [147,148]. The phosphorylation reactions of chitin and chitosan in phosphorus pentoxide–methanesulfonic acid were found to be very efficient [149–152]. In this method, MSA is a good solvent for chitin or chitosan but also acts as an efficient catalyst for the esterification reaction. However, in this case it was found that only the P-chitosan with low DS was water soluble. The incorporation of methylene phosphonic groups into chitosan allowed solubility in water under neutral conditions [153]. A water-soluble N-methylene phosphonic chitosan (NMPC) was also synthesized using chitosan, phosphorous acid, and formaldehyde.

Chitosan-O-ethyl phosphonate can be prepared using KOH/methanol and 2-chloroethyl phosphonic acid under mild conditions as reported earlier [154]. The preparation of new types of phosphorylated chitosan using NaOH, n-hexane with diethyl chlorophosphate (phosphorylating agent) under a heterogeneous system has been reported [155]. The main difference in this reaction is that the reaction was carried out in n-hexane, an inert solvent, because the 2-propanol usually employed could be attacked by chlorophosphate, yielding undesired products. In these systems alkali chitosan is being used to prepare the chitosan alkyl phosphate/chitosan-O-ethyl phosphonate, in order to increase the reactivity of hydroxyl groups and to favor the coupling reaction with diethyl chlorophosphate/2-chloro ethyl phosphonic acid.

The introduction of a hydrophobic alkyl chain into free amino groups of N-methylenephosphonic chitosan by a reductive amine reaction leads to new amphiphilic chitosan

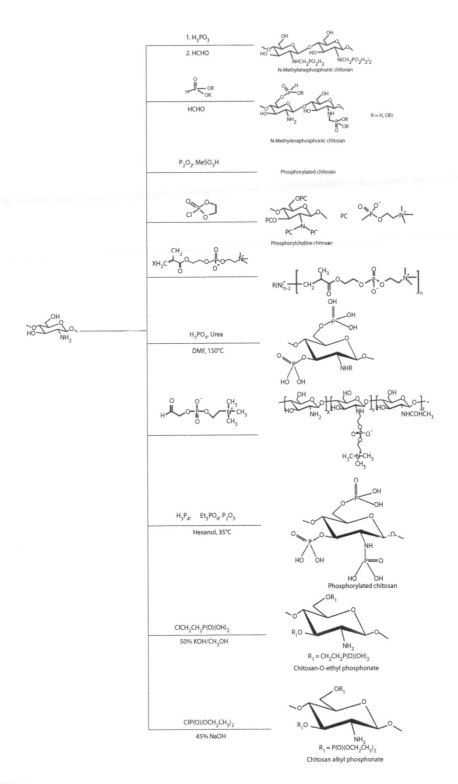

FIGURE 2.16
Synthesis of phosphorylated chitosan.

derivatives with the potential to act as surfactants. N-Lauryl-N-methylenephosphonic chitosan is one such surfactant reported [156]. Phosphorylated chitosans are synthesized in the phosphorus pentoxide–methanesulfonic acid system also [149].

To impart good anti-blood-coagulation properties to chitosan, modifications are carried out with phosphorylcholine (PC) compounds. Reaction with 2-chloro-1,3,2-dioxaphospholane in homogeneous or heterogeneous conditions yields PC chitosan [157]. Modification of chitosan with 2-methacryloyloxyethyl phosphorylcholine through the Michael addition reaction has been carried out with cell adhesion studies, indicating that cell attachment could be easily controlled by adjusting the concentration of 2-methacryloyloxyethyl phosphorylcholine bound to chitosan [158].

To achieve regiospecific functionalization of chitosan, Winnik and coworkers [159,160] chose to introduce PC groups via chemical modification of the C2 amine group, thus leaving intact all the hydroxyl groups that play an important role in the biological activity of chitosan derivatives. The synthetic strategy involves two reactions carried out in sequence, without isolation of the intermediate: (1) reductive amination of phosphorylcholine-glyceraldehyde by the C2 primary amine groups of chitosan and (2) reduction of the resulting imine groups with NaCNBH$_3$, a reagent extensively used in various modifications of chitosan. Note that, overall, the reaction path converts primary amines into secondary amines, a transformation that will affect, yet maintain, the polyelectrolyte properties of native chitosan. These PC-substituted chitosans (PC-CH) exhibit remarkable solubility in water under physiological pH conditions and demonstrate that the introduction of zwitterionic PC moieties into chitosan, even with modest DSs, provides a new and effective route toward nontoxic chitosan, while remaining soluble under neutral and even slightly alkaline conditions. Moreover, the cytotoxicity of the polymers was evaluated, confirming the nontoxic nature of chitosan and its PC derivatives.

The premodified chitosan can also be extended with Phosphorus-containing groups; for example, the –COOH group of carboxymethyl chitosan was made to react with –NH$_2$ of phosphatidylethanolamine giving an amphiphilic polymer [161]. This polymer was investigated for its feasibility as a delivery carrier for the transfection of hydrophobic model drug ketoprofen by forming beads on ionic cross-linking by sodium tripolyphosphate.

P-chitosan was used for the preparation of gel beads using TPP to improve the controlled release system in a gastrointestinal fluid [162]. This work included the *in vitro* drug release profiles monitored at various pH media at 37°C using Ib as a model drug. The release percentages of Ib from P-chitosan gel beads were found to increase with increasing pH of the dissolution medium. This behavior indicated that the drug release profile is pH sensitive. The release rate of Ib at pH 7.4 was noticeably higher than the release rate at pH 1.4 due to the ionization of phosphorus groups and the high solubility of Ib at pH 7.4 [163,164] and also the electrostatic repulsion between negatively ionized carboxyl groups of Ib and phosphate groups in P-chitosan molecules. The release rate in simulated intestinal fluid (pH 7.4) was higher than that in simulated gastric fluid (pH 1.4), enabling drug delivery or release to take place preferentially in the intestine while simultaneously avoiding drug leakage in the stomach. All of these interesting features indicated that the P-chitosan gel beads could be used as a successful drug carrier for controlled drug delivery in oral administration.

In polymeric implants used in orthopedics, the presence of a calcium phosphate overlayer is often desirable to promote osteoconduction and to ensure bone bonding. Grafting negatively charged functionalities, such as phosphates, is a well-known strategy for inducing the deposition of apatite-like layers under simulated physiological conditions [165–168]. Recently, Amaral et al. [169] applied this approach to chitosan membranes, using the

$H_3PO_4/Et_3PO_4/P_2O_5$/butanol phosphorylation reaction system, at 30°C, for periods up to 48 h [170]. The phosphorylation method is based on the $H_3PO_4/Et_3PO_4/P_2O_5$/hexanol reaction route optimized by Granja et al. [171] for the synthesis of highly phosphorylated cellulose derivatives and originally proposed by Touey and Kingsport [172] in 1956 for the synthesis of water-soluble and nondegraded cellulose phosphates. This method has the advantage of being carried out at room temperature, with low degradation of the polymer thus resulting. The $H_3PO_4/Et_3PO_4/P_2O_5$/butanol method is an alternative to the H_3PO_4/urea/dimethylformamide method described for the phosphorylation of chitin and chitosan [146,173], which is the phosphorylation pathway usually followed to introduce phosphate functionalities into chitin fibers and chitosan films/sponges and which involves the use of high temperatures, typically higher than 120°C [174–176].

The influence of two water-soluble anionic derivatives, namely sodium carboxymethylchitin (CM-chitin) and P-chitin, on the crystallization of calcium phosphate by seeded growth and turbidity was studied in [177]. Macroporous scaffolds were obtained through a freeze-drying technique using both NMPC and CS [178]. Biomimetic mineralization was carried out in different media, that is, simulated body fluid (SBF) or $CaCl_2$ and Na_2HPO_4 solutions [116]. NMPC with phosphonic groups led to clear differences in the ability of scaffold wall surface to support heterogeneous calcium phosphate nucleation and growth. Chitosan scaffold incubated in SBF for 20 days did not display mineral growth, whereas NMPC scaffold showed increasing mineral particulates, surface coverage with an essential continuous mineral layer. The biomineralization behavior of NMPC was superior to that of chitosan at higher soaking cycle number. Moreover, these scaffolds only deposit apatite slightly in SBF. This result provided NMPC derivatives constituting the biocomposite scaffold with improved compressive stiffness. Similarly, it has been reported that calcium phosphate mineral was formed on P-chitosan membranes after soaking with $Ca(OH)_2$ [179].

2.8 Thiolated Chitosan

Thiomers are hydrophilic macromolecules bearing free thiol groups on their backbone. Due to the immobilization of thiol groups on already well-established polymers, their mucoadhesive, enzyme-inhibitory, permeation-enhancing, and efflux pump-inhibiting properties are strongly improved. Thiol-bearing ligands can be covalently immobilized on the primary amino groups at the C-2 position of the glucosamine subunits of chitosan. According to this, chitosan-cysteine [180], chitosan-glutathione [181], chitosan-thioethylamidine [182], chitosan-thioglycolic acid [183], chitosan-4-thio-butyl-amidine [184], chitosan-*N*-acetyl cysteine conjugates [185], and chitosan-6-mercaptonicotinic acid conjugate [186] as well as other thiolated chitosans [187,188] have been synthesized (*cf.* Figure 2.17).

The primary amino group at the 2-position of the glucosamine subunits of chitosan is the main target for the immobilization of thiol groups. As outlined in Figure 2.17, sulfhydryl-bearing agents can be covalently attached to this primary amino group via the formation of amide or amidine bonds. In the case of the formation of amide bonds, the carboxylic acid group of the ligands cysteine and thioglycolic acid reacts with the primary amino group of chitosan mediated by a water-soluble carbodiimide. The formation of disulfide bonds by air oxidation during the synthesis is avoided by performing the process at a pH below 5. At this pH range, the concentration of thiolate anions, representing the reactive form for oxidation of thiol groups, is low, and the formation of disulfide bonds can be

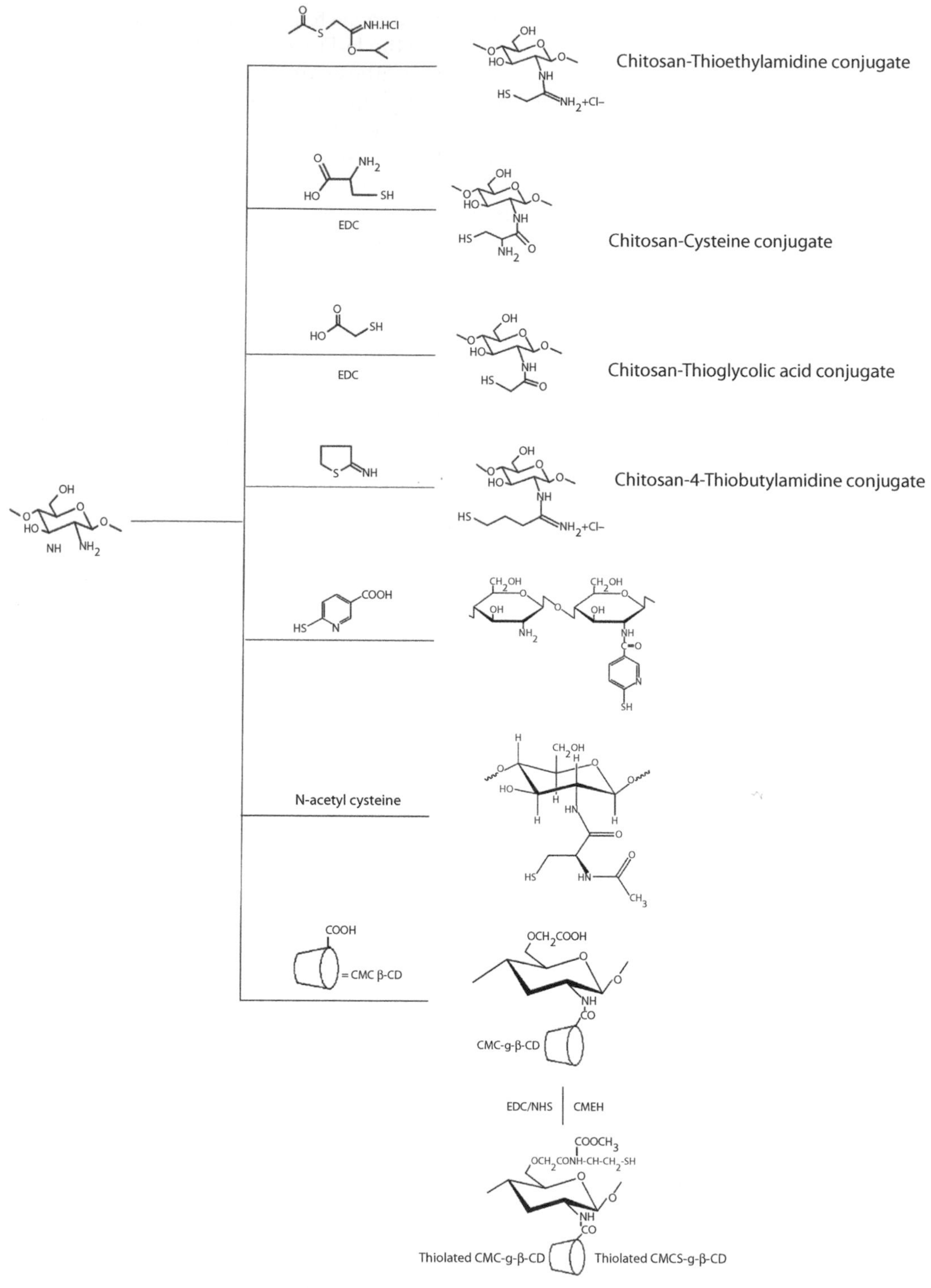

FIGURE 2.17
Synthesis of thiolated chitosan.

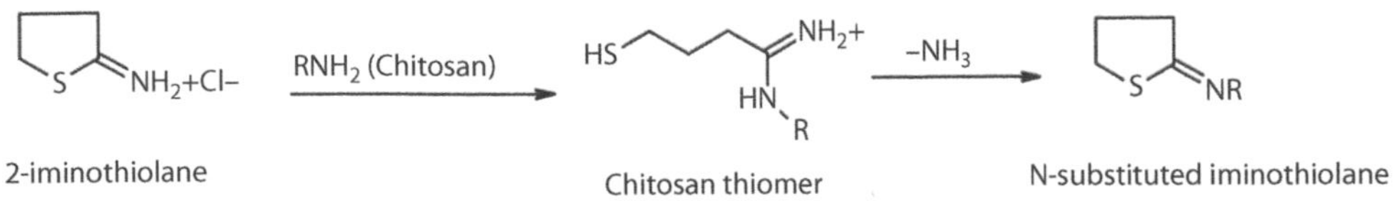

FIGURE 2.18
Instability of the chitosan-4-thiobutylamidine conjugate.

almost excluded. Alternatively, the coupling reaction can be performed under inert conditions. In the case of the formation of amidine bonds, 2-iminothiolane is used as a coupling reagent. It offers the advantage of a simple one-step coupling reaction. In addition, the thiol group of the reagent is protected from oxidation because of the chemical structure of the reagent. However, storage stability studies under nitrogen showed an insufficient stability of thiomer, which resulted in a decrease of free thiol moieties. This might be due to the formation of N-chitosanyl-substituted 2-iminothiolane structures. This undesired side-reaction occurs after the derivatization of different amines with 2-imino-thiolane. It involves the loss of ammonia and yields recyclized N-substituted 2-iminothiolane (Figure 2.18) [189]. To achieve the same properties as chitosan-4-thiobutyl-amidine and to overcome at the same time its insufficient stability, chemical modification of chitosan can be done with isopropyl-S-acetylthioacetimidate HCl (i-PATAI), resulting in chitosan-thioethylamidine conjugate [182]. The nucleophilicity of amino groups is dictated by the protonation state making the reaction pH dependent. The reactions can be carried out at pH 6.5–7.0, at which pH value the oxidation process of thiol groups is decreased and chitosan is soluble as well [190]. This imidoester reacts rapidly with an amine—maximum for 1.5 h in comparison with the reaction with 2-iminothiolane, which ends after 24 h under continuous stirring at room temperature [184]. The short chain of i-PATAI excludes theoretically the possibility of yielding cyclic nonthiol products. Various properties of chitosan are improved by this immobilization of thiol groups allocating it to a promising new category of thiomers used in particular for the noninvasive administration of hydrophilic macromolecules.

A drawback of the thiomers developed so far is their pH-dependent reactivity. The reactive form of thiomers is the thiolate anion. The pK_a of alkyl thiols is in the range of 8–10. This means that thiomers will be most reactive in a pH range slightly above the physiological intestinal pH. 6-Mercaptonicotinic acid was chosen to develop a novel thiomer with a pH-independent action mechanism. Due to its particular structure, this compound has two tautomeric structures: thiol (S–H) and thione (C=S). In polar solvents such as water, the thione form (C=S) is the most predominant structure. This structure can react with a disulfide bond both as a nucleophile and as a proton donor. Therefore, disulfide bonds can be formed even without thiol groups being available on the polymer in the form of thiolate anions. The newly synthesized chitosan-6-mercaptonicotinic acid conjugate showed excellent *in situ* gelling properties without the addition of any oxidizing species. Moreover, in contrast to all other thiolated polymers, the gelling properties are pH independent. This property might be of considerable advantage for drug delivery applications requiring *in situ* gelling properties where the pH could be different according to age or individual differences, such as the vagina.

Thiolated chitosans have recently emerged as new biomaterials for delivering drugs throughout the body. The covalent attachment of various compounds bearing sulfhydryl groups to chitosan leads to a powerful modification. Thiolated chitosans exhibit comparatively strong mucoadhesive and *in situ* gelling properties, enabling controlled drug release.

In addition, they further proved to be effective as efflux pump inhibitors and permeation enhancers. The potential of thiolated chitosans to transfect plasmid DNA proposes a new perspective for gene liberation to a targeted site. Along with thiolated chitosans as new emerging biomaterials with promising properties, the combination of thiolated chitosans with innovative technologies such as micro/nanotechnology is an optional choice as a drug delivery system [191].

2.9 Sugar-Modified Chitosan

The first report on the modification of chitosan with sugars was by Hall and Yalpani (*cf.* Figure 2.19) in 1980 [192,193]. They synthesized sugar-bound chitosan by reductive N-alkylation using NaCNBH$_3$ and unmodified sugar (1: method A) or a sugar-aldehyde derivative (2: method B).

Sashiwa and Shigemasa [194] reported N-alkylation of chitosan performed in aqueous methanol with various aldehydes, monosaccharides, and disaccharides (glycolaldehyde, DL-glyceraldehyde, D-ribose, D-arabinose, D-xylose, 2-deoxy-D-ribose, D-glucose, 2-deoxy-D-glucose, 3-O-Me-D-glucose, D-galactose, D-mannose, L-fucose, L-rhamnose, and GlcNAc).

Since the specific recognition of cells, viruses, and bacteria by sugars was discovered, this type of modification has generally been used to introduce cell-specific sugars into chitosan. Morimoto et al. [195, 196] and Morimoto and coworkers [197–198] reported the synthesis of sugar-bound chitosans, such as those with D- and L-fucose, and their specific

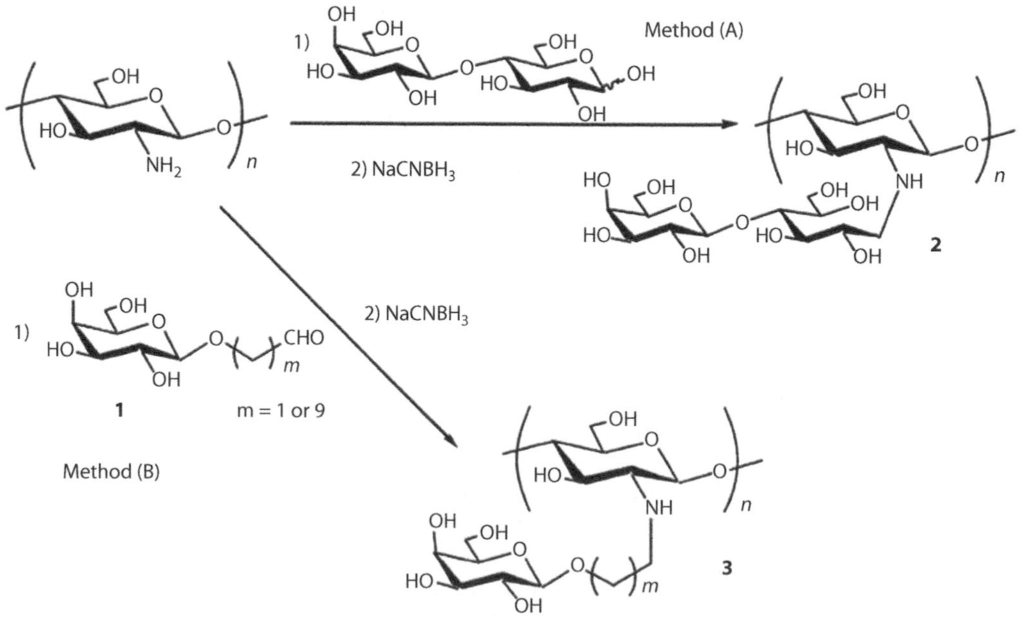

FIGURE 2.19
Strategy for the substitution of sugars to chitosan by reductive N-alkylation.

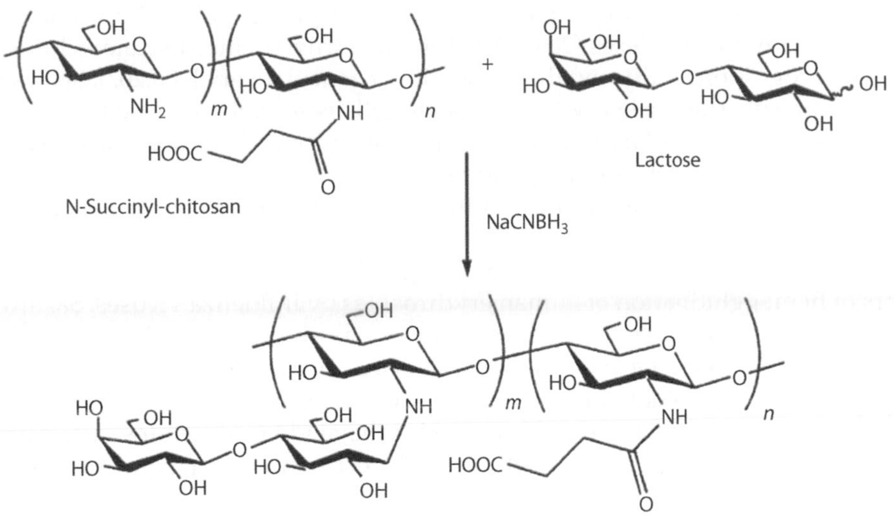

FIGURE 2.20
Synthesis of lactosaminated NSCS.

interactions between lectin and cells. Stredanska and coworkers [199] synthesized lactose-modified chitosan for a potential application in the repair of articular cartilage by the same mode. Kato et al. [200] also prepared lactosaminated NSCS (Figure 2.20) and its fluorescein thiocarbanyl derivative as a liver-specific drug carrier in mice through asialoglycoprotein receptor. Moreover, lactosaminated N-succinylchitosan was found to be a good drug carrier for mitomycin C in the treatment of liver metastasis [201].

Galactosylated chitosan prepared from lactobionic acid and chitosan with EDC and N-hydroxysuccinimide (Figure 2.21) showed promise as a synthetic extracellular matrix for hepatocyte attachment [202]. Furthermore, graft copolymers of galactosylated chitosan with PEG or poly(vinyl pyrrolidone) and dextran were useful as hepatocyte-targeting

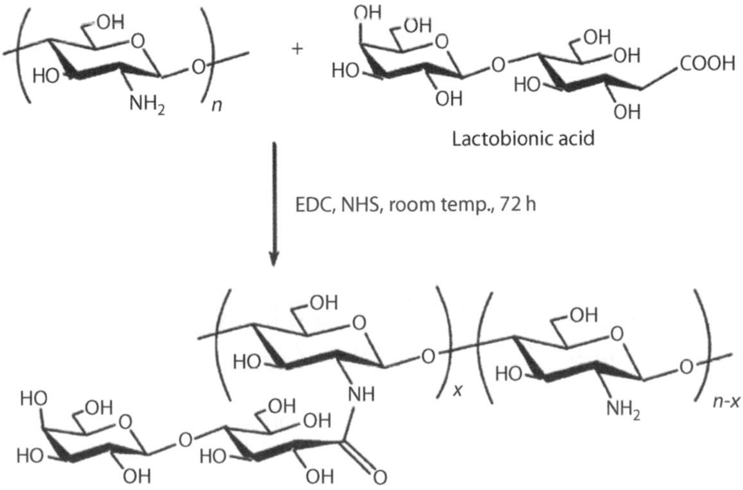

FIGURE 2.21
Synthesis of galactosylated chitosan.

DNA carriers because PEG reduces particle sizes of complexes and PVP prevents albumin from interaction with complexes [203–205]. The quaternized galactosylated chitosan also has cellular recognition ability and the possibility of gene delivery [206,207]. Such selective targeting of the substrate delivery to hepatocyte cells is feasible because hepatocytes are the only cells that possess large numbers of high-affinity cell-surface asialoglycoprotein receptors that can bind to asialoglycoproteins.

Sialic acid is the most prevalent sugar of the glycolipids and glycoproteins on the mammalian cell surface and is the key epitope recognized as essential for a number of pathogenic infections. Moreover, sialic acid-containing polymers have been shown to be potent inhibitors of hemagglutination of human erythrocytes by influenza viruses. Sashiwa et al. [209] prepared sialic acid-bound chitosan as a new family of sialic acid-containing polymers using *p*-formylphenyl-*a*-sialoside [208] by reductive N-alkylation. Since sialic acid-bound chitosan was insoluble in water, successive N-succinylations were carried out to obtain the water-soluble derivative *N*-succinyl-sialic acid-bound chitosan (Figure 2.22). Specific binding of wheat germ agglutinin with lectin was shown in the presence of

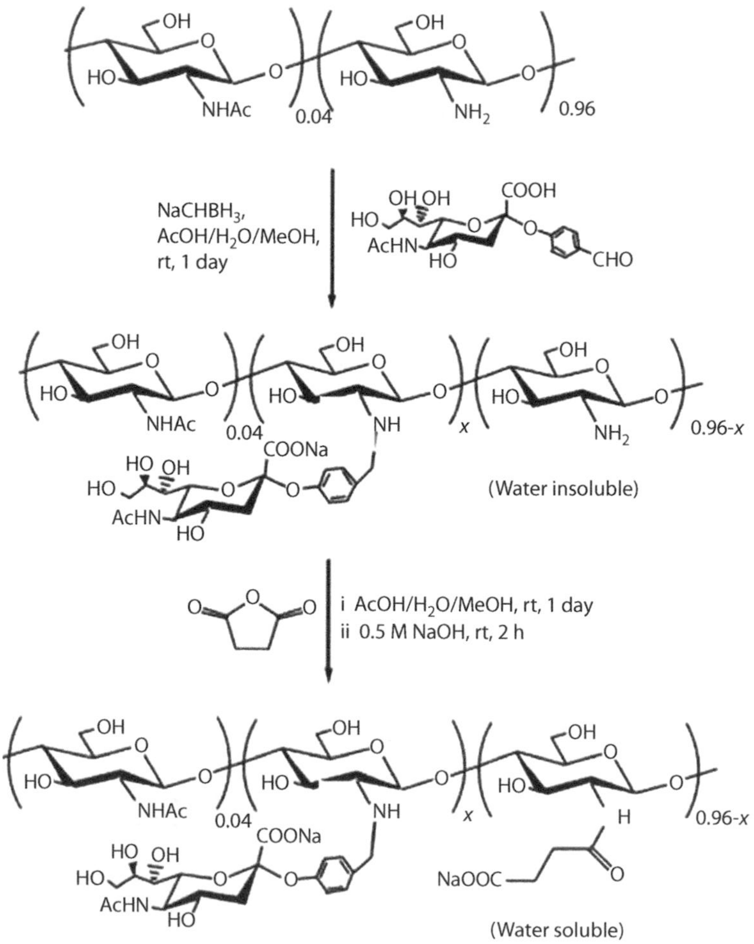

FIGURE 2.22
Synthesis of sialic acid–chitosan and its *N*-succinylation.

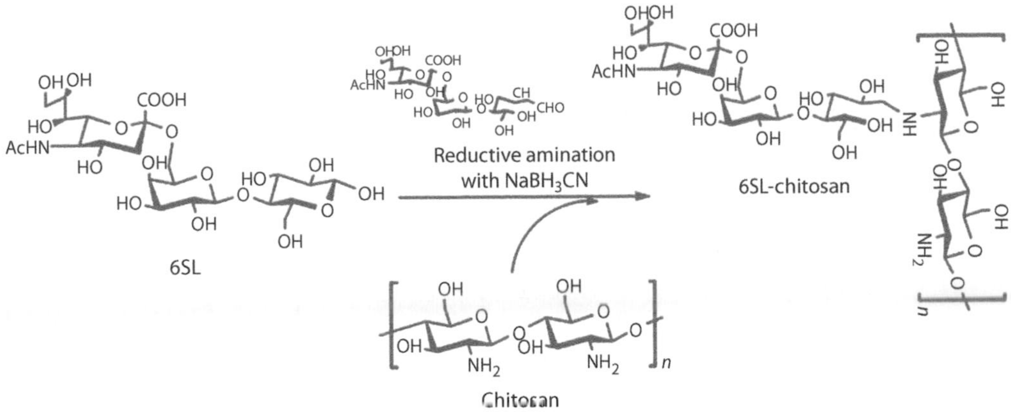

FIGURE 2.23
Synthesis of 6SL-chitosan.

N-succinyl-sialic acid-bound chitosan. Water-soluble α-galactosyl chitosan prepared by the same strategy as sialic acid showed specific binding against a galactosyl-specific lectin (*Griffonia simplicifolia*) [210]. Different types of spacers have been prepared on sialic acid or α-galactosyl epitope-bound chitosans [211]. These epitope-bound chitosans may be useful as potent inhibitors of influenza viruses or blocking agents for acute rejection [210,212].

Umemura et al. [213] modified chitosan with multiple sialyl saccharides, α-2,6-sialyllactose or free sialyl glycan, using reductive amination reaction. After only one step of the procedure, the binding inhibitor of influenza virus, 6SL-chitosan, was obtained that has multiple Neu5Acα2, 6Gal components recognized by the viral hemagglutinin (Figure 2.23). It might be difficult to add 6SL to chitosan with a DS of more than 40% owing to the chitosan structure. It is interesting that the DS values of 6SL-chitosan were in inverted order of the amount of 6SL in the reaction solution. It is considered that the 0.5 equivalent of 6SL was sufficient for this synthesis, and excessive amounts of 6SL might have caused too crowded a condition for the reductive amination of chitosan glucosamine.

To compare with the inhibitory activity of 6SL-chitosan, another binding inhibitor, FSG-chitosan, by substituting FSG for 6SL (Figure 2.24), was synthesized. Free sialyl glycan (FSG) is a biantennary decasaccharide that contains two sialic acids at each nonreducing terminal. The highest DS value reached only 4.4% with the resulting compound. The resulting inhibitors showed sufficient inhibitory activity against influenza virus infection in MDCK cells compared to that of α-2, 6-sialyllactose, or free sialyl glycan.

2.10 CD-Linked Chitosan

CDs are cyclic oligosaccharides built from six to eight (α = 6, β = 7, γ = 8) D-glucose units and are formed during the enzymatic degradation of starch and related compounds. CD has the merit of a hydrophobic cavity, which is easy to assemble with other molecules. Chitosan has the merit of degradation slowly in an organism. Therefore, grafting CD molecules into chitosan-reactive sites may lead to a molecular carrier that possesses the cumulative effects of inclusion, size specificity, and transport properties of CDs as well as the controlled release ability of the polymeric matrix [214]. The products obtained by CD

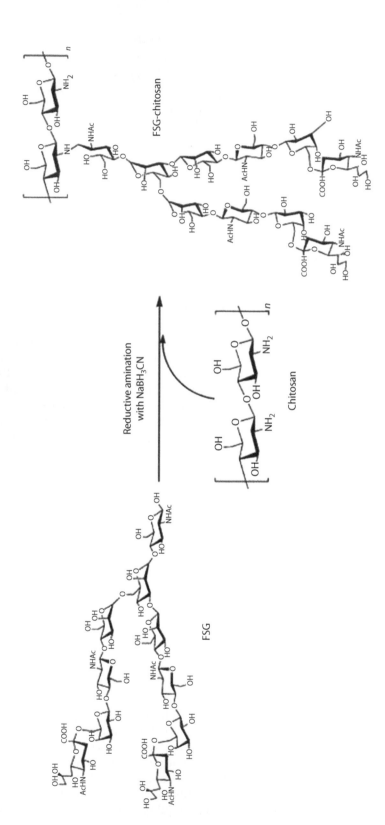

FIGURE 2.24
Synthesis of FSG-chitosan.

grafting to chitosan using different methods and their inclusion ability, sorption, and controlled release properties have been studied extensively [215].

2.10.1 Grafting of CD onto Chitosan by Using EDC

EDC reacts with the carboxyl group of carboxymethylated β-CD to form an active ester intermediate. The intermediate can react with a primary amine of chitosan to form an amide linkage. Furusaki et al. [216] described the preparation of a β-CD-grafted chitosan by coupling carboxymethylated β-CD and a partially deacetylated chitin oligomer using water-soluble EDC. An insoluble cross-linked chitosan bearing CD moieties was prepared by a one-step procedure with N-succinylated chitosan and mono-6-amino-mono-6-deoxy-β-cyclodextrin in the presence of water-soluble EDC under homogeneous conditions (Figure 2.25) [217]. It was considered that the product obtained in this study was cross-linked between the carboxyl groups and amino groups on the succinyl chitosan skeleton. DS by the CD moiety achieved 0.27 with the addition of *N,N*-dimethylformamide (DMF) to the reaction solution.

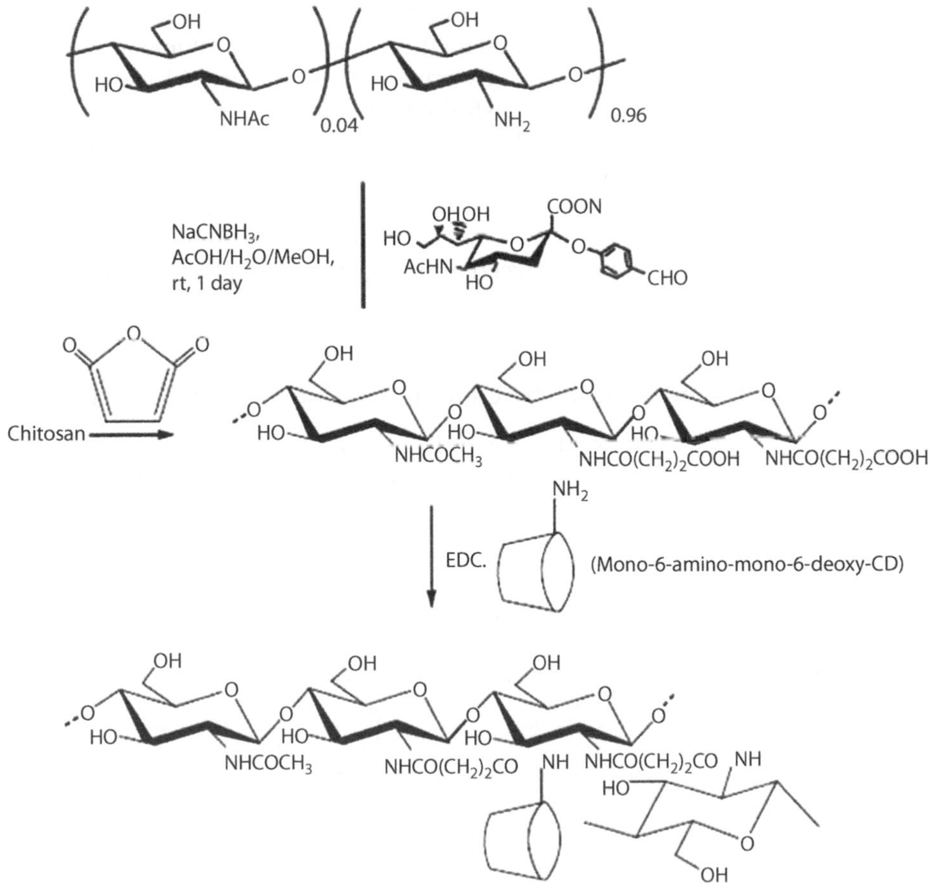

FIGURE 2.25
Preparation of chitosan-graft-β-CD from *N*-succinyl chitosan. (From Aoki, N., Nishikawa, M., and Hattori, K. 2003. *Carbohydr Polym* 52: 219–223. With permission.)

2.10.2 Grafting of CD onto Chitosan by Nucleophilic Substitution

Monochlorotriazinyl groups are often encountered in textile chemistry, where they are used as functional groups of reactive dyes for the finishing of wool and cellulose. Their reactivity is based on the ready nucleophilic displacement of the chlorine atom by the amino or hydroxyl groups carried by the polymer that builds the fiber. Martel et al. [218] used a monochlorotriazinyl derivative of β-CD as a reagent for the grafting of β-CD onto chitosan. In this approach, as shown in Figure 2.26, β-CD was coupled to chitosan by the intermediate of its monochlorotriazinyl derivative through the nucleophilic substitution of the chloride atom by the amino groups. The resulting products were not soluble, but did swell, in water, nor were they soluble in the numerous organic solvents. Because the average DS of the monochlorotriazinyl derivative of β-CD was 2.8, the reaction yielded cross-linked insoluble products due to both intra- and intermolecular bondings occurring with the polymer chains.

2.10.3 Grafting of CD onto Chitosan by Using Tosylated β-CD

Chen and Wang [219] synthesized β-CD-graft-2-chitosan by reacting β-CD with *p*-toluene-sulfonyl chloride and then grafting with chitosan. The reaction scheme for the synthesis is shown in Figure 2.27. The products obtained by this method were soluble in water, methanol, DMSO, and DMF. The polymer inclusion complex of β-CD-graft-2-chitosan with iodine was prepared and its inclusion ability was studied. The experimental results showed that a substantial amount of iodine was included with β-CD-graft-2-chitosan and formed a stable inclusion complex, while chitosan alone had little ability to absorb iodine. The stronger inclusion ability of β-CD-graft-2-chitosan with iodine was caused by the special hydrophobic cavity structure of β-CD-graft-2-chitosan. The absorption of iodine was considered to be caused by n-δ charge transfer between amino groups of chitosan and iodine molecules [220].

2.10.4 Grafting of CD onto Chitosan by Using 1,6-Hexamethylene Diisocyanate

6-Hexamethylene diisocyanate (HMDI) is generally utilized as a strong cross-linker of amino or hydroxyl groups because it possesses two isocyanate groups (–N=C=O). Under suitable conditions (pH < 6), the hydroxyl groups of chitosan react with an isocyanate to form a

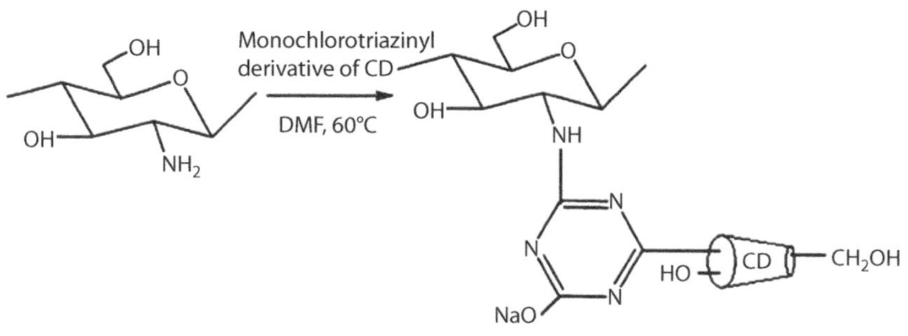

FIGURE 2.26
Reaction scheme for the synthesis of β-CD-graft-chitosan by the nucleophilic substitution reaction. (From Martel, B. et al. 2001. *J Polym Sci A-Polym Chem* 39: 169–176. With permission.)

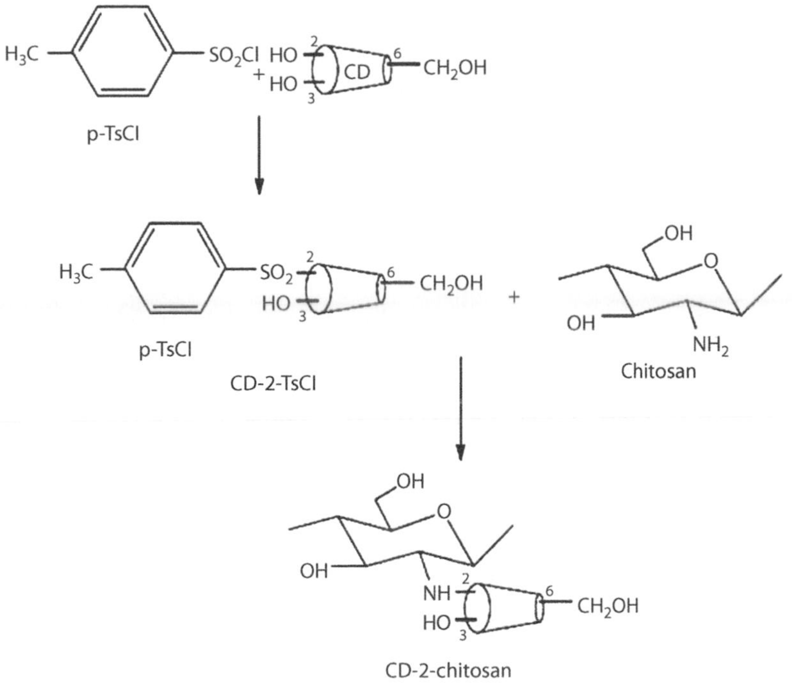

FIGURE 2.27
Reaction scheme for the synthesis of β-CD-graft-chitosan. (From Chen, S. and Wang, Y. 2001. *J Appl Polym Sci* 82: 2414–2421. With permission.)

urethane product (–NH–COO–) due to the transfer of a proton from the hydroxyl group to the nitrogen atom of isocyanate. In addition, isocyanate reacts with the hydroxyl groups of β-CD to form a product similar to urethane [221]. It is assumed that the cross-linking of the hydroxyl groups of chitosan with HMDI resulted in a chitosan–HMDI complex, which then binds with the hydroxyl groups of β-CD to form β-CD-graft-chitosan. HMDI cannot bind to the amino groups of chitosan due to the lower affinity for amino groups as compared to hydroxyl groups under low pH value [221]. For these reasons, Sreenivasan [222] reported an adsorbent matrix synthesized by coupling β-CD to chitosan using HMDI. The matrix obtained in this study was found to be insoluble in organic as well as acidic or alkali media. The extent of cholesterol removal by this matrix from the solution was studied. The results indicated that nearly 21% of cholesterol was removed from the solution.

2.10.5 Grafting of CD onto Chitosan by Reductive Amination

Reductive amination is one of the major reactions applicable to the modification of chitosan. Introduction of CD residue into chitosan has been successfully attained in a homogeneous system through a reductive amination strategy. CD derivatives with aldehyde functional groups are useful to graft CD into chitosan by the formation of Schiff's base. Tanida et al. [223] reported the synthesis of β-CD-grafted chitosan by the formation of Schiff's base between 2-*O*-formylmethyl-β-cyclodextrin and chitosan in acetate buffer at pH 4.4, followed by reduction with NaBH$_3$CN. The product, which had a DS of 37%, was found to be soluble in water at neutral and alkaline conditions. 2-*O*-formylmethyl-α-CD was linked to chitosan by reductive amination. 2-O-formylmethyl-α-CD was prepared by selective allylation of α-CD and subsequent ozonolysis of the C–C double bond in the resulting mono-allylated derivative [224]. The reaction scheme and conditions are given in Figure 2.28. All the derivatives obtained were found to be soluble in water and in alkaline solvents such as aqueous ammonia and aqueous sodium hydroxide, except for that with a DS of 11%, which was soluble only in acidic solution.

2.10.6 Grafting of CD onto Chitosan via Epoxy-Activated Chitosan

Recently, a new synthetic route was reported to graft β-CD onto chitosan using epoxy-activated chitosan as shown in Figure 2.29 [225]. The adsorption properties of this product for *p*-dihydroxybenzene were studied and compared with that of chitosan and β-CD-graft-6-chitosan that was synthesized by the reaction of mono [6-O-(*p*-toluenesulfonyl)]-6-β-CD with chitosan. The grafting of β-CD onto chitosan resulted in higher adsorption capacities for *p*-dihydroxybenzene than for chitosan.

2.10.7 Grafting of CD onto Chitosan by Using a Redox Initiator

β-CD-graft-chitosan was prepared by reacting β-CD itaconate vinyl monomer with chitosan using ceric ammonium nitrate (CAN) [226]. In this work, β-CD itaconate was prepared

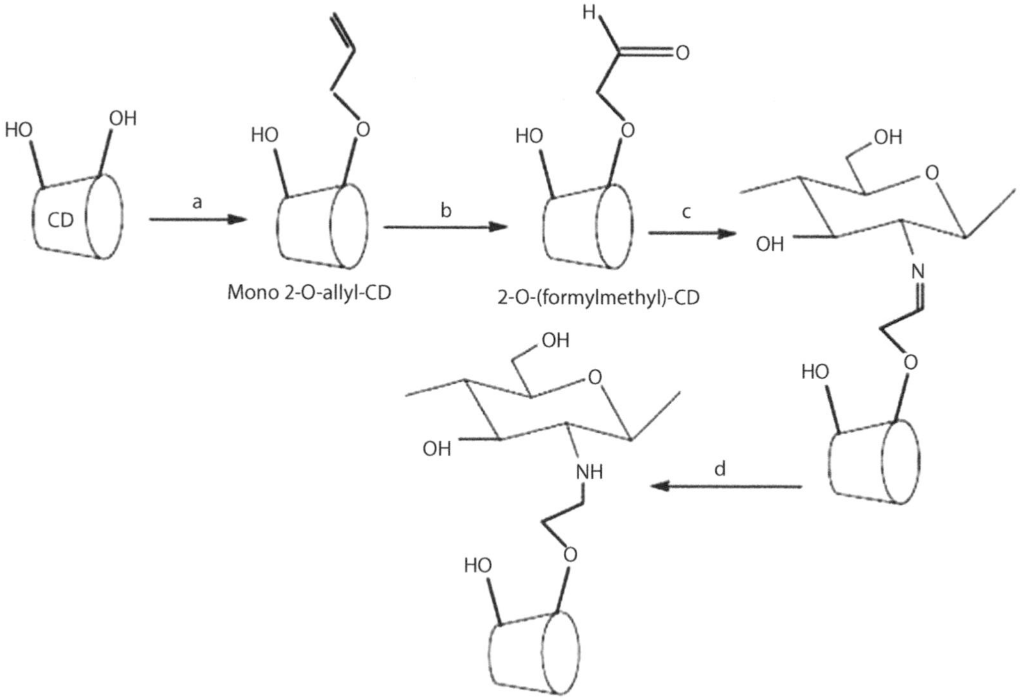

FIGURE 2.28
Reaction scheme and conditions for the synthesis of α-CD-graft-chitosan: (a) LiH-LiI, DMSO, and then allyl bromide, 60°C, overnight; (b) O₃ in 50% aqueous MeOH, 0°C, 4 h, and then Me₂S, 25°C, overnight; (c) chitosan in acetate buffer (pH 4.4), 25°C, 1 h; and (d) NaBH₃CN in acetate buffer (pH 4.4), 25°C, 4 days. (From Tojima, T. et al. 1998. *J Polym Sci A-Polym Chem* 36: 1965–1968. With permission.)

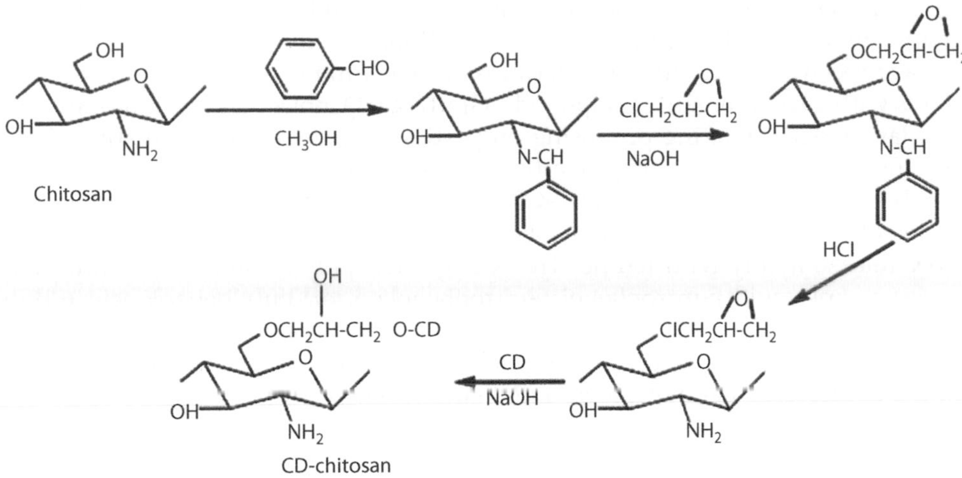

FIGURE 2.29
Reaction scheme for the synthesis of β-CD-graft-chitosan via epoxy-activated chitosan. (From Zhang, X., Wang, Y., and Yi, Y. 2004. *J Appl Polym Sci* 94: 860–864. With permission.)

by esterification of β-CD with itaconic acid in a semidry process and then the pendant double bonds of β-CD itaconate were utilized in graft copolymerization onto chitosan (Figure 2.30). The resultant product was then subjected to cross-linking using different concentrations of glutaraldehyde. This cross-linked chitosan derivative was evaluated as a new adsorbent for three classes of dyes (acid, basic, and hydrolyzed reactive), because it has three different active groups such as carboxyl groups, amino groups, and CD-ring

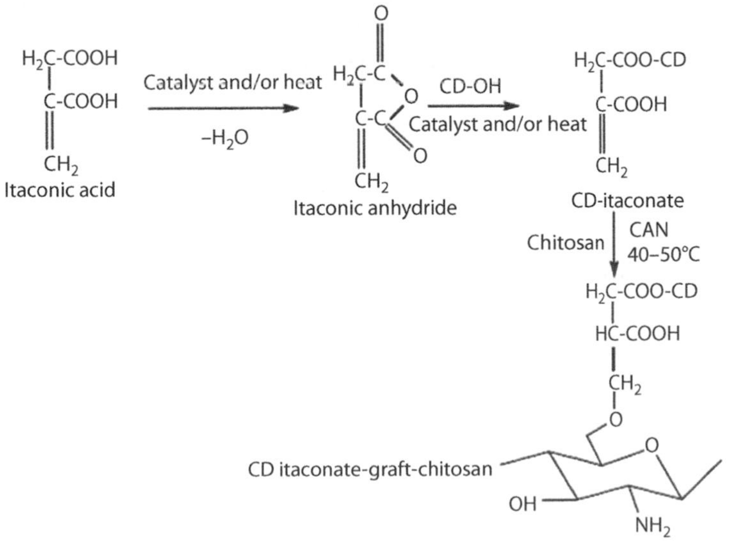

FIGURE 2.30
Reaction scheme for the synthesis of β-CD itaconate-graft-chitosan using CAN. (From Gaffar, M. A., Rafie, S. M. E., and Tahlawy, K. F. E. 2004. *Carbohydr Polym* 56: 387–396. With permission.)

hosting molecules. The adsorption experiments were conducted under different conditions with a view to establishing appropriate conditions for dye adsorption.

CDs have received much attention because of their unique ability to form host–guest complexes with various organic compounds. Grafting CD molecules into chitosan leads to a molecular carrier exhibiting promising properties because of the cumulative effects of size specificity and the transport properties of CDs. Due to the CD moiety present in the chitosan backbone, it was found that β-CD-grafted chitosan has some selectivity for the adsorption of TNS, bisphenol A, p-nonylphenol, and cholesterol and has stronger inclusion and slow release ability with iodine. This CD-grafted polymer has also confirmed the host–guest complex with p-nitrophenol, p-nitrophenolate, tert-butylbenzoic acid, 6-thiopurine, p-dihydroxybenzene, and copper ions. Due to the inclusion properties, the CD-grafted chitosan was found to be useful in drug delivery, cosmetics, decontamination of water containing textile dyes and metal ions, and analytical chemistry.

2.11 Graft Copolymers of Chitosan

Graft copolymerization is the main method used to modify chitosan chemically. In recent years, a number of initiator systems such as ammonium persulfate (APS), potassium persulfate (PPS), CAN, thiocarbonationpotassium bromate (TCPB), potassium diperiodatocuprate(III) (PDC), 2,2-azobisisobutyronitrile (AIBN), and ferrous ammonium sulfate (FAS) have been developed to initiate grafting copolymerization [227–230]. Graft copolymerization can also be initiated by irradiation and enzymes. Grafting parameters such as grafting percentage and grafting efficiency are greatly influenced by several parameters such as the type and concentration of initiator, monomer concentration, reaction temperature, and time. The properties of the resulting graft copolymers are widely controlled by the characteristics of the side chains, including molecular structure, length, and number. To date, many researchers have studied the effects of these variables on the grafting parameters and the properties of the resultant grafted chitosan (Table 2.3).

TABLE 2.3

Different Graft Copolymers of Chitosan and Ways of Grafting

Initiator		Monomers Grafted
Copolymerization via radical-induced radical generation	CAN $(NH_4)_2Ce(NO_3)_6$	Acrylonitrile [231,232]
		N-isopropyl acrylamide [233]
		Acrylic, methylacrylic acid [234]
		Methyl methacrylate, 2-hydroxyethylmethacrylate [235–237]
		Vinyl acetate [235]
		Vinyl pyridine [229]
		N,N0-dimethyl-N-methacryloxyethyl-N-(3-sulfopropyl)ammonium [238]
		Dimethylamino ethyl methacrylate [239]
		Acrylamide [240]
		Triethylene glycol dimethacrylate [241]
		N-vinylimidazole [242]

TABLE 2.3   (continued)

Different Graft Copolymers of Chitosan and Ways of Grafting

Initiator	Monomers Grafted
Potassium persulfate $K_2S_2O_8$	Acrylic acid [229]
	2-Hydroxyethyl acrylate [243]
	Acrylonitrile and methyl methacrylate [244,245]
	Acrylic acid and acrylamide [246]
	Methyl methacrylate [247]
	Maleic acid [248]
	2-Acrylamide-methylpropanesulfonic acid [249]
	Vinyl pyrrolidone [250]
	Acrylamide [251]
APS $(NH_4)_2S_2O_8$	Methacrylic acid [252]
	(*N,N*-dimethylamino)ethylmethacrylate [253]
	Maleic acid [254]
	Acrylamide [255]
Fenton's reagent ($Fe^{2+} + H_2O_2$)	Methyl methacrylate [256]
2,2-Azobis(2-methylpropionitrile) (AMPN)	MAA [257]
2,2-Azobisisobutyro nitrile (AIBN)	HEMA [258]
	Vinyl monomers [259]
Tributyl borane	Methylmethacrylate [260]
TCPB	HEMA [261]
PDC	Methyl acrylate [262]
Potassium diperiodatonickelate(IV)	Acrylonitrile [263]
Potassium ditelluratocuprate(III)	Methyl methacrylate [264]
γ-Rays	Styrene [265]
	2-Hydroxyethylmethacrylate [266]
	NIPAAm [267]
	N,N-dimethylaminiethylmethacrylate [266]
	Butyl acrylate [268]
UV radiation	Methylmethacrylate [269]
	2-Hydroxyethyl methacrylate [270,271]
	NIPAAm [272]
Microwave radiation	Acrylonitrile [273]
Copolymerization via polycondensation	LA [274]
	Peptide [275]
Copolymerization via oxidative coupling	Aniline [276]
Copolymerization of cyclic monomer via ring opening	D,L-alanine NCAs [277]
	c-methyl L-glutamate NCAs [277]
	L-alanine NCAs [278]
	Caprolactone [279]
	Poly(2-methyl-2-oxazoline) [280]
	Octamethylcyclotetrasiloxane [281]
	L-lactide [282]
	Aziridine [283]
Copolymerization of preformed polymer or grafting onto	PEG and derivatives (PEGylation) [284]
	Poly(ethylene imine) [285]
	Polyurethane [286]
	Poly(dimethylsiloxane) [287]
	Polylactide [288,289]

Chitosan has two types of reactive groups that can be grafted. First, the free amino groups on deacetylated units and, second, the hydroxyl groups on the C-3 and C-6 carbons on acetylated or deacetylated units. Grafting of chitosan allows the formation of functional derivatives by covalent binding of a molecule, the graft, onto the chitosan backbone. Recently, researchers have also shown that after primary deviation followed by graft modification, chitosan would obtain much improved water solubility and bioactivities such as antibacterial and antioxidant properties [290]. Grafting chitosan is a common way to improve chitosan properties such as increasing chelating [291] or complexation properties [219], bacteriostatic effect, or enhancing adsorption properties [292]. Although the grafting of chitosan modifies its properties, it is possible to maintain some interesting characteristics such as mucoadhesivity, biocompatibility, and biodegradability. Many investigations have been carried out on the graft copolymerization of chitosan in view of preparing polysaccharide-based advanced materials with unique bioactivities and thus widening their applications in biomedicine and environmental fields.

2.11.1 Graft Copolymerization by Radical Generation

Polyvinylic and polyacrylic synthetic materials are the most frequently grafted polymers on polysaccharides. These copolymers are frequently prepared by radical polymerization wherein free radicals are generated first on the biopolymer backbone and then these radicals serve as macroinitiators for the vinyl or acrylic monomer. The generation of radicals can be achieved by chemical or radiation initiation. Among the variety of chemical reagents reported for initiating graft copolymerization onto chitin/chitosan, CAN, potassium or ammonium persulfate, and Fenton's reagent are the most important redox systems. Grafting parameters such as grafting percentage and grafting efficiency are greatly influenced by type and concentration of the initiator, monomer concentration, reaction temperature, and time. The obtained grafts were studied for all or some of the parameters such as optimization of reaction conditions, and properties such as solubility, water absorption, swelling, thermal property, pH dependence, adsorption capacity, and so on. Researchers have also performed graft copolymerization of chitosan after its primary derivatization. The different predesignated chitosans subjected to graft copolymerization include carboxymethyl, N-carboxyethyl, maleoyl and hydroxypropyl trimethyl chitosan, and so on. This simple method of grafting is plagued with difficulties such as radical-induced depolymerization and degradation of the polysaccharide itself, lack of a well-defined initiating site and structures of the resulting copolymers as well as homopolymerization.

N-Isopropylacrylamide (NIPAAm) has a lower critical solution temperature (LCST) of around 32°C, and this is an advantage in the design of drug delivery systems due to its ability to form hydrogels with liquid–gel transition occurring at temperatures that are similar to that of the human body. Grafting NIPPAm onto chitosan provides an increase in water content on exposure to aqueous media and improvement in mechanical properties and temperature-responsive properties [293]. Kim and coworkers synthesized a chitosan-g-NIPAAm copolymer using Ce(IV) ammonium nitrate as the initiator. The copolymer was then cross-linked with glutaraldehyde. The efficiency and percentage of copolymerization increased as the monomer concentration (NIPAAm) increased. The resulting copolymer exhibited pH-responsive behavior and temperature-responsive behavior, with swelling ratios higher at pH 4 than at pH 7. At 35°C, above the LCST (32°C), the equilibrium water content was lower in comparison with the one at 25°C [228].

Sun et al. [252] prepared carboxymethyl chitosan-grafted methacrylic acid (MAA) by using APS as an initiator in aqueous solution. The effects of APS, MAA, reaction

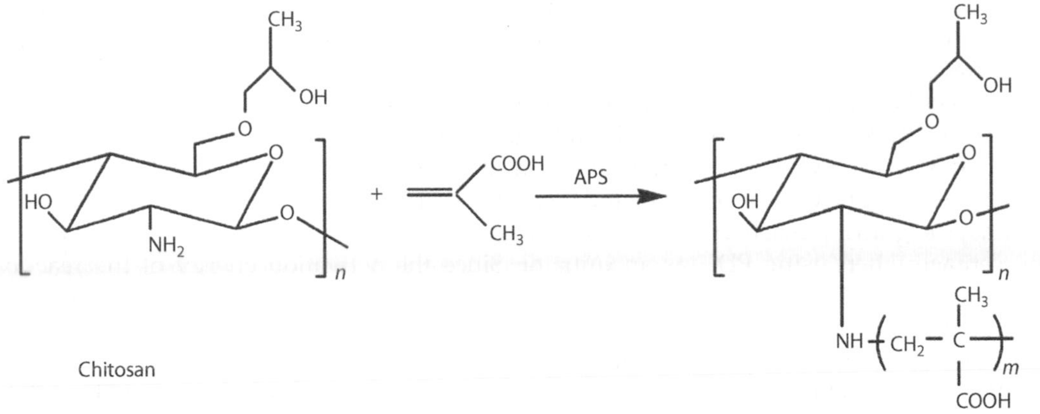

FIGURE 2.31
Graft copolymerization of MAA on hydroxypropyl chitosan.

temperature, and time on graft copolymerization were analyzed by determining grafting percentage and grafting efficiency. After grafting, the chitosan derivatives had improved water solubility. Similarly, Xie et al. [253] prepared hydroxypropyl chitosangrafted MAA by using APS initiator (Figure 2.31), obtaining a derivative that also presented good solubility in water.

Graft copolymerization of maleic acid sodium onto carboxymethyl chitosan and hydroxypropyl chitosan using APS initiator has been reported [248, 294]. Compared with chitosan, the graft chitosan derivatives were found to have improved scavenging ability against superoxide anion. Graft chitosan derivatives with hydroxypropyl groups had relatively higher superoxide anion scavenging ability owing to the incorporation of hydroxyl groups. Acylation of chitosan with maleic anhydride furnishes carbon–carbon double bonds, which are available for subsequent polymerization. The copolymerization of the derivative with acrylamide in water in the presence of APS has been used to obtain three-dimensional cross-linked products [255]. The resulting copolymers swelled highly in water with a volume increase of 20–150 times.

Graft copolymerization of vinyl monomers onto chitosan can also be carried out using redox initiator systems, such as CAN and PPS. Poly(vinyl acetate) (PVAc) is known as a leathery and water-resistant polymer, which may improve the properties of chitosan material, and hence the graft polymerization of vinyl acetate onto chitosan by using CAN as an initiator was reported. Experimental results indicated that chitosan molecules not only took part in the graft copolymerization but also acted as a surfactant, providing stability of the dispersed particles. The data also showed that the incorporation of PVAc into chitosan chains increased the toughness and decreased the water absorption of chitosan. CAN was also found to be a suitable initiator for grafting N,N-dimethyl-N-methacryloxyethyl-N-(3-sulfopropyl)ammonium [238], poly(acrylonitrile) (PAN) [232], polyacrylamide, poly(acrylic acid), and poly(4-vinylpyridine) [295] onto chitosan.

Chitosan was modified with poly(acrylic acid), a well-known hydrogel-forming polymer, using a grafting reaction in a homogeneous phase [229]. Grafting was carried out in the presence of PPS and FAS as the combined redox initiator system. It was observed that the level of grafting could be controlled to some extent by varying the amount of ferrous ion as a cocatalyst in the reaction. Tahlawy and Hudson [261] have discussed the effects of the reaction conditions and temperature on the grafting efficiency of 2-hydroxyethyl methacrylate (HEMA) onto chitosan in the presence of redox initiators, in this case TCPB. Here, the total conversion of HEMA monomer was found to be up to 75%. The resulting material was found to increase the hydrophilicity and therefore may be used as textile finishes enhancing the hydrophilicity of synthetic fibers.

A novel redox system, PDC [Cu(III)-chitosan], was employed to initiate the graft copolymerization of methyl acrylate onto chitosan in an alkali aqueous solution [262]. In this work, Cu(III) was employed as an oxidant and chitosan as a reductant in the redox system used to initiate the grafting reaction. The result showed that there is a high grafting efficiency and percentage when using PDC as an initiator. Since the activation energy of the reaction employing Cu(III)-chitosan as an initiator is low, graft copolymerization is carried out at a mild temperature of 35°C and in an alkali aqueous medium, which makes it superior to other initiators. Graft copolymerization onto chitosan has also been attempted by using AIBN. Some vinyl monomers such as acrylonitrile, methyl methacrylate, methyl acrylate, and vinyl acetate were grafted onto chitosan with AIBN in aqueous acetic acid solutions or in aqueous suspensions [230]. Here, the grafting percentages were generally low [230]. Fenton's reagent (Fe^{2+}/H_2O_2) was also successfully used as a redox initiator for grafting methyl methacrylate onto chitosan [256]. Although chitosan is an effective flocculating agent only in acidic media, the derivatives having side-chain carboxyl groups showed zwitterionic characteristics with high flocculation abilities in both acidic and basic media.

2.11.2 Grafting by Using Radiation

Recently, great effort has been made to graft natural polymers using the radiation method. Grafting of polystyrene onto chitin and chitosan using ^{60}Co γ-irradiation at room temperature was investigated [265]. Grafting yield was controlled by changing the grafting conditions. It was found that grafting yield increased with an increase in adsorbed dose. Singh and Ray [266] have also reported the radiation grafting of chitosan with *N,N'*-dimethylaminoethylmethacrylate (DMAEMA). Parameters such as solvent composition, monomer concentration, radiation dose rate, and total dose/time were found to affect the rate of grafting and homopolymerization. The degree of swelling, crystallinity, and tensile strength decreased by 51%, 43%, and 37%, respectively, at a 54% graft level of DMAEMA, whereas modified films showed improved thermal stability.

Yu et al. [268] have reported the graft copolymerization of butyl acrylate onto chitosan by using γ-irradiation. In this study, grafting percentage was observed to increase when monomer concentration and total dose were increased or when chitosan concentration and reaction temperature were decreased. Under lower dose rates, grafting percentage has no significant change, whereas above 35 Gy/min (dose rate), grafting percentage exhibits a sharp decrease. Compared with pure chitosan film, the chitosan graft poly(butyl acrylate) films have enhanced hydrophobic and impact strength.

Similar work has also been reported on grafting poly(hydroxyethyl methacrylate) with chitosan in the presence of UV light [271]. Here, the sulfite oxidase enzyme was covalently immobilized onto the matrix of the grafted polymer. After the completion of photo-induced polymerization reaction, *p*-benzoquinone (an electron transfer mediator) was coupled onto the polymer network for activation of the chitosan-poly(hydroxyethyl methacrylate) copolymer. This study demonstrated the feasibility of using chitosan in electrochemical biosensor fabrication.

Singh et al. [296] grafted PAN onto chitosan using the microwave irradiation technique under homogeneous conditions. They obtained 170% grafting yield within 1.5 min. The effects of reaction variables such as monomer or chitosan concentration, microwave power, and exposure time on graft copolymerization were studied. Grafting was found to increase with an increase in the initial concentration of monomer. Grafting was also found to increase up to 80% microwave power and thereafter decrease. Grafted chitosan showed good solubility at higher pH than chitosan.

2.11.3 Copolymerization via Polycondensation

Condensation polymerization has not been widely used for preparing graft copolymers of polysaccharides, usually due to susceptibility of the saccharide backbone to high temperature and harsh conditions of the typical polycondensation reactions. However, lactic acid (LA) was successfully graft copolymerized onto chitosan through condensation polymerization of D,L lactic acid in the absence of a catalyst [274,297], which forms a pH-sensitive hydrogel (Figure 2.32). The condensation of polylactide has also been achieved by using the catalyst 4-dimethylaminopyridine, where polylactide was grafted through the hydroxyl groups phthaloylchitosan. A carbodiimide process of condensation too is used to link the amino group of chitosan to polylactic acid surface or to a peptide to improve cell compatibility and adhesion [298] and support the proliferation of human endothelial cells [274,299].

2.11.4 Cationic Graft Polymerization

Some years ago, Yoshikawa et al. [300] showed that grafting reactions onto chitosan can also be performed by using living cationic polymerization. These authors grafted chitosan with living poly(isobutylvinyl ether) and poly(2-methyl-2-oxazoline) cation with controlled molecular weight distribution. In this study, the effect of the molecular weight of living polymer cation on the mole number of grafted polymer was analyzed. The mole number of grafted polymer chains was found to decrease with increasing molecular weight of

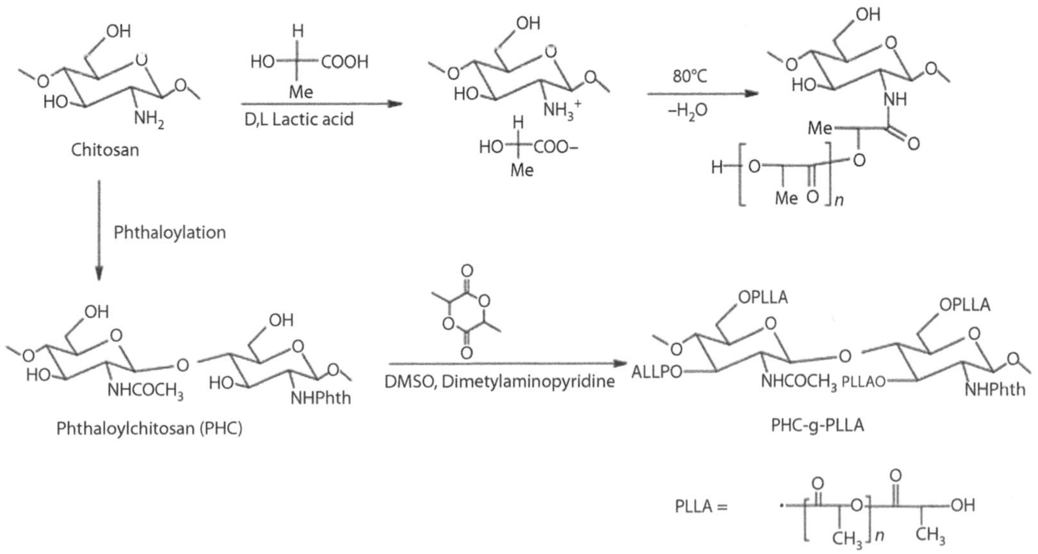

FIGURE 2.32
Grafting of LA on chitosan.

living polymer cation, due to the steric hindrance of the functional groups of chitosan with increasing molecular weight of living polymer. The viscosity of the resulting polymer was found to increase with increasing percentage of grafting. This grafted polymer was also found to be soluble in water.

2.11.5 Copolymerization via Oxidative Coupling

With an aim to prepare conductive polymers, polyaniline was grafted onto chitosan by the method of oxidative coupling (Figure 2.33) [325].

2.11.6 Cyclic Monomer Copolymerization via Ring Opening

In general, four groups of cyclic monomers have been mainly used for graft copolymerization onto polysaccharides: α-amino acid, N-carboxy anhydrides (NCAs), lactones, oxiranes (epoxides), and 2-alkyl oxazolines. An NCA ring can undergo nucleophilic attack to open and polymerize with evolution of CO_2 to yield a polypeptide chain. The free amine of chitosan is believed to initiate graft copolymerization by means of attack upon carbonyl, ultimately creating the grafted chitosan derivative. The advantages of this method are a low level of homopolymer formation and the possibility of side chain length control through the regulation of NCA concentration under proper conditions. DP, however, is not usually higher than 20 [231]. The resulting copolymers are new types of hybrid materials composed of both a polysaccharide and polypeptides.

The novel artificial glycoprotein, chitosan-poly(L-tryptophan) copolymers with two-dimensional structure side chains, has been synthesized successfully under homogeneous conditions with ring-opening graft polymerization between L-tryptophan NCA and the water-soluble chitosan [301] (*cf.* Figure 3.34). With increased DP, the conformation of side chains on glycopeptides starts to convert from β-sheet to α-helix. The copolymers have a strong fluorescence emission at 360 nm, and emission intensities can be adjusted by DP and quenched by coordination with copper ions within 30 min. Significantly enhanced mechanical rigidity has been achieved by graft polymerization, in comparison with that by chitosan. The solubility of graft copolymers depends strongly on the length and conformation of the poly-L-tryptophan side chains.

Living poly(2-alkyl oxazolines) telechelic polymers have been grafted onto partially deacetylated chitins in DMSO by Aoi et al. [280] and studied for process optimization and solubility profile (*cf.* Figure 2.35). In this solvent, the water-soluble chitin swells to some extent; thus the amino group was used to terminate the living polyoxazolines (synthesized by cationic ring-opening polymerization of the corresponding 2-alkyloxazolines with

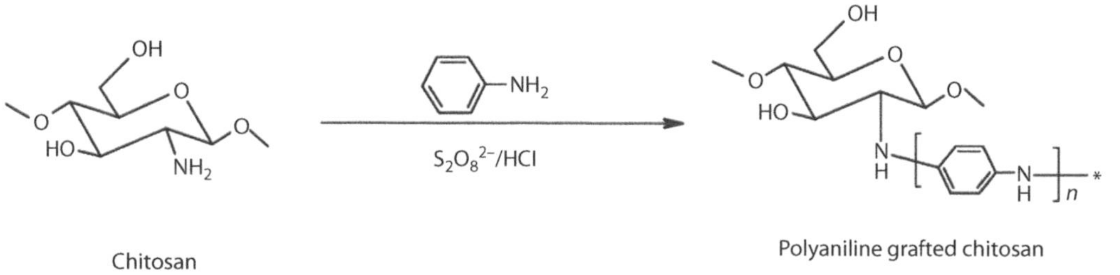

Chitosan   Polyaniline grafted chitosan

FIGURE 2.33
Grafting of polyaniline on chitosan.

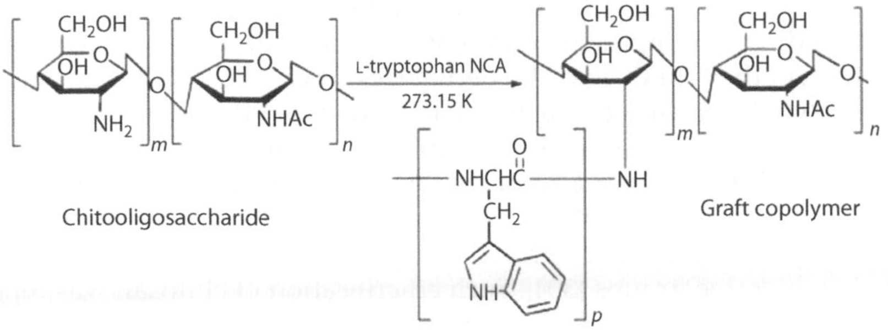

FIGURE 2.34
Preparation scheme of chitosan-poly-L-tryptophan.

methyl trifluoromethanesulfonate). Living poly(2-methyl-2-oxazoline) and poly(isobutyl-vinyl ether) cation was successfully terminated by surface amino groups on chitosan powder to give the corresponding polymer-grafted chitosan [302].

Cationic chitosan-graft-polycaprolactone (CS-g-PCL) copolymers were synthesized using the facile one-pot method via ring-opening polymerization of ε-CL onto the hydroxyl groups of chitosan by using MSA as solvent and catalyst. These graft copolymers could form spherical nanomicelles with controllable sizes and positive zeta potentials. The water-insoluble antitumor drug 7-ethyl-10-hydroxy-camptothecin (SN-38) was successfully encapsulated into these nanomicelles [303]. Their entrapment efficiency, DL, and accumulative drug release could also be controlled by adjusting the grafting PCL content in CS-g-PCL. In comparison with free SN-38, the SN-38-loaded CS-g-PCL nanomicelles showed prolonged drug release profiles, improved drug stability against hydrolysis under physiological conditions, and decreased cytotoxicity against the L929 cell line. These results indicated that nanomicelles based on cationic CS-g-PCL might be a candidate as drug carrier for SN-38 and other hydrophobic drugs.

2.11.7 Copolymerization of Preformed Polymer by the Grafting onto Method

Telechelic polymers have been defined as those containing one or more functional end groups that have the capacity for selective reaction to form bonds with another molecule. Unlike the classic grafting techniques where the grafted chain is grown from the trunk polymer by the continual addition of monomer to the growing chain end, grafting onto

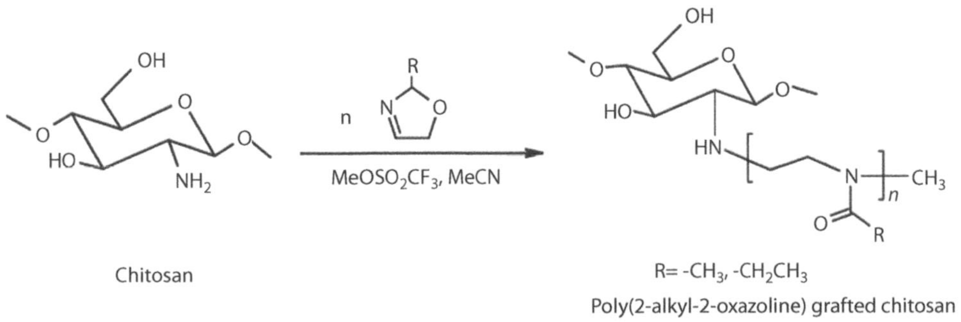

FIGURE 2.35
Synthesis of chitosan–polypeptide bioconjugate via grafting of living poly(2-alkyl-2-oxazoline) onto chitosan.

connects preformed telechelic polymer chains and the trunk polymer at a particular site by covalent bonding. Examples of different polymers grafted onto chitosan include poly(isobutylvinyl ether), PEG, and the derivatives PEO–PPO–PEO (pluronic polyols or poloxamers), poly(ethyleneimine), polyurethane, poly(dimethylsiloxane), and polylactide (Figure 2.36). Of these, PEG is an important hydrophilic polymer commonly grafted (PEGylated) onto chitin–chitosan. Several methods have been reported on the PEGylation of chitin–chitosan using PEGs with various terminal reactive groups (Table 2.4). PEG can be regioselectively grafted to obtain chitosan-*O*-poly(ethylene glycol) graft copolymers by prior protection of amino groups [304]. Such etherification of chitosan was reported with poly(ethylene glycol) monomethyl ether (MPEG) using triazine derivative as coupler and with MPEG iodide without coupler [239] (Figure 2.37). Regioselective modification of chitosan through the C-6 position of glucosamine units by PEG has been reported for the first time using 6-oxo-2-*N*-phthaloylchitosan, 6-*O*-dichlorotriazine-2-*N*-phthaloylchitosan, and 3-*O*-acetyl-2-*N*-phthaloylchitosan intermediates with high DS [305].

Methods of immobilizing adhesive peptide ligands on nonfouling surfaces are important because they allow us to study the effect of individual factors on cell adhesion, proliferation, and differentiation without the confounding influence of protein adsorption from the serum or the extracellular matrices produced by the cells themselves. Ying and coworkers [306] engineered the RGD peptide on chitosan PEC using a three-tiered system (*cf.* Figure 2.38). The three-tiered system described in this work offers unique advantages. First, the three-tiered system enabled the isolation of the effect of the ligand from the effect of chitosan by interposing a nonfouling second tier between the underlying substrate (first

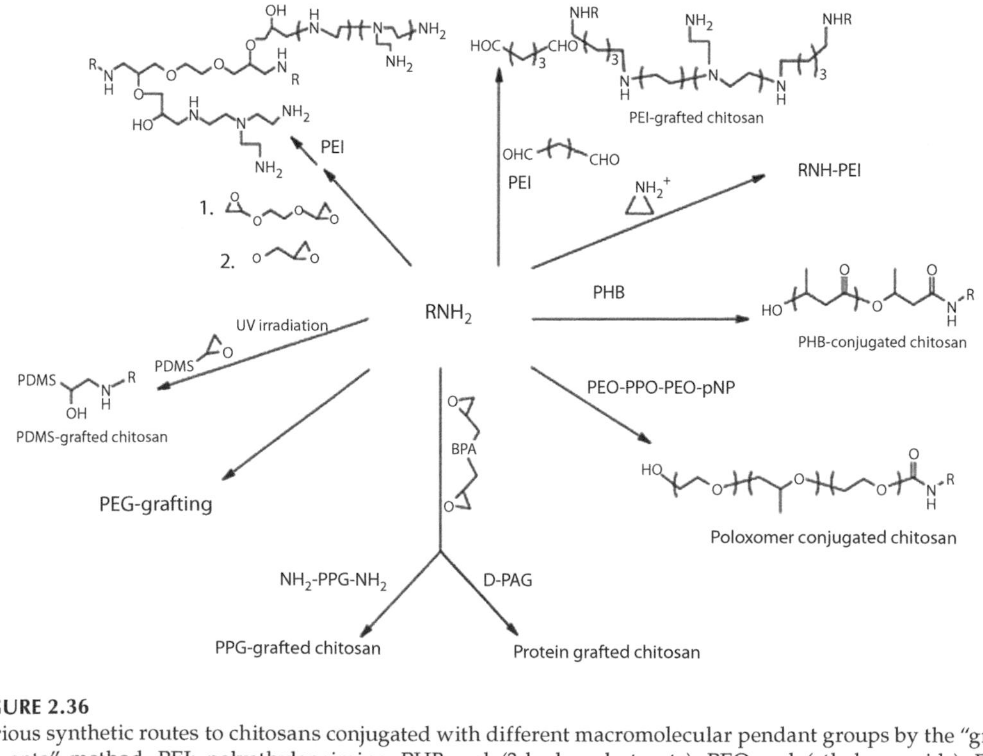

FIGURE 2.36
Various synthetic routes to chitosans conjugated with different macromolecular pendant groups by the "grafting onto" method. PEI: polyethyleneimine, PHB: poly(3-hydroxybutyrate), PEO: poly(ethylene oxide), PPO: poly(propylene oxide), pNP: *p*-nitrophenyl, G-APG: gluadin APG (a partially hydrolyzed wheat gluten protein, $M_W = 5000$), PPG: poly(propylene glycol), BPA: bisphenol A residue, PDMS: poly(dimethylsiloxane).

TABLE 2.4

Approaches for PEGylating Chitosan: Grafting of a Preformed Polymer onto Chitosan

Chitosan (RNH$_2$)	Reactants and Reaction Condition	Chitosan-g-PEG
	MPEGCOOH, WSC, BtOH 6-*O*-triphenyl methylation MPEGCOOH, WSC, BtOH	

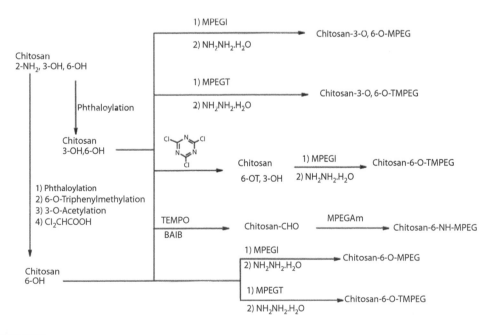

Note: The chitosan-g-PEG graft copolymer is often referred to as "PEGylated chitosan." MPEG: methoxy-terminated PEG, PNP: *p*-nitrophenyl, WSC: water-soluble carbodiimide, and BtOH: hydroxybenzotriazole.

FIGURE 2.37

Approaches for regioselective PEGylating chitosan: grafting of a preformed polymer onto chitosan. The chitosan-g-PEG graft copolymer is often referred to as "PEGylated chitosan." In chitosan, only free groups are denoted; TEMPO radical: 2,2,6,6-tetramethylpiperidin-1-oxyl; BAIB: [bis(acetoxy) iodo]benzene; MPEGAm: MPEGamine; MPEGI: MPEG iodide; MPEGT: MPEG dichlortriazine.

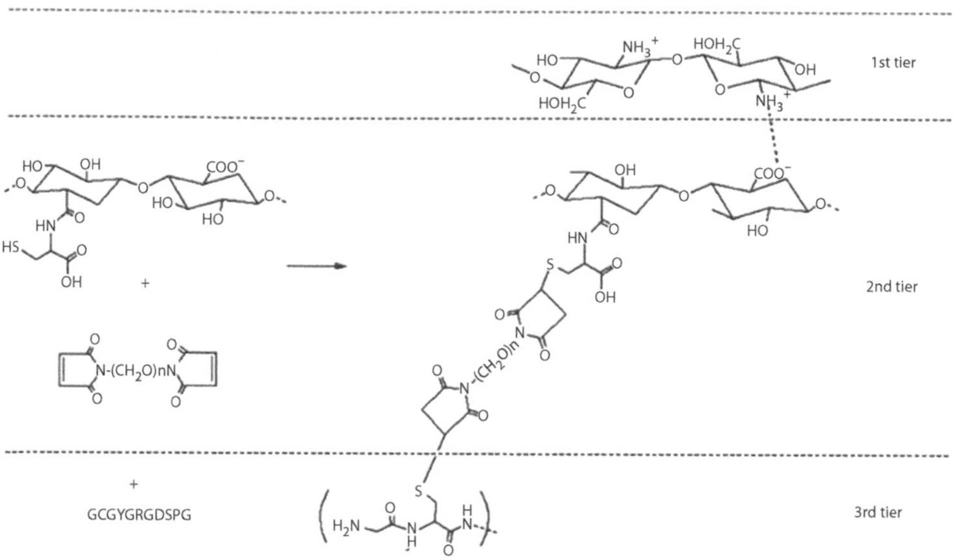

FIGURE 2.38

Three-tiered membrane/coating structure and their respective chemistries. First tier: chitosan membrane/coating; second tier: polyanion–PEG conjugate (e.g., alginate-PEG conjugate), which forms a polyelectrolyte complex with the first tier. Third tier: ligand (e.g., RGD) conjugated to the second tier by maleimidyl chemistry. (From Wan, A. C. A. et al. 2008. *Langmuir* 24: 2611–2617. With permission.)

tier) and the ligand (third tier). Human marrow stromal cells (hMSCs) seeded onto RGD-modified chitosan membranes exhibit good adhesion and spreading of cells and could be further endowed with signals to affect stem cell proliferation and/or differentiation. The RGDS sequence is immobilized on chitosan scaffolds by the formation of imide bonds between amino groups on chitosan and carboxyl groups on peptides. The concentration of the immobilized RGDS in chitosan is measured to be on the order of 10^{-12} mol/cm^2 [307]. The GRGDS sequence is a very intriguing member of the RGD family. $R_V\beta_3$, $R_V\beta_5$, and RIIbβ_3 are integrins most reported to be involved in bone function [308]. They can be immobilized on the chitosan film surface with 10^{-9} mol/cm^2. Using photochemical immobilization technology, RGDS sequences can be immobilized onto chitosan films with 10^{-7} mol/cm^2 of relatively higher concentrations (as shown in Figure 2.39). Nishimura and coworkers [309] established a facile and efficient method for the conjugation of chitosan with sulfhydryl-containing synthetic peptide on the basis of 2-iminothiolane-mediated selective cross-linking in a mild and homogeneous solution (*cf.* Figure 2.40). Chitosan-RGDSGGC conjugates exhibited excellent cell adhesion and proliferation activity for chondrocytes and fibroblasts.

2.11.8 Graft Copolymerization Based on Living Radical Polymerization

Great progress has been made in the last decade on the development of controlled/living radical polymerization methods [310,311]. The most widely used controlled/living radical polymerization (CLRP) methods are nitroxide-mediated polymerization, atom transfer radical polymerization (ATRP), and degenerative-based methods such as reversible addition fragmentation transfer (RAFT) and iodine transfer. These methods are applicable to a wide range of monomers, solvents, and end functionalities. CLRP methods allow the synthesis of

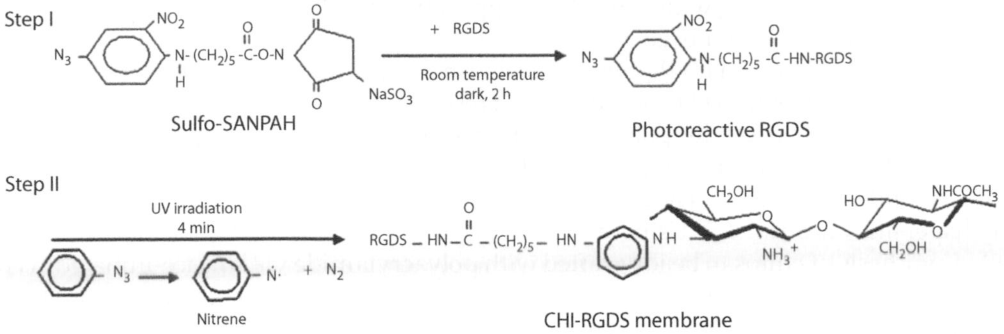

FIGURE 2.39
Schematic of chitosan surface modification with RGDS by photochemical immobilization technique. (From Schaffner P. and Dard, M. M. 2003. *Cell Mol Life Sci* 60: 119–132. With permission.)

polymers with predetermined molecular weight, narrow molecular weight distribution, chain end functionality, topology, and complex architecture and composition.

The application of these techniques to the graft-controlled polymerization of natural polymers, such as chitosan, could open a new door to the synthesis of a wide variety of molecular structures, affording the precise synthesis of tailor-made hybrid materials based on natural polymers. It will be possible to develop new materials to mimic the complexity of natural structures made by the conjunction of different natural and synthetic polymers, by designing new molecular architectures with controlled topologies and graft-controlled

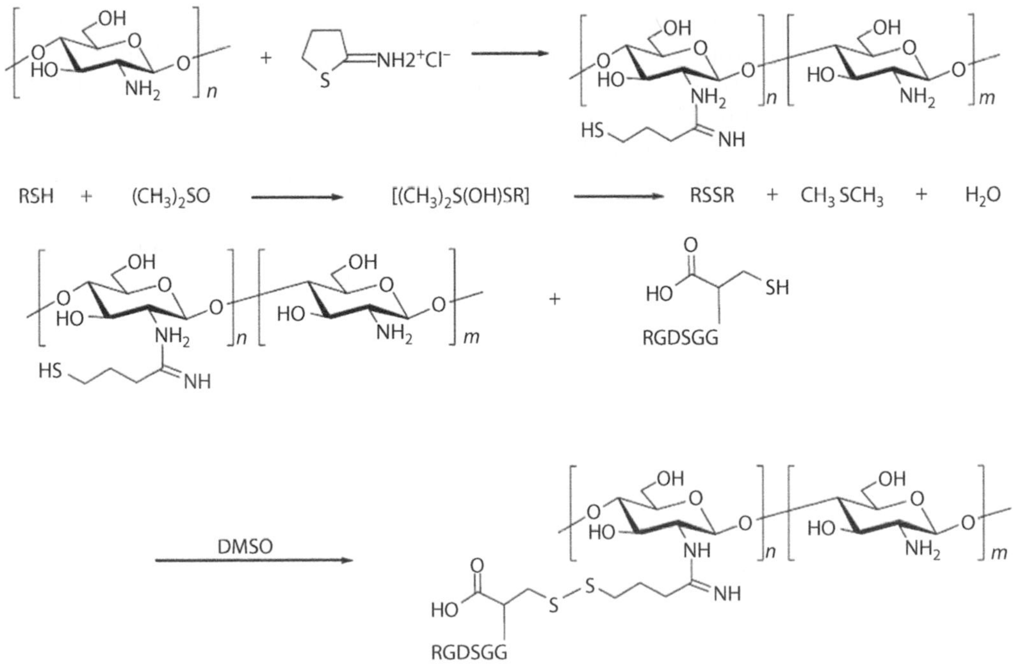

FIGURE 2.40
Coupling reaction of sulfhydryl-chitosan with RGDSGGC in the presence of DMSO. (From Masuko, T. et al. 2005. *Biomaterials* 26: 5339–5347. With permission.)

segments. In spite of being widely used, the application of CLRP techniques to the modification of chitosan is seldom used.

El Tahlawy and Hudson [312] prepared chitosan macroinitiators by acetylation of chitosan with 2-bromo-isobutyryl bromide in the presence of pyridine as a base. The chitosan macroinitiator was used to polymerize a methoxy-poly(ethylene glycol)methacrylate (MeO(PEG)MA) monomer using the Cu(I)Br–bipyridyl complex under heterogeneous aqueous conditions at 25°C. The kinetics studies revealed a first-order polymerization and polydispersities around 1.5. Using a similar approach, Li et al. [313] proposed the controlled synthesis of chitosan beads grafted with polyacrylamide via surface-initiated ATRP (SI-ATRP). The bromide end groups were immobilized on the surfaces of chitosan beads through reaction of –NH$_2$ or –OH groups of 2-bromo-isobutryl bromide using triethylamine as the trapping agent in dry tetrahydrofuran (THF) (Figure 2.41).

Tang et al. [314] proposed the graft copolymerization of poly(methyl methacrylate) (PMMA) and amphiphilic block copolymer PMMA-b-poly(ethylene glycol) methyl ether methacrylate on the surface of chitosan nanospheres, The proposed method used iron(III)-mediated ATRP with activators generated by electron transfer (AGET). This work explores the use of an iron(III)-mediated catalytic system, instead of copper(I)/copper(II) salts, due to the possible toxic effects of copper on human health, when the materials are intended to be used for *in vivo* biomedical applications. The use of the AGET initiating method can overcome an important drawback of ATRP, because transition metal compound in lower oxidation can be easily oxidized leading to uncontrolled polymerization.

Regarding the other widely used CLRP methods RAFT and nitroxide-mediated polymerization, to the best of our knowledge there are only three reports available in the literature, all from the same laboratory. As for the RAFT approach, Zhu and coworkers proposed the synthesis of chitosan-g-PNIPAM [315] and chitosan-g-PAA [316] using *S*-1-dodecyl-*S′*-(α,α′-dimethyl-α″-acetic acid) trithiocarbonate as the RAFT agent. Chitosan-RAFT agents were synthesized in dry DMF by reacting *N*-phthaloylchitosan with *S*-1-dodecyl-*S′*-(α,α′-dimethyl-α″-acetic acid)trithiocarbonate in the presence of 1,3-dicyclohexylcarbodiimide and 4-(*N,N*-dimethylamino)pyridine. Both graft copolymerizations (chitosan-g-PINPAM and chitosan-g-PAA) were carried out in dry DMF, using AIBN as the initiator and reaction temperatures ranging from 60°C to 80°C [315], leading to polymers with living features.

It is expected that in the next few years, improvement in the graft copolymerization of natural polymers techniques based on CLRP will take place, leading to the preparation of

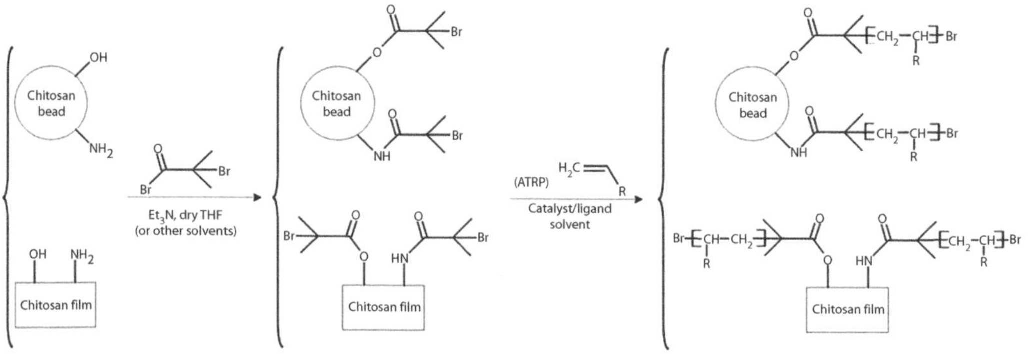

FIGURE 2.41
General scheme used to prepare chitosan macroinitiator for ATRP.

smart polymers based on chitosan. Grafted copolymerization, by CLRP methods, of monomers such as NIPAM and acrylic acid (AA) (among others) will enable the preparation of a variety of responsive graft copolymers with precise structure and molecular design to give materials made up of tailored chitosan and synthetic polymers.

2.12 Chitosan–Dendrimer Hybrid

Dendrimers are attractive molecules owing to their multifunctional properties and have useful applications as viral and pathogenic cell adhesion inhibitors. Increasing scientific efforts have gone into the design and synthesis of dendrimers. Dendronized polymers, on the other hand, are also attractive because of their rod-like conformation and nanostructure. Dendrimer-like hyperbranched polymers, a new class of topological macromolecules, have recently been grafted onto chitosan. Tsubokawa and Takayama [317] reported the surface modification of chitosan powder by the grafting of hyperbranched dendritic polyamidoamine (PAMAM). They found that PAMAM was propagated from the surface of chitosan by the repetition of two processes: (1) Michael addition of methyl acrylate to the surface amino groups and (2) amidation of the resulting esters with ethylenediamine to give PAMAM dendrimer-grafted chitosan powder (Figure 2.42).

Sashiwa established the synthesis of a variety of chitosan–dendrimer hybrids, mainly by two procedures (Figure 2.43) [318–320]. In method A, corresponding dendrimers bearing aldehyde and a spacer are synthesized, and then these are reacted with chitosan by reductive N-alkylation. This procedure has the advantage of no cross-linking during the reaction.

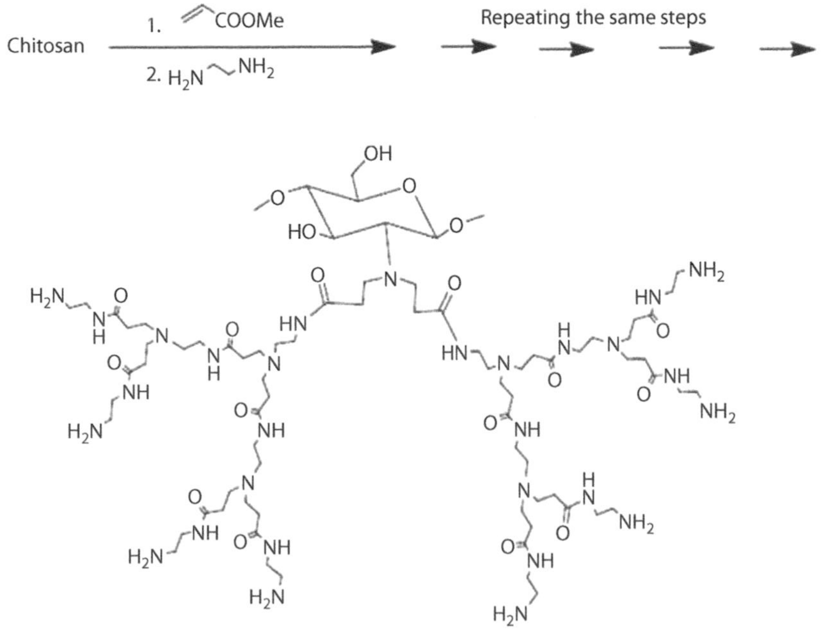

FIGURE 2.42
Polyamidiamine dendrimer-grafted chitosan surface.

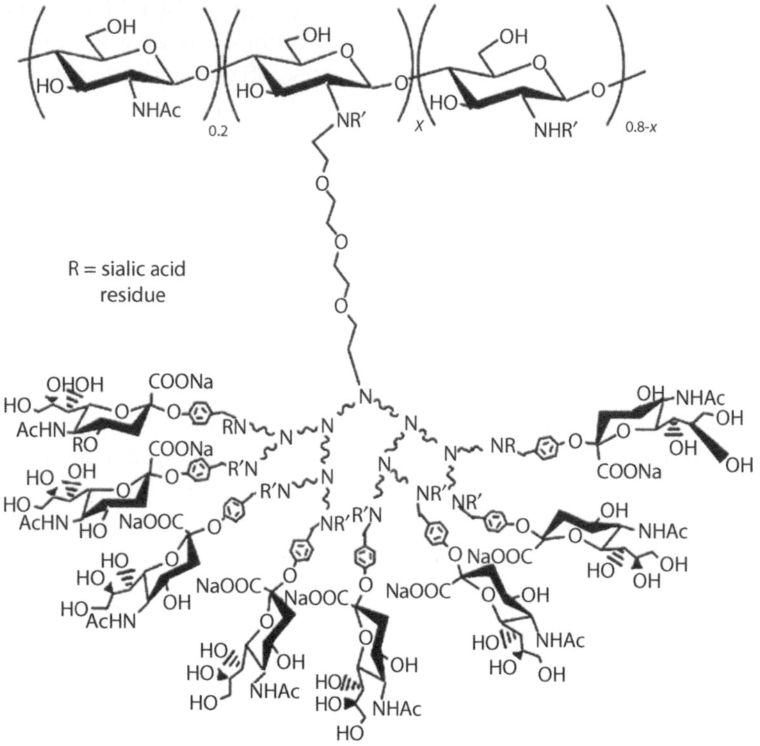

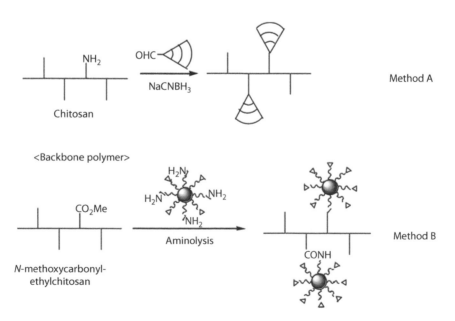

FIGURE 2.43
Chemical structure of chitosan–sialodendrimer hybrid.

FIGURE 2.44
Synthetic strategy on chitosan–dendrimer hybrid.

However, the generation of reactive dendrimer is limited owing to steric hindrance. On the other hand, method B, with binding of chitosan to the dendrimer surface, allows the use of commercially available amino-dendrimers such as PAMAM or poly(ethylene imine) dendrimers; and binding is possible even for high generations. One weak point in method B is that it has two or more binding points that may sometimes cause cross-linking. A typical example of a hybrid obtained by methods A and B is shown in Figure 2.44 [318,320]. In this case, tetraethylene glycol was modified in 5–7 steps, to synthesize the scaffold of the dendrimer. PAMAM dendrimers of generations (G) from 1 to 3 bearing tetraethylene glycol spacers were attached to sialic acid by reductive N-alkylation, and finally attached to chitosan. The DS of dendrimer per sugar unit decreased with increasing generation [0.08 ($G = 1$), 0.04 ($G = 2$), and 0.02 ($G = 3$)] owing to steric hindrance of the dendrimers. Figure 2.45 shows a different type of chitosan–dendrimer hybrid [319]. A sialic acid dendron bearing a focal aldehyde end group was synthesized by a reiterative amide bond strategy. Trivalent ($G = 1$) and nanovalent ($G = 2$) dendrons having gallic acid as the branching unit and triethylene glycol as the spacer arm were prepared and initially attached to a sialic acid p-phenylisothiocyanate derivative. The focal aldehyde sialodendrons were then convergently attached to chitosan. The DS values of sialodendrimer were 0.13 ($G = 1$) and 0.06 ($G = 2$). The water solubility of these novel hybrids was further improved by N-succinylation of the remaining amine functionality.

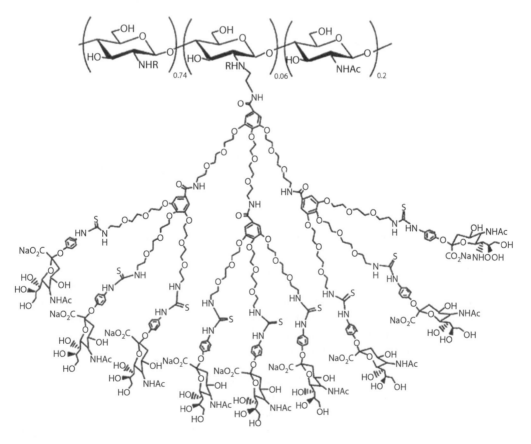

FIGURE 2.45
Hybridization of chitosan with sialodendrimer, composed of gallic acid as junction point.

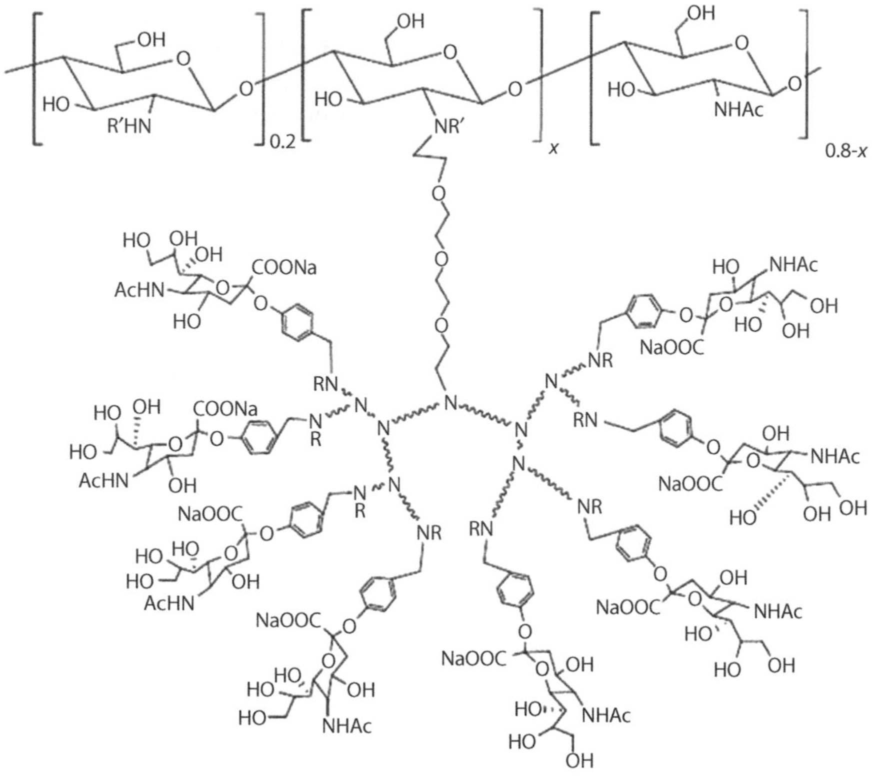

FIGURE 2.46
Chemical structure of chitosan–sialodendrimer hybrid.

In another convergent approach taken by the team of Sashiwa et al. [318–320], first tetra-ethylene glycol was modified in five or seven steps to synthesize the scaffold of dendrimer. PAMAM dendrimers of generation (G) from 1 to 3 bearing tetraethylene glycol spacer were prepared, attached to sialic acid by reductive N-alkylation, and finally attached to chitosan (Figure 2.46). The DS of dendrimer decreased with increasing generation as 0.08 (G1), 0.04 (G2), and 0.02 (G3) owing to the steric hindrance of dendrimer.

A chitosan–dendrimer hybrid prepared by method B is shown in Figure 2.47 [321]. As the construction of the hybrid was difficult from the original chitosan, a derivative, N-methoxycarbonylethylchitosan (NMCC), was used as the chitosan backbone. PAMAM dendrimers ($G = 1$–5) having a 1,4-diaminobutane core were attached to NMCC by amidation under conditions that prevented cross-linking. The hybrids could be prepared even at high generations ($G = 4$ or 5), although the DS of dendrimer was decreased with increasing generation of dendrimer from 0.53 ($G = 1$) to 0.17 ($G = 4$) or 0.11 ($G = 5$). Because this hybrid was soluble in acidic solutions, undesired cross-linking did not occur. However, two or more intermolecular binding points were observed. Finally, sialic acid was successfully attached to the primary amine of the dendrimer with DS ranging from 0.7 to 1.4 per glucosamine unit, which indicates a highly convergent synthesis of sialic acid in the chitosan backbone. Given the fact that flu virus hemagglutinins exist as clusters of trimers (200–300/virions), it is likely that the novel dendronized chitosan–sialic acid hybrids prepared by method B will present added beneficial architectures not present in previously reported sialodendrimers [322,323].

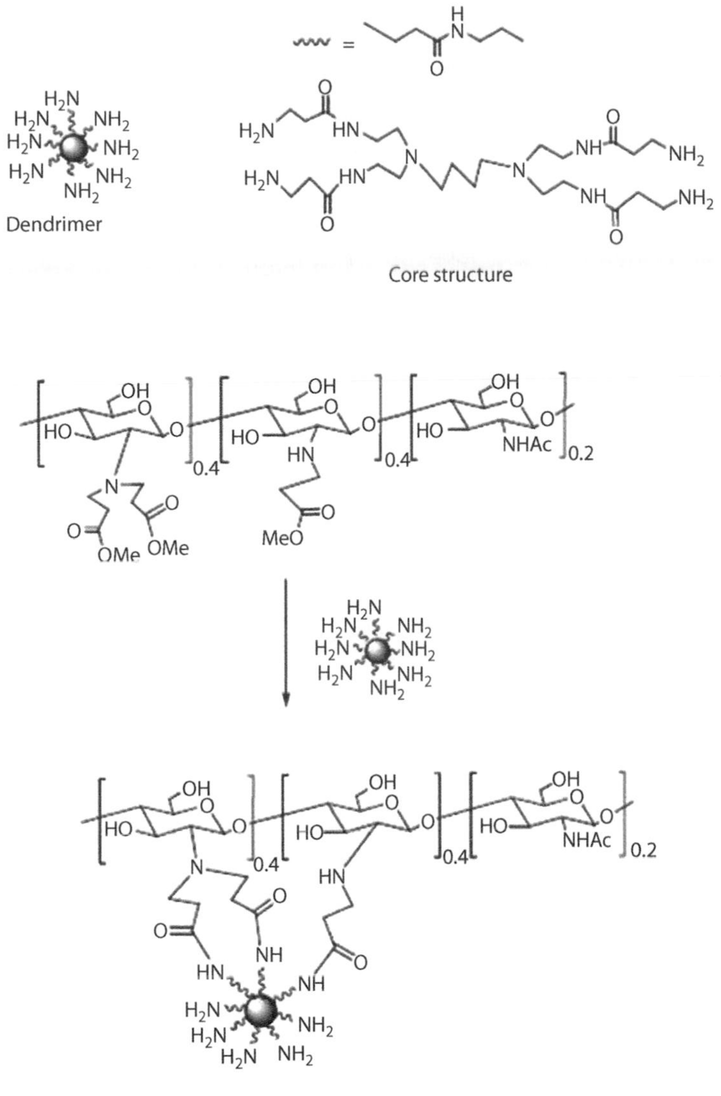

FIGURE 2.47
Reaction of NMCC with PAMAM dendrimer.

The cationic hyperbranched dendritic PAMAM containing terminal methyl ester end groups was synthesized and then employed for modifying flake chitosan [324]. The synthesis was achieved using repetitive reactions between Michael addition and amidation to obtain the methyl ester group-terminated hyperbranched PAMAM, and then the methyl ester-terminated hyperbranched dendritic PAMAM (PAMAM-ester) was methylated with dimethyl sulfate. The subsequent modification of chitosan with the cationic hyperbranched PAMAM-ester was carried out at room temperature for 5 days. As a result, cationic hyperbranched PAMAM-modified chitosan was achieved (Figure 2.48).

The cationic hyperbranched PAMAM-chitosan was applied onto cotton fabric at 1 wt% add-on by using a padding method and was found to have good antimicrobial performance against *Staphylococcus aureus* compared to that obtained with unmodified chitosan.

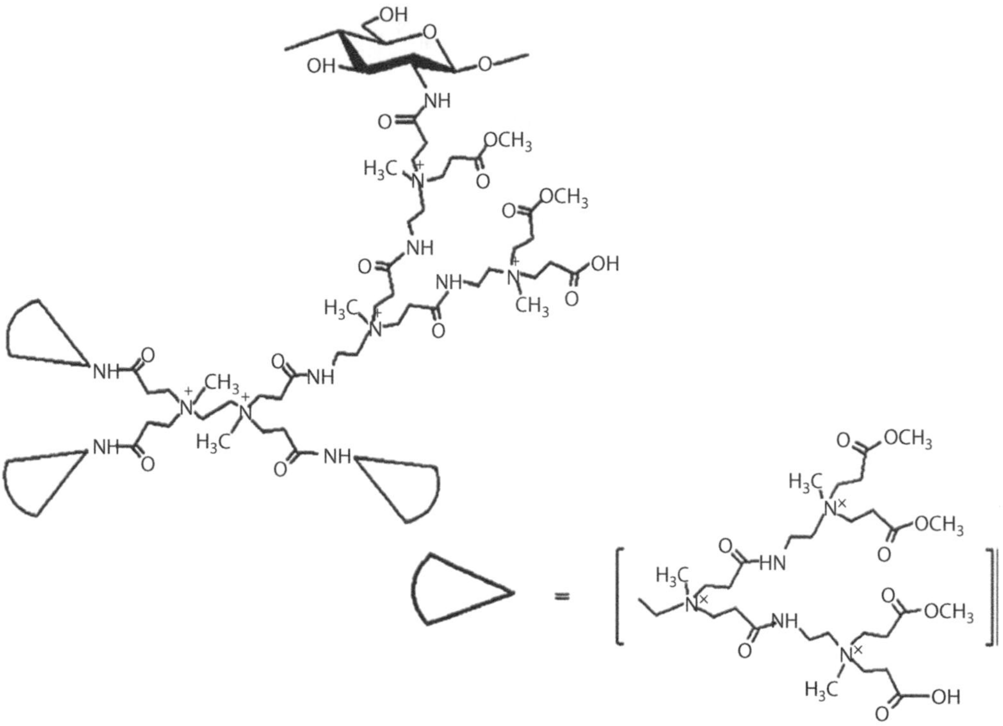

FIGURE 2.48
Putative structure of the G2.5 cationic hyperbranched PAMAM-chitosan.

References

1. Desbrières, J., Martinez, C., and Rinaudo, M. 1996. Hydrophobic derivatives of chitosan: Characterization and rheological behaviour. *Int J Biol Macromol* 19: 21–28.
2. Desbrières, J. 2004. Autoassociative natural polymer derivatives: The alkylchitosans. Rheological behaviour and temperature stability. *Polymer* 45: 3285–3295.
3. Rinaudo, M., Auzely, R., Vallin, C., and Mullagaliev, I. 2005. Specific interactions in modified chitosan systems. *Biomacromolecules* 6: 2396–2407.
4. Klotzbach, T., Watt, M., Ansari, Y., and Minteer, S. D. 2006. Effects of hydrophobic modification of chitosan and Nafion on transport properties, ion-exchange capacities, and enzyme immobilization. *J Membr Sci* 282: 276–283.
5. Klotzbach, T. L., Watt, M., Ansari, Y., and Minteer, S. D. 2008. Improving the microenvironment for enzyme immobilization at electrodes by hydrophobically modifying chitosan and Nafion® polymers. *J Membr Sci* 311: 81–88.
6. Xiangyang X., Ling, L., Jianping, Z., Shiyue, L., Jie, Y., Xiaojin, Y., and Jinsheng, R. 2007. Preparation and characterization of N-succinyl-N-octyl chitosan micelles as doxorubicin carriers for effective anti-tumor activity. *Colloid Surf B* 55: 222–228.
7. Cano-Cebrian, M. J., Zornoza, T., Granero, L., and Polache. A. 2005. Intestinal absorption enhancement via the paracellular route by fatty acids, chitosans and others: a target for drug delivery. *Curr Drug Delivery* 2: 9–22.
8. Muzzarelli, R. A. A. and Tanfani, F. 1985. The N-permethylation of chitosan and the preparation of N-trimethyl chitosan iodide. *Carbohydr Polym* 5: 297–307.

9. Domard, A., Rinaudo, M., and Terrassin, C. 1986. New method for the quaternization of chitosan. *Int J Biol Macromol* 8: 105–107.

10. Domard, A., Gey, C., Rinaudo, M., and Terrassin, C. 1987. ^{13}C and ^{1}H-NMR spectroscopy of chitosan and N-trimethyl chloride derivatives. *Int J Biol Macromol* 9: 233–327.

11. Sieval, A. B., Thanou, M., Kotźe, A. F., Verhoef, J. C., Brussee, J., and Junginger, H. E. 1998. Preparation and NMR characterization of highly substituted N-trimethyl chitosan chloride. *Carbohydr Polym* 36: 157–165.

12. Hamman, J. H. and Kotźe, A. F. 2001. Effect of the type of base and number of reaction steps on the degree of quaternization and molecular weight of N-trimethyl chitosan chloride. *Drug Dev Ind Pharm* 27: 373–380.

13. Snyman, D., Hamman, J. H., Kotze, J. S., Rollings, J. E., and Kotźe, A. F. 2002. The relationship between the absolute molecular weight and the degree of quaternization of N-trimethyl chitosan chloride. *Carbohydr Polym* 50: 145–150.

14. Curiti, E., Britto, D., and Campana-Filho, D. P. 2003. Methylation of chitosan with iodomethane: Effect of reaction conditions on chemoselectivity and degree of substitution. *Macromol Biosci* 3: 571–576.

15. Polnok, A., Borchard, G., Verhoef, J. C., Sarisuta, N., and Junginger, H. E. 2004. Influence of methylation process on the degree of quaternization of N-trimethyl chitosan chloride. *Eur J Pharm Biopharm* 57: 77–83.

16. Runarsson, O. V., Holappa, J., Nevalainen, T., Hjalmarsdottir, M., Jarvinen, T., Loftsson, T. Einarsson, J. M. Josdottir, S. Valdimarsdottir, M., and Masson, M. 2007. Antibacterial activity of methylated chitosan and chitooligomer derivatives: Synthesis and structure activity relationships. *Eur Polym J* 43: 2660–2671.

17. Runarsson, O. V., Holappa, J., Jonsdottir, S., Steinsson, H., and Masson, M. 2008. N-selective "one pot" synthesis of highly N-substituted trimethyl chitosan (TMC). *Carbohydr Polym* 74: 740–744.

18. Verheul, R. J., Amidi, M., Wal, S., Riet, E., Jiskoot, W., and Hennink, W. 2008. Synthesis, characterization and *in vitro* biological properties of O-methyl free N,N,N-trimethylated chitosan. *Biomaterials* 29: 3642–3649.

19. Loubaki, E., Ourevitch, M., and Sicsic, S. 1991. Chemical modification of chitosan by glycidyl trimethylammonium chloride: Characterization of modified chitosan by 13C- and 1H-NMR spectroscopy. *Eur Polym J* 27: 311–317.

20. Daly, W. H. and Manuszak-Guerrini, M. A. 2001. Biocidal chitosan derivatives for cosmetics and pharmaceuticals. US Patent, Pat. No. 6 306 835.

21. Geresh, S., Dawadi, R. P., and Arad, S. M. 2000. Chemical modifications of biopolymers: Quaternization of the extracellular polysaccharide of the red microalga *Porphyridium* sp. *Carbohydr Polym* 63: 75–80.

22. Song, Y., Sun, Y., Zhang, X., Zhou, J., and Zhang, L. 2008. Homogeneous quaternization of cellulose in NaOH/urea aqueous solutions as gene carriers. *Biomacromolecules* 9: 2259–2264.

23. Sajomsang, W., Tantayanon, S., Tangpasuthadol, V., and Daly, W. H. 2009. Quaternization of N-aryl chitosan derivatives: Synthesis, characterization, and antibacterial activity. *Carbohydr Res* 344: 2502–2511.

24. De Britto, D. and Assis, O. B. G. 2007. A novel method for obtaining a quaternary salt of chitosan. *Carbohydr Polym* 69: 305–310.

25. Kim, C. H. and Choi, K. S. 2002. Synthesis and antibacterial activity of quaternized chitosan derivatives having different methylene spacers. *J Ind Eng Chem* 8: 71–76.

26. Kim, C. H., Choi, J. W., Chun, H. J., and Choi, K. S. 1997. Synthesis of chitosan derivatives with quaternary ammonium salt and their antibacterial activity. *Polym Bull* 38: 387–393.

27. Sadeghi, A. M. M., Amini, M., Avadi, M. R., Siedi, F., Rafiee-Tehrani, M., and Junginger, H. E. 2008. Synthesis, characterization, and antibacterial effects of trimethylated and triethylated 6-NH$_2$-6-deoxy chitosan. *J Bioact Compat Pol* 23: 262–275.

28. Holappa, J., Nevalainen, T., Savolainen, J., Soininen, P., Elomaa, M., Safin, R., Suvanto, S. Pakkanen, T. Masson, M., Loftsson, T., and Jarvinen, T. 2004. Synthesis and characterization of chitosan N-betainates having various degrees of substitution. *Macromolecules* 37: 2784–2789.

29. Holappa, J., Nevalainen, T., Soininen, P., and Jarvinen, T. 2006. Synthesis of novel quaternary chitosan derivatives via *N*-chloroacyl-6-*O*-triphenylmethylchitosans. *Biomacromolecules* 7: 407–863.

30. Holappa, J., Nevalainen, T., Safin, R., Soininen, P., Asplund, T., Luttikhedde, T., Masson, M., and Jarvinen, T. 2006. Novel water-soluble quaternary piperazine derivatives of chitosan: Synthesis and characterization. *Macromol Biosci* 6: 139–144.

31. Sajomsang, W., Gonil, P., and Saesoo, S. 2009. Synthesis and antibacterial activity of methylated *N*-(4-*N*,*N*-dimethylaminocinnamyl) chitosan chloride. *Eur Polym J* 45: 2319–2328.

32. Sajomsang, W., Tantayanon, S., Tangpasuthadol, V., and Daly, W. H. 2008. Synthesis of methylated chitosan containing aromatic moieties: Chemoselectivity and effect on molecular weight. *Carbohydr Polym* 72: 740–750.

33. Aranaz, I., Harris, R., and Heras, A. 2010. Chitosan amphiphilic derivatives. Chemistry and applications. *Curr Org Chem* 14: 308–330.

34. Zhu, A. P., Yuan, L. H., Chen, T., Wu, H., and Zhao, F. 2007. Interactions between *N* succinyl–chitosan and bovine serum albumin. *Carbohydr Polym* 69: 363–370.

35. Liu, K. H., Chen, S. Y., Liu, D. M., and Liu, T. Y. 2008. Self-assembled hollow nanocapsule from amphiphatic carboxymethyl-hexanoyl chitosan as drug carrier. *Macromolecules* 41: 6511–6516.

36. Jiang, G. B., Quan, D., Liao, K., and Wang, H. 2006. Novel polymer micelles prepared from chitosan grafted hydrophobic palmitoyl groups for drug delivery. *Mol Pharm* 3: 152–160.

37. Zhang, J., Chen, X. G., Li, Y. Y., and Liu, C. S. 2007. Self-assembled nanoparticles based on hydrophobically modified chitosan as carriers for doxorubicin. *Nanomed Nanotechnol Biol Med* 3: 258–265.

38. Hu, J., Huang, L., Zhuang, X., Zhang, P., Lang, L., and Chen, X. 2008. Electroactive aniline pentamer cross-linking chitosan for stimulation growth of electrically sensitive cells. *Biomacromolecules* 9: 2637–2644.

39. Qu, X., Khutoryanskiy, V. V., Stewart, A., Rahman, S., Papahadjopoulos-Sternberg, B., and Dufes, C. 2006. Carbohydrate-based micelle clusters which enhance hydrophobic drug bioavailability by up to 1 order of magnitude. *Biomacromolecules* 7: 3452–3459.

40. Liu, C. G., Chen, X. G., and Park, H. J. 2005. Self-assembled nanoparticles based on linoleic-acid modified chitosan: Stability and adsorption of trypsin. *Carbohydr Polym* 62: 293–298.

41. Liu, C., Fan, W., Chen, X., Liu, C., Meng, X., and Park, H. J. 2007. Self-assembled nanoparticles based on linoleic-acid modified carboxymethyl-chitosan as carrier of adriamycin (ADR). *Curr Appl Phys* 7(Suppl.1): 25–29.

42. Hu, F. Q., Ren, G. F., Yuan, H., Du, Y. Z., and Zeng, S. 2006. Shell cross-linked stearic acid grafted chitosan oligosaccharide self-aggregated micelles for controlled release of paclitaxel. *Colloid Surf B* 50: 97–103.

43. Hu, F. Q., Meng, P., Dai, Y. Q., Du, Y. Z., You, J., and Wei, X. H. 2008. PEGylated chitosan-based polymer micelle as an intracellular delivery carrier for antitumor targeting therapy. *Eur J Pharm Biopharm* 70: 749–757.

44. Ye, Y. Q., Yang, F. L., Hu, F. Q., Du, Y. Z., Yuan, H., and Yu, H. Y. 2008. Core modified chitosan-based polymeric micelles for controlled release of doxorubicin. *Int J Pharm* 352: 294–301.

45. Wu, Y., Li, M., and Gao, H. 2009. Polymeric micelle composed of PLA and chitosan as a drug carrier. *J Polym Res* 16: 11–18.

46. Bian, F., Jia, L., Yu, W., and Liu, M. 2009. Self-assembled micelles of *N*-phthaloylchitosan-g-polyvinylpyrrolidone for drug delivery. *Carbohydr Polym* 76: 454–459.

47. Hu, Y., Du, Y., Yang, J., Tang, Y., Li, J., and Wang, X. 2007. Self-aggregation and antibacterial activity of N-acylated chitosan. *Polymer* 48: 3098–3106.

48. Chae, S. Y., Son, S., Lee, M., Jang, M. K., and Nah, J. W. 2005. Deoxycholic acid conjugated chitosan oligosaccharide nanoparticles for efficient gene carrier. *J Control Release* 109: 330–344.

49. Hu, F. Q., Zhao, M. D., Yuan, H., You, J., Du, Y. Z., and Zeng, S. 2006. A novel chitosan oligosaccharide-stearic acid micelles for gene delivery: Properties and *in vitro* transfection studies. *Int J Pharm* 315: 158–166.

50. Tikhonov, V. E., Stepnova, E. A., Babak, V. G., Krayukhina, M. A., Berezin. B. B., and Yamskov, I. A. 2008. Amphiphilic *N*-[2(3)-(dodec-2'-en-1'-yl)succinoyl]chitosan: Synthesis and properties. *React Funct Polym* 68: 436–445.

51. Zhu, A., Yuan, L., and Dai, S. 2008. Preparation of well-dispersed superparamagnetic iron oxide nanoparticles in aqueous solution with biocompatible *N*-succinyl-*O*-carboxymethylchitosan. *J Phys Chem C* 112: 5432–5438.

52. Nandanan, E., Jana, N. R., and Ying, J. Y. 2008. Functionalization of gold nanospheres and nanorods by chitosan oligosaccharide derivatives. *Adv Mater* 20: 2068–2073.

53. Félix, L., Hernández, J., Argüelles, W. M., and Goycoolea, F. M. 2005. Kinetics of gelation and thermal sensitivity of *N*-isobutyryl chitosan hydrogels. *Biomacromolecules* 6: 2408–2415.

54. You, J., Hu, F. Q., Du, Y. Z., and Yuan, H. 2007. Polymeric micelles with glycolipidlike structure and multiple hydrophobic domains for mediating molecular target delivery of paclitaxel. *Biomacromolecules* 8: 2450–2456.

55. You, J., Hu, F. Q., Du, Y. Z., Yuan, H., and Ye, B. F. 2007. High cytotoxicity and resistant-cell reversal of novel paclitaxel loaded micelles by enhancing the molecular-target delivery of the drug. *Nanotechnology* 18: 495101.

56. You, J., Hu, F. Q., Du, Y. Z., and Yuan, H. 2008. Improved cytotoxicity of doxorubicin by enhancing its nuclear delivery mediated via nanosized micelles. *Nanotechnology* 19: 255103.

57. Uygun, D. A., Uygun, M., Karagözler, A., Öztürk, N., Akgöl, S., and Denizli, A. 2009. A novel support for antibody purification: Fatty acid attached chitosan beads. *Colloid Surf B* 70: 266–270.

58. Tong, Y., Wang, S., Xu, J., Chua, B., and He, C. 2005. Synthesis of *O,O'*-dipalmitoyl chitosan and its amphiphilic properties and capability of cholesterol absorption. *Carbohydr Polym* 60: 229–233.

59. Wu, Y., Hisada, K., Maeda, S., Sasaki, T., and Sakurai, K. 2007. Fabrication and structural characterization of the Langmuir–Blodgett films from a new chitosan derivative containing cinnamate chromophores. *Carbohydr Polym* 68: 766–772.

60. Shigemasa, Y., Usui, H., Morimoto, M., Saimoto, H., Okamoto, Y., Minami, S., and Sashiwa, H. 1999. Chemical modification of chitin and chitosan 1: Preparation of partially deacetylated chitin derivatives via a ring-opening reaction with cyclic acid anhydrides in lithium chloride/*N,N*-dimethylacetamide. *Carbohydr Polym* 39: 237.

61. Hirano, S., Yamaguchi, Y., and Kamiya, M. 2002. Novel N-saturated-fatty-acyl derivatives of chitosan soluble in water and in aqueous acid and alkaline solutions. *Carbohydr Polym* 48: 203.

62. Seo, T., Hagura, S., Kanbara, T., and Iijima, T. 1989. Interaction of dyes with chitosan derivatives. *J Appl Polym Sci* 37: 3011–3027.

63. Tien, C. L., Lacroix, M., Ispas-Szabo, P., and Mateescu, M. A. 2003. N-acylated chitosan: Hydrophobic matrices for controlled drug release. *J Controlled Release* 93: 1–13.

64. Sashiwa, H., Kawasaki, N., Nakayama, A., Muraki, E., Yamamoto, N., and Zhu, H. 2002. Chemical modification of chitosan. 13.1: Synthesis of organosoluble, palladium adsorbable, and biodegradable chitosan derivatives toward the chemical plating on plastics. *Biomacromolecules* 3: 1120–1125.

65. Grant, S., Blair, H. S., and Mckay, G. 1990. Deacetylation effects on the dodecanoyl substitution. *Polym Commun* 31: 267–268.

66. Seo, T., Ikeda, Y., Torada, Y., Nakata, Y., and Shimomura, Y. 2001. Synthesis of N,O-acylated chitosan and its sorptivity. *Chitin Chitosan Res* 7: 212–213.

67. Wu, Y., Seo, T., Maeda, S., Sasaki, T., Irie, S., and Sakurai, K. 2005. Circular dichroism induced by the helical conformations of acylated chitosan derivatives bearing cinnamate chromophores. *J Polym Sci Part B: Polym Phys* 43: 1354–1364.

68. Zong, Z., Kimura, Y., Takahashi, M., and Yamane, H. 2000. Characterization of chemical and solid state structures of acylated chitosans. *Polymer* 41: 899–906.

69. Martin, L., Wilson, C. G., Koosha, F., Tetley, L., Gray, A. I., Senel, S., and Uchegbu, I. F. 2002. The release of model macromolecules may be controlled by the hydrophobicity of palmitoyl glycol chitosan hydrogels. *J Controlled Release* 80: 87–100.

70. Wang, W., McConaghy, A. M., Tetley, L., and Uchegbu, I. F. 2001. Controls on polymer molecular weight may be used to control the size of palmitoyl glycol chitosan polymeric vesicles. *Langmuir* 17: 631–636.

71. Nishimura, S. Miura, Y., Ren, L., Sato, M., Yamagishi, A., Nishi, N., Tokura, S., Kurita, K., and Ishii, S. 1993. An efficient method for the syntheses of novel amphiphilic polysaccharides by regio- and thermoselective modifications of chitosan. *Chem Lett* 22: 1623–1626.

72. Xu, J., McCarthy, S. P., and Gross, R. A. 1996. Chitosan film acylation and effects on biodegradability. *Macromolecules* 29: 3436–3440.

73. Rout, D. K., Pulapura, S. K., and Gross, R. A. 1993. Gel–sol transition and thermotropic behavior of a chitosan derivative in lyotropic solution. *Macromolecules* 26: 6007–6010.

74. Wu, Y., Dong, Y. Zhou, F., Ruan, Y., Wang, H., and Zhao, Y. 2003. Studies on the critical phase-transition behavior of cholesteric N-phthaloyl chitosan/dimethyl sulfoxide solutions by five techniques. *J Appl Polym Sci* 90: 583–586.

75. Seo, T., Ohtake, H., Unishi, T., and Iijima, T. 1995. Permeation of solutes through chemically modified chitosan membranes. *J Appl Polym Sci* 58: 633–644.

76. Hirano, S., Zhang, M., Chung, B. G., and Kim, S. K. 2000. The N-acylation of chitosan fibre and the N-deacetylation of chitin fibre and chitin–cellulose blended fibre at a solid state. *Carbohydr Polym* 41: 175–179.

77. Hirano, S. and Moriyasu, T. 2004. Some novel *N*-(carboxyacyl)chitosan filaments. *Carbohydr Polym* 55: 245–248.

78. Aiping, Z., Tian, C., Lanhua, Y., Hao, W., and Ping, L. 2006. Synthesis and characterization of N-succinyl-chitosan and its self-assembly of nanospheres. *Carbohydr Polym* 66: 274–279.

79. Jiang, G. B., Quan, D., Liao, K., and Wang, H. 2006. Preparation of polymeric micelles based on chitosan bearing a small amount of highly hydrophobic groups. *Carbohydr Polym* 66: 514–520.

80. Nishimura, S., Kohgo, O., Ishii, S., Hurita, K., Mochida, K., and Kuzuhara, H. 1992. New trends in bioactive chitosan derivatives: Use of "standardized intermediates" with excellent solubility in common organic solvents. In *Advances in Chitin and Chitosan*, Brine, C. J., Sandford, P. A., and Zikakis, J. P., eds, London: Elsevier, pp. 533–542.

81. Dong, Y. M., Mao, W., Wang, H. W., Zhao, Y. Q., Bi, D. X., and Yang, L. L. 2006. Electron microscopic studies on planar texture and disclination of cholesteric mesophases in acyloyl chitosan/acrylic acid composite films. *Carbohydr Polym* 65: 42–48.

82. Dong, Y. M., Mao, W., Wang, H. W., Zhao, Y. Q., Li, X. J., and Bi, D. X. 2006. Measurement of critical concentration for mesophase formation of chitosan derivatives in both aqueous and organic solutions. *Polym Int* 55: 1444–1449.

83. Xu, C., Pan, H., Jiang, H., Tang, G., and Chen, W. 2008. Biocompatibility evaluation of N,O-hexanoyl chitosan as a biodegradable hydrophobic polycation for controlled drug release. *J Mater Sci-Mater Med* 19: 25–32.

84. Muzzarelli, R. A. A. 1988. Carboxymethylated chitins and chitosans. *Carbohydr Polym* 8: 1–21.

85. Chen, S. C., Wu, Y. C., Mi, F. L., Lin, Y. H., Yu, L. C., and Sung, H. W. 2004. A novel pH-sensitive hydrogel composed of N,O-carboxymethyl chitosan and alginate cross-linked by genipin for protein drug delivery. *J Control Release* 96: 285–300.

86. Thanou, M., Nihot, M. T., Jansen, M., Verhoef, J. C., and Junginger, H. E. 2001. Mono-N-carboxymethyl chitosan (MCC), a polyampholytic chitosan derivative, enhances the intestinal absorption of low molecular weight heparin across intestinal epithelia *in vitro* and *in vivo*. *J Pharm Sci* 90: 38–46.

87. Chen, Y. and Tan, H. M. 2006. Cross-linked carboxymethylchitosan-g-poly(acrylic acid) copolymer as a novel superabsorbent polymer. *Carbohydr Res* 341: 887–896.

88. Sui, W., Wang, S., Chen, G., and Xu, G. 2004. Surface and aggregate properties of an amphiphilic derivative of carboxymethylchitosan. *Carbohydr Res* 339: 1113–1118.

89. Zhu, A. P., Liu, J. H., and Ye, W. H. 2006. Effective loading and controlled release of camptothecin by O-carboxymethylchitosan aggregates. *Carbohydr Polym* 63: 89–96.

90. Mourya, V. K. and Inamdar, N. N. 2008. Chitosan-modifications and applications: Opportunities galore. *React Funct Polym* 68: 1013–1051.

91. Sun, T., Yao, Q., Zhou, D. X., and Mao, F. 2008. Antioxidant activity of *N*-carboxymethyl chitosan oligosaccharides. *Bioorg Med Chem Lett* 18: 5774–5776.
92. Marguerite, R., Pham Le, D., Claude, G., and Michel, M. 1992. Substituent distribution on *O,N*-carboxymethylchitosans by ^{1}H and ^{13}C n.m.r. *Int J Biol Macromol* 14: 122–128.
93. Pavlov, G. M., Korneeva, E. V., Harding, S. E., and Vichoreva, G. A. 1998. Dilute solution properties of carboxymethylchitins in high ionic-strength solvent. *Polymer* 39: 6951–6961.
94. Yin, L. C., Fei, L. K., Cui, F. Y., Tang, C., and Yin, C. H. 2007. Superporous hydrogels containing poly(acrylic acid-*co*-acrylamide)/*O*-carboxymethyl chitosan interpenetrating polymer networks. *Biomaterials* 28: 1258–1266.
95. Chen, L. Y., Tian, Z. G., and Du, Y. M. 2004. Synthesis and pH sensitivity of carboxymethyl chitosan-based polyampholyte hydrogels for protein carrier matrices. *Biomaterials* 25: 3725–3732.
96. Lin, Y. H., Liang, H. F., Chung, C. K., Chen, M. C., and Sung, H. W. 2005. Physically cross-linked alginate/*N,O*-carboxymethyl chitosan hydrogels with calcium for oral delivery of protein drugs. *Biomaterials* 26: 2105–2113.
97. Chen, S. C., Wu, Y. C., Mi, F. L., Lin, Y. H., Yu, L. C., and Sung, H. W. 2004. A novel pH-sensitive hydrogel composed of *N,O*-carboxymethyl chitosan and alginate cross-linked by genipin for protein drug delivery. *J Control Release* 96: 285–300.
98. Peng, X. and Zhang, L. 2007. Formation and morphologies of novel self-assembled micelles from chitosan derivatives. *Langmuir* 23: 10493–10498.
99. Peng, X. and Zhang, L. 2009. Self-assembled micelles of *N*-phthaloylcarboxymethylchitosan for drug delivery. *Colloid Surf. A* 337: 21–25.
100. Sashiwa, H., Yamamori, N., Ichinose, Y., Sunamoto, J., and Aiba, S. 2003. Michael reaction of chitosan with various acryl reagents in water. *Biomacromolecules* 4: 1250–1254.
101. Sashiwa, H., Kawasaki, N., Nakayama, A., Muraki, E., Yajima, H., Yamamori, N., Ichinose, Y., Sunamoto, J., and Aiba, S. 2003. Chemical modification of chitosan. Part 15: Synthesis of novel chitosan derivatives by substitution of hydrophilic amine using *N*-carboxyethylchitosan ethyl ester as an intermediate. *Carbohydr Res* 338: 557–561.
102. Alban, S., Schauerte, A., and Franz, G. 2002. Anticoagulant sulfated polysaccharides: Part I. Synthesis and structure–activity relationships of new pullulan sulfates. *Carbohydr Polym* 47: 267–276.
103. Huang, R. H., Du, Y., Zhang, L. S., Liu, H., and Fan, L. H. A new approach to chemically modified chitosan sulfates and study of their influences on the inhibition of *Escherichia coli* and *Staphylococcus aureus* growth. *React Funct Polym* 59: 41–51.
104. Desai, U. R. 2004. New antithrombin-based anticoagulants. *Med Res Rev* 24: 151–181.
105. Drozd, N. N., Sher, A. I., Makarov, V. A., Vichoreva, G. A., Gorbachiova, I. N., and Galbraich, L. S. 2001. Comparison of antithrombin activity of the polysulphate chitosan derivatives *in vitro* and *in vivo* system. *Thromb Res* 102: 445–455.
106. Maculotti, K., Tira, E. M., Sonaggere, M., Perugini, P., Conti, B., Modena, T., and Pavanetto, F. 2009. *In vitro* evaluation of chondroitin sulphate-chitosan microspheres as carrier for the delivery of proteins. *J Microencapsul* 26: 535–543.
107. Vikhoreva, G., Bannikova, G., Stolbushkina, P., Panov, A., Drozd, N., Makarov, V., Varlamov, V., and Gal'braikh, L. 2005. Preparation and anticoagulant activity of a low-molecular-weight sulfated chitosan. *Carbohydr Polym* 62: 327–332.
108. Cushing, I. B., Davis, R. V., Kratovil, E. J., and MacCorquodale, D. W. 1954. The sulfation of chitin in chlorosulfonic acid and dichloroethane. *J Am Chem Soc* 76: 4590–4591.
109. Wolfrom, M. L. and Shen-Han, T. M. 1959. The sulfonation of chitosan. *J Am Chem Soc* 81: 1764–1766.
110. Horton, D. and Just, E. K. 1973. Preparation from chitin of (1,4)-2-amino-2-deoxyb-D-glucopyranuronan and its 2-sulfoamino analog having blood-anticoagulant properties. *Carbohydr Res* 29: 173–179.
111. Nishimura, S. I., Nishi, N., Tokura, S., Okiei, W., and Somorin, O. 1986. Inhibition of the hydrolytic activity of thrombin by chitin heparinoids. *Carbohydr Res* 156: 286–292.

112. Terbojevich, M., Carraro, C., Cosani, A., Focher, B., Naggi, A. M., and Torri, G. 1989. Solution studies of chitosan 6-O-sulfate. *Macromol Chem Phys* 190: 2847–2855.
113. Gamzazade, A., Sklyar, A., Nasibov, S., Sushkov, I., Shashkov, A., and Knirel, Y. 1997. Structural features of sulfated chitosans. *Carbohydr Polym* 34: 113–116.
114. Vongchan, P., Sajomsang, W., Subyen, D., and Kongtawelert, P. 2002. Anticoagulant activity of a sulfated chitosan. *Carbohydr Res* 337: 1239–1242.
115. Hirano, S., Hasegawa, M., and Kinugawa, J. 1991. ^{13}C-NMR analysis of some sulphate derivatives of chitosan. *Int J Biol Macromol* 13: 316–317.
116. Hirano, S., Tanaka, Y., Hasegawa, M., Tobetto, K., and Nishioka, A. 1985. Effect of sulfated derivatives of chitosan on some blood coagulant factors. *Carbohydr Res* 137: 205–215.
117. Nishimura, S. I. and Tokura, S. 1987. Preparation and antithrombogenic activities of heparinoid from 6-O-(carboxymethyl) chitin. *Int J Biol Macromol* 9: 225–232.
118. Holme, K. R. and Perlin, A. S. 1997. N-sulfate. A water-soluble polyelectrolyte. *Carbohydr Res* 302: 7–12.
119. Kinzo, N., Yasuo, T., Yuko, I., and Noriko, T. 1971. Reaction between carbohydrates and sulfuric acid: Part I. Depolymerization and sulfation of polysaccharides by sulfuric acid. *Carbohydr Res* 18: 95–102.
120. Vikhoreva, G., Bannikova, G., Stolbushkina, P., Panov, A., Drozd, N., Makarov, V., Varlamov, V., and Gal'braikh, L. 2005. Preparation and anticoagulant activity of a low-molecular-weight sulfated chitosan. *Carbohydr Polym* 62: 327–332.
121. Holme, K. R. and Perlin, A. S. 1997. Chitosan N-sulfate. A water-soluble polyelectrolyte. *Carbohydr Res* 302: 7.
122. Yin, Q., Li, Y., Yin, Q. J., Miao, X., and Jiang, B. 2009. Synthesis and rheological behavior of a novel N-sulfonate ampholyte chitosan. *J Appl Polym Sci* 2009, 113: 3382–3387.
123. Muzzarelli, R. A. A. 1992. Modified chitosans carrying sulfonic acid groups. *Carbohydr Polym* 19: 231–236.
124. Nishimura, S., Kai, H., Shinada, K., Yoshida, T., Tokura, S., Kurita, K., Nakashima, H., Yamamoto, N., and Uryu, T. 1998. Regioselective syntheses of sulfated polysaccharides: Specific anti-HIV-1 activity of novel chitin sulfates. *Carbohydr Res* 306: 427–433.
125. Yao, Z., Zhang, C., Ping, Q. N., and Yu, L. L. L. 2007. A series of novel chitosan derivatives: Synthesis, characterization and micellar solubilization of paclitaxel. *Carbohydr Polym* 68: 781–792.
126. Can, Z., Ping, Q. N., Zhang, H. J., and Jian, S. 2003. Preparation of N-alkyl-O-sulfate chitosan derivatives and micellar solubilization of taxol. *Carbohydr Polym* 54: 137–141.
127. Xing, R. E., Liu, S., Yu, H. H., Guo, Z. Y., Li, Z., and Li, P. C. 2005. Preparation of high-molecular weight and high-sulfate content chitosans and their potential antioxidant activity *in vitro*. *Carbohydr Polym* 61: 148–154.
128. Xing, R. E., Liu, S., Yu, H. H., Zhang, Q. B., Li, Z., and Li, P. C. 2004. Preparation of low-molecular-weight and high-sulfate-content chitosans under microwave radiation and their potential antioxidant activity *in vitro*. *Carbohydr Res* 339: 2515–2519.
129. Zou, Y. Q. and Khor, E. 2009. Preparation of sulfated-chitins under homogeneous conditions. *Carbohydr Polym* 77: 516–525.
130. Jung, B. O., Na, J., and Kim, C. H. 2007. Synthesis of chitosan derivatives with anionic groups and its biocompatibility *in vitro*. *J Ind Eng Chem* 13: 772–776.
131. Tsai, H. S., Wang, Y. Z., Lin, J. J., and Lien, W. F. 2010. Preparation and properties of sulfopropyl chitosan derivatives with various sulfonation degree. *J Appl Polym Sci* 116: 1686–1693.
132. Baumann, H. and Faust, V. 2001. Concepts for improved regioselective placement of O-sulfo, N-sulfo, N-acetyl, and N-carboxymethyl groups in chitosan derivatives. *Carbohydr Res* 331: 43–57.
133. Focher, B., Massoli, A., Torri, G., Gervasini, A., and Morazzoni, F. 1986. High molecular weight chitosan 6-O-sulfate. Synthesis, ESR and NMR characterization. *Macromol Chem Phys* 187: 2609–2620.

134. Takano, R., Ye, Z., Ta, T. V., Hayashi, K., Kariya, Y., and Hara, 1998. S. Specific 6-O-desulfation of heparin. *Carbohydr Lett* 3: 71–77.

135. Suwan, J., Zhang, Z. Q., Li, B. Y. Z., Vongchan, P., Meepowpan, P., Zhang, F. M., Mousa, S. A., Mousa, S., Premanode, B., Kongtawelert, P., and Linhardt, R. J. 2009. Sulfonation of papain-treated chitosan and its mechanism for anticoagulant activity. *Carbohydr Res* 344: 1190–1196.

136. Whistler, R. J. and Kosik, M. 1971. Anticoagulant activity of oxidized and N- and O-sulfated chitosan. *Arch Biochem Biophys* 142: 106.

137. Muzzarelli, R. A. A., Tanfani, F., Emanuelli, M., Pace, D. P., Chiurazzi, E., and Piani, M. 1986. *Chitin in Nature and Technology.* New York, NY: Plenum Press, pp. 469–476.

138. Hirano, S. 1999. Chitin and chitosan as novel biotechnological materials. *Polym Int* 48: 732–734.

139. Zhang, C., Ping, Q. N., and Zhang, H. J. 2004. Self-assembly and characterization of paclitaxel-loaded N-octyl-O-sulfate chitosan micellar system. *Colloid Surf B* 39: 69–75.

140. Berth, G., Voigt, A., Dautzenberg, H., Donath, E., and Mohwald, H. 2002. Polyelectrolyte complexes and layer-by-layer capsules from chitosan/chitosan sulfate. *Biomacromolecules* 3: 579–590.

141. Hendrickson, H. S. 1967. Comparison of the metal-binding properties of nitrilotri(methylene-phosphonic) acid and nitrilotriacetic acid: Calcium(II), nickel(II,), iron(III), and thorium(IV) complexes. *Anal Chem* 27: 998–1000.

142. Westerback, S., Rajan, K. S., and Martell, A. E. 1965. New multidentate ligands. III. Amino acids containing methylenephosphonate groups. *J Am Chem Soc* 87: 2567.

143. Schwarzenbach, G., Ackermann, H., and Ruckstuhl, P. 1949. Komplexone XV. Neue Derivate der Imino-diessigsäure und ihre Erdalkalikomplexe. Beziehungen zwischen Acidität und Komplexbildung. *Helv Chim Acta* 32: 1175.

144. Hamodrakas, S. J., Jones, C. W., and Kafatos, F. C. 1982. Secondary structure predictions for silkmoth chorion proteins. *Biochim Biophys Acta* 700: 42–51.

145. Hamodrakas, S. J., Asher, S. A., Mazur, G. D., Regier, J. C., and Kafatos, K. C. 1982. Laser Raman studies of protein conformation in the silkmoth chorion. *Biochim Biophys Acta* 703: 216–222.

146. Sakaguchi, T., Hirokoshi, T., and Nakajima, A. 1981. Adsorption of uranium by chitin phosphate and chitosan phosphate. *Agric Biol Chem* 45: 2191–2195.

147. Nishi, N., Nishimura, S., Ebina, A., Tsutsumi, A., and Tokura, S. 1984. Preparation and characterization of water-soluble chitin phosphate. *Int J Biol Macromol* 6: 53–54.

148. Nishi, N., Ebina, A., Nishimura, S., Tsutsumi, A., Hasegawa, O., and Tokura, S. 1986. Highly phosphorylated derivatives of chitin, partially deacetylated chitin and chitosan as new functional polymers: Preparation and characterization. *Int J Biol Macromol* 8: 311–317.

149. Somorin, O., Nishi, N., Tokura, S., and Naguchi, J. 1979. Studies on chitin. II. preparation of benzyl and benzoylchitins. *Polym J* 11: 391–395.

150. Kaifu, K., Nishi, N., Komai, T., Tokura, S., and Somorin, O. 1983. Studies on chitin. V. Formylation, propionylation, and butyrylation of chitin. *Polym J* 13: 241–245.

151. Nishi, N., Ohnuma, H., Nishimura, S., Somorin, O., and Tokura, S. 1982. Studies on chitin. VII. Preparations of p-substituted benzoylchitins. *Polym J* 14: 919–923.

152. Nishi, N., Noguchi, J., Tokura, S., and Noguchi, J. 1979. Studies on chitin. I. Acetylation of chitin. *Polym J* 11: 27–32.

153. Heras, A., Rodriguez, N. M., Ramos, V. M., and Agullo, E. 2001. N-methylene phosphonic chitosan: A novel soluble derivative. *Carbohydr Polym* 44: 1–8.

154. Palma, G., Casals, P., and Cardenas, G. 2005. Synthesis and characterization of new chitosan-o-ethyl phosphonate. *J Chile Chem Soc* 50: 719–724.

155. Cardenas, G., Cabrera, G., Taboada, E., and Rinaudo, M. 2006. Synthesis and characterization of chitosan alkyl phosphate. *J Chile Chem Soc* 51: 815–820.

156. Ramos, V. M., Rodryguez, N. M., Rodryguez, M. S., Heras, A., and Agullo, E. 2003. Modified chitosan carrying phosphonic and alkyl groups. *Carbohydr Polym* 51: 425–429.

157. Meng, S., Liu, Z., Zhong, W., Wang, Q., and Du, Q. 2007. Phosphorylcholine modified chitosan: Appetent and safe material for cells. *Carbohydr Polym* 70: 82–88.

158. Zhu, A. P., Wang, S. Q., Yuan, Y. L., and Shen, J. 2002. Cell adhesion behavior of chitosan surface modified by bonding 2-methacryloyloxyethyl phosphorylcholine. *J Biomater Sci Polym Ed* 13: 501–510.
159. Tiera, M. J., Qiu, X. P., Bechaouch, S., Shi, Q., Fernandes, J. C., and Winnik, F. M. 2009. Synthesis and characterization of phosphorylcholine-substituted chitosans soluble in physiological pH conditions. *Biomacromolecules* 7: 3151–3156.
160. Case, A.H., Picola, I. P. D., Zaniquelli, M. E. D., Fernandes, J. C., Taboga, S. R., Winnik, F. M., and Tiera, M. J. 2009. Physicochemical characterization of nanoparticles formed between DNA and phosphorylcholine substituted chitosans. *J Colloid Interface Sci* 336: 125–133.
161. Prabaharan, M., Reis, R. L., and Mano, J. F. 2007. Carboxymethyl chitosan-graft-phosphatidyle-thanolamine: Amphiphilic matrices for controlled drug delivery. *React Funct Polym* 67: 43–52.
162. Win, P. P., Ya, Y. S., Hong, K. J., and Kajiuchi, T. 2003. Formulation and characterization of pH sensitive drug carrier based on phosphorylated chitosan (PCS). *Carbohydr Polym* 53: 305–310.
163. Hadgraft, J. and Valenta, C. 2000. pH, pK(a) and dermal delivery. *Int J Pharm* 200: 243–247.
164. Sorlier, P., Denuziere, A., Viton, C., and Domard, A. 2001. Relation between the degree of acetylation and the electrostatic properties of chitin and chitosan. *Biomacromolecules* 2: 765–772.
165. Mucalo, M. R., Yokogawa, Y., Suzuki, T., Kawamoto, Y., Nagata, F., and Nishizawa, K. 1995. Further studies of calcium phosphate growth on phosphorylated cotton fibres. *J Mater Sci-Mater Med* 6: 658–669.
166. Tanahashi, M. and Matsuda, T. 1997. Surface functional group dependence on apatite formation on self-assembled monolayers in a simulated body fluid. *J Biomed Mater Res* 34: 305–315.
167. Yokogawa, Y., Reyes, J. P., Mucalo, M. R., Toriyama, M., Kawamoto, Y., Suzuki, T., Nishizawa, K., Nagata, F., and Kamayama, T. 1997. Growth of calcium phosphate on phosphorylated chitin fibres. *J Mater Sci-Mater Med* 8: 407–412.
168. Granja, P. L., Barbosa, M. A., Pouysegu, L., De Jeso, B., Rouais, F., and Baquey, C. 2001. Cellulose phosphates as biomaterials. Mineralization of chemically modified regenerated cellulose hydrogels. *J Mater Sci* 36: 2163–2172.
169. Amaral, I. F., Granja, P. L., Melo, L. V., Saramago, B., and Barbosa, M. A. 2006. Functionalization of chitosan membranes through phosphorylation: Atomic force microscopy, wettability, and cytotoxicity studies. *J Appl Polym Sci* 102: 276–284.
170. Amaral, I. F., Granja, P. L., and Barbosa, M. A. 2005. Chemical modification of chitosan by phosphorylation: An XPS, FT-IR and SEM study. *J Biomater Sci Polym Ed* 16: 1575–1593.
171. Granja, P. L., Pouysegu, L., Petraud, M., De Jeso, B., Baquey, C., and Barbosa, M. A. 2001. Cellulose phosphates as biomaterials. I. Synthesis and characterization of highly phosphorylated cellulose gels. *J Appl Polym Sci* 82: 3341–3353.
172. Touey, G. P. and Kingsport, T. 1956. (to Eastman Kodak Co.). U.S. Pat. 2,759,924.
173. Sakairi, N., Shirai, A., Miyazaki, S., Tashiro, H., Tsuji, Y., Kawahara, H., Yoshida, T., Nishi, N., and Tokura, S. 1998. Synthesis and properties of chitin phosphate. *Kobunshi Ronbunshu* 55: 212–216.
174. Lee, Y. M. and Shin, E. M. 1991. Pervaporation separation of water–ethanol through modified chitosan membranes. IV. phosphorylated chitosan membranes. *J Membr Sci* 64: 145–152.
175. Varma, H. K., Yokogawa, Y., Espinosa, F. F., Kawamoto, Y., Nishizawa, K., Nagata, F., and Kameyama, T. 1999. Porous calcium phosphate coating over phosphorylated chitosan film by a biomimetic method. *Biomaterials* 20: 879–884.
176. Yokogawa, Y., Nishizawa, K., Nagata, F., and Kamayama, T. 1999. In *Bioceramics*, Ohgushi, H., Hastings, G. W., and Yoshikawa, T., eds. Singapore: World Scientific, pp. 129–134.
177. Aoba, T. and Moreno, E. C. 1985. Adsorption of phosphoserine onto hydroxyapatite and its inhibitory activity on crystal growth. *J Colloid Interface Sci* 106: 110–121.
178. Amaral, I. F., Granja, P. L., and Barbosa, M. A. 2004. *In vitro* mineralisation of chitosan membranes carrying phosphate functionalities. *Key Eng Mater* 254–256: 577–580.
179. Damien, J. C. and Parson, J. R. 1991. Bone graft and bone graft substitutes: A review of current technology and applications. *J Appl Biomater* 2: 187–208.

180. Bernkop-Schnurch, A., Brandt, U. M., and Clausen, A. E. 1999. Synthesis and *in vitro* evaluation of chitosan–cysteine conjugates. *Sci Pharm* 67: 96–208.
181. Kafedjiiski, K., Foger, F., Werle, M., and Bernkop-Schnurch, A. 2005. Synthesis and *in vitro* evaluation of a novel chitosan–glutathione conjugate. *Pharm Res* 22: 1480–1488.
182. Kafedjiiski, K., Krauland, A. H., Hoffer, M. H., and Bernkop-Schnurch, A. 2005. Synthesis and *in vitro* evaluation of a novel thiolated chitosan. *Biomaterials* 26: 819–826.
183. Kast, C. E. and Bernkop-Schnurch, A. 2001. Thiolated polymers-thiomers: Development and *in vitro* evaluation of chitosan–thioglycolic acid conjugates. *Biomaterials* 22: 2345–2352.
184. Bernkop-Schnurch, A., Hornof, M., and Zoidl, T. 2003. Thiolated polymers–thiomers: Synthesis and *in vitro* evaluation of chitosan-2-iminothiolane conjugates. *Int J Pharm* 260: 229–237.
185. Schmitz, T., Grabovac, E., Palmberger, T. E., Hoffer, M. H., and Bemkop-Schnurch, A. 2008. Synthesis and characterization of a chitosan-N-acetyl cysteine conjugate. *Int J Pharm* 347: 79–85.
186. Millotti, G., Samberger, C., Frohlich, E., and Bernkop-Schnurch, A. 2009. Chitosan-*graft*-6-mercaptonicotinic acid: Synthesis, characterization, and biocompatibility. *Biomacromolecules* 10: 3023–3027.
187. Jayakumar, R., Reis, R. L., and Mano, J. F. 2007. Synthesis and characterization of pH-sensitive thiol-containing chitosan beads for controlled drug delivery applications. *Drug Deliv* 14: 9–17.
188. Prabaharan, M. and Shaoquin, G. 2008. Novel thiolated carboxymethyl chitosan-g-β-cyclodextrin as mucoadhesive hydrophobic drug delivery carriers. *Carbohydr Polym* 73: 117–125.
189. Singh, R., Kats, L., Blattler, W. A., and Lambert, J. M. 1996. Formation of N-substituted 2-iminothiolanes when amino groups in proteins and peptides are modified by 2-iminothiolane. *Anal Biochem* 236: 114–125.
190. Delprino, L., Giacomotti, M., Dosio, F., Brusa, P., Ceruti, M., Grosa, G., and Cattel, L. 1993. Toxin-targeted design for anticancer therapy. I: Synthesis and biological evaluation of new thio-imidate heterobifunctional reagents. *J Pharm Sci* 82: 506–512.
191. Sakloetsakun, D. and Bernkop-Schnurch, A. 2010. Thiolated chitosans. *J Drug Deliv Sci Technol* 20: 63–69.
192. Hall, L. D. and Yalpani, M. 1980. Formation of branched-chain, soluble polysaccharides from chitosan. *J Chem Soc Chem Commun* 1980: 1153–1154.
193. Yalpani, M. and Hall, L. D. 1984. Some chemical and analytical aspects of polysaccharide modifications. 3. Formation of branched chain, soluble chitosan derivatives. *Macromolecules* 17: 272–281.
194. Sashiwa, H. and Shigemasa, Y. 1999. Chemical modification of chitin and chitosan—2: Preparation and water soluble property of N-acylated or N-alkylated partially deacetylated chitins. *Carbohydr Polym* 39: 127–138.
195. Morimoto, M., Saimoto, H., Usui, H., Okamoto, Y., Minami, S., and Shigemasa, Y. 2001. Biological activities of carbohydrate-branched chitosan derivatives. *Biomacromolecules* 2: 1133–1136.
196. Morimoto, M., Saimoto, H., and Shigemasa, Y. 2002. Control of functions of chitin and chitosan by chemical modification. *Trends Glycosci Glycotechnol* 14: 205–222.
197. Li, X. B., Tushima, Y., Morimoto, M., Saimoto, H., Okamoto, Y., Minami, S., and Shigemasa, Y. 2000. Biological activity of chitosan–sugar hybrids: Specific interaction with lectin. *Polym Adv Technol* 11: 176–179.
198. Li, X. B., Morimoto, M., Sashiwa, H., Saimoto, H., Okamoto, Y., Minami, S., and Shigemasa, Y. 1999. Synthesis of chitosan–sugar hybrid and evaluation of its bioactivity. *Polym Adv Technol* 10: 455–458.
199. Donati, I., Stredanska, S., Silvestrini, G., Vetere, A., Marcon, P., Marsich, E., Mozetic, P., Gamini, A., Paoletti, S., and Vittur, F. 2005. The aggregation of pig articular chondrocyte and synthesis of extracellular matrix by a lactose-modified chitosan. *Biomaterials* 26: 987–998.
200. Kato, Y., Onishi, H., and Machida, Y. 2001. Biological characteristics of lactosaminated N-succinyl-chitosan as a liver-specific drug carrier in mice. *J Control Release* 70: 95–307.

201. Kato, Y., Onishi, H., and Machida, Y. 2001. Lactosaminated and intact *N*-succinyl-chitosans as drug carriers in liver metastasis. *Int J Pharm* 226: 93–106.
202. Park, I. K., Yang, J., Jeong, H.J., Bom, H.S., Harada, I., Akaike, T., and Cho, C.S. 2003. Galactosylated chitosan as a synthetic extracellular matrix for hepatocytes attachment. *Biomaterials* 24: 2331-2337.
203. Park, I. K., Kim, T. H., Park, Y. H., Shin, B. A., Choi, E. S., Chowdhury, E. H. Akaike, T., and Cho, C.S. 2001. Galactosylated chitosan-graft-poly(ethylene glycol) as hepatocyte-targeting DNA carrier. *J Control Release* 76: 349–362.
204. Park, I. K., Ihm, J. E., Park, Y. H., Choi, Y. J., Kim, S. I., Kim, W. J., Akaike, T., and Cho, C. S. 2003. Galactosylated chitosan (GC)-graft-poly(vinyl pyrrolidone) (PVP) as hepatocyte-targeting DNA carrier: Preparation and physicochemical characterization of GC-graft-PVP/DNA complex (1). *J Control Release* 86: 349–359.
205. Park, Y. K., Park, Y. H., Shin, B. A., Choi, E. S., Park, Y. R., Akaike, T., and Cho, C. S. 2000. Actosylated chitosan–graft–dextran as hepatocyte-targeting DNA carrier. *J Control Release* 69: 97–108.
206. Murata, J., Ohya, Y., and Ouchi, T. 1996. Possibility of application of quaternary chitosan having pendant galactose residues as gene delivery tool. *Carbohyd Polym* 29: 69–74.
207. Murata, J., Ohya, Y., and Ouchi, T. 1997. Design of quaternary chitosan conjugate having antennary galactose residues as a gene delivery tool. *Carbohyd Polym* 32: 105–109.
208. Roy, R., Tropper, D. F., Romanowska, A., Letellier, M., Cousineau, L., Meunier, S. J., and Boratynski, J. 1991. Expedient syntheses of neoglycoproteins using phase transfer catalysis and reductive amination as key reactions. *Glycoconjugate J* 8: 75–81.
209. Sashiwa, H., Makimura, Y., Shigemasa, Y., and Roy, R. 2000. Chemical modification of chitosan: Preparation of chitosan-sialic acid branched polysaccharide hybrids. *Chem Commun* 11: 909–910.
210. Sashiwa, H., Thompson, J. M., Das, S. K., Shigemasa, Y., Tripathy, S., and Roy, R. 2000. Chemical modification of chitosan: Preparation and lectin binding properties of α-galactosyl-chitosan conjugates. Potential inhibitors in acute rejection following xenotransplantation. *Biomacromolecules* 1: 303–305.
211. Sashiwa, H., Shigemasa, Y., and Roy, R. 2001. Preparation and lectin binding property of chitosan–carbohydrate conjugates. *Bull Chem Soc Jpn* 74: 937–943.
212. Gamian, A., Chomik, A., Laferriere, C. A., and Roy, R. 1991. Inhibition of influenza A virus hemagglutinin and induction of interferon by synthetic sialylated glycoconjugates. *Can J Microbiol* 37: 233–237.
213. Umemura, M., Makimura, Y., Itoh, M., Yamamoto, T., Mine, T., Mitani, S., Simizu, I., Ashida, H., and Yamamoto, K. 2010. One-step synthesis of efficient binding-inhibitor for influenza virus through multiple addition of sialyloligosaccharides on chitosan. *Carbohyd Polym* 81: 330–334.
214. Auzely, R. and Rinaudo, M. 2001. Chitosan derivatives bearing pendant cyclodextrin cavities: Synthesis and inclusion performance. *Macromolecules* 34: 3574–3580.
215. Prabaharan, M. and Mano, J. F. 2006. Chitosan derivatives bearing cyclodextrin cavities as novel adsorbent matrices. *Carbohyd Polym* 63: 53–166.
216. Furusaki, E., Ueno, Y., Sakairi, N., Nishi, N., and Tokura, S. 1996. Facile preparation and inclusion ability of a chitosan derivative bearing carboxymethyl-β-cyclodextrin. *Carbohyd Polym* 29: 29–34.
217. Aoki, N., Nishikawa, M., and Hattori, K. 2003. Synthesis of chitosan derivatives bearing cyclodextrin and adsorption of *p*-nonylphenol and bisphenol A. *Carbohyd Polym* 52: 219–223.
218. Martel, B., Devassine, M., Crini, G., Weltrowski, M., Bourdonneau, M., and Morcellet, M. 2001. Preparation and sorption properties of a β-cyclodextrin-linked chitosan derivative. *J Polym Sci A-Polym Chem* 39: 169–176.
219. Chen, S. and Wang, Y. 2001. Study on β-cyclodextrin grafting with chitosan and slow release of its inclusion complex with radioactive iodine. *J Appl Polym Sci* 82: 2414–2421.
220. Shigeno, Y. and Takemot, K. 1980. Functional monomers and polymers on the adsorption of iodine onto chitosan. *J Appl Polym Sci* 25: 731–738.

221. Wade, L. G. 1999. *Organic Chemistry*. Englewood Cliffs, NJ: Prentice-Hall International, p. 822.
222. Sreenivasan, K. 1998. Synthesis and preliminary studies on a β-cyclodextrin coupled chitosan as a novel adsorbent matrix. *J Appl Polym Sci* 69: 1051–1055.
223. Tanida, F., Tojima, T., Han, S. M., Nishi, N., Tokura, S., Sakairi, N., Haruyoshi Seino, H., and Hamada, K. 1998. Novel synthesis of a water-soluble cyclodextrin-polymer having a chitosan skeleton. *Polymer* 39: 5261–5263.
224. Tojima, T., Katsura, H., Han, S. M., Tanida, F., Nishi, N., Tokura, S., and Sakairi, N. 1998. Preparation of an α-cyclodextrin-linked chitosan derivative via reductive amination strategy. *J Polym Sci A-Polym Chem* 36: 1965–1968.
225. Zhang, X., Wang, Y., and Yi, Y. 2004. Synthesis and characterization of grafting α-cyclodextrin with chitosan. *J Appl Polym Sci* 94: 860–864.
226. Gaffar, M. A., Rafie, S. M. E., and Tahlawy, K. F. E. 2004. Preparation and utilization of ionic exchange resin via graft copolymerization of β-CD itaconate with chitosan. *Carbohydr Polym* 56: 387–396.
227. Don, T. M., King, C. F., and Chiu, W. Y. 2002. Synthesis and properties of chitosan-modified poly(vinyl acetate) . *J Appl Polym Sci* 86: 3057–3063.
228. Kim, S. Y., Cho, S. M., Lee, Y. M., and Kim, S. J. 2000. Thermo- and pH-responsive behaviors of graft copolymer and blend based on chitosan and *N*-isopropylacrylamide. *J Appl Polym Sci* 78: 1381–1391.
229. Pedram, M. Y., Retuert, J., and Quijada, R. 2000. Hydrogels based on modified chitosan, 1. Synthesis and swelling behavior of poly(acrylic acid) grafted chitosan. *Macromol Chem Phys* 201: 923–930.
230. Blair, H. S., Guthrie, J., Law, T. K., and Turkington, P. 1987. Chitosan and modified chitosan membranes I. Preparation and characterization. *J Appl Polym Sci* 33: 641–656.
231. Jenkins, D. W. and Hudson, S. M. 2001. Review of vinyl graft copolymerization featuring recent advances toward controlled radical-based reactions and illustrated with chitin/chitosan trunk polymers. *Chem Rev* 101: 3245–3274.
232. Pourjavadi, A., Mahdavinia, G. R., Zohuriaan-Mehr, M. J., and Omidian, H. 2003. Modified chitosan. I. Optimized cerium ammonium nitrate-induced synthesis of chitosan-*graft*-polyacrylonitrile. *J Appl Polym Sci* 88: 2048–2054.
233. Kim, S. Y., Cho, S. M., Lee, Y. M., and Kim, S. J. 2000. Thermo- and pH-responsive behaviors of graft copolymer and blend based on chitosan and *N*-isopropylacrylamide. *J Appl Polym Sci* 78: 1381–1391.
234. Huacai, G., Wan, P., and Dengke, L. 2006. Graft copolymerization of chitosan with acrylic acid under microwave irradiation and its water absorbency. *Carbohydr Polym* 66: 372–378.
235. Don, T. M., King, C. F., and Chiu, W. Y. 2002. Synthesis and properties of chitosan-modified poly(vinyl acetate). *J Appl Polym Sci* 86: 3057–3063.
236. Don, T. M., King, C. F., and Chiu, W. Y. 2002. Preparation of Chitosan-*graft*-poly(vinyl acetate) copolymers and their adsorption of copper ion. *Polym J* 34: 418.
237. Radhakumary, C., Divya, G., Nair, P. D., Mathew, S., and Nair, C. P. R. 2003. Graft copolymerization of 2-hydroxy ethyl methacrylate onto chitosan with cerium (IV) ion. I. Synthesis and characterization. *J Macromol Sci Part A: Pure Appl Chem* A40: 715–730.
238. Zhang, J., Yuan, Y., Shen, J., and Lin, S. 2003. Synthesis and characterization of chitosan grafted poly(*N;N*-dimethyl-*N*-methacryloxyethyl-*N*-(3-sulfopropyl)ammonium) initiated by ceric (IV) ion. *Eur Polym J* 39: 847–850.
239. Liang, J., Ni, P. H., Zhang, M. Z., and Yu, Z. Q. 2004. Graft copolymerization of (dimethylamino) ethyl methacrylate onto chitosan initiated by ceric ammonium nitrate. *J Macromol Sci Part A: Pure Appl Chem* 416: 685–696.
240. Joshi, M. and Sinha, V. K. 2007. Ceric ammonium nitrate induced grafting of polyacrylamide onto carboxymethyl chitosan. *Carbohydr Polym* 67: 427–435.
241. Yilmaz, E., Adali, T., Yilmaz, O., and Bengisu, M. 2007. Grafting of poly(triethylene glycol dimethacrylate) onto chitosan by ceric ion initiation. *React Funct Polym* 67: 10–18.

242. Caner, H., Yilmaz, E., and Yilmaz, O. 2007. Synthesis, characterization and antibacterial activity of poly(*N*-vinylimidazole) grafted chitosan. *Carbohydr Polym* 69: 318–325.

243. Mun, G. A., Nurkeeva, Z. S., Dergunov, S. A., Nam, I. K., Maimakov, T. P., Shaikhutdinov, E. M., Lee, S. C., and Park, K. 2008. Studies on graft copolymerization of 2-hydroxyethyl acrylate onto chitosan. *React Funct Polym* 28: 389–395.

244. Harish Prashanth, K. V. and Tharanathan, R. N. 2003. Studies on graft copolymerization of chitosan with synthetic monomers. *Carbohydr Polym* 54: 343–351.

245. Harish Prashanth, K. V., Lakshman, K., Shamala, T. R., and Tharanathan, R. N. 2005. Biodegradation of chitosan-graft-polymethylmethacrylate films. *Int Biodeterior Biodegrad* 56: 115–120.

246. Mahdavinia, G. R., Pourjavadi, A., Hosseinzadeh, H., and Zohuriaan, M. J. 2004. Modified chitosan 4. Superabsorbent hydrogels from poly(acrylic acid-*co*-acrylamide) grafted chitosan with salt- and pH-responsiveness properties. *Eur Polym J* 40: 1399.

247. Hsu, S. C., Don, T. M., and Chiu, W. Y. 2002. Synthesis of chitosan-modified poly(methyl methacrylate) by emulsion polymerization. *J Appl Polym Sci* 86: 3047–3056.

248. Hasipoglu, H. N., Yilmaz, E., Yilmaz, O., and Caner, H. 2005. Preparation and characterization of maleic acid grafted chitosan. *Int J Polym Anal Charact* 10: 313–327.

249. Najjar, A. M. K., Yunus, W. M. Z. W., Ahmad, M. B., and Rahman, M. Z. A. 2000. Preparation and characterization of poly(2-acrylamido-2-methylpropane-sulfonic acid) grafted chitosan using potassium persulfate as redox initiator. *J Appl Polym Sci* 77: 2314–2318.

250. Yazdani-Pedram, M. and Retuert, J. 1997. Homogeneous grafting reaction of vinyl pyrrolidone onto chitosan. *J Appl Polym Sci* 63: 1321–1326.

251. Yazdani-Pedram, M., Lagos, A., and Retuert, P. J. 2002. Study of the effect of reaction variables on grafting of polyacrylamide onto chitosan. *Polym Bull* 48: 93–98.

252. Sun, T., Xu, P., Liu, Q., Xue, J., and Xi, W. 2003. Graft copolymerization of methacrylic acid onto carboxymethyl chitosan. *Eur Polym J* 39: 189–192.

253. Xie, W., Xu, P., Wang, W., and Liu, Q. 2002. Preparation and antibacterial activity of a water-soluble chitosan derivative. *Carbohydr Polym* 50: 35–40.

254. Kang, H. M., Cai, Y. L., and Liu, P.S. 2006. Synthesis, characterization and thermal sensitivity of chitosan-based graft copolymers. *Carbohydr Res* 341: 2851–2857.

255. Berkovich, L. A., Tsyurupa, M. P., and Davankov, V. A. 1983. The synthesis of cross-linked copolymers of maleilated chitosan and acrylamide. *J Polym Sci Part A Polym Chem* 21: 1281–1287.

256. Lagos, A. and Reyes, J. 1988. Grafting onto chitosan. I. Graft copolymerization of methyl methacrylate onto chitosan with Fenton's reagent ($Fe^{2+} - H_2O_2$) as a redox initiator. *J Polym Sci Part A Polym Chem* 26: 985–991.

257. El-Tahlawy, K. F., El-Raie, S. M., and Sayed, A. A. 2006. Preparation and application of chitosan/poly(methacrylic acid)graft copolymer. *Carbohydr Polym* 66: 176–183.

258. Bayramoglu, G., Yılmaz, M., and Arica, M. Y. 2003. Affinity dye–ligand poly(hydroxyethyl methacrylate)/chitosan composite membrane for adsorption lysozyme and kinetic properties. *Biochem Eng J* 13: 35–42.

259. Blair, H. S., Guthrie, D. J., Law, T. K., and Turkington, P. 1987. Chitosan and modified chitosan membranes I. Preparation and characterisation. *J Appl Polym Sci* 33: 641–645.

260. Kojima, K., Yoshikuni, M., and Suzuki, T. 1979. Tributylborane-initiated grafting of methyl methacrylate onto chitin. *J Appl Polym Sci* 24: 1587–1593.

261. El-Tahlawy, K. and Hudson, S. M. 2001. Graft copolymerization of hydroxyethyl methacrylate onto chitosan. *J Appl Polym Sci* 82: 683–702.

262. Liu, Y. H., Liu, Z. H., Zhang, Y. Z., and Deng, K. L. 2003. Graft copolymerizaztion of methyl acrylate onto chitosan initiated by potassium diperiodatocuprate (III). *J Appl Polym Sci* 89: 2283–2289.

263. Liu, Y., Liu, Z., Zhang, Y., and Deng, K. 2000. Graft copolymerization of acrylonitrile onto chitosan initiated by potassium diperiodatonickelate (IV). *Chem J Internet* 4: 27. (www.chemistrymag.org/cji/2002/046027pe.htm).

264. Liu, Y. H., Li, Y. X., Lv, J., Wu, G., D., and Li, J. B. 2005. Graft copolymerization of methyl methacrylate onto chitosan initiated by potassium ditelluratocuprate(III). *J Macromol Sci Part A Pure Appl Chem* 42: 1169–1180.

265. Liu, P. F., Zhai, M. L., and Wu, J. L. 2001. Study on radiation-induced grafting of styrene onto chitin and chitosan. *Radiat Phys Chem* 61: 149–153.

266. Singh, D. K. and Ray, A. R. 1997. Radiation-induced grafting of *N,N'*-dimethylaminoethylmethacrylate onto chitosan films. *J Appl Polym Sci* 66: 869–877.

267. Cai, H., Zhang, Z. P., Sun, P. C., He, B. L., and Zhu, X. X. 2005. Synthesis and characterization of thermo- and pH- sensitive hydrogels based on Chitosan-grafted N-isopropylacrylamide via γ-radiation. *Radiat Phys Chem* 74: 26–30.

268. Yu, L., He, Y., Bin, L., and Yuee, F. 2003. Study of radiation-induced graft copolymerization of butyl acrylate onto chitosan in acetic acid aqueous solution. *J Appl Polym Sci* 90: 2855.

269. Morita, Y., Sugahara, Y., Takahashi, A., and Ibonai, M. 1997. Non-catalytic photo-induced graft copolymerization of methyl methacrylate onto O-acetyl-chitin. *Eur Polym J* 33: 1505.

270. Takahshi, A., Sugahara, Y., and Hirano, Y. 1989. Studies on graft copolymerization onto cellulose derivatives. XXIX. Photo-induced graft copolymerization of methyl methacrylate onto chitin and oxychitin. *J Polym Sci A—Polym Chem* 27: 3817.

271. Ng, L. T., Guthrie, J. T., Yuan, Y. J., and Zha, H. J. 2001. UV-cured natural polymer-based membrane for biosensor application. *J Appl Polym Sci* 79: 466–472.

272. Don, T. M. and Chen, H. R. 2005. Synthesis and characterization of AB-cross-linked graft copolymers based on maleilated chitosan and N-isopropylacrylamide. *Carbohydr Polym* 61: 334–347.

273. Singh, V., Tripathi, D. N., Tiwari, A., and Sanghi, R. 2006. Microwave synthesized chitosan-graft-poly(methylmethacrylate): An efficient Zn^{2+} ion binder. *Carbohydr Polym* 65: 35–41.

274. Feng, H. and Dong, C. M. 2007. Synthesis and characterization of phthaloyl-chitosan-g-poly-(L-lactide) using an organic catalyst. *Carbohydr Polym* 70: 258–264.

275. Chung, T. W., Lu, Y. F., Wang, S. S., Lin, Y. S., and Cho, S. H. 2002. Growth of human endothelial cells on photochemically grafted Gly–Arg–Gly–Asp (GRGD) chitosans. *Biomaterials* 23: 4803.

276. Yang, S., Tirmizi, S. A., Burns, A., Barney, A. A., and Risen, W. M. 1989. Chitaline materials: soluble chitosan-poly-pyrrole copolymers and their conductive doped forms. *Synth Met* 32: 191–200.

277. Kurita, K. 1996. Chitin and chitosan graft copolymers. In *Polymeric Materials Encyclopedia*. Salamone, J. C., ed., Boca Raton, FL: CRC Press. 2: 1205–1208.

278. Kurita, K., Iwawaki, S., Ishi, S., and Nishimura, S. I. 1992. Introduction of poly(L-alanine) side chains into chitin as versatile spacer arms having a terminal free amino group and immobilization of NADH active sites. *J Polym Sci A-Polym Chem* 30: 685.

279. Detchprohm, S., Aoi, K., and Okada, M. 2001. Synthesis of a novel chitin derivative having oligo(ε-caprolactone) side chains in aqueous reaction media. *Macromo Chem Phys* 202: 3560–3570.

280. Aoi, K., Takasu, A., and Okada, M. 1994. Synthesis of novel chitin derivatives having poly(2-alkyl-2-oxazoline) side chains. *Macromo Chem Phys* 195: 3835–3844.

281. Rutnakornpituk, M., Ngamdee, P., and Phinyocheep, P. 2006. Preparation and properties of polydimethylsiloxane-modified chitosan. *Carbohydr Polym* 63: 229–237.

282. Luckachan, G. E. and Pillai, C. K. S. 2006. Chitosan/oligo L-lactide graft copolymers: Effect of hydrophobic side chains on the physico-chemical properties and biodegradability. *Carbohydr Polym* 64: 254–266.

283. Wong, K., Sun, G. B., Zhang, X. Q., Dai, H., Liu, Y., He, C. B., and Leong, K. W. 2006. PEI-g-chitosan, a novel gene delivery system with transfection efficiency comparable to polyethylenimine *in vitro* and after liver administration *in vivo*. *Bioconjugate Chem* 17: 152–158.

284. Hiroshi, S., Wu, X., Harris, J. M., and Hoffman, A. S. 1997. Graft copolymers of poly(ethylene glycol) (PEG) and chitosan. *Macromol Rapid Commun* 18: 547–550.

285. Yalpani, M., Marchessault, R. H., Morin, F. G., and Monasterios, C. J. 1991. Synthesis of poly(3-hydroxyalkanoate) (PHA) conjugates: PHA–carbohydrate and PHA–synthetic polymer conjugates. *Macromolecules* 24: 6046–6049.

286. Silva, S. S., Menezes, S. M. C., and Garcia, R. B. 2003. Synthesis and characterization of polyurethane-g-chitosan. *Eur Polym J* 39: 1515–1519.

287. Kim, I. Y., Kim, S. J., Shin, M. S., Lee, Y.M., Shin, D.I., and Kim, S. I. 2002. pH- and thermal characteristics of graft hydrogels based on chitosan and poly(dimethylsiloxane). *J Appl Polym Sci* 85: 2661–2666.

288. Yao, F. L., Chen, W., Wang, H., Liu, H. F., Yao, K. D., Sun, P. C., and Lin, H. 2003. A study on cytocompatible poly (chitosan-g-L-lactic acid). *Polymer* 44: 6435–6441.

289. Yao, F. L., Liu, C., Chen, W., Bai, Y., Tang, Z. Y., and Yao, K. D. 2003. Synthesis and characterization of chitosan grafted oligo(L-lactic acid). *Macromol Biosci* 3: 653–656.

290. Xie, W. M., Xu, P. X., Wang, W., and Lu, Q. 2001. Antioxidant activity of water-soluble chitosan derivatives. *Bioorg Med Chem Lett* 11: 1699–1701.

291. Yang, Z. K. and Yuan, Y. 2001. Studies on the synthesis and properties of hydroxyl azacrown ether-grafted chitosan. *J Appl Polym Sci* 82: 1838–1843.

292. Thanou, M., Verhoef, J. C., and Junginger, H. E. 2001. Oral drug absorption enhancement by chitosan and its derivatives. *Advan Drug Delivery Rev* 52: 117–126.

293. Zhang, H. F., Zhong, H., Zhang, L. L., Chen, S. B., Zhao, Y. J., and Zhu, Y. L. 2009. Synthesis and characterization of thermosensitive graft copolymer of N-isopropylacrylamide with biodegradable carboxymethylchitosan. *Carbohydr Polym* 77: 785–790.

294. Sun, T., Xie, W., and Xu, P. 2004. Superoxide anion scavenging activity of graft chitosan derivatives. *Carbohydr Polym* 58: 379–382.

295. Caner, H., Hasipoglu, H., Yilmaz, O., and Yilmaz, E. 1998. Graft copolymerization of 4-vinylpyridine on to chitosan—I. By ceric ion initiation. *Eur Polym J* 34: 493–497.

296. Singh, V., Tripathi, D. N., Tiwari, A., and Sanghi, R. 2005. Microwave promoted synthesis of chitosan-graft-poly(acrylonitrile). *J Appl Polym Sci* 95: 820–825.

297. Qu, X., Wirsen, A., and Albertsson, A. C. 1999. Structural change and swelling mechanism of pH-sensitive hydrogels based on chitosan and D,L-lactic acid. *J Appl Polym Sci* 74: 3186–3192.

298. Cai, K. Y., Yao, K. D., Cui, Y. L., Lin, S. B., Yang, Z. M., Li, X. Q., Xie, H. Q., Qing, T. W., and Luo, J. 2002. Surface modification of poly (D,L-lactic acid) with chitosan and its effects on the culture of osteoblasts *in vitro*. *J Biomed Mater Res* 60: 398–404.

299. Chung, T. W., Yang, J., Akaike, T., Cho, K. Y., Nah, J. W., Kim, S., and Cho, C. S. 2002. Preparation of alginate/galactosylated chitosan scaffold for hepatocyte attachment. *Biomaterials* 23: 2827–2834.

300. Yoshikawa, S., Takayama, T., and Tsubokawa, N. 1998. Grafting reaction of living polymer cations with amino groups on chitosan powder. *J Appl Polym Sci* 68: 1883–1889.

301. Xiang, Y., Si, J. J., Zhang, Q., Liu, Y., and Guo, H. 2009. Homogeneous graft copolymerization and characterization of novel artificial glycoprotein: Chitosan-poly(L-tryptophan) copolymers with secondary structural side chains. *J Polym Sci A-Polym Chem* 47: 925–934.

302. Aoi, K., Takasu, A., Okada, M., and Imae, T. 1999. Synthesis and assembly of novel chitin derivatives having amphiphilic polyoxazoline block copolymer as a side chain. *Macromol Chem Phys* 200: 1112–1120.

303. Duan, K. R., Zhang, X. L., Tang, X. X., Yu, J. H., Liu, S. Y., Wang, D. X., Li, Y. P., and Huang, J. 2010. Fabrication of cationic nanomicelle from chitosan-graft-polycaprolactone as the carrier of 7-ethyl-10-hydroxy-camptothecin. *Colloid Surf B* 76: 475–482.

304. Makuska, R. and Gorochovceva, N. 2006. Regioselective grafting of poly(ethylene glycol) onto chitosan through C-6 position of glucosamine units. *Carbohydr Polym.* 64: 319–327.

305. Liu, L., Li, F. Z., Fang, Y. E., and Guo, S. R. 2006. Regioselective grafting of poly(ethylene glycol) onto chitosan and the properties of the resulting copolymers. *Macromol Biosci* 6: 855–861.

306. Wan, A. C. A., Tai, B. C. U., Schumacher, K. M., Schumacher, A., Chin, S. Y., and Ying, J. Y. 2008. Polyelectrolyte complex membranes for specific cell adhesion. *Langmuir* 24: 2611–2617.

307. Ho, M. H., Wang, D. M., Hsieh, H. J., Liu, H. C., Hsien, T. Y., Lai, J. Y., and Hou, L. T. 2005. Preparation and characterization of RGD-immobilized chitosan scaffolds. *Biomaterials* 26: 3197–3206.

308. Schaffner P. and Dard, M. M. 2003. Structure and function of RGD peptides involved in bone biology. *Cell Mol Life Sci* 60: 119–132.

309. Masuko, T., Iwasaki, N., Yamane, S., Funakoshi, T., Majima, T., Minami, A., Ohsuga, N., Ohta, T., and Nishimura, S. I. 2005. Chitosan–RGDSGGC conjugate as a scaffold material for musculoskeletal tissue engineering. *Biomaterials* 26: 5339–5347.

310. Cunningham, M. F. 2008. Controlled/living radical polymerization in aqueous dispersed systems. *Prog Polym Sci* 33: 365–398.

311. Matyjaszewski, K. and Tsarevsky, N. V. 2009. Nanostructured functional materials prepared by atom transfer radical polymerization. *Nat Chem* 1: 276–288.

312. El Tahlawy, K. and Hudson, S. M. 2003. Synthesis of a well-defined chitosan graft poly(methoxy polyethyleneglycol methacrylate) by atom transfer radical polymerization. *J Appl Polym Sci* 89: 901–912.

313. Li, N., Bal, R. B., and Liu, C. K. 2005. Enhanced and selective adsorption of mercury ions on chitosan beads grafted with polyacrylamide via surface-initiated atom transfer radical polymerization. *Langmuir* 21: 11780–11787.

314. Tang, F., Zhang, L. F., Zhu, J., Cheng, Z. P., and Zhu, X. L. 2009. Surface functionalization of chitosan nanospheres via surface-initiated AGET ATRP mediated by iron catalyst in the presence of limited amounts of air. *Ind Eng Chem Res* 48: 6216–6223.

315. Tang, J., Hua, D. B., Cheng, J. X., Jiang, J., and Zhu, X. I. 2008. Synthesis and properties of temperature-responsive chitosan by controlled free radical polymerization with chitosan–RAFT agent. *Int J Biol Macromol* 43: 383–389.

316. Hua, D. B., Tang, J., Cheng, J. X., Deng, W. C., and Zhu, M. L. 2008. A novel method of controlled grafting modification of chitosan via RAFT polymerization using chitosan–RAFT agent. *Carbohydr Polym* 73: 98–104.

317. Tsubokawa, N. and Takayama, T. 2000. Surface modification of chitosan powder by grafting of "dendrimer-like" hyperbranched polymer onto the surface. *React Funct Polym* 43: 341–350.

318. Sashiwa, H., Shigemasa, Y., and Roy, R. 2000. Chemical modification of chitosan. 3. Hyperbranched chitosan–sialic acid dendrimer hybrid with tetraethylene glycol spacer. *Macromolecules* 33: 6913–6915.

319. Sashiwa, H., Shigemasa, Y., and Roy, R. 2001. Chemical modification of chitosan. 10. Synthesis of dendronized chitosan–sialic acid hybrid using convergent grafting of preassembled dendrons built on gallic acid and tri(ethylene glycol) backbone. *Macromolecules* 34: 3905–3909.

320. Sashiwa, H., Shigemasa, Y., and Roy, R. 2002. Chemical modification of chitosan 11: Chitosan–dendrimer hybrid as a tree like molecule. *Carbohydr Polym* 49: 195–205.

321. Sashiwa, H., Shigemasa, Y., and Roy, R. 2001. Hyghly convergent synthesis of dendrimerized chitosan–sialic acid hybrid. *Macromolecules* 34: 3211–3214.

322. Msmmen, M., Choi, S., and Whiteside, G. M. 1998. Polyvalent interactions in biological systems: Implications for design and use of multivalent ligands and inhibitors. *Angew Chem Int Ed* 37: 2754–2757.

323. Kamitakahara, H., Suzuki, T., Nishigori, N., Suzuki, Y., Kanie, O., and Whong, C. H. 1998. A lysoganglioside/poly-L-glutamic acid conjugate as a picomolar inhibitor of influenza hemagglutinin. *Angew Chem Int Ed* 37: 1524–1527.

324. Klaykruayat, B., Siralertmukul, K., and Srikulkit, K. 2010. Chemical modification of chitosan with cationic hyperbranched dendritic polyamidoamine and its antimicrobial activity on cotton fabric. *Carbohydr Polym* 80: 197–207.

325. Aoi, K., Takasu, A., and Okada, M. 1997. New Chitin-Based Polymer Hybrids. 2. Improved Miscibility of Chitin Derivatives Having Monodisperse Poly(2-methyl-2-oxazoline) Side Chains with Poly(vinyl chloride) and Poly(vinyl alcohol). *Macromolecules* 30: 6134–6138.

3

Bioactivities of Chitosan and Its Derivatives

Aiping Zhu and Jian Shen

CONTENTS

3.1 Cytocompatibility

3.1.1 Immunocyte

The efficacy of orally administered vaccines is generally low due to factors such as degradation of the antigen in the gastrointestinal (GI) tract and low uptake by gut-associated lymphoid tissue (GALT). Peyer's patches (PPs) are the main target for oral vaccines, which are present in the lower ileum. The intestinal epithelium overlying PPs is specialized to allow the transport of pathogens into the lymphoid tissue. This sampling function is carried out by M-cells [1]. Association of the vaccine with microparticulate drug carrier systems may prevent its degradation in the stomach and the gut and may stimulate M-cells to transport the vaccine to the dome of PPs [2–7]. After transport of the microparticles to the dome of PPs, the microparticles are degraded and the vaccine is released into the lymphoid tissue. Following stimulation by an antigen in PPs and its presentation to B- and T-cells, the antigen induces B- and T-cell proliferation and these cells subsequently leave PPs via efferent lymphatics and reach the systemic circulation through the thoracic duct. The uptake efficiency by PPs is mainly dependent on the size of microparticles: particles larger than 10 μm are not internalized by M-cells [8].

In the nasal-associated lymphoid tissue, morphologically and functionally similar cells have been described [9]. Although vaccine degradation is not as drastic as in the gut, for this route also a carrier system is needed [10]. Since the half-time of clearance in the human nasal cavity is only about 15 min and protein-like agents are hardly transported over the epithelial barrier, vaccine encapsulation in microparticles may enhance the uptake by M-cells or coadministering the antigen with an absorption enhancer may increase the induction of immune responses after nasal application.

3.1.1.1 Vaccine Encapsulation Matrix

Chitosan, the deacetylated form of chitin, is able to open the tight junctions and in this way allows paracellular transport across the epithelium. Both nasal and oral drug delivery research has demonstrated that significantly higher amounts of macromolecular drugs can be transported after coadministration with chitosan. Besides its ability to facilitate paracellular transport, chitosan can also be used to prepare microparticles or nanoparticles. In contrast to chitosan formulations, which are able to open the tight junctions, particulate vaccine delivery systems are taken up by M-cells and subsequently biodegraded. Only then the lymphoid tissue will be targeted efficiently. Particulate systems for macromolecular and hydrophilic drug delivery need to be smaller than 200 nm to be taken up by epithelial cells or to release the drug upon arrival at the mucosae [11].

Molecular weight (MW) and degree of acetylation determine the properties of chitosan. Because of its biocompatibility, biodegradability, low cost, and ability to open intercellular tight junctions, this polymer is a valuable excipient for oral drug delivery systems. Recently, numerous studies on chitosan as a drug absorption enhancer have been published. Chitosan formulations are used for ocular, oral, parenteral, and nasal delivery. Furthermore, chitosan can easily form microparticles. Advances in microparticulate drug delivery researches have opened up the way to apply these techniques in oral vaccination. Due to the high protein-binding properties of some types of chitosan microparticles, they are also potential candidates for oral delivery of antigens [12]. Mild preparation can protect the proteins when they are incorporated during preparation of the microparticles [12]. In order to circumvent protein denaturation conditions, chitosan microparticles can be loaded passively. Such a mild loading procedure has been described by Jameela et al. [13].

Chitosan microparticles, 4.3 ± 07 μm in size and positively charged (20 ± 1 mV), have a suitable size and zeta potential to be taken up by the M-cells of PPs. These microparticles show a high loading capacity and loading efficacy for the model antigen ovalbumin. About 90% of the ovalbumin remained in the microparticles after release studies for 4 h in phosphate-buffered saline (PBS). Because the chitosan microparticles are biodegradable, this entrapped ovalbumin will be released after intracellular digestion in PPs. Initial studies *in vivo* demonstrated that fluorescently labeled chitosan microparticles can be taken up by the epithelium of murine PPs. Since uptake by PPs is an essential step in oral vaccination, these results show that the presently developed porous chitosan microparticles are a very promising vaccine delivery system [14].

Systemic (IgG) and local (IgA) immune responses against diphtheria toxoid associated with chitosan microparticles were strongly enhanced after oral delivery in mice. Furthermore, dose-dependent systemic immune responses could be elicited and enough antitoxin was produced to protect against the harmful effects of the diphtheria toxin [15]. Chitosan–alginate microcapsules are found to be an effective means of protecting immunoglobulin (IgY) from gastric inactivation, allowing its use for the widespread prevention and control of enteric diseases [16].

Cancer is a disease state in which the cells in our body undergo mutations at the genetic level and are transformed, acquiring the ability to replicate limitlessly. Conventional cancer treatment involves the use of surgery and cytotoxic chemotherapy and/or radiotherapy, which have the potential for harming normal, otherwise healthy, nonneoplastic cells. Newer forms of therapy such as immunotherapy and gene therapy have shown initial promise due to the treatment of a wide range of diseases, both inherited and acquired [17], but still require better ways to limit exposure to cancerous lesions in the body.

3.1.1.2 Chitosan as a Gene Vector

The basic concept underlying gene therapy is that human disease may be treated by the transfer of genetic material into specific cells of a patient in order to correct or supplement defective genes responsible for disease development. Gene therapy is currently being applied in many different health problems such as cancer, AIDS, and cardiovascular diseases. Recently, the key research aim of gene therapy is to search for effective and safe vector systems. The main systems for gene delivery are both viral and nonviral vectors. Although viral vectors show high transfection efficiency, many drawbacks limit their applications, such as oncogenic effects, nonspecificity, immunogenicity to the target cells, and degradation by enzymes [18]. Nonviral vectors for gene therapy are preferred as safer alternatives to viral vectors. They have many advantages, including safety, stability, and lower immunogenicity [19]. Currently, the two main types of nonviral gene delivery vectors are cationic liposomes and cationic polymers [20,21].

Cationic liposomes have potential as a gene delivery vector. However, their applications are limited to local delivery due to low stability and rapid degradation in the body [22,23]. Cationic polymers have been used to deliver DNA both *in vitro* and *in vivo* in terms of biocompatibility, low cytotoxicity, and cost-effectiveness [24]. As a natural cationic polymer, chitosan has been widely employed in gene delivery due to its biocompatibility, biodegradability, low immunogenicity, and nontoxic material [25]. Chitosan protonated in acidic conditions can form complex nanoparticles with anionic DNA by electrostatic interactions [26] and protect it against nuclease degradation [27]. Also, the mucoadhesive property of chitosan potentially permits a sustained interaction between the macromolecules and an efficient uptake [28–30]. Chitosan has the ability to open intercellular tight junctions, facilitating its transport into the cells [31]. It has the advantage of not requiring sonication and organic solvents for its preparation, therefore minimizing possible damage to DNA during complexation. However, chitosan as a gene vector still has some disadvantages such as relative inefficiency and low specificity [32].

The first report suggesting the probable candidature of chitosan as a gene delivery agent was published in the year 1998 [33]. Chitosan self-aggregate–DNA complexes achieved an efficient transfection of chitooligosaccharide-1 (COS-1) cells and the level of expression with plasmid–chitosan was observed to be no less than that with plasmid–lipofectin complexes in SOJ cells. A few years later, Mao et al. [34] reported the preparation of chitosan–DNA nanoparticles using a complex cooperation process. They investigated important parameters for nanoparticle synthesis, including concentrations of DNA, chitosan, and sodium sulfate, temperature of the solutions, pH value of the buffer, and MWs of chitosan and DNA. At an amino group to phosphate group ratio (N/P ratio) between 3 and 8 and a chitosan concentration of 100 mg/mL, the size of particles was optimized to 100–250 nm with a narrow distribution, with a composition of 35.6% and 64.4% by weight for DNA and chitosan, respectively. The surface charge of these particles was slightly positive with a zeta potential of 112–118 mV at pH lower than 6.0, and became nearly neutral at pH 7.2. In this system, the transfection efficiency of chitosan–DNA nanoparticles was cell type dependent. They also developed three different schemes to conjugate transferrin or knob protein to the nanoparticle surface. Transferrin conjugation only yielded a maximum 4-fold increase in transfection efficiency in HEK293 cells and HeLa cells, whereas knob-conjugated nanoparticles could improve the gene expression level in HeLa cells by 130-fold. Conjugation of polyethylene glycol (PEG) on the nanoparticles allowed lyophilization without aggregation and without loss of bioactivity for at least 1 month in storage. The clearance of PEGylated nanoparticles in mice following intravenous (i.v.) administration was slower than unmodified nanoparticles at 15 min, and with higher depositions in kidney and liver. However, no difference was observed at the 1 h time point.

A study of the condensation of depolymerized chitosans with DNA was carried out. High-molecular-weight (HMW) chitosan was depolymerized by oxidative degradation with $NaNO_2$ at room temperature to obtain 11 samples of chitosan derivatives of varying MWs with a view to assessing their effective MW range for gene delivery applications. The results showed that chitosans with very low MWs and high charge density exhibited a strong binding affinity to DNA compared to HMW chitosans [35–36].

Chitosan was used to transfer luciferase plasmid into tumor cells. Chitosan largely enhanced the transfection efficiency of luciferase plasmid (pGL3). Transfection efficiencies of the pGL3–chitosan complexes were dependent on pH of the culture medium, stoichiometry of pGL3, chitosan, serum, and molecular mass of chitosan. The transfection efficiency at pH 6.9 was higher than that at pH 7.6. The optimum charge ratio of pGL3:chitosan was 1:5. Chitosan of 15 and 52 kDa largely promoted luciferase activities. The transfection efficiency mediated by chitosan of >100 kDa was less than that mediated by chitosan of 15 and 52 kDa. Heptamer (1.3 kDa) did not show any gene expression. Chitosan showed resistance to serum [37].

In an approach to study the transfection mechanism of plasmid–chitosan complexes as well as the relationship between transfection activity and cell uptake, Ishii et al. [38] used fluorescein isothiocyanate-labeled plasmid and Texas Red-labeled chitosan. They observed that there are several factors that contribute to transfection activity, MW of chitosan, stoichiometry of the complex, as well as serum concentration and pH of the transfection medium. The level of transfection with plasmid–chitosan complexes was found to be highest when the molecular mass of chitosan was 40 or 84 kDa, the ratio of chitosan nitrogen to DNA phosphate (N/P ratio) was 5, and the transfection medium contained 10% serum at pH 7.0. While investigating the transfection mechanism, they found that plasmid–chitosan complexes most likely condense to form large aggregates, which adsorb on the cell surface. After this, plasmid–chitosan complexes are endocytosed, and possibly released from endosomes due to the swelling of lysosomes along with the swelling of the plasmid–chitosan complex, causing the endosome to rupture. Finally, these complexes were observed to accumulate in the nucleus.

Probing for a solution to track the efficiency of DNA delivery, Lee et al. [39] used fluorescence resonance energy transfer (FRET) to monitor the molecular dissociation of a chitosan–DNA complex with different MWs of chitosan. Chitosan with different MWs was complexed with plasmid DNA and complex formation was monitored using dynamic light scattering (DLS) and a gel retardation assay. Plasmid DNA and chitosan were separately labeled with quantum dots and Texas Red, respectively, and the dissociation of the complex was subsequently monitored using confocal microscopy and fluorescence spectroscopy. As the chitosan MW in the chitosan–DNA complex increased, the Texas Red-labeled chitosan gradually lost FRET-induced fluorescence light. This observation was noted when HEK293 cells incubated with the chitosan–DNA complex were examined with confocal microscopy. This suggested that the dissociation of the chitosan–DNA complex was more significant in the HMW chitosan–DNA complex. Fluorescence spectroscopy also determined the molecular dissociation of the chitosan–DNA complex at pH 7.4 and 5.0 and confirmed that the dissociation occurred in acidic environments. This finding suggested that the HMW chitosan–DNA complex can more easily be dissociated in lysosomes compared to a low-molecular-weight (LMW) complex. Furthermore, the HMW chitosan–DNA complex showed superior transfection efficiency in relation to the LMW complex. Therefore, it could be concluded that the dissociation of the chitosan–DNA complex is a critical event in obtaining the high transfection efficiency of the gene carrier–DNA complex [39].

3.1.1.3 Chitosan Derivatives as a Gene Delivery Matrix

Although chitosan has been widely used in gene delivery, further developed applications of chitosan for gene delivery are limited because of its poor water solubility and low transfection efficiency. Its low transfection efficiency problem remains to be solved. For this target, various modifications of the side chains of chitosan and optimizations of chitosan formulation have been performed.

Chitosan modified with betaine could increase its ability to facilitate DNA uptake and its cytotoxicity, both of which showed an influence on transfection efficiency. It was able to increase the cellular uptake and transfection efficiency of complex nanoparticles in COS-7 cells to increase betaine substitution of CsB; however, the higher sensitivity of MDA-MB-468 cells to CsBs led to decreased transfection efficiency because of the increased cytotoxicity with increasing betaine substitution [40].

Quaternized modifications of chitosan are another technique with characteristics that might be useful in DNA condensing and efficient gene delivery [41]. The transfection efficiency was compared with DOTAP (*N*-[1-(2,3-dioleoyloxy)propyl]-*N,N,N*-trimethylammonium sulfate) lipoplexes. Additionally, their effect on the viability of respective cell cultures was investigated using the 3-[4,5-dimethylthiazol-2-yl]-2, 5-diphenyl tetrazolium bromide (MTT) assay. Their observations suggested that quaternized chitosan oligomers were able to condense DNA and form complexes with a size ranging from 200 to 500 nm. Chitoplexes proved to transfect COS-1 cells, but to a lesser extent than DOTAP–DNA lipoplexes. The quaternized oligomer derivatives appeared to be superior to oligomeric chitosan.

Chitosan, trimethyl chitosan, or polyethyleneglycol-graft-trimethyl chitosan–DNA complexes were characterized with respect to physicochemical properties such as hydrodynamic diameter, condensation efficiency, and DNA release [42–44]. Further, the cytotoxicity of these polymers and the uptake and transfection efficiency of polyplexes *in vitro* were evaluated. Under conditions found in cell culture, the formation of aggregates and strongly decreased DNA condensation efficiency were observed in the case of chitosan polyplexes. These characteristics resulted in only 7% cellular uptake in NIH/3T3 cells and low transfection efficiencies in four different cell lines. By contrast, quaternization of chitosan strongly reduced aggregation tendency and pH dependency of DNA complexation. Accordingly, cellular uptake was increased 8.5-fold compared to chitosan polyplexes, resulting in up to 678-fold increased transfection efficiency in NIH/3T3 cells. Apart from reduction of cytotoxicity, PEGylation led to improved colloidal stability of polyplexes and significantly increased cellular uptake compared to unmodified trimethyl chitosan. These improvements resulted in a significant, up to 10-fold increase of transfection efficiency in NIH/3T3, L929, and MeWo cells compared to trimethyl chitosan, which not only highlights the importance of investigating polyplex stability under different pH and ionic strength conditions, but also elucidates correlations between physicochemical characteristics and biological efficacy of the studied polyplexes.

A self-assembled nanoparticle using a hydrophobically modified glycol chitosan (HGC) for gene delivery has been prepared [45]. Here a primary amine of glycol chitosan was modified with 5-cholanic acid to prepare an HGC. The modified chitosan was found to form DNA nanoparticles spontaneously by a hydrophobic interaction between HGC and hydrophobized DNA. As the HGC content increased, the encapsulation efficiencies of DNA increased while the size of HGC nanoparticles decreased. Upon increasing HGC contents, HGC nanoparticles became less cytotoxic. The increased HGC contents also facilitated endocytic uptakes of HGC nanoparticles by COS-1 cells. The HGC nanoparticles showed increasing *in vitro* transfection efficiencies in the presence of serum. *In vivo* results also showed that the HGC nanoparticles had superior transfection efficiencies compared to naked DNA and a commercialized transfection agent.

Stearic acid (SA)-grafted chitosan oligosaccharide COSs (COS-SA) could self-aggregate to form a micelle-like structure in aqueous solution [46]. In particular, SA, an endogenous long-chain saturated fatty acid, was widely accepted for pharmaceutical use. As a main composition of fat, SA is biocompatible with low cytoxicity. COS-SA has efficient ability to condense the plasmid DNA to form COS complex nanoparticles, which can efficiently protect the condensed DNA from enzymatic degradation by DNase I. The *in vitro* transfection experiments showed that the optimal transfection efficiency of COS–SA micelle in A549 cells was higher than that of COS, and comparable with Lipofectamine™ 2000. The presence of 10% fetal bovine serum increased the transfection ability of COS–SA. On the other hand, the cytotoxicity of COS–SA was highly lower than that of Lipofectamine 2000.

Another group used the reverse microemulsion technique as a template to fabricate chitosan–alginate core-shell nanoparticles encapsulated with enhanced green fluorescent protein-encoded plasmids [47]. These alginate-coated chitosan nanoparticles endocytosed by NIH 3T3 cells were found to trigger swelling of transport vesicles, which render gene escape before entering the digestive endolysosomal compartment, and concomitantly promote gene transfection rate. The results indicate that DNA-encapsulated chitosan–alginate nanoparticles with an average size of 64 nm (N/P ratio of 5) could achieve the level of gene expression comparable with the one obtained by using polyethyleneimine–DNA complexes.

Chitosan–alginate microcapsules were evaluated as a method of oral delivery of IgY antibodies. Small and monodispersed nanoparticles with high *in vitro* transfection capabilities were obtained by the complexation of these two polyelectrolytes. Chitosan (<10 kDa) presents more advantageous characteristics over the HMW chitosan for clinical applications, namely increased solubility at physiological pH and improved DNA release. Consequently, after incorporating γ-polyglycolic acid (γ-PGA) into CS–DNA complexes, a significant increase in their transfection efficiency was found [48].

An approach for the enhancement of cellular uptake and transfection efficiency of chitosan–DNA complexes through modifying the internal structure by incorporating a negatively charged poly(γ-glutamic acid) was reported recently [49]. The aforementioned results indicated that γ-PGA plays multiple important roles in enhancing the cellular uptake and transfection efficiency of CS/DNA/γ-PGA nanoparticles. This high transfection efficiency of the nonviral gene delivery system could be attributed to the synergic effect of ultra-low molecular weight chitosan (ULMWCh) and the low charge density of the sodium hyaluronate (HA) chain for easy release of DNA, which makes the system suitable for targeted gene delivery [50].

Chitosan/trimeric sodium phosphate (TPP) nanoparticles showed high encapsulation efficiencies for both plasmid DNA and dsDNA oligomers (20-mers), independent of chitosan MW. LMW chitosan (LMWC)/TPP nanoparticles gave high gene expression levels in HEK293 cells already 2 days after transfection, reaching a plateau of sustained and high gene expression between 4 and 10 days. The inclusion of BSA into the nanostructures did not alter the inherent transfection efficiency of nanoparticles. Confocal studies suggest endocytotic cellular uptake of the nanoparticles and subsequent release into the cytoplasm within 14 h. LMWC/TPP nanoparticles mediated a strong β-galactosidaseexpression *in vivo* after intratracheal administration. That is to say, ionically cross-linked chitosan/TPP nanoparticles serve as a biocompatible nonviral gene delivery system and generate a solid ground for further optimization studies, for example with regard to steric stabilization and targeting [51].

3.1.1.4 Clinical Applications of Chitosan–DNA Systems

To test the chitosan–DNA system as a potential DNA vaccine candidate, Kumar et al. [52] utilized a strategy involving an intranasal gene transfer, referred to as IGT, complexed with chitosan–DNA nanospheres containing a cocktail of DNA encoding nine immunogenic respiratory syncytial virus (RSV) antigens. This system was tested against acute RSV infection in a BALB/c mouse model. The effectiveness and mechanism of this IGT strategy were investigated, and the results demonstrated that IGT was safe and effective against RSV and significantly attenuates the pulmonary inflammation induced by RSV infection. A single dose of about 1 mg/kg body weight was capable of decreasing viral titers by two orders of magnitude (100-fold) on primary infection. This therapy works by induction of high levels of both serum IgG and mucosal IgA antibodies, generation of effective control response, and elevated lung-specific production of interferon-γ (IFN-γ)-antiviral action. Also, IGT significantly decreased pulmonary inflammation and did not alter airway hyperresponsiveness, making it safe for *in vivo* use.

Another application of chitosan–DNA gene therapy is against Coxsackie virus B3 infections, which cause acute and chronic myocarditis [53]. Intranasal delivery of the chitosan–DNA complex prepared by vortexing DNA with chitosan resulted in transgenic DNA expression in mouse nasopharynx and also induced mucosal SIgA secretion. Sun et al. [54] constructed a eukaryotic expression vector pVAX1-pZP3a as an oral zona pellucida (ZP) DNA contraceptive and successfully encapsulated in nanoparticles with chitosan to target ZP, the extracellular matrix surrounding oocytes. After 5 days of feeding to mice, the transcription and expression of pZP3 were found in mouse alvine chorion. Okamoto et al. [55] investigated the potential of chitosan in the form of inhaled powder for gene delivery purposes by preparing powders using pCMV-Luc as a reporter gene and LMWC (3–30 kDa) as a cationic vector with supercritical CO_2. This powder was administered to the lungs of mice and their transfection efficiency was compared to that of DNA solution and DNA powder without the cationic vector. The gene powder with the cationic vector was found to be an excellent gene delivery system to the lungs.

Chitosan/small interfering RNA (siRNA) nanoparticle-mediated tumor necrosis factor-α (TNF-α) knockdown in peritoneal macrophages was used for antiinflammatory treatment in a murine arthritis model [56].

3.1.2 Target Cell

3.1.2.1 Hepatocyte-Targeting Gene Delivery

In the body, the liver is an attractive target tissue for gene therapy due to its large size and metabolic capacity [57]. Research on hepatocyte-targeting gene delivery is much more attractive. Since Gref mentioned that galactose-modified oligosaccharides showed a high affinity for asialoglycoprotein (ASGR) receptors in hepatocyte [58], a number of synthetic approaches for galactosylate compounds have been reported. Chung et al. [59] synthesized galactosylated chitosan (GC) through the covalent coupling of lactobionic acid with chitosan. Park et al. [60,61] reported that galactosylated chitosan-graft-dextran and chitosan-graft-PEG (GCP) were synthesized and characterized as hepatocyte-targeting gene carriers, respectively. The complexes were only transfected with cells having ASGR. Chitosan-*O*-PEG-galactose as a targeting ligand for glycoprotein receptor was prepared through several steps [58].

As a novel technique, Dai et al. [62] studied gene delivery by chitosan–DNA nanoparticles through retrograde intrabiliary infusion (RII) and examined the efficacy of liver-specific targeting. The transfection efficiency of chitosan–DNA nanoparticles, as compared with polymine (PEI)–DNA nanoparticles, was evaluated in Wistar rats by infusion into the common bile duct, portal vein, or tail vein. Chitosan–DNA nanoparticles administrated through the portal vein or tail vein did not produce detectable luciferase expression. In contrast, rats that received chitosan–DNA nanoparticles showed more than 500 times higher luciferase expression in the liver 3 days after RII, and transgene expression levels decreased gradually over 14 days. Luciferase expression in the kidney, lung, spleen, and heart was negligible compared with that in the liver. RII of chitosan–DNA nanoparticles did not yield significant toxicity and damage to the liver and biliary tree as evidenced by liver function analysis and histopathological examination. Luciferase expression by RII of PEI–DNA nanoparticles was 17-fold lower than that of chitosan–DNA nanoparticles on day 3, but increased slightly over time. These results suggest that gene delivery by chitosan–DNA nanoparticles through RII is a promising routine to achieve liver-targeted gene delivery, and both gene carrier characteristics and mode of administration significantly influence gene delivery efficiency.

3.1.2.2 Macrophage-Targeting Therapy

In an approach to target the pDNA–chitosan complex using cell-specific receptors, mannose-modified chitosan (man-chitosan) was used to target macrophages expressing a mannose receptor [63]. The cellular uptake of pDNA–man-chitosan complexes through mannose recognition was then observed. The pDNA–man-chitosan complexes showed no significant cytotoxicity in mouse peritoneal macrophages, while pDNA–man-PEI complexes showed strong cytotoxicity. The pDNA–man-chitosan complexes showed much higher transfection efficiency than pDNA–chitosan complexes in mouse peritoneal macrophages. Observation with a confocal laser microscope suggested differences in the cellular uptake mechanism between pDNA–chitosan complexes and pDNA–man-chitosan complexes. Mannose receptor-mediated gene transfer thus enhances the transfection efficiency of pDNA–chitosan complexes.

Chitosan was modified with mannose to target primary APCs such as dendritic cells (DCs) owing to the high density of mannose receptors expressed on the surface of immature DCs. After (i.m.) immunization, the microspheres induced significantly enhanced serum antibody and cytotoxic T lymphocyte responses in comparison with naked DNA [64].

The mean particle diameter and average zeta potential of the galactosylated chitosan (GC)/DNA complex were 350 nm and +22.1 mV, respectively. The GC–DNA nanoparticle was tested to transfect HEK293 cells, and the viability of HEK293 cells was not affected by the GC–DNA nanoparticle compared to that of the control [65].

Recently, some peptide sequences known as protein transduction domains or membrane translocalization signals were identified and introduced for the delivery of plasmid DNA [66,67]. Interestingly, it is known that these sequences usually contain positively charged amino acid residues such as arginine and lysine, which have been reported to be able to enhance transportation into cells by several groups [68,69]. Oligo-arginine conjugates demonstrated characteristics similar to cell-penetrating peptides in cell translocation, and the transfection efficiency in HeLa cells could be highly improved by conjugating oligo-arginine to PEGylated lipids [70]. The polyamidoamine dendrimer conjugated with L-arginine was also found to enhance gene delivery potency compared with native dendrimer [71].

Arginine-rich peptides have attracted considerable attention due to their distinct internalization mechanism. It was reported that arginine and guanidino moieties were able to translocate through cell membranes and played a critical role in the process of membrane permeation. Arginine was conjugated to the backbone of chitosan to form a novel chitosan derivative, arginine-modified chitosan (Arg-CS). Arg-CS–DNA complexes were prepared according to the method of the coacervation process. Arg-CS was characterized by FTIR and ^{13}C NMR. Arg-CS–DNA polyelectrolyte complexes were investigated by agarose gel retardation, DLS, and atomic force microscopy (AFM). Arg-CS–DNA complexes started to form at an N:P ratio of 2:1, and the size of particles varied from 100 to 180 nm. The cytotoxicities of Arg-CS and their complexes with plasmid DNA were determined by the MTT assay for HeLa cells, and the results suggested that Arg-CS–DNA complexes were slightly less toxic than Arg-CS. Moreover, the derivative alone and their complexes showed significantly lower toxicity than PEI and PEI–DNA complexes, respectively. Taking HeLa cells as target cells and using pGL3-control as reporter gene, the luciferase expression mediated by Arg-CS was greatly enhanced by about 100-fold compared with the luciferase expression mediated by chitosan in different pH media. These results suggest that Arg-CS is a promising candidate as a safe and efficient vector for gene delivery and transfection [72].

Arg-CS/DNA self-assembled nanoparticles (ACSNs) showed that particle size and zeta potential were 200–400 nm and 0.23–12.25 mV, respectively. The transfection efficiency of ACSNs was much higher than that of CS/DNA self-assembled nanoparticles. The average cell viability of ACSNs was over 90% [73].

Folic acid (FA) is appealing as a ligand for targeting the cell membrane and allowing nanoparticle endocytosis via the folate receptor (FR) for higher transfection yields. The high affinity of folate to bind its receptor (1 nM) [72] and folate's small size allow its use in specific cell targeting. Moreover, the ability of FA to bind its receptor to allow endocytosis is not altered by covalent conjugation of small molecules [74]. FR is overexpressed on many human cancer cell surfaces [75], and the nonepithelial isoform of FR (FRX) is expressed on activated synovial macrophages present in large numbers in arthritic joints [76]. Many researchers have used FA as a ligand with cationic liposome and other polymers to target cells expressing FRs. FA–chitosan–DNA nanoparticles were synthesized using reductive amidation and a complex coacervation process [77]. FA–chitosan–DNA shows very low cytotoxicity. Moreover, the FA linkage to chitosan did not affect the properties of nanoparticles. Nanoparticle–FA aggregates are promising candidates for nonviral gene therapy in cancer and inflammatory diseases such as rheumatoid arthritis, where FA receptors are overexpressed at the cell membrane.

3.1.3 Conclusions

Chitosan has been widely used in pharmaceutical and medical areas because of favorable biological properties such as biodegradability, biocompatibility, low toxicity, hemostatic, bacteriostatic, fungistatic, anticarcinogen, and anticholesteremic properties, as well as reasonable cost. Owing to its unique cationic nature, chitosan is able to interact electrostatically with negatively charged polyions such as indomethacin, sodium hyaluronate, pectin, and acacia polysaccharides; it has been found to interact with negatively charged DNA in a similar fashion. The development of water-soluble chitosan is a prerequisite to successful implementation in gene delivery. A polycationic carrier that incorporates cell-specific ligands such as galactose has been shown to improve transfection efficiency. Bioactive molecule-conjugated chitosan would make a promising nonviral vector for targeted gene delivery.

References

1. Lydyard, P. and Grossi, C. 1998. The lymphoid system. In: Roitt, I, Brostoff, J, Male, D. eds. *Immunology*. London: Mosby, pp. 31–42.
2. Alpar, H. O., Ward, K. R., and Williamson, E. D. 2000. New strategies in vaccine delivery. *STP Pharma Sci* 10: 269–278.
3. Van der Lubben, I. M., Konings, F. A. J., Borchard, G., Verhoef, J. C., and Junginger, H. E. 2001. *In vivo* uptake of chitosan microparticles by murine Peyer's patches: Visualization studies using confocal laser scanning microscopy and immunohistochemistry. *J Drug Target* 9: 39–47.
4. Barackman, J. D., Singh, M., Ugozolli, M., Ott, G.S., and OHagan, D. T. 1998. Oral immunization with poly(lactide-co-glycolide) microparticles containing an entrapped recombinant glycoprotein (gD2) from Herpes simplex type 2 virus. *STP Pharma Sci* 8: 41–46.
5. Igartua, M., Hernandez, R. M., Esquisabel, A., Gascon, A. R., Calvo, M. B., and Pedraz, J. L. 1998. Enhanced immune response after subcutaneous and oral immunization with biodegradable PLGA microspheres. *J Control Release* 56: 63–73.
6. Cho, N. H., Seong, S. Y., Chun, K. H., Kim, Y. H., Kwon, I., Ahn, B. Y., and Jeong, S. Y. 1998. Novel mucosal immunization with polysaccharide–protein conjugates entrapped in alginate microspheres. *J Control Release* 53: 215–224.
7. Heritage, P. L., Underdown, B. J., Brook, M. A., and McDermott, M. R. 1998. Oral administration of polymer-grafted starch microparticles activates gut-associated lymphocytes and primes mice for a subsequent systemic antigen challenge. *Vaccine* 16: 2010–2017.
8. Eldridge, J. H., Hammond, C. J., Meulbroek, J. A., Staas, J. K., Gilley, R. M., and Rice, T. R. 1990. Controlled vaccine release in the gut associated lymphoid tissues. I. Orally administered biodegradable microspheres target the Peyer's patches. *J Control Release* 11: 205–214.
9. Kuper, C. F., Koornstra, P. J., Hameleers, D. M. H., Biewenga, J., Spit, B. J., Duijvestijn, A. M., van Breda Vriesman, P. J. C., and Taede Sminia, T. 1992. The role of nasopharyngeal lymphoid tissue. *Immunol Today* 13: 219–224.

10. Illum, L. 1998. Chitosan and its use as a pharmaceutical excipient. *Pharm Res* 15: 1326–1331.

11. van der Lubben, I. M., Verhoef, J. C., Borchard, G., and Junginger, H. E. 2001. Chitosan and its derivatives in mucosal drug and vaccine delivery. *Eur J Pharm Sci* 14: 201–207.

12. Calvo, P., Remunan-Lopez, C., Vila-Jato, J. L., and Alonso, M. J. 1997. Novel hydrophilic chitosan–polyethylene oxide nanoparticles as protein carriers. *J Appl Polym Sci* 16: 125–132.

13. Jameela, S. R., Kumary, T. V., Lal, A. V., and Jayakrishnan, A. 1998. Progesterone-loaded chitosan microspheres: A long acting biodegradable controlled delivery system. *J Control Release* 52: 17–24.

14. van der Lubben, I. M., Verhoef, J. C., van Aelst, A. C., Borchard, G., and Junginger, H. E. 2001. Chitosan microparticles for oral vaccination: Preparation, characterization and preliminary *in vivo* uptake studies in murine Peyer's patches. *Biomaterials* 22: 687–694.

15. van der Lubben, I. M., Kersten, G., Fretz, M. M., Beuvery, C., Verhoef, J. C., and Junginger, H. E. 2003. Chitosan microparticles for mucosal vaccination against diphtheria: Oral and nasal efficacy studies in mice. *Vaccine* 21: 1400–1408.

16. Li, X. Y., Jin, L. J., Uzonna, J. E., Li, S. Y., Liu, J. J., Li, H. Q., Lu, Y. N., Zhen, Y. H., and Xu, Y. P. 2009. Chitosan–alginate microcapsules for oral delivery of egg yolk immunoglobulin (IgY): *In vivo* evaluation in a pig model of enteric colibacillosis. *Vet Immuno Immunop* 129: 132–136.

17. Kim, T. H., Jiang, H. L., Jere, D., Park, I. K., Cho, M. H., Nah, J. W., Choi, Y. J., Akaike, T., and Cho, C. S. 2007. Chemical modification of chitosan as a gene carrier *in vitro* and *in vivo*. *Prog Polym Sci* 32: 726–753.

18. Verma, I. M., and Somia, N. 1997. Gene therapy—Promises, problems and prospects. *Nature* 389: 239–242.

19. Munier, S., Messai, I., Delair, T., Verrier, B., and Ataman-Onal, Y. 2005. Cationic PLA nanoparticles for DNA delivery: Comparison of three surface polycations for DNA binding, protection and transfection properties. *Colloids Surf B* 43: 163–173.

20. Baker, A., Saltik M., Lehrmann, H., Killisch, I., Mautner, V., Lamm, G., Christofori, G., and Cotten, M., 1997. Polyethylenimine (PEI) is a simple, inexpensive and effective reagent for condensing and linking plasmid DNA to adenovirus for gene delivery. *Gene Ther* 4: 773–782.

21. Byk, T., Haddada, H., Vainchenker, W., and Louache, F. 1998. Lipofectamine and related cationic lipids strongly improve adenoviral infection efficiency of primitive human hematopoietic cells. *Hum Gene Ther* 9: 2493–2502.

22. Lew, D., Oarker, S. E., Latimer, T., Abai, A. M., Kuwahara-Rundell, A., Doh, S. G., Yang, Z. Y., Laface, D., Gromkowski, S. H., Nabel, G. J., Manthorpe, M., and Norman, J. 1995. Cancer gene therapy using plasmid DNA: pharmacokinetic study of DNA following injection in mice. *Hum Gene Ther* 6: 553–564.

23. Lee, K. Y., Kwon, I. C., Jo, W. H., and Jeong, S. Y. 2005. Complex formation between plasmid DNA and self-aggregates of deoxycholic acid-modified chitosan. *Polymer* 46: 8107–8112.

24. Thanou, M., Florea, B. I., Geldof, M., Junginger, H. E., and Borchard, G. 2002. Quaternized chitosan oligomers as novel gene delivery vectors in epithelial cell lines. *Biomaterials* 23: 153–159.

25. Thanou, M., Verhoef, J. C., and Junginger, H. E. 2001. Oral drug absorption enhancement by chitosan and its derivatives. *Adv Drug Deliv Rev* 52 : 117–126.

26. Zhu, A. P., Fang, N., Chan-Park, M. B., and Chan, V. 2005. Interaction between O-carboxymethylchitosan and dipalmitoyl-*sn*-glycero-3-phosphocholine bilayer. *Biomaterials* 26: 6873–6879.

27. Illum, L., Jabbal-Gill, I., Hinchcliffe, M., Fisher, A. N., and Davis, S. S. 2001. Chitosan as a novel nasal delivery system for vaccines. *Adv Drug Deliv Rev* 51: 81–96.

28. Takeuchi, H., Yamamoto, H., Niwa, T., Hino, T., and Kawashima, Y. 1996. Enteral absorption of insulin in rats from mucoadhesive chitosan-coated liposomes. *Pharm Res* 13: 896–901.

29. Richardson, S. C. W., Kolbe, H. V. J., and Duncan, R. 1999. Potential of low molecular mass chitosan as a DNA delivery system: biocompatibility, body distribution and ability to complex and protect DNA. *Int J Pharm* 178: 231–243.

30. Hejazi, R. and Amiji, M. 2003. Chitosan-based gastrointestinal delivery systems. *J Control Release* 89: 151–65.
31. Illum, L., Gill, I. J., Hinchcliffe, M., Fisher, A. N., and Davis, S. S. 2001. Chitosan as a novel nasal delivery system for vaccines. *Adv Drug Deliver Rev* 51: 81–96.
32. Liu, F., and Huang, L. 2002. Development of non-viral vectors for systemic gene delivery. *J Control Release* 78: 259–266.
33. Lee, K. Y., Kwon, I. C., Kim, Y. H., Jo, W. H., and Jeong, S. Y. 1998. Preparation of chitosan self-aggregates as a gene delivery system. *J Control Release* 51: 213–220.
34. Mao, H. Q., Roy, K., Troung-Le, V. L., Janes, K. A, Lin, K. Y. Wang, Y., August, J. T., and Leong, K. W. 2001. Chitosan–DNA nanoparticles as gene carriers: Synthesis, characterization and transfection efficacy. *J Control Release* 2001; 70: 399–421.
35. Morris, V. B., Neethu, S., Abraham, E. T., Pillai, C. K. S., and Sharma, C. P. 2008. Studies on the condensation of depolymerized chitosans with DNA for preparing chitosan–DNA nanoparticles for gene delivery applications. *J Biomed Mater Res B Appl Biomater* 89B: 282–292.
36. Morris, V. B., Emilia, A., and Pillai, C. K. S. 2006. Studies on dispersive stability of DNA–chitosan complexes on varying the molecular weight and degree on deacetylation of chitosan. *Asian Chitin J* 2: 39–44.
37. Sato T., Ishii T., and Okahata, Y. 2001. *In vitro* gene delivery mediated by chitosan. Effect of pH, serum, and molecular mass of chitosan on the transfection efficiency. *Biomaterials* 22: 2075–2080.
38. Ishii, T., Okahata, Y., and Sato, T. 2001. Mechanism of cell transfection with plasmid/chitosan complexes. *Biochimica et Biophysica Acta* 15: 51–64.
39. Lee, J. M., Ha, K. S., and Yoo, H. S. 2008. Quantum-dot-assisted fluorescence resonance energy transfer approach for intracellular trafficking of chitosan/DNA complex. *Acta Biomater* 4: 791–798.
40. Gao, Y., Zhang, Z. W., Chen, L. L., Gu, W. W., and Li, Y. P. 2009. Chitosan *N*-betainates/DNA self-assembly nanoparticles for gene delivery: *In vitro* uptake and transfection efficiency. *Int J Pharm* 371: 156–162.
41. Thanou, M., Florea, B. I., Geldof, M., Junginger, H. E., and Borchard, G. 2002. Quaternized chitosan oligomers as novel gene delivery vectors in epithelial cell lines. *Biomaterials* 23: 153–159.
42. Germershaus, O., Mao, S., Sitterberg, J., Bakowsky, U., and Kissel, T. 2008. Gene delivery using chitosan, trimethyl chitosan or polyethyleneglycol-graft-trimethyl chitosan block copolymers: Establishment of structure–activity relationships *in vitro*. *J Control Release* 125: 145–154.
43. Mao, S. R., Shuai, X. T., Unger, F., Wittmar, M., Xie, X. L., and Kissel, T. 2005. Synthesis, characterization and cytotoxicity of poly(ethylene glycol)-graft-trimethyl chitosan block copolymers. *Biomaterials* 26: 6343–6356.
44. Kean, T., Roth, S., and Thanou, M. 2005. Trimethylated chitosans as non-viral gene delivery vectors: cytotoxicity and transfection efficiency. *J Control Release* 103: 643–653.
45. Yoo, H. S., Lee, J. E., Chung, H., Kwon, I. C., and Jeong, S. Y. 2005. Self-assembled nanoparticles containing hydrophobically modified glycol chitosan for gene delivery. *J Control Release* 103: 235–243.
46. Hu, F. Q., Zhao, M. D., Yuan, H., You, J., Du, Y. Z., and Zeng, S. 2006. A novel chitosan oligosaccharide–stearic acid micelles for gene delivery: Properties and *in vitro* transfection studies. *Int J Pharm* 315: 158–166.
47. You, J. O., Liu, Y. C., and Peng, C. A. 2006. Efficient gene transfection using chitosan–alginate core-shell nanoparticles. *Int J Nanomed* 1: 173–180.
48. Li, X. Y., Jin, L. J., and Mcallister, T. A. 2007. Chitosan–alginate microcapsules for oral delivery of egg yolk immunoglobulin (IgY). *J Agr Food Chem* 55: 2911–2917.
49. Peng, S. F., Yang, M. J., Su, C. J., Chen, H. L., Lee, P. W., Wei, M. C., and Sung, H. W. 2009. Effects of incorporation of poly(γ-glutamic acid) in chitosan/DNA complex nanoparticles on cellular uptake and transfection efficiency. *Biomaterials* 30: 1797–1808.

50. Duceppe, N. and Tabrizian, M. 2009. Factors influencing the transfection efficiency of ultra low molecular weight chitosan/hyaluronic acid nanoparticles. *Biomaterials* 30: 2625–2631.

51. Csaba, O., Köping-Höggård, M., and Alonso, M. J. 2009. Ionically cross-linked chitosan/trip-olyphosphate nanoparticles for oligonucleotide and plasmid DNA delivery. *Int J Pharm* 382: 205–214.

52. Kumar, M., Behera, A. K., Lockey, R. F., Zhang, J., Bhullar, G., de la Cruz, C. P., Chen, L. C., Leong, K. W., Huang, S. K., and Mohapatra, S. S. 2002. Intranasal gene transfer by chitosan–DNA nanospheres protects BALB/c mice against acute respiratory syncytial virus infection. *Hum Gene Ther* 13: 1415–1425.

53. Xu, W., Shen, Y., Jiang, Z., Wang, Y., Chu, Y., and Xiong, S. 2004. Intranasal delivery of chitosan–DNA vaccine generates mucosal SIgA and anti-CVB3 protection. *Vaccine* 22: 3603–3612.

54. Sun, C. J., Pan, S. P., Xie, Q. X., and Xiao, L. J. 2004. Preparation of chitosan–plasmid DNA nanoparticles encoding zona pellucida glycoprotein-mouse. *Mol Reprod Dev* 68: 182–188.

55. Okamoto, H., Nishida, S., Tod, H., Sakabura, Y., Iida, K., and Danjo, K. 2003. Pulmonary gene delivery by chitosan–pDNA complex powder prepared by a supercritical carbon dioxide process. *J Pharm Sci* 92: 371–380.

56. Howard, K. A., Paludan, S. R., Behlke, M. A., Besenbacher, F., Deleuran, B., and Kjems, J. 2008. Chitosan/siRNA nanoparticle-mediated TNF-α knockdown in peritoneal macrophages for anti-inflammatory treatment in a murine arthritis model. *Mol Ther* 17: 162–168.

57. Kim, T. H., Kim, S. I., Akaike, T., and Cho, C. S. 2005. Synergistic effect of poly (ethylenimine) on the transfection efficiency of galactosylated chitosan/DNA complexes. *J Control Release* 105: 354–366.

58. Lin, W. J. and Chen, M. H. 2007. Synthesis of multifunctional chitosan with galactose as a targeting ligand for glycoprotein receptor. *Carbohydr Polym* 67: 474–480.

59. Chung, T. W., Yang, J., Akaike, T., Cho, K. Y., Nah, J. W., Kim, S. I., and Cho, C. S. 2002. Preparation of alginate/galactosylated chitosan scaffold for hepatocyte attachment. *Biomaterials* 23: 2827–2834.

60. Park, Y. K., Park, Y. H., Shin, B. A., Choi, E. S., Park, Y. R., Akaike, T., and Cho, C. S. 2000. Galactosylated chitosan-graft-dextran as hepatocyte-targeting DNA carrier. *J Control Release* 69: 97–108.

61. Park, I. K., Kim, T. H., Park, Y. H., Shin, B. A., Choi, E. S., Chowdhury, E. H., Akaike, T., and Cho, C. S. 2001. Galactosylated chitosan-graft-poly(ethylene glycol) as hepatocyte-targeting DNA carrier. *J Control Release* 76: 349–362.

62. Dai, H., Jiang, X., Tan, G. C. Y., Chen, Y., Torbenson, M., Leong, K. W., and Mao, H. Q. 2006. Chitosan–DNA nanoparticles delivered by intrabiliary infusion enhance liver-targeted gene delivery. *Int J Nanomed* 1: 507–522.

63. Hashimoto, M., Morimoto, M., Saimoto, H., Shigemasa, Y., Yanagie, H., Eriguchi, M., and Sato, T. 2006. Gene transfer by DNA/mannosylated chitosan complexes into mouse peritoneal macrophages. *Biotechnol Lett* 28: 815–821.

64. Zhou, X. F., Liu, B., Yu, X. H., Zha, X., Zhang, X. Z., Chen, Y., Wang, X. Y., Jin, Y. H., and Wu, Y. G. 2007. Controlled release of PEI/DNA complexes from mannose-bearing chitosan microspheres as a potent delivery system to enhance immune response to HBV DNA vaccine. *J Control Release* 121: 200–207.

65. Song, B. F., Zhang, W., Peng, R., Huang, J., Nie, T., Li, Y., Jiang, Q., and Gao, R. 2009. Synthesis and cell activity of novel galactosylated chitosan as a gene carrier. *Colloid Surf B* 70: 181–186.

66. Tung, C. H. and Weissleder, R. 2003. Arginine containing peptides as delivery vectors. *Adv Drug Deliv Rev* 55: 281–294.

67. Futaki, S. 2005. Membrane-permeable arginine-rich peptides and the translocation mechanisms. *Adv Drug Deliv Rev* 57: 547–558.

68. Eguchi, A., Akuta, T., Okuyama, H., Senda, T., Yokoi, H., Inokuchi, H., Fujita, S., Hayakawa, T., Takeda, K., Hasegawa, M., and Nakanishi, M. 2001. Protein transduction domain of HIV-1Tat protein promotes efficient delivery of DNA into mammalian cells. *J Biol Chem* 276: 26204–26210.

69. Nakanishi, M., Eguchi, A., Akuta, T., Nagoshi, E., Fujita, S., Okabe, J., Senda, T., and Hasegawa, M. 2003. Basic peptides as functional components of non-viral gene transfer vehicles. *Curr Prot Pept Sci* 4: 141–150.

70. Furuhata, M., Kawakami, H., Toma, K., Hattori, Y., and Maitani, Y. 2006. Design, synthesis and gene delivery efficiency of novel oligo-arginine-linked PEG-lipids: Effect of oligo-arginine length. *Int J Pharm* 316: 109–116.

71. Choi, J. S., Nam, K., Park, J. Y., Kim, J. B., Lee, J. K., and Park, J. S. 2004. Enhanced transfection efficiency of PAMAM dendrimer by surface modification with l-arginine. *J Control Release* 99: 445–456.

72. Zhu, D. W., Zhang, H. L., Bai, J. G., Liu, W. G., Leng, X. G., Song, C. X. Yang, J., Li, X. W., Jin, X., Song, L. P., Liu, L. X., Li, X. L., Zhang, Y., and Yao, K. D. 2007. Enhancement of transfection efficiency for HeLa cells via incorporating arginine moiety into chitosan. *Chinese Sci Bull* 52: 3207–3215.

73. Gao, Y., Xu, Z. H., Chen, S. W., Gu, W. W., Chen, L. L., and Li, Y. P. 2008. Arginine-chitosan/DNA self-assemble nanoparticles for gene delivery: *In vitro* characteristics and transfection efficiency. *Int J Pharm* 359: 241–246.

74. Lee, R. J., and Low, P. S. 1994. Delivery of liposomes into cultured KB cells via folate receptor-mediated endocytosis. *J Biol Chem* 4: 3198–3204.

75. Antony, A. C. 1996. Folate receptors. *Annu Rev Nutr* 16: 501–521.

76. Turkm, M. J., Breur, G. J., Widmer, W. R., Paulos, C. M., Xu, L. C., Grote, L. A., and Low, P. S. 2002. Folate-targeted imaging of activated macrophages in rats with adjuvant-induced arthritis. *Arthritis Rheum* 46: 1947–1955.

77. Mansouri, S., Cuie, Y., Winnik, F., Shi, Q., Lavigne, P., Benderdour, M., Beaumont, E., and Fernandes, J. C. 2006. Characterization of folate–chitosan–DNA nanoparticles for gene therapy. *Biomaterials* 27: 2060–2065.

3.2 Blood Compatibility

3.2.1 Hemolytic Potential

Chitosan microspheres were found to have great utility in drug carrier and delivery systems [78]. More recent research published in the major biomaterial journals has focused on the area of implantable applications of chitosan, including orthopedic/periodontal applications, tissue engineering, and wound healing [79]. Chitosan microspheres are potentially useful as bone and periodontal filling materials [80,81]. Li et al. [82] reported that chitosan–alginate microspheres had excellent short- and long-term effects on renal arterial embolization. The preceding section highlighted the principal implantable application of chitosan microspheres, among which chitosan microspheres have the opportunity to make contact with blood. Therefore, the blood coagulation property seems to be important for the safe use of chitosan microspheres.

3.2.1.1 Preparation of Chitosan Microspheres

Chitosan microspheres were prepared by following a patented procedure [83]. Chitosan was dissolved in an acetic acid aqueous solution (1%, v/v) and dropped into toluene (oil phases) containing 1% (v/v) Tween-80 and 1% Span-80 through a nozzle. The mixture was stirred vigorously for 30 min and formaldehyde (15 mL) was added into the reaction system for 1 h; then chitosan microspheres were separated, washed with deionized water, and further cross-linked chemically with glutaraldehyde (0.025 wt%) for 2 h. Next, chitosan microspheres were treated with H_2O_2, washed repeatedly and dehydrated successively with ethanol (30%, 50%, 80%, 95%, and 100%), and finally vacuum dried overnight.

3.2.1.2 Blood Collection and Platelet Isolation

Swine blood was collected from a cannulated femoral artery under nonactivation conditions and anticoagulated with acid citrate dextrose (20 mM citric acid, 110 mM sodium citrate and 5 mM d-glucose) at a v/v ratio of 9:1 or 1 U/mL heparin, as per the protocol approved by the DSO Institutional Animal Care and Use Committee. To isolate platelet solutions, whole blood was centrifuged at 180 g for 20 min, and platelet-rich plasma was separated from the red blood cell (RBC) fraction and further centrifuged at 1500 g for 15 min to pellet and concentrate the platelets. The platelet pellet was removed and resuspended in a buffer (140 mM NaCl, 3 mM KCl, 12 mM $NaHCO_3$, 0.4 mM NaH_2PO_4 and 0.1% glucose, pH 7.4, adjusted with 4% HEPES). The concentration of the platelet suspension was measured using the Cell-Dyn 500 hemostasis analyzer (Abbott Laboratories, IL, USA). Only suspensions with >100,000 platelets/mL were used in experiments.

3.2.1.3 Dynamic Blood Clotting Test

For clotting time measurement, a kinetic method similar to the work described by K. Y. Lee [84] was used. Microspheres were put into beakers and placed in a thermostat at 37°C for 5 min; then ACD whole blood stay focused on the prepositions (0.25 mL) was dropped onto the surface of these microspheres, followed by the addition of 0.02 mL $CaCl_2$ solution (0.2 mol/L). The blood clotting test was carried out by spectrophotometric measurement at 540 nm. The relative absorbency of 0.25 mL ACD whole blood diluted in 50 mL distilled water was assumed to be 100. The blood clotting index (BCI) of a biomaterial can be quantified by using the following equation:

$$\text{BCI (\%)} = \frac{\text{Absorbency of blood in contact with the sample}}{\text{Absorbency of the solution of distilled water and ACD blood}} \times 100$$

The platelet suspensions (0.5 mL) were spread over the microspheres and incubated at 37°C. After the specified incubation period, the platelet suspensions were counted using a cytometer.

$$\text{Adhesion ratio (\%)} = \frac{\text{Total platelets} - \text{Suspension plates}}{\text{Total platelets}} \times 100$$

3.2.1.4 Platelet Adhesion and Aggregation

The microspheres after incubation were gently and uniformly washed with 0.1 M PBS (pH 7.4), fixed with 2.5% glutaraldehyde solution in saline at 4°C for 2 days, washed with saline and dehydrated with a series of graded ethanol–water solutions (0, 30, 50, 70, 90, and 100%), and dried under vacuum conditions overnight. The dried microspheres after gold coating were examined with a scanning electron microscope.

3.2.1.5 Hemolysis Test

The hemolytic activity of microspheres was investigated according to Singhal's method [85]. Fresh rabbit blood was diluted using saline water (1:1.25, v/v). Microspheres with different concentrations were suspended in 10 mL of 0.9% NaCl solution and incubated for 1 h at 37°C in a shaking water bath. Diluted blood (0.2 mL) was added into microsphere suspensions and incubated for 1 h. The release of hemoglobin was determined after centrifugation (700 g for 10 min) by photometric analysis of the supernatant at 545 nm. Positive and negative controls were produced by adding 0.2 mL of diluted blood to 10 mL of distilled water and saline water. Percentage hemolysis was calculated as follows:

$$\text{Hemolysis (\%)} = \frac{AS - AN}{AP - AN} \times 100$$

where AS, AP, and AN are the absorbencies of sample, positive control, and negative control. Less than 10% hemolysis was regarded as the nontoxic effect level.

3.2.1.6 Sodium Dodecyl Sulfate-Polyacrylamide Gel Electrophoresis

Sodium dodecyl sulfate-polyacrylamide gel electrophoresis (SDS-PAGE) was performed on vertical slab gels (18 × 13 × 0.1 cm³). Resolving and stacking gel conditions were 8% and 5% acrylamine, respectively. Protein extract samples were mixed in a 1:1 ratio with sample buffer and heated at 100°C for 5 min; then 20 mL of protein–buffer solution was applied to the gel. The protein was visualized by staining with Coomassie Brilliant Blue R-250. MWs were estimated using the linear relationship between the lag of the MW of the standards and relative mobility.

3.2.1.7 Hemolytic Properties

Figure 3.1 shows the dynamic blood clotting profiles for chitosan microspheres. The absorbance of the hemolyzed hemoglobin solution varied with time. Chitosan microspheres showed a rapid decrease of BCI at 5 min, while the control exhibited the same phenomenon at 10 min. The time at which absorbance equals 0.01 was generally defined as the clotting time, and the slower the decrease of BCI value with time, the longer the clotting

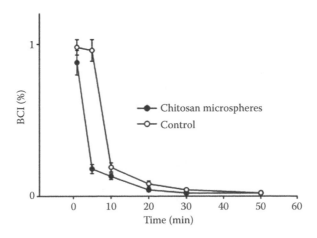

FIGURE 3.1
BCI of chitosan microspheres.

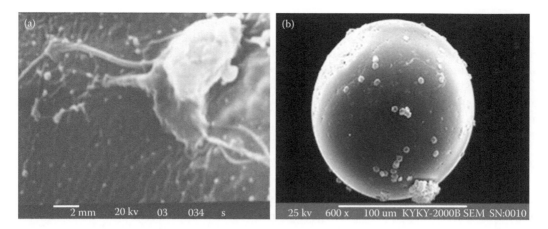

FIGURE 3.2
Scanning electron micrographs of platelets and erythrocytes on chitosan microsphere surfaces. (a) Platelets with pseudopodia and (b) erythrocyte aggregation.

time [86]. The clotting time for chitosan microspheres was 30 min compared to 50 min for the control, indicating that chitosan microspheres can induce blood coagulation.

The morphology of aggregated platelets in each microsphere was investigated using scanning electron microscopy (SEM) (Figure 3.2a). Platelets adhered strongly on the surface with pseudopodia. Furthermore, platelets were bound to each other and formed the aggregated mass. Erythrocytes considerably adhered on the surface of chitosan microspheres. The surface thus tended to enhance erythrocyte agglutination or agglomeration (Figure 3.2b). Table 3.1 shows the results obtained for hemolysis of rabbit blood with chitosan microspheres. It was observed that hemolysis was less than 5% at the concentration of 1 mg/mL chitosan microspheres, which was well within the permissible limit. When the concentration of microspheres changed to 100 mg/mL, chitosan showed a little hemolysis, with the value 7.99%.

To examine the specific interactions of protein with microspheres, adsorption for plasma was studied using SDS-PAGE. Figure 3.3 shows gels of proteins adsorbed to microspheres from 4% plasma. It can be seen that by comparing the microsphere gels (lane 3) to the gel of the plasma (lane 2), the surface of chitosan microspheres bound a large amount of plasma proteins, a fact that may explain the observed coagulation behavior of chitosan microspheres.

When blood is in contact with a foreign material surface, adsorption of plasma proteins occurs first, followed by platelet adhesion and deformation. These platelets release substrates that start the coagulation process, resulting in thrombosis. Blood compatibility

TABLE 3.1

Hemolytic Activity of Chitosan Microspheres with Different Concentration

Sample	Optical Density at 545 nm	Hemolysis (%)
Distilled water	0.866 ± 0.041	+ve control
Normal saline	0.035 ± 0.010	−ve contol
Chitosan microspheres (500 mg/mL)	0.103 ± 0.020	7.99%
Chitosan microspheres (500 mg/mL)	0.044 ± 0.009	1.20%

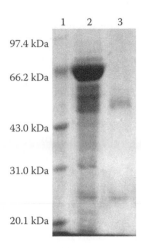

FIGURE 3.3
SDS-PAGE gel stained by Coomassie Blue. Lane 1, marker; lane 2, 4% of the plasma before adsorption; lane 3, supernatant after adsorption of chitosan.

is reached when there is not too much interaction of platelets with the material surface. Therefore, platelet adhesion on microspheres from blood is an important test for the evaluation of blood compatibility of microspheres. Platelet adhesion and activation are two important steps that regulate the formation of the thrombus and medical device rejection. During the initial stage of surface activation, the change in conformation of adsorbed proteins exposes RGD sequences that are sensitive to the platelet GPIIb/III receptor. When platelets are surface activated, they progress through a sequence of morphological changes. The surface activation contributes to the change in the organization of the cytoskeleton, and thus increases the surface area of platelets by the formation of pseudopods. The platelets thus, adhered and activated, go through a sequence of cytoskeletal events and increase in endoplasmic Ca^{2+} concentration, polymerization of action filaments, thrombin activation, and release of cytoskeletal granule contents, as well as platelet aggregation. The extent of shape change and spread area has been related to the surface energy of polymer materials [87]. Chitosan microspheres make them activated. Chou et al. [88] demonstrated that chitosan is an effective inducer of rabbit platelet adhesion and aggregation, and explained that the mechanisms of action of chitosan may be associated with the increase of Ca^{2+} mobilization and the enhancement of expression of the GPIIb–IIIa complex. It has also been reported that chitosan and chitin enhance platelet aggregation due to their amino residues [89]. In acidic solution, the amine groups of chitosan are protonated to $-NH_3^+$, which makes chitosan cationic in nature, allowing for electrostatic interactions with the negatively charged biological molecules on the platelet surface [90].

The shortening of clotting time by chitosan may be related to not only platelet aggregation but also erythrocyte aggregation [89]. Earlier it was observed that the procoagulation properties of chitosan were partly due to erythrocytes [91]. Chitosan may induce the adhesion of erythrocytes with its amino groups or by forming a three-dimensional network structure in blood that captures the erythrocytes and then makes them aggregates [92]. In this system [93], chitosan microspheres were directly immersed into erythrocyte suspension without any blood proteins. The surface of chitosan microspheres greatly enhanced erythrocyte agglutination or agglomeration, which indicated that chitosan can directly induce erythrocyte adhesion without forming any dimensional network structure or adsorbing any plasma proteins at first. The reason for the promotion of erythrocyte aggregation may be due to its cationic nature. Furthermore, it can also adsorb various plasma proteins, which may enhance procoagulation.

Hemolysis of blood is the problem associated with bioincompatibility [94]. Previous studies indicated that chitosan promoted surface-induced hemolysis, which can be attributed in part to electrostatic interactions [90,95]. In the literature [93], when the concentration of microspheres adds up to 100 mg/mL, chitosan showed a little hemolysis. However, the largest hemolytic activity was lower than 10%, which indicated a wide safety margin in blood contacting applications and suitability for i.v. administration [96,97]. Furthermore, by comparing the low hemolytic activity with the high erythrocyte agglutination, it was shown that chitosan only induces the adhesion of erythrocytes but does not seriously damage the cell membrane.

The procoagulation properties of chitosan microspheres give them the potential for use as thrombospheres. Most thrombospheres (Hemosphere, Irvine, CA) are composed of cross-linked human albumin with human fibrinogen bound to the surface. A similar product, Synthocytes (Andaris Group Ltd, Nottingham, UK), has just entered clinical trials in Europe [98].

3.2.2 Hemostatic Potential

3.2.2.1 Characterization

Whole-blood clotting: The blood clotting test was adapted from Shih et al. [99]. Dressings were placed in polypropylene (PP) tubes and prewarmed to 37°C. Citrated whole blood (0.2 mL) was then dispensed onto the dressings, and 20 mL of 0.2 M $CaCl_2$ solution was added to start coagulation. The tubes were incubated at 37°C and shaken at 30 rpm. After 10 min, RBCs that were not trapped in the clot were hemolyzed with 25 mL of water, and the absorbance of the resulting hemoglobin solution was measured at 540 nm.

Platelet adhesion: The platelet adhesion assay was adapted from Vanickova et al. [100]. Before the start of the test, platelets were reconstituted to 2.5 mM $CaCl_2$ and 1.0 mM $MgCl_2$. Then 1.5 mL of the platelet suspension was added to each dressing. After incubation at 37°C for 1 h, the dressings were removed and dip rinsed twice in PBS to remove platelets that were not attached. Samples were then placed in PBS containing 0.9% Triton-X100 for 1 h at 37°C to lyse the adhered platelets. The lactate dehydrogenase (LDH) enzyme that was released was measured using a kit (Promega, USA) as per the manufacturer's instructions. A platelet calibration curve was generated by serially diluting a known number of platelets, followed by lysis with 0.9% Triton-X100 and measurement of LDH. Samples were also fixed in 4% paraformaldehyde and 0.5% glutaraldehyde for electron microscopy studies.

Thrombin generation: Thrombin–antithrombin complex (TAT), a marker of thrombin neutralization, is an indicator of how much thrombin was formed over a period of time [101]. Dressings were incubated with 1 mL of heparinized whole blood for 30 min at 37°C and then 20 mL of sodium citrate (0.633 M) was added to stop thrombin generation. TAT levels in blood samples were measured by an ELISA kit (DadeBehring, Germany) as per the manufacturer's instructions.

Blood and simulated body fluid (SBF) absorption: The absorption efficiency of dressings was determined in citrated whole blood and SBF, a solution with ion concentrations similar to that of human plasma. SBF consists of 142 mM Na^+, 5.0 mM K^+, 2.5 mM Ca^{2+}, 148 mM Cl^-,

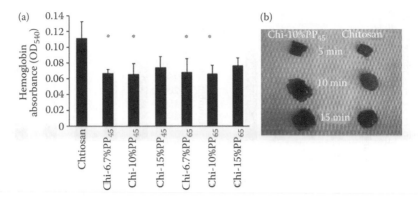

FIGURE 3.4
(a) Effect of the proportion and type of PP in chitosan on blood clotting rates, as measured by absorbance of hemoglobin from lyzed uncoagulated RBCs. $*p < 0.05$ compared to chitosan, analyzed by one-way ANOVA with the post-hoc Scheffe test, $n = 4$. (b) Photograph showing more rapid clot formation on chitosan–10% PP compared to chitosan. (From Park, C. J. et al. 2009. *Acta Biomater* 5: 1926–1936. With permission.)

4.2 mM HCO_3^-, 1.0 mM HPO_4^{2-}, and 5.0 mM SO_4^{2-}, and was buffered at pH 7.4 with tris(hydroxymethyl)aminomethane and 1 M hydrochloric acid at 37°C. Weighed dry dressings (*Wini*) were placed in tissue culture plate wells containing 1.5 mL of SBF or citrated whole blood. Plates were sealed and incubated in a humidified chamber at 37°C. At the end of 2 h, the dressings were removed, placed on absorbent paper towel for 3 s to remove surface water and freely draining liquid, and weighed to determine wet weight (*Wwet*). Fluid uptake (g/g) was calculated as (*Wwet – Win*)/*Wini*.

3.2.2.2 Hemostatic Potential of Chitosan and Its Derivatives

Hemorrhage remains a leading cause of early death after trauma, and infectious complications in combat wounds continue to challenge caregivers. Chitosan and its derivatives were developed to address these problems, chitosan containing different amounts and types of polyphosphate polymers was fabricated, and their hemostatic efficacies were evaluated *in vitro*.

Figure 3.4a shows the effect of the proportion and type of PP in chitosan on blood clotting rates, as measured by absorbance of hemoglobin from lyzed uncoagulated blood. A higher absorbance value of the hemoglobin solution thus indicates a slower clotting rate. Chitosan with 6.7% w/w or 10% w/w PP65 or PP45 led to significantly lower absorbance values than chitosan (Figure 3.4a). The clots formed on chitosan–10% PP45 were also visibly larger than those on chitosan at 10 min (Figure 3.4b). Blood clotting rates on gauze were significantly slower than on chitosan ($p < 0.05$), while the absorbance value of no-sample controls was significantly higher than that of chitosan-based materials ($p < 0.001$) but not gauze ($p = 0.362$). This indicates that gauze was not able to cause significant blood clotting within 10 min. Significantly more platelets adhered on chitosan–10% PP45 ($p < 0.01$) and chitosan–10% PP65 ($p < 0.05$) than on chitosan (Figure 3.5a), while significantly fewer platelets adhered on gauze than on chitosan ($p < 0.001$). More platelets were also observed on chitosan–10% PP45 than on chitosan under SEM (Figures 3.5c and f). In addition, larger platelet aggregates and more extensive platelet pseudopod formation can be observed on chitosan–10% PP45 compared to

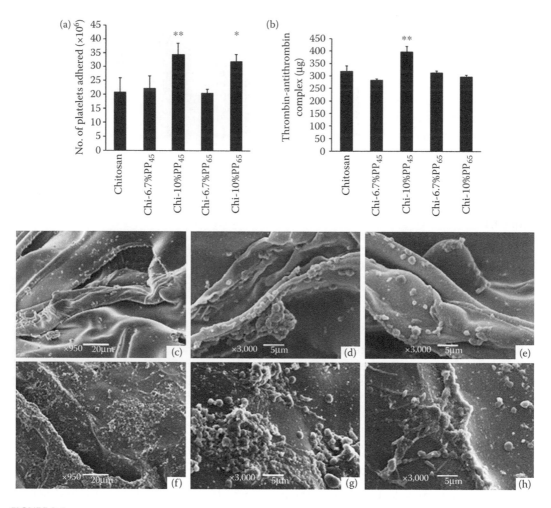

FIGURE 3.5
Effect of the proportion and type of PP in chitosan on (a) platelet adhesion and (b) thrombin generation over time, as measured by the levels of the TAT complex. $*p < 0.05$ and $**p < 0.005$ compared to chitosan, analyzed by one-way ANOVA with the post-hoc Scheffe test, $n = 4$. SEM micrographs show that more platelets adhered on chitosan–10% PP (f) than on chitosan (c); the scale bar represents 20 μm. Platelets also formed more aggregates and pseudopods on chitosan–10% PP (g, h) than on chitosan (d, e); the scale bar represents 5 μm.

chitosan (Figures 3.5d, e, g, and h). Only bloodcontacted with chitosan–10% PP45 had significantly higher TAT levels than chitosan after 30 min (Figure 3.5b). The level of TAT in blood contacted with hitosan–10% PP45 was 100-fold higher than baseline no-sample controls. Significantly lower levels of TAT were measured in blood contacted with gauze ($p < 0.05$) than in blood contacted with chitosan-based biomaterials. After immersion for 2 h in respective fluids, chitosan–10% PP45 (coded as ChiPP) absorbed about two times as much blood as chitosan (16.3 ± 1.8 g/g compared to 8.2 ± 0.8 g/g, $p < 0.001$, one-way ANOVA with the post-hoc Scheffe test, $n = 5$). Both chitosan and chitosan PP absorbed about the same amount of SBF ($w = 17.5$ g/g, not significant). Gauze absorbed about 5.2 g/g of both blood and SBF, which was significantly less than both chitosan-based materials ($p < 0.001$, $n = 5$).

3.2.2.3 Hemostatic Mechanism

Protonated amine groups of chitosan can attract negatively charged residues on RBC membranes, causing strong hemagglutination [103–106]. Chitosan also adsorbed fibrinogen and plasma proteins, enhancing platelet aggregation [107,108].

On the other hand, polyphosphate specifically activated the contact pathway, which shortened both the time lag for initial thrombin generation and the time to peak thrombin generation. Polyphosphate in the dressing would accelerate the production of sufficient amounts of thrombin to support earlier fibrin generation. At the same time, chitosan would recruit RBCs to enlarge and solidify the growing thrombus, leading to a stable clot that stops bleeding. While chitosan containing 6.7% w/w and 10% w/w PP accelerated whole-blood clotting compared to chitosan, the benefits of PP were negated at higher concentrations (15% w/w). One possible explanation is the following: At lower PP levels, the accelerated thrombin generation and resultant fibrin formation could trap more RBCs that were aggregated on chitosan into the clot. However, at higher PP levels, free cationic amine groups of chitosan were reduced to an extent that significantly reduced its ability to electrostatically attract and bring RBCs in close proximity with fibrin. The dressing's ability to adhere RBCs was significant, not only because RBCs provided bulk to the clot, but more importantly because adhered RBCs have been shown to deform and expose procoagulant phospholipids (phosphatidylserine) on the membrane surface, similar to activated platelets [109]. These procoagulant sites allowed the assembly of prothrombinase complexes that catalyze the conversion of prothrombin to thrombin [110].

PP may be required above a critical level to significantly shorten the lag time for initial thrombin generation and lead to faster platelet activation and adhesion [109]. Alternatively, complexes containing different proportions of PP may have different surface charge distributions, which affected electrostatic interactions between plasma proteins and in turn affected platelet binding and subsequent activation [110].

The type of polyphosphate polymer in the complex may also affect hemostatic activity. Chitosan–10% PP45 induced significantly faster thrombin generation than chitosan, while chitosan–10% PP65 dressings containing the same amount of polyphosphate did not. Since there were a greater number of polyphosphate chains (albeit 20 units shorter) in the chitosan–10% PP45 complex compared with the chitosan–10% PP65 complex, the frequency of complexed segments, rather than the size of complexed segments, may be more critical for increasing the number of procoagulant sites on the material, which accelerated coagulation cascade turnover and led to faster thrombin formation.

3.2.3 Blood Compatibility

In recent years, various biomaterials that are natural or synthetic polymeric materials have been widely used for manufactory biomedical applications such as artificial organs, medical devices, and disposable clinical apparatus [111]. These include vascular prostheses, blood pumps, artificial kidneys, heart valves, pacemaker lead wire insulation, intra-aortic balloons, artificial hearts, dialyzers, and plasma separators, which could be used in contact with blood. However, the polymers currently used are conventional materials, such as cellulose, chitosan, poly(tetrafluoroethylene) (PTFE), poly(vinyl chloride) (PVC), segmented polyetherurethane (SPU), polyethylene (PE), silicone rubber (SR), nylon, and polysulfone (PSf). When in direct contact with blood, they are still prone to initiating the formation of clots, as platelets and other components of the blood coagulation system are activated. It is well known that the formation of a thrombus is dependent on the behavior of platelets at or near the surface and/or on the protein-based coagulation cascade, whereas these are harmful for maintaining a well-balanced function even the life during the treatment of patients. For example, thrombogenicity of artificial organs, such as artificial heart valves (AHVs), is a serious problem. Many of the deaths in animals given AHVs were caused not by the malfunction of the artificial organ but by blood clot formation. Hence patients with mechanical heart values must undergo lifelong anticoagulation therapy. Even so, the incidence of thrombogenic complications and bleeding complications has been 1.5–3% per year in the USA, and 58% of implanted mechanical heart valves have failed within the past 12 years in China [112]. Improving the hemocompatibility of this kind of device has become a very important task for biomedical material scientists [112].

Chitosan exhibits properties that make it a desirable candidate for biocompatible and blood-compatible biomaterials [113–115]. *N*-acyl chitosans have already been reported as blood-compatible materials [84].

3.2.3.1 Platelet Adhesion

Samples were rinsed with PBS and contacted at 37°C during 1 h with freshly prepared platelet-rich plasma (PRP) of human blood. Samples were rinsed with PBS and then treated with 2.5% glutaraldehyde for 30 min at room temperature. The samples were washed with PBS again and subsequently dehydrated by systemic immersion in a series of ethanol–water solutions (50%, 60%, 70%, 80%, 90%, 95%, and 100% v/v) for 30 min each and allowed to evaporate at room temperature. Blood platelet adhesion *in vitro* was observed through SEM. The platelet-attached surfaces were coated with gold prior to being observed by SEM.

3.2.3.2 Protein Adsorption

Bovine fibrinogen (BFG, Sigma, F-8630) was obtained as lyophilized powder. The buffer solution used in the protein adsorption experiments was PBS, pH 7.4. Quantification of adsorbed protein on the polymer surfaces was performed using ^{125}I-labeled protein. ^{125}I-labeled protein was added to unlabeled protein solution in order to obtain a final activity of about 10^7 cpm/mg. The samples were immersed in 1 mL of buffer solution at 37°C, and then 1 mL of fibrinogen solution (0.2 mg/mL) was added and mixed. Adsorption tests were carried out at 37°C during 1 h. After protein adsorption, samples were rinsed three times with 2 mL of buffer solution. Gamma activities were counted with the samples placed in radio-immunoassay tubes by a Gamma Counter. Four replicates were used. The counts from each sample were averaged and the surface concentration was calculated by the equation

$$\text{BFG}\,(\mu g/cm^2) = \frac{\text{Counts}\,(\text{cpm}) \cdot C_{\text{solution}}\,(\mu g/mL)}{A_{\text{solution}}\,(\text{cpm}/mL) \cdot S_{\text{samples}}\,(cm^2)}$$

where the count measures the radioactivity, S_{samples} measures the surface area of the samples, and C_{solution} and A_{solution} are the concentration and specific activity of the protein solution, respectively.

3.2.3.3 Blood-Compatible Chitosan Derivatives

O-Butyrylchitosan (OBCS) was prepared as follows [116,117]. Chitosan (2.1 g) was added to methanesulfonic acid (11 mL) and the mixture was stirred at 0°C for 15 min until a

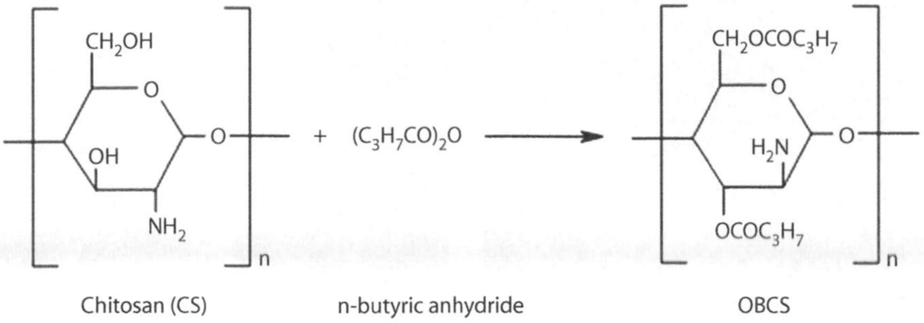

FIGURE 3.6
Scheme of OBCS synthesis.

homogeneous solution was obtained. Butyric anhydride (20 mL) was added dropwise and the total mixture was stirred at between 0°C and 5°C for 2 h. The resulting gel was stored at 15°C overnight. Pouring into acetone precipitated the thawed product, after which the acylated chitosan was dried *in vacuo*. The synthesis of OBCS is shown in Figure 3.6.

OBCS [118], a kind of water-soluble derivative of chitosan, can be covalently immobilized onto PE film surface using the photosensitive heterobifunctional cross-linking reagent 4-azidobenzoic acid, which was previously bonded to OBCS by reaction between an acid group of the cross-linking reagent and a free amino group of OBCS, as seen in Figure 3.7.

Platelet adhesion results are shown in Figure 3.8. The blank PE film showed high platelet adhesion; most of the adhered platelets were distorted with pseudopodia. However, the surfaces of OBCS surface-modified films have nearly no platelets adhered. The platelet adhesion test revealed that films immobilized by OBCS show excellent antiplatelet adhesion. It is considered that the improved antithrombogenicity can be attributed to OBCS.

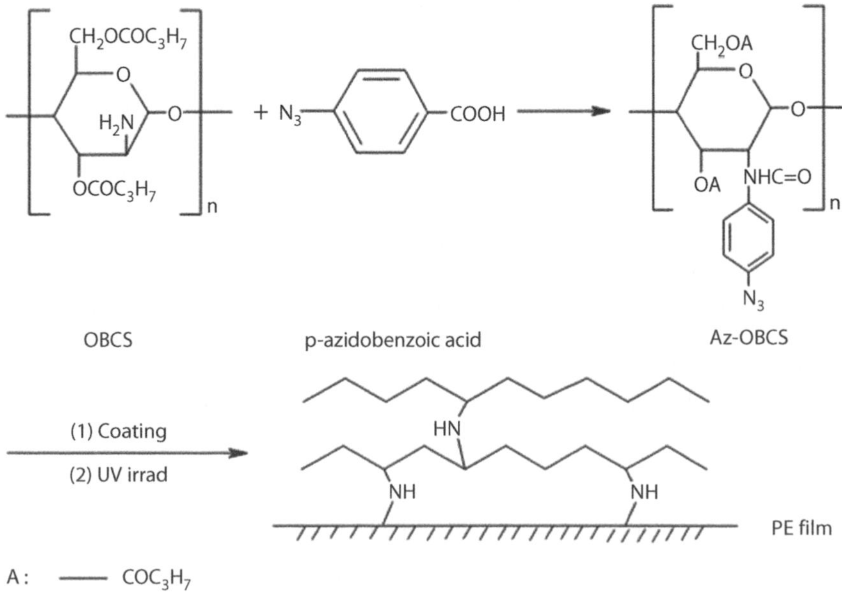

FIGURE 3.7
Reaction scheme of Az-OBCS and immobilization scheme of OBCS on PE film surface.

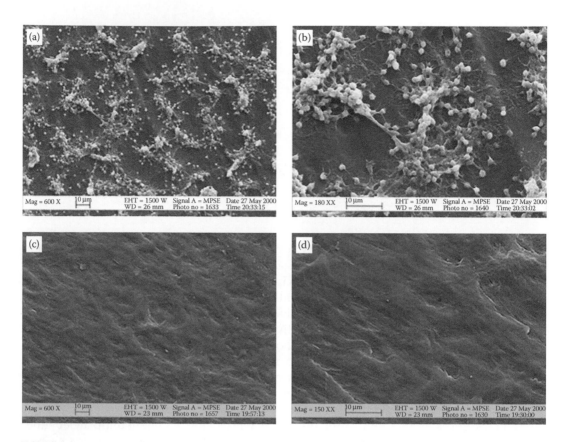

FIGURE 3.8
SEM images of the morphology of PRP contacted surfaces: (a) blank PE-1 h (×600), (b) blank PE-1 h (×1500), (c) OBCS-grafted PE-1 h (×600), and (d) OBCS-grafted PE-1 h (×1500).

Material biocompatibility is generally considered to have a relation with the protein adsorption process, because adsorbed proteins may trigger the coagulation sequence [119]. In the present work, the PE surface and the OBCS-modified PE surface were studied in relation to adsorption of BFG *in vitro*. Table 3.2 shows the adsorption of BFG onto PE surfaces from the protein solution (0.1 mg/mL). These results demonstrate that grafting OBCS onto the PE surface decreases fibrinogen adsorption.

O-Carboxymethylchitosan (OCMCS) is another blood-compatible chitosan derivative. It was prepared as follows. Chitosan (2 g) was immersed into a 25 mL 50 wt% NaOH solution to swell and alkalize for 24 h. Alkalized chitosan was crushed into a filtration cake and then transferred into a flask. Monochloroacetic acid (5 g) was first dissolved in isopropanol (25 mL), the solution was added dropwise into a flask for 20 min, and the reaction was allowed to

TABLE 3.2

BFG Adsorption onto Blank PE and OBCS-Immobilized PE Film

Polymer Film	BFG Adsorption (µg/cm²)
Blank PE	2.116 ± 0.077
OBCS-immobilized PE	1.315 ± 0.097

proceed for 8 h at room temperature. The reaction mixture was filtered to remove solvent. The filtrate was dissolved in 100 mL of water and then 2.5 M HCl was added to adjust the pH to 7. After centrifugation and removal of the insoluble precipitate, 150 mL of anhydrous ethanol was slowly added into the solution and the product was precipitated. The solid was filtered and rinsed three times with anhydrous ethanol and vacuum dried at room temperature.

A simple and effective method for the coupling of OCMCS to the polyethylene terephthalate (PET) surface was developed through surface grafting PAA treated by plasma treatment. In contrast to the PET surface, platelet adhesion and protein-adsorptive resistance of PET–OCMCS were greatly improved. The blood compatibility of PET–OCMCS is believed to be related to its zeta potential, the balance of hydrophilicity/hydrophobicity, and low adsorption of protein [120,121].

Vascular grafts made of expanded PTFE (ePTFE) are widely used in vascular reconstructive surgery. Although successful as replacements for large-diameter blood vessels, they are unsuitable for small-diameter ones because when the internal diameters of the graft are less than 6 mm, they fail (without exception) due to blood clot formation. To reduce platelet adhesion onto the ePTFE vascular graft, a novel method for binding the chitosan–heparin (CS–Hp) complex to the surface of the vascular graft was developed. The binding of chitosan was achieved by irradiating the azide-modified chitosan that was coated on the ePTFE surface with ultraviolet light. By forming a complex with this coating of chitosan, heparin was then bonded to the ePTFE surface. *In vitro* blood-compatibility experiments showed that CS–Hp surface-modified ePTFE vascular grafts showed markedly reduced platelet adhesion (Figure 3.9). The outstanding performance of these grafts was further demonstrated by *in vivo* experiments, in which grafts were found to be still unclogged two weeks postimplantation into dog veins (Figures 3.10 and 3.11) [122].

3.2.4 Conclusions

Although chitosan does possess the necessary properties for biomedical product development, for those applications that involve blood contact, chitosan promotes thrombosis and

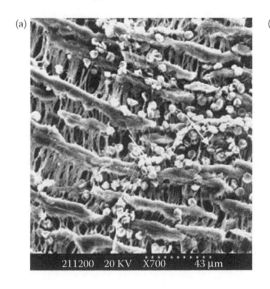
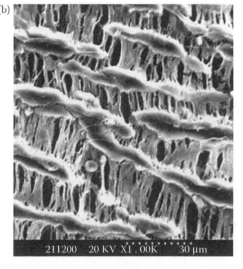

FIGURE 3.9
SEM images of vascular grafts after being contacted with blood *in vitro*: (a) ePTFE (×700) and (b) ePTFE/CS/Hp (×1000).

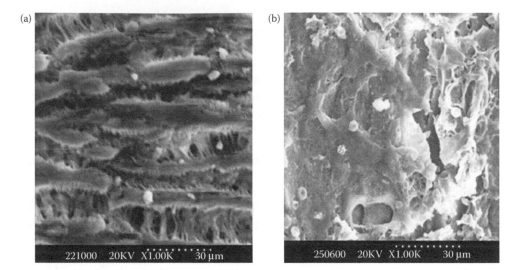

FIGURE 3.10
SEM images of ePTFE/CS/Hp vascular grafts after being implanted into veins of a dog: (a) implanted for a week
and (b) implanted for 2 weeks.

embolization. Surface-induced thrombosis on polymeric biomaterials is initiated by the
adsorption of plasma proteins, followed by adhesion and activation of platelets. Attempts
have been made to improve the blood compatibility of chitosan with physical blends,
surface modification, and synthesis of blood-compatible derivatives.

References

78. Roberts, G. A. F. and Taylor, K. E. 1989. Chitin chitosan: Sources, chemistry, biochemistry, physical properties and applications. Proceedings of the 4th International Conference, London, p. 577.
79. Khor, E. and Lim, L. Y. 2003. Implantable applications of chitin and chitosan. *Biomaterials* 24: 2339–2349.
80. Sunny, M. C., Ramesh, P., and Varma, H. K. 2002. Microstructured microspheres of hydroxy-apatite bioceramic. *J Mater Sci Mater Med* 13: 623–632.
81. Sivakumar, M., Manjubala, I., and Rao, K. P. 2002. Preparation, characterization and *in-vitro* release of gentamicin from coralline hydroxyapatite-chitosan composite microspheres. *Carbohydr Polym* 49: 281–288.
82. Li, S., Wang, X. T., Zhang, X. B., Yang, R. J., Zhang, H. Z., Zhu, L. Z., and Hou, X. P. 2002. Studies on alginate-chitosan microcapsules and renal arterial embolization in rabbits. *J Control Release* 84: 87–98.
83. Chen, X.G., Liu, W.S., Lang, G, H., Liu, C.S., and Cong, R.S. 2002. Chinese Patent No. ZL 96115714.3.
84. Lee, K. Y., Ha, W. S., and Park, W. H. 1995. Blood compatibility and biodegradability of partially *N*-acylated chitosan derivatives. *Biomaterials* 16: 1211–1216.
85. Singhal, J. P. and Ray, A. R. Synthesis of blood compatible polyamide block copolymers. *Biomaterials* 23: 1139–1145.
86. Sharma, C. P. 1984. LTI carbons: blood compatibility. *J Colloid Interf Sci* 97: 585–586.
87. Baier, R. E., Depalma, V. A., Goupil, D. W., and Cohen, E. J. 1985. Human platelet spreading on substrata of known surface chemistry. *Biomed Mater Res* 19: 1157–1167.

88. Chou, T. C., Fu, E., Wu, C. J., and Yeh, J. H. 2003. Chitosan enhances platelet adhesion and aggregation. *Biochem Biophys Res Comm* 302: 480–483.

89. Okamoto, Y., Yano, R., Miyatake, K., Tomobiro, I., Shigemasa, Y., and Minami, S. 2003. Effects of chitin and chitosan on blood coagulation. *Carbohydr Polym* 53: 337–342.

90. Hirano, S., Zhang, M., Nakagawa, M., and Miyata, T. 2000. Wet spun chitosan–collagen fibers, their chemical N-modifications, and blood compatibility. *Biomaterials* 21: 997–1003.

91. Malette, W. G., Quigley, H., Gaines, R. D., Johnso, N. D., and Rainer, W. G. 1983. Chitosan: A new hemostatic. *Ann Thorac Surg* 36: 55–58.

92. Klokkevold, P. R., Lew, D. S., Ellis, D. G., and Bertolami, C. N. 1991. Effect of chitosan on lingual hemostasis in rabbits. *J Oral Maxillofac Surg* 9: 858–863.

93. Wang, O. Z., Chen, X. G., Li, Z. X. Wang, S., Liu, C. S. Meng, X. H., Liu, C. G., Lv, Y. H., and Yu, L. J. 2008. Preparation and blood coagulation evaluation of chitosan microspheres. *J Mater Sci Mater Med* 19: 1371–1377.

94. Shim, D., Wechsler, D. S., Lloyd, T. R., and Beekman, R. H. 1996. Hemolysis following coil embolization of a patent ductus arteriosus. *Catheter Cardiovasc Diagn* 39: 287–290.

95. Amiji, M. M. 1998. Platelet adhesion and activation on an amphoteric chitosan derivative bearing sulfonate groups. *Colloid Surf B* 10: 263–271.

96. Jumaa, M., Furkert, F. H., and Muller, B. W. 2002. A new lipid emulsion formulation with high antimicrobial efficacy using chitosan. *Eur J Pharm Biopharm* 53: 115–123.

97. Richardson, S. C. W., Koler, H. V. J., and Duncan, R. 1999. Potential of low molecular mass chitosan as a DNA delivery system: Biocompatibility, body distribution and ability to complex and protect DNA. *Int J Pharm* 178: 231–243.

98. Kresie, L. 2001. Artificial blood: An update on current red cell and platelet substitutes. *Proc (Bayl Univ Med Cent)* 14: 158–161.

99. Shih, M. F., Shau, M. D., Chang, M. Y., Chiou, S. K., Chang, J. K., and Cherng, J. Y. 2006. Platelet adsorption and hemolytic properties of liquid crystal/composite polymers. *Int J Pharm* 327: 117–125.

100. Vanickova, M., Suttnar, J., and Dyr, J. E. 2006. The adhesion of blood platelets on fibrinogen surface: Comparison of two biochemical microplate assays. *Platelets* 17: 470–476.

101. Diquelou, A., Lemozy, S., Dupouy, D., Boneu, B., Sakariassen, K., and Cadroy, Y. 1994. Effect of blood flow on thrombin generation is dependent on the nature of the thrombogenic surface. *Blood* 84: 2206–2213.

102. Ong, S. Y., Wu, J., Moochhala, S. M., Tan, M. H., and Lu, J. 2008. Development of a chitosan-based wound dressing with improved hemostatic and antimicrobial properties. *Biomaterials* 29: 4323–4332.

103. Klokkevold, P. R., Fukayama, H., Sung, E. C., and Bertolami, C. N. 1999. The effect of chitosan (poly-N-acetylglucosamine) on lingual hemostasis in heparinized rabbits. *J Oral Maxillofac Surg* 57: 49–52.

104. Okamoto, Y., Yano, R., Miyatake, K., Tomohiro, I., Shigemasa, Y., and Minami, S. 2003. Effects of chitin and chitosan on blood coagulation. *Carbohydr Polym* 53: 337–342.

105. Rao, S. B. and Sharma, C. P. 1997. Use of chitosan as a biomaterial: Studies on its safety and hemostatic potential. *J Biomed Mater Res* 34: 21–28.

106. Yang, J., Tian, F., Wang, Z., Wang, Q., Zeng, Y. J., and Chen, S. Q. 2008. Effect of chitosan molecular weight and deacetylation degree on hemostasis. *J Biomed Mater Res B Appl Biomater* 84: 31–37.

107. Chou, T. C., Fu, E., Wu, C. J., and Yeh, J. H. 2003. Chitosan enhances platelet adhesion and aggregation. *Biochem Biophys Res Commun* 302: 480–483.

108. Benesch, J. and Tengvall, P. 2002. Blood protein adsorption onto chitosan. *Biomaterials* 23: 2561–2568.

109. Fischer, T. H., Valeri, C. R., Smith, C. J., Scull, C. M., Merricks, E. P., Nichols, T. C., Demcheva, M., and Vournakis, J. N. 2008. Non-classical processes in surface hemostasis: mechanisms for the poly-N-acetyl glucosamine-induced alteration of red blood cell morphology and surface prothrombogenicity. *Biomed Mater* 3: 15009.

110. Peyrou, V., Lormeau, J. C., Herault, J. P., Gaich, C., Pfliegger, A. M., and Herbert, J. M. 1999. Contribution of erythrocytes to thrombin generation in whole blood. *Thromb Haemost* 8: 400–406.

111. Hong, J., Larsson, A., Ekdahl, K. N., Elgue, G., Larsson, R., and Nilsson, B. 2001. Contact between a polymer and whole blood: Sequence of events leading to thrombin generation. *J Lab Clin Med* 138: 139–145.

112. Yancheva, E., Paneva, D., Danchev, D., Mespouille, L., Dubois, P., Manolova, N., and Rashkov, I. 2007. Polyelectrolyte complexes based on (quaternized) poly[(2-dimethylamino)ethyl methacrylate]: Behavior in contact with blood. *Macromol Biosci* 7: 940–954.

113. Popowicz, P., Kurzyca, J., Dolinska, B., and Popowicz, J. 1985. Cultivation of MDCK epithelial cells on chitosan membranes. *J Biomed Biochim Acta* 44: 1329–1333.

114. Chuang, W. Y., Young, T. H., Yao, C. H., and Chiu, W. Y. 1999. Properties of the poly (vinyl alcohol)/chitosan blend and its effect on the culture of fibroblast *in vitro*. *Biomaterials* 20: 1479–1487.

115. Foster, A. and Matthew, H. W. T. 1998. Growth of vascular cells on bioactive polysaccharide surface. *Proc NOBCChE* 25: 127–129 (Eng).

116. Grant, S., Blair, H. S., and Mckay, G. 1988. Water-soluble derivatives of chitosan. *Polym Commun* 29: 342–344.

117. Zhu, A. P., Wu, H., and Shen, J. 2004. Preparaion and characterization of a novel Si-containing cross-linkable O-butyrylchitosan. *Colloid Polym Sci* 282: 1222–1227.

118. Zhu, A. P., and Shen, J. 2003. Covalent Immobilization of O-butyrylchitosan with a photosensitive hetero-bifunctional cross-linking reagent on biopolymer substrate surface and blood-compatibility characterization. *J Biomater Sci Polym Edn* 14: 411–421.

119. Chin, J. A., Horbett, T. A., and Ratner, B. D. 1991. Baboon fibrinogen adsorption and platelet adhesion to polymeric materials. *Thromb Haemost* 65: 608–617.

120. Zhu, A. P., and Chen, T. 2006. Blood compatibility of surface-engineered poly(ethyleneterephthalate) via o-carboxymethylchitosan. *Colloid Surf B* 50: 120–112.

121. Zhu, A. P., Zhang, M., and Zhang, Z. 2004. Surface modification of ePTFE vascular grafts with O-carboxymethylchitosan. *Polym Int* 53: 15–19.

122. Zhu, A. P., Jian, S., and Zhang, M. 2005. Blood compatibility of chitosan/heparin complex surface modified ePTFE vascular graft. *Appl Surf Sci* 241: 485–492.

3.3 Antimicrobial Activity

Chitosan is made up of two monomers: glucosamine and *N*-acetyl glucosamine. The amino groups of chitosan have cationic properties that are believed to have electrostatic interactions with anionic systems. This property has been found to be quite valuable in using chitosan as an antibacterial agent [123–125]. It has been proposed that the interaction between the anionic cell surface of bacteria and the cationic amino group of chitosan weakens the cell membrane of the bacteria. In order to optimize chitosan's antibacterial properties at physiological pH, the amine group must remain cationic at pH 7.4. This poses a challenge as chitosan's amine group has a pK_a of 6.3, which implies that optimal protonation occurs at an acidic pH (~5.3) [126]. Alteration of the pKa of the amine group is therefore a necessary goal to increase the bioactivity of chitosan.

Quaternized chitosan, which has quaternary amino groups introduced into the chitosan chain, is both a facile and effective method to render it soluble in water. Moreover, quaternized chitosan has cationic activity, bioadhesive properties, permeation enhancing effects, and high efficacy against bacteria and fungi even under neutral conditions [127].

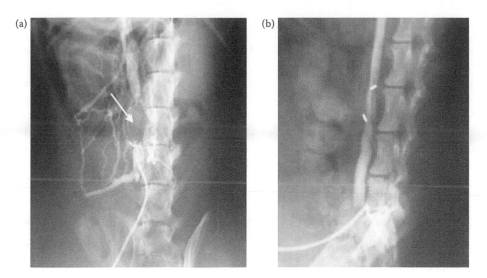

FIGURE 3.11
Angiograph image of vascular graft: (a) ePTFE and (b) ePTFE/CS/Hp.

3.3.1 Evaluation Index of Antimicrobial Activity

3.3.1.1 Bacterial Strains and Growth Conditions

The reference bacteria strains that represented the oral microbiota included two strict anaerobes and two facultative anaerobic bacteria: *Porphyromonas gingivalis* (*P. gingivalis* ATCC33277), *Prevotella intermedia* (*P. intermedia* ATCC 25611), *Actinobacillus actinomycetem-comitans* (*A. actinomycetemcomitans* Y4), and *Streptococcus mutans* (*S. mutans* Ingbritt C). Bacterial cells were grown in BHI culture media supplemented with hemin (5 g/mL), menadione (1%), and defibrinated goat blood (5%) before the medium was transferred into sterilized Petri dishes at about 50°C. The agar plates were incubated in an anaerobic chamber (Thermo, USA) with an atmosphere of 80% N_2, 10% H_2, and 10% CO_2 with deoxidized palladium for 72 h (*P. gingivalis*, *P. intermedia*) or 48 h (*A. actinomycetemcomitans*, *S. mutans*). A few singular colonies of each organism were picked from the blood agar plate and diluted into sterile physiological saline. The suspension was adjusted spectrophotometrically at 800 nm (OD_{800}) to match a turbidity of 1.5×10^8 CFU mL (equivalent to 0.5 McFarland standard), and used for further antibacterial activity testing.

3.3.1.2 Test of Minimum Inhibitory Concentration

The minimum inhibitory concentration (MIC) method was carried out *in vitro* using a 2-fold dilution technique approved by CLSI (Clinical and Laboratory Standard Institute) [127]. The concentrations of the samples ranged from 5 to 0.00122 mg/mL. A serial sample was obtained by mixing 1 mL of the standard sample with 9 mL of anaerobic medium. A total of 100 µL of 0.5 McFarland standard organism suspension was dropped onto the surface of the blood agar medium plate. The blood plates were incubated in the anaerobic chamber (Thermo Life Science, USA) under an atmosphere of 80% N_2, 10% H_2, and 10% CO_2 with deoxidized palladium for 72 h. Control tests were simultaneously run to ensure reliable results. Each assessment was performed three times to ensure the reproducibility of the experiments. MIC was defined as the lowest concentration of the tested sample at which the bacterial colonies were not visible to the naked eye.

3.3.1.3 Determination of Inhibitory Zone Diameters [128]

A total of 150 μL of 0.5 McFarland standard bacterial suspensions was spread onto the agar plate. Sterilized stainless steel tubes of $8.0 \times 1.0 \times 10$ mm (inner diameter 6 mm) were added to the surfaces of the media and filled with 100 μL of sterilized antimicrobial solution. The blood plates were incubated in an anaerobic chamber under an atmosphere of 80% N_2, 10% H_2, and 10% CO_2. The inhibitory zone was considered to be the shortest distance (mm) between the outer margin of the cylinder and the initial point of microbial growth. Six replicates were made for each microorganism. Each assessment was performed three times to ensure the reproducibility of the results.

3.3.2 Antimicrobial Chitosan Derivatives

3.3.2.1 Preparation of N-[1-hydroxy-3-(trimethylammonium)propyl] Chitosan Chloride

N-[1-hydroxy-3-(trimethylammonium)propyl] chitosan chloride (HTCC) was synthesized by reacting chitosan with glycidyltrimethylammonium chloride (GTMAC) [129]. Briefly, 6 g of chitosan was mixed and dispersed in 225 mL of 2-PrOH. The reaction was carried out with stirring at 80–90°C for 1 h. GTMAC was dissolved in deionized water (30% w/v) to form a solution. The GTMAC solution was added to the chitosan suspension slowly under continuous stirring. The molar ratio of GTMAC to the amino groups of chitosan was 4:1. After 4 h of reaction at 80°C, any precipitate that formed was filtered. The product was then poured into EtOH and washed three times. Quaternized CS was obtained by drying at 80°C for 48 h. The degree of quaternization (DQ) was determined by titrating the amount of Cl ions on HTCC with 0.1 M $AgNO_3$ [130].

3.3.2.2 Antibacterial Activities of HTCC

P. gingivalis, *P. intermedia*, and *A. actinomycetemcomitans* are Gram-negative strains, and *S. mutans* is a Gram-positive strain. MIC was quantified for all the standard bacterial strains selected, and the results are shown in Table 3.3 and Figure 3.12. MIC values for each bacteria strain ranged from 0.25 to 2.5 mg/mL. The lactic acid (LA) solution of HTCC exerted higher antibacterial activities against *P. intermedia*, *A. actinomycetemcomitans*, and *S. mutans* (MICs were 1, 1 and 0.5 mg/mL, respectively) than the LA solution of chitosan (MIC 2.5 mg/mL). However, the LA solution of chitosan and HTCC had the same MIC value against *P. gingivalis* (MIC 0.5 mg/mL). The aqueous solution of HTCC exhibited relatively lower antibacterial activity against *P. gingivalis* and *S. mutans* than the LA solution of HTCC. In addition, Gram-negative and Gram-positive strains were all susceptible to chitosan and HTCC, and there was no significant difference between them.

TABLE 3.3

MIC Values of CS and HTCC for Four Oral Bacterial Strains (mg/mL)

Samples	*P. gingivalis*	*P. intermedia*	*A. actinomycetemcomitans*	*S. mutans*
HTCC(LA)	0.5	1	1	0.5
HTCC(H_2O)	1	1	1	1
CS(LA)	0.5	2.5	2.5	2.5
CS + HTCC	0.25	0.25	0.25	0.25

Note: (LA): lactic acid solution, (H_2O): aqueous solution.

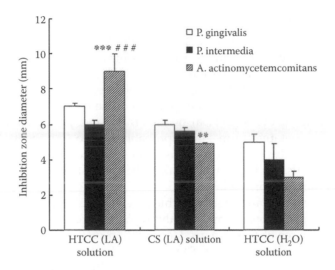

FIGURE 3.12
Inhibition zone diameter for different samples.

The effect of MW on antifungal activity was investigated [131]. Experiments were conducted to test their antifungal activities against *Botrytis cinerea* Pers. (*B. cinerea* Pers.) and *Colletotrichum lagenarium* (Pass) Ell.et halst (*C. lagenarium* (Pass) Ell.et halst). The results indicate that quaternized chitosan derivatives have stronger antifungal activities than chitosan. Furthermore, quaternized chitosan derivatives with high MW are shown to have even stronger antifungal activities than those with low MW.

3.3.3 Mechanism of Inhibition

3.3.3.1 Antibacterium Mechanism of Chitosan and HTCC

To date, the mechanism of inhibition of chitosan on bacteria is not clear. One possibility is that, due to the interaction between the two charges, the bacterial cell wall breaks, leading to cytoplasmic leakage, which eventually causes cell death [132–134]. In addition, stacking of chitosan molecules over the microbial cell surface may block the transport of nutrients [135] or binding to DNA, thus inhibiting transcription or permeabilization of the microbial cell wall/membrane. Helander et al. [133] showed that the binding of chitosan to the outer membrane of a Gram-negative bacteria resulted in a vesicular structure, causing disruption and extensive alteration to the outer membrane surface, resulting in the loss of its barrier properties.

No et al. [136] found that the antibacterial activities of chitosan are strain dependent. Other investigators have shown that an increase in the MW and degree of deacetylation (DD) of chitosan enhances antibacterial activity [137]. A higher DQ of HTCC should enhance antibacterial activity. In the experiments, HTCC exerted more potent antibacterial activities than chitosan in the same solution against *P. intermedia*, *A. actinomycetemcomitans*, and *S. mutans*. This was probably due to the introduction of quaternary ammonium salts onto the chitosan backbone, which enhanced the water solubility of chitosan and increased the antimicrobial activity of HTCC over the entire pH range.

3.3.3.2 AFM Characterization

AFM was used to assess the relationship between the MW of chitosan and its antimicrobial activity on both the vegetative and resistance forms of *Bacillus cereus* (*B. cereus*). Higher MW chitosan (628 and 100 kDa) surrounded both forms of *B. cereus* cells by forming a polymer layer. This eventually led to the death of the vegetative form by preventing the uptake of nutrients, yet did not affect the spores because these can survive for extended periods without nutrients. COSs (<3 kDa), on the other hand, produced more visible damage in the *B. cereus* vegetative form—most probably due to the penetration of the cells by COS. The use of COS by itself on *B. cereus* spores was not enough for the destruction of a large number of cells, but it may well weaken the spore structure and its ability to contaminate, by inducing exosporium loss [138].

The effect of low, medium, and high MW chitosan was evaluated on the development of three isolates of *Rhizopus stolonifer*. Image analysis and electronic microscopy observations were performed in spores of this fungus. Germination of *R. stolonifer* in potato dextrose broth with chitosan was also evaluated. The results indicated that LMWC was more effective in the inhibition of mycelial growth whereas HMW chitosan affected spore shape, sporulation, and germination. Studies with scanning and transmission electron microscopy revealed numerous and deeper ridge ornamentations of the chitosan-treated spore [139].

The antibacterial activity of chitosan was investigated by assessing the mortality rates of *Escherichia coli* and *Staphylococcus aureus* based on the extent of damaged or missing cell walls and the degree of leakage of enzymes and nucleotides from different cellular locations. Chitosan was found to react with both the cell wall and the cell membrane, but not simultaneously, indicating that the inactivation of *E. coli* by chitosan occurs by a two-step sequential mechanism: an initial separation of the cell wall from its cell membrane, followed by destruction of the cell membrane. The similarity between the antibacterial profiles and patterns of chitosan and those of two control substances, polymyxin and EDTA, verified this mechanism. The antibacterial activity of chitosan could be altered by blocking the amino functionality through coupling of the chitosan to active agarose derivatives. These results verify the status of chitosan as a natural bactericide.

3.3.3.3 Antibacterium Activity of the Schiff Base of Chitosan and Metallic Ion-Loaded Chitosan Nanoparticles

The Schiff base of chitosan was synthesized by the reaction of chitosan with citral working under high-intensity ultrasound. The antimicrobial activities of chitosan and the Schiff base of chitosan were investigated against *E. coli*, *S. aureus*, and *Aspergillus niger*. The results indicate that the antimicrobial activity of Schiff base increases with an increase in the concentration. It was also found that the antimicrobial activity of Schiff base was stronger than that of chitosan [140].

Chitosan nanoparticles were prepared based on ionic gelation between chitosan and sodium tripolyphosphate. Then, Ag^+, Cu^{2+}, Zn^{2+}, Mn^{2+}, or Fe^{2+} was individually loaded onto chitosan nanoparticles. Their antibacterial activities were evaluated by the determination of MIC and minimum bactericidal concentration (MBC) against *E. coli* 25922, *Salmonella choleraesuis* ATCC 50020, and *S. aureus* 25923 *in vitro*. The results showed that antibacterial activity was significantly enhanced by the metal ions loaded, except for Fe^{2+}. Especially for chitosan nanoparticle-loaded Cu^{2+}, the MIC and MBC against *E. coli* 25922, *S. choleraesuis* ATCC 50020, and *S. aureus* 25923 were 21–42 times lower than that of Cu^{2+}, respectively. Moreover, it was found that antibacterial activity was directly proportional to zeta potential [141].

3.3.4 Conclusions

Chitosan has shown high antimicrobial activity against a wide variety of pathogenic and spoilage microorganisms, including fungi, and Gram-positive and Gram-negative bacteria. The presence of an amino group at the C2 position of chitosan provides major functionality toward biotechnological needs.

References

123. Ikinci, G., Senel, S., Akincibay, H., Kas, S., Ercis, S., Wilson, C. G., and Hincal, A. A. 2002. Effect of chitosan on a periodontal pathogen *Porphyromonas gingivalis*. *Int J Pharm* 235: 121–127.

124. Chung, Y. C., Wang, H. L., Chen, Y. M., and Li, S. L. 2003. Effect of abiotic factors on the antibacterial activity of chitosan against waterborne pathogens. *Bioresour Technol* 88: 179–184.

125. Li, B., Wang, X., Chen, R. X., Huang, W. G., and Xie, G. L. 2008. Antibacterial activity of chitosan solution against *Xanthomonas* pathogenic bacteria isolated from *Euphorbia pulcherrima*. *Carbohydr Polym* 72: 287–292.

126. Madihally, S. V. and Matthew, H. W. 1999. Porous chitosan scaffolds for tissue engineering. *Biomaterials* 20: 1133–1142.

127. Sandri, G., Rossi, S., Bonferoni, M. C., Ferrari, F., Zambito, Y., Di Colo, G., and Caramella, C. 2005. Buccal penetration enhancement properties of *N*-trimethyl chitosan: Influence of quaternization degree on absorption of a high molecular weight molecule. *Int J Pharm* 297: 146–155.

128. Milazzo, I., Blandino, G., Caccamo, F., Musumeci, R., Nicoletti, G., and Speciale, A. 2003. Faropenem, a new oral penem: Antibacterial activity against selected anaerobic and fastidious periodontal isolates. *J Antimicrob Chemother* 51: 721–725.

129. Zhang, Y.Y., Ma, Q.M., and Jiang, Z.H. 2005 *J. Ocean Univ. Qingdao* 35: 459–462.

130. Xu, H., Kaar, J. L., Russell, A. J., and Wagner, W. R. 2006. Characterizing the modification of surface proteins with poly (ethylene glycol) to interrupt platelet adhesion. *Biomaterials* 27: 3125–3135.

131. Guo, Z. Y., Xing, R., Liu, S., Zhong, Z. M., Ji, X., Wang, L., and Li, P. C. 2008. The influence of molecular weight of quaternized chitosan on antifungal activity. *Carbohydr Polym* 71: 694–697.

132. Choi, B. K., Kim, K. Y., Yoo, Y. J., Oh, S. J., Choi, J. H., and Kim, C. Y. 2001. *In vitro* antimicrobial activity of a chitooligosaccharide mixture against *Actinobacillus actinomycetemcomitans* and *Streptococcus mutans*. *Int J Antimicrob Agents* 18: 553–557.

133. Helander, I. M., Nurmiaho-Lassila, E. L., Ahvenainen, R., Rhoades, J., and Roller, S. 2001. Chitosan disrupts the barrier properties of the outer membrane of Gram-negative bacteria. *Int J Food Microbiol* 71: 235–244.

134. Qi, L., Xu, Z., Jiang, X., Hu, C., and Zou, X. 2004. Preparation and antibacterial activity of chitosan nanoparticles. *Carbohydr Res* 339: 2693–2700.

135. Vishu Kumar, A. B., Varadaraj, M. C., Gowda, L. R., and Tharanathan, R. N. 2007. Low molecular weight chitosans—Preparation with the aid of pronase, characterization and their bactericidal activity towards *Bacillus cereus* and *Escherichia coli*. *Biochim Biophys Acta* 1770: 495–505.

136. No, H. K., Lee, S. H., Park, N. Y., and Meyers, S. P. 2003. Comparison of physicochemical, binding, and antibacterial properties of chitosans prepared without and with deproteinization process. *J Agric Food Chem* 51: 7659–7663.

137. Chen, Y. M., Chung, Y. C., Wang, L. W., Chen, K. T., and Li, S. Y. 2002. Antibacterial properties of chitosan in waterborne pathogen. *J Environ Sci Health Part A: Toxic/Hazard Subst Environ Eng* 37: 1379–1390.

138. Fernandes, J. C., Eaton, P., Gomes, A. M., Pintado, M. E., and Malcata, F. X. 2009. Study of the antibacterial effects of chitosans on *Bacillus cereus* (and its spores) by atomic force microscopy imaging and nanoindentation. *Ultramicroscopy* 109: 854–860.

139. Hernández-Lauzardo, A. N., Bautista-Baños, S., Velázquez-del Valle, M. G., Méndez-Montealvo, M. G., Sánchez-Rivera, M. M., and Bello-Pérez, L. A. 2008. Antifungal effects of chitosan with different molecular weights on *in vitro* development of *Rhizopus stolonifer* (Ehrenb.: Fr.) Vuill. *Carbohydr Polym* 73: 541–547.
140. Jin, X. X., Wang, J. T., and Bai, J. 2009. Synthesis and antimicrobial activity of the Schiff base from chitosan and citral. *Carbohydr Res* 344: 825–829.
141. Du, W. L., Niu, S. S., Xu, Y. L., Xu, Z. R., and Fan, C. L. 2009. Antibacterial activity of chitosan tripolyphosphate nanoparticles loaded with various metals. *Carbohydr Polym* 75: 385–383.

3.4 Pharmacological Activity

3.4.1 Antiinflammatory Activity

3.4.1.1 Cytokine and Chemical Substances Correlated with Inflammatory Activity

Chitosan is a linear polymer of N-acetyl-D-glucosamine and deacetylated glucosamine that shares some characteristics of glucosaminoglycan and hyaluronic acid, suggesting related bioactivities [142]. Chitosan enhances the functions of inflammatory cells such as polymorphonuclear leukocytes, macrophages (MU), and fibroblasts [143–146]. TNF-α was an inflammatory cytokine, which was produced by the various cells including macrophages, lymphocytes, neutrophils, and mast cells. TNF-α is known to be a key mediator for the induction of apoptosis and development of humoral immune response. However, at high concentrations, TNF-α has disadvantageous effects, such as inducing tissue injury and potentiating septic shock. TNF-α may have a homeostatic effect in limiting the extent of an inflammatory response as well as acting as an antimalarial agent and being functional in intramembranous bone repair.

Interleukin-6 (IL-6) is a multifunctional cytokine that plays important roles in host defense, acute-phase reactions, immune responses, nerve cell functions, and hematopoiesis. It is expressed by a variety of normal and transformed lymphoid and nonlymphoid cells. The production of IL-6 is upregulated by numerous signals such as mitogenic or antigenic stimulation, lipopolysaccharides (LPSs), calcium ionophores, cytokines, and viruses. Elevated serum IL-6 levels have been observed in a number of pathological conditions, including bacterial and viral infections, trauma, autoimmune diseases, and inflammations.

Nitric oxide (NO) is a highly reactive free radical involved in a number of physiological and pathological processes. NO may play an important role in the pathophysiology of numerous diseases. In numerous mammalian cells and tissues, the oxidation of the terminal guanidino nitrogen of L-arginine (Arg), yielding NO and citrulline, is catalyzed by different NO synthases. The role of NO is well established in the relaxation of vascular smooth muscle, in the inhibition of mitogenesis and growth of glomerular mesangial cells, and in macrophage toxicity. NO acts immunologically as a cytotoxic agent on invading microorganisms in macrophages or on tumor cells.

LPS is one of the major constituents of the outer membrane of Gram-negative bacteria, and LPS recognition and signal transmission are among the key events in the host defense reaction toward Gram-negative bacteria. Humans are constantly exposed to low levels of LPS through infection. Many different cell types such as neutrophils and macrophages can respond to LPS by releasing potent inflammatory mediators such as IL-8 and TNF-α to destroy invading bacteria. Additionally, epithelial and endothelial cells as well as smooth muscle cells have also been shown to be targets for LPS stimulation, and activation of these cells by LPS has been linked to the pathogenesis of a variety of diseases. These imply the possibility that in case of an abnormal condition, LPS has also been known to induce endotoxemia and acute renal failure. However, the exact mechanism of LPS-induced toxicity remains unclear.

3.4.1.2 Characterization

Measurement of nitrite: An aliquot of the incubation supernatant (100 μL) was transferred to 96-well plates and nitrite was determined spectrophotometrically using Griess reagent (0.8% sulfanilamide and 0.75% N-(naphthylethylene) diamine in 0.5 N HCl) by mixing 100 μL of the Griess reagent. After 15 min incubation at room temperature, the nitrite concentrations were measured at 540 nm using a microplate reader. Sodium nitrate (0.5–100 μM) was used as nitrite standards and nitrite was linear over this concentration range.

Reverse transcriptase polymerase chain reaction (RT-PCR) RAW264.7 cells were treated with 1 μg/mL LPS for 6 or 12 h. The cells were harvested and total RNA was isolated by Trizol according to the manufacturer's instructions. For amplification of IL-6 and TNF-α, the following primers were used: TNF-α forward primer was 5′CCC AAA TGG CCT CCC TCT C3′, reverse primer was 5′CAA ATC GGC TGA CGG TGT GTC C3′; IL-6 primer sense was 5′ATG AAG TTC CTC TGC AAG AGA CT3′,antisense was 5′CAC TAG GTT TGC CGA GTA GAT CTC3′. For PCR amplification, the following conditions were used: 94°C for 30 s (denaturation), 55°C for 1 min (annealing), and 72°C for 1 min (extension) for one cycle and 72°C for 1 min for 30 cycles. The amplified PCR products were separated with 2% agarose gel, and then stained with ethidium bromide.

Western blotting: Proteins (20 μg) in incubation media were separated by 15% SDS-PAGE and transferred to polyvinylidene fluoride (PVDF) membrane. The membrane was blocked with 5% skim milk in TPBS for 1 h at room temperature and incubated with anti-mouse TNF-α antibody or anti-mouse IL-6 antibody for 3 h at room temperature or overnight at 4°C. After washing in TPBS three times, the blot was incubated with secondary antibody (horseradish peroxidase-conjugated anti-goat antiserum) for 1 h at room temperature. The antibody-specific proteins were detected by using West-ZOL (plus).

3.4.1.3 Function of Chitosan in Antiinflammatory Activity

Upon stimulation with increasing concentrations of chitosan, LPS-stimulated TNF-α secretion was significantly recovered within the incubation media of RAW264.7 cells. The effect of chitosan on LPS-stimulated TNF-α secretion was similar in 6 h and 12 h incubation media. The effective concentration range of chitosan was 0.05–0.5 wt% and, at higher concentrations, TNF-α secretion plateaued. Also, above 1% concentration, chitosan was toxic *in vitro*. Consistently, RT-PCR with mRNA of TNF-α and Western blot with anti-TNF-α antiserum showed that the amount of TNF-α secretion in the incubation media recovered with the concentration of chitosan. These results suggest that chitosan may have an antiinflammatory effect in LPS-stimulated inflammation and may affect LPS-stimulated TNF-α secretion within 6 h.

Upon stimulation with increasing concentrations of chitosan, LPS-stimulated IL-6 secretion was also significantly recovered within the incubation media of RAW264.7 cells. However, the effect of chitosan on LPS-stimulated IL-6 secretion was different in 6 h and 12 h incubation media. In 0.05% concentration of chitosan, the effect of chitosan on IL-6 secretion was late, compared with TNF-α secretion. Consistently, RT-PCR with mRNA of IL-6 and Western blot with anti-IL-6 antiserum showed that the amount of

TNF-α secretion in the incubation media recovered with the concentration of chitosan. These results and reports once again suggest that chitosan may have an antiinflammatory effect on LPS-stimulated inflammation and the effect of chitosan on IL-6 secretion may be induced via the stimulus of TNF-α in RAW264.7 cells. In the experiment [147], upon stimulation with increasing concentrations of chitosan, LPS-stimulated NO secretion was also significantly recovered within the 6 h and 12 h incubation media of RAW264.7 cells. These results once again suggest that chitosan may have an antiinflammatory effect on LPS-stimulated inflammation.

In the TNF-α-treated group, chitosan did not affect LPS-stimulated IL-6 and NO secretion in RAW264.7 cells. These results again confirmed that the recovery effect of chitosan on IL-6 and NO secretion might be induced via the stimulus of TNF-α in RAW 264.7 cells.

3.4.1.4 Antiinflammatory Activity of COSs

Chitosan has been used as a source of potential bioactive material in the past few decades. However, in the biomedical field, COSs are more widely applicable due to their water solubility and higher absorption profiles at the intestinal level, quickly getting into the blood flow and having systemic biological effects on the organism. To explore the antiinflammatory activities of COS, two COS mixtures (obtained via enzymatic activity, with MW < 3 and <5 kDa) at several concentrations were tested, by carrageenan-induced pawedema methodology, in mice. The inflammatory response was quantified by increase in paw size (edema), which is maximal around 5 h post-carrageenan injection, and is modulated by inhibitors of specific molecules within the inflammatory cascade. COS showed antiinflammatory action, which increased with increasing MW. COS < 5 kDa even showed a higher effect than the control, indomethacin, after 2 h, with no harmful secondary effects. The data suggest that COS possesses antiinflammatory effect, and is dose and MW dependent.

3.4.1.5 Sustained Release Matrix of Chitosan Microspheres

Chitosan has been used for sustained release systems, preparation of mucoadhesive formulations, and improvement of the dissolution rate of poorly soluble drugs, drug targeting, and enhancement of peptide drug absorption. So far, studies on the preparation of chitosan microspheres have been carried out. Microspheres were prepared by using a cross-linking agent such as glutaraldehyde combined with an emulsion technique. Other approaches used an emulsion/solvent evaporation technique and spray drying. In general, chitosan microspheres can be prepared as follows [148]. Chitosan (0.25% w/v) was dissolved in an aqueous solution of acetic acid (2% v/v) containing 1% polysorbate 80. A solution of sodium sulfate (20% w/v) was added dropwise (5 mL/min) during stirring with a blade stirrer at 400 rpm and ultrasonication. The formation of microspheres was indicated by turbidity and examined by transmission measurements at 500 nm. After the addition of sodium sulfate, stirring and sonication were continued for another 1 h. The microspheres were purified by centrifugation for 15 min at 3000 rpm. The obtained sediment was then suspended in water. These two purification steps were repeated twice. All purified microspheres were then lyophilized.

The production process of the present microspheres is based on the solubility behavior of chitosan, which is poorly soluble in water. Addition of an acid improves the solubility as a result of the protonation of the amino groups. The solubility is also dependent on other anions present in the solution. In the presence of acetate, lactate, or glutamate, chitosan shows good solubility, whereas phosphate, polyphosphates, and sulfate decrease the solubility. For this reason, sulfate was taken for microsphere formulation. Sulfate leads to a poorly soluble chitosan derivative, whereby microsphere formulation becomes possible.

Chitosan was always employed at a concentration of 0.25% (w/v). Higher concentrations were not practical, because the viscosity became too high. As a consequence, a homogeneous distribution of the added sodium sulfate was not possible, which would have led to the formation of agglomerates. The addition of polysorbate 80 was necessary to stabilize the suspensions. Without polysorbate 80 the formation of agglomerates occurred.

SEM studies confirm that the MW of chitosan has no influence on the size and appearance of microspheres. Microspheres are spherical and regular, with a size between 1.5 and 2.5 μm revealed by the scanning electron micrograph. The surface is smooth.

The chitosan microspheres were charged positively, although sulfate ions were used as the precipitant. This indicates that only a part of the amino groups are neutralized during microsphere formation. The residual amino groups would be responsible for the positive zeta potential. Moreover, these groups are freely accessible for interaction with drugs as well. The zeta potential was higher at low pH than at high pH. The pH dependence was strongest between pH 3 and 6, leveling off at pH values above 6. This correlated with the dissociation constant of chitosan, which is about 6. MW had no effect on zeta potential. This was expected because the deacetylation grade of chitosan was not dependent on MW.

The adsorption of prednisolone sodium phosphate (PSP) was 10 times greater than that of prednisolone. PSP is a hydrophilic drug; therefore, ethanol addition during loading was not necessary. In addition and probably most importantly, PSP has a negatively charged phosphate group. This phosphate group presumably led to a powerful interaction of the drug with chitosan and facilitated the formation of an ion pair. Figure 3.13 shows the adsorption isotherms of PSP onto microspheres with different MWs. During these adsorption experiments, the pH of the medium was kept at 4.0 ± 0.2. At this pH, PSP is present in an anionic form and protonation of the amino groups of chitosan is still considerable. These conditions lead to an optimal interaction between PSP and chitosan. At lower and

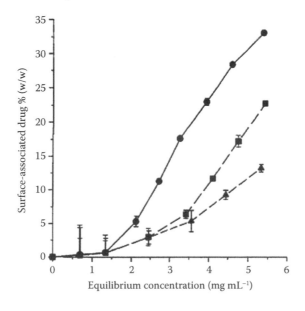

FIGURE 3.13
Adsorption isotherms of PSP onto chitosan microspheres: (●) LMWC; (■) medium-molecular-weight chitosan; and (▲) HMW chitosan (mean ± SD; $n = 3$).

higher pH values, the drug loading efficacy was decreased. One problem in these equilibrium experiments was the flocculation of microspheres at high drug concentrations. Probably due to binding of the charged drug, the positive charge of the microspheres was neutralized. This in turn decreased the repulsive forces between the microspheres. In the experiments displayed in Figure 3.13, only those drug concentrations that did not lead to flocculation were used. The adsorbed amount of drug depended on the MW of the chitosan. Adsorption increased with decreasing MWs. Probably due to the lower amount of sodium sulfate required for microsphere preparation with LMWC, more amino groups in LMWC were available for drug binding.

Differential scanning calorimetry (DSC) is a possible method to determine the modification of a drug. Figure 3.14 shows the DSC thermoanalysis of blank microspheres, drug-loaded microspheres, physical mixture, and PSP. PSP crystals show an endothermic peak at 341.5°C due to decomposition of PSP. Blank microspheres showed two peaks, one at 233.4°C and the other at 271.9°C corresponding to the α- and β-form of glucosamine. The DSC curve of a physical mixture of microspheres with PSP showed three peaks at 235.9°C, 275.4°C, and 341.9°C, demonstrating no interactions of the drug with chitosan. In contrast, in the case of microspheres with adsorbed PSP, only two peaks at 235.2°C and 263.9°C appeared. No PSP peak was observable. This leads to the assumption that PSP is present on the microsphere surface in amorphous form. Furthermore, one peak of chitosan sulfate was shifted from 271.9°C to 263.9°C. These observations indicate an interaction between the amino group of chitosan and the phosphate group of the drug such as the formation of an ion pair.

The model antiinflammatory drug prednisolone (PS) was retained in chitosan gel beads, which were prepared in a 10% aqueous amino acid solution (pH 9.0). Sustained release of PS from the chitosan gel beads was observed. Carrageenan solution was injected into air

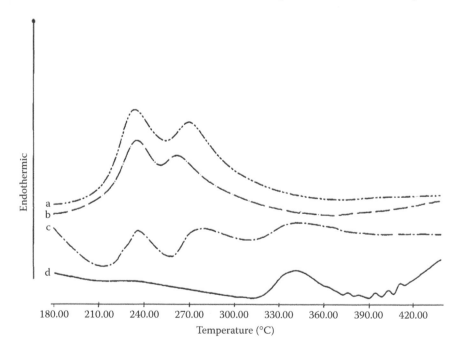

FIGURE 3.14
(a) DSC thermoanalysis of blank microspheres, (b) drug-loaded microspheres, (c) physical mixture, and (d) PSP.

pouches, which were prepared subcutaneously on the dorsal surface of mice, in order to induce local inflammation. Chitosan gel beads retaining PS were then implanted into the APs to investigate the therapeutic efficacy of sustained PS release against local inflammation. *In vivo* PS release from chitosan gel beads was governed by both diffusion of the drug and degradation of the gel matrix. Sustained drug release by chitosan gel beads allowed the supply of the minimum effective dose and facilitated prolonged periods of local drug presence. Inflammation indexes were significantly reduced after implantation of chitosan gel beads when compared with injection of PS suspension. Thus, extension of the duration of drug activity by chitosan gel beads resulted in improved therapeutic efficacy. These observations indicate that chitosan gel beads are a promising biocompatible and biodegradable vehicle for the treatment of local inflammation [149].

3.4.2 Antiulcer

3.4.2.1 Antiulcer Function of Chitosan

An ulcer is a sore or hole in the lining of the stomach or duodenum (the first part of the small intestine). It occurs as a result of a disturbance of the natural balance between aggressive acid–pepsin and mucosal defence–mucosal turnover. Ulcers induced by a mixture of HCl and ethanol has been reported to show many metabolic and morphological aberrations in the gastric mucosa of experimental animals similar to those observed in human peptic ulcer [150]. Chitosan and their oligomers have been found to promote antiulcer, especially in the phases of proliferation and matrix formation. It has been demonstrated that chitosan has numerous pharmacological actions, and it can be prepared as membrane, scaffold, powder, and so on. Histological findings indicate that chitosan membrane stimulates the migration of inflammatory cells and promotes cellular organization. Since 1980, chitosan and its derivatives have been used in skin ulcer management products in Japan [151]. It is well established that chitosan attracts neutrophils *in vitro* and *in vivo* [152,153] and that neutrophils accelerate ulcer healing by inciting a quicker, more aggressive inflammation. Azad et al. [154] used chitosan membrane as a wound-healing dressing and found that the chitosan mesh membrane showed a positive effect on re-epithelialization and regeneration of the granular layer. Figure 3.15 confirms that the chitosan mesh membrane is a potential substitute for human wound dressing. In the chitosan mesh membrane area, collagen fibers started to mature and consolidate in thicker and more mature fibers, and were oriented and distributed more regularly. In the control Bactigras, the fibers remained in a young, less-pronounced form.

3.4.2.2 Promoting Ulcer Healing of Chitosan

The quality of ulcer healing is closely related to growth factors, local blood circulation, prostaglandin, and *Helicobacter pylori* (*H. pylori*) infection. The administration of basic fibroblast growth factor (bFGF), a potent angiogenic and fibroblastic growth factor, to pressure ulcers may especially benefit those of advanced age because of the biological deficiencies associated with aging. Guo et al. [155] administered chitosan, chitosan with sucralfate, and chitosan with ranitidine as oral drugs, to investigate the effect of chitosan on the quality of ulcer healing of gastric ulcer in rats and its possible mechanism. After 14 days, the size of the ulcer decreased significantly, and the expressions of EGF and bFGF in the three experimental groups were significantly higher than those in the placebo and ranitidine groups (Figures 3.16 and 3.17). It was concluded that chitosan has a synergistic effect with sucralfate and ranitidine in promoting the quality of ulcer healing.

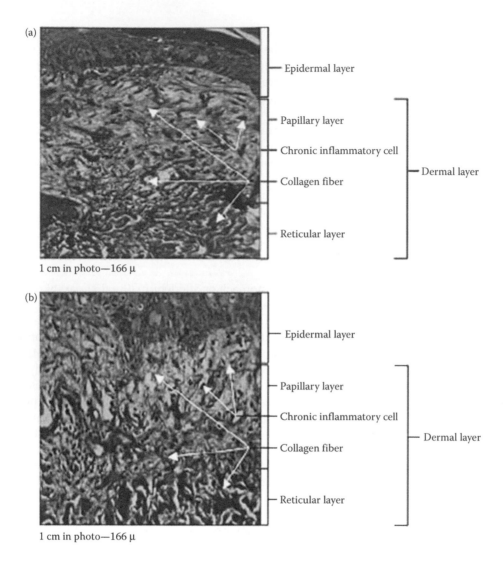

FIGURE 3.15
Histological findings (Masson's trichrome stain) of wounded skin tissue treated with (a) control Bactigras and (b) chitosan mesh membrane.

Some studies have shown chitosan as an oral drug healing gastric ulcer. Ito et al. [156] compared the effects of LMWC (MW: 25–50 kDa) and HMW chitosan (MW: 500–1000 kDa). From Figure 3.18, it is obvious that oral administration of LMWC (250, 500, and 1000 mg/kg) dose dependently prevented ethanol-induced gastric mucosal injury. However, the effects of HMW chitosan on gastric mucosal injury formation and gastric ulcer healing were less potent than those of LMWC. These results indicate that LMWC has the most potent gastric cytoprotective and ulcer healing-promoting actions.

3.4.2.3 Accelerating Pressure Ulcer Cure of Growth Factor-Loaded Chitosan

Pressure ulcers are a significant healthcare problem that affects up to 23% of bedridden patients in long-term care [157]. Each year, pressure ulcers afflict up to 3 million people in

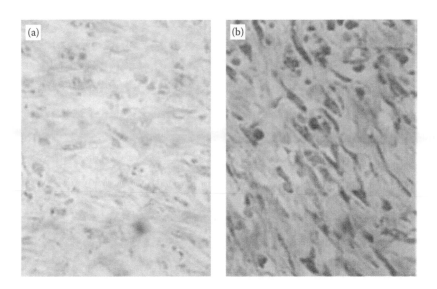

FIGURE 3.16
bFGF expression in granulation tissue in the control group and in the chitosan group (bFGF-positive product was brown, located in the cytoplasm). (a) Granulation tissue in the control group expressed less bFGF. (b) Granulation tissue in the chitosan group expressed more bFGF.

the United States, and the costs associated with these ulcers have been estimated at $3.3 billion [158,159]. The material used for wound treatment is critical since material–wound interactions may significantly influence healing prognoses. Chitosan was chosen because of its acute wound-healing properties [160–164], Park et al. [165] developed chitosan scaffolds loaded with basic fibroblast growth factors (bFGFs) contained in gelatin microparticles and tested for clinical relevance in an aged mouse model (Figures 3.19 and 3.20). These

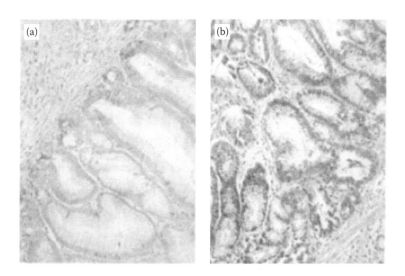

FIGURE 3.17
EGF expression in regenerative mucosa in the control group and in the chitosan group (EGF-positive product was brown, located in the cytoplasm and cell membrane). (a) Regenerative mucosa in the control group expressed less bFGF. (b) Granulation tissue in the chitosan group expressed more bFGF.

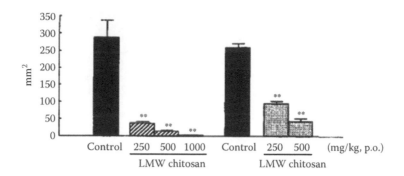

FIGURE 3.18
Effects of LMWC and HMW chitosan on ethanol-induced gastric mucosal injury in rats.

results suggest that chitosan is an effective material for growth factor delivery and can help in healing chronic ulcers. The data show that chitosan–bFGF scaffolds are effective in accelerating wound closure of pressure ulcers in aged animals.

3.4.3 Fat and Hypocholesteremic Lowering

3.4.3.1 *Function of Chitosan in Fat and Hypocholesteremic Lowering*

Chitosan is a natural dietary fiber and is made from the shell of shrimps that were harvested from the northern Atlantic Ocean, which has the least level of pollution. The unique property of chitosan makes it an effective fat blocker. Chitosan can bind dietary fat and cholesterol. Each gram of chitosan can bind an equal amount of fat. By binding with cholesterol, chitosan can reduce the reabsorption of cholesterol of the bile acid. Chitosan-bound dietary fats and cholesterol are excreted from the body. Chitosan also reduces the micelle formation of fat in the intestine and interferes with the enzymatic interaction of pancreatic lipase with fat.

In early studies on the properties of chitosan, several investigators demonstrated that chitosan is capable of binding dietary fats and can prevent their absorption through the

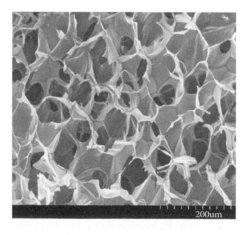

FIGURE 3.19
SEM micrograph of a porous chitosan scaffold.

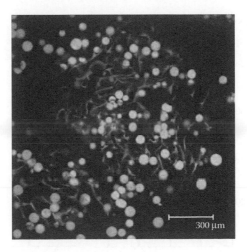

FIGURE 3.20
Confocal micrograph of gelatin microparticles in a chitosan scaffold.

gut [166]. Several other related studies showed that chitosan has the unique ability of absorbing fat from the body: that is, chitosan can absorb fat up to five times its weight. Chitosan was also shown to lower the level of low-density lipoprotein (LDL) cholesterol while boosting the high-density lipoprotein (HDL) cholesterol level. Some studies have shown that chitosan can decrease blood cholesterol levels by more than 50%, and it was considered to be an effective hypocholesterolemic agent. Further, in a preliminary human study, intake of 3–6 g of chitosan in a day for 2 weeks could decrease the blood cholesterol level by 6% and increase the HDL level by 10% [167]. In addition to chitosan, the chitosan oligosaccharides (COSs) also lead to control of blood cholesterol level. COSs are capable of decreasing the cholesterol level in the liver. Unlike HMW chitosan, COS application does not lead to an increase in compensatory cholesterol synthesis and a decrease in essential fatty acids, fat-soluble vitamins, and microelements from the organisms [168]. In particular, COSs prevent the development of fatty liver caused by the action of hepatotrope poisons.

Despite some research carried out to search for the ability of chitosan and COSs to bind with bile salts and lipids, the exact mechanism by which they lower blood cholesterol level has not been completely elucidated. However, several hypotheses have been suggested to explain the possible action of COS in reducing blood cholesterol levels. One hypothesis suggests that ionic binding of COS with bile salts and bile acids may inhibit micelle formation during lipid digestion in the digestive track [169]. Another hypothesis suggests that chitosan and its oligomers can directly trap lipids and fatty acids [170]. However, contradictory results have been observed with regard to ionic interactions of COS, and thus the fat-binding and cholesterol-lowering effects of chitosan cannot be explained using only the ion binding hypothesis [171]. Moreover, some other evidence from animal studies suggests that the effective lowering of cholesterol level can be explained in relation to the ability of COSs to increase the excretion of neutral sterol and indigestion of dietary fats. Sugano et al. [172] employed a series of experiments with male rats that clearly demonstrated the hypocholesterolemic activity of dietary chitosan. On feeding a high-cholesterol diet for 20 days, the addition of 2–5% chitosan resulted in a significant reduction, by 25–30%, of plasma cholesterol without influencing food intake

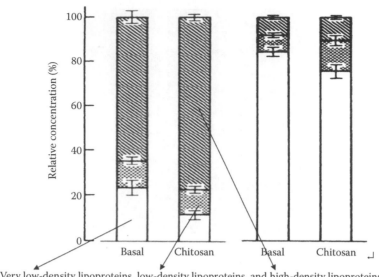

Very low-density lipoproteins, low-density lipoproteins, and high-density lipoproteins.

FIGURE 3.21
Relative concentration of LDLs, very low-density lipoproteins, and HDLs.

and growth. The concentration of liver cholesterol and triglyceride also decreased significantly. Plasma, but not liver cholesterol-lowering effect, was roughly comparable with that of cholestyramine. Chitosan at the 10% level further reduced plasma cholesterol, but depressed growth. Also, finer chitosan particles tended to restrain growth even at the 2% level. In rats fed a cholesterol-free diet containing 0.5% chitosan for 81 days, the concentration of serum cholesterol was the same as that of the corresponding control, but relatively more cholesterol existed as HDLs and less as very low-density lipoproteins (Figure 3.21). Dietary chitosan increased the fecal excretion of cholesterol, both exogenous and endogenous, while that of bile acids remained unchanged. There was no constipation or diarrhea. A proper supplementation of chitosan to the diet seemed to be effective in lowering plasma cholesterol.

Helgason et al. [173] investigated the effect of molecular characteristics of chitosan on its ability to bind fat in an *in vitro* simulation model for digestion. It was concluded that physicochemical properties of chitosan and environmental conditions greatly influenced the interaction between chitosan and oil micelles (Figures 3.22 and 3.23).

3.4.3.2 Characterization

Cholesterol absorption efficiency: Cholesterol absorption was measured by a modification of the fecal dual isotope ratio method. Rats were gavaged on two consecutive days at 100 h with 5.0 kBq ^{14}C-bsitosterol (2.05 GBq/mmol; Amersham Life Sciences, Arlington Hills, IL) and 34.7 kBq ^{3}H-cholesterol (130 GBq/mmol, Amersham Life Sciences) using soybean oil as the vehicle. Two consecutive 24-h fecal collections were taken beginning at 1800 h of gavage day 1. Collections were individually lyophilized and stored at 220°C until analysis. Fecal lipids were extracted from each collection by homogenizing ground feces with chloroform/methanol (2:1). The homogenate was filtered and then rinsed twice with normal saline. The filtrate was dried under nitrogen gas and reconstituted with chloroform/

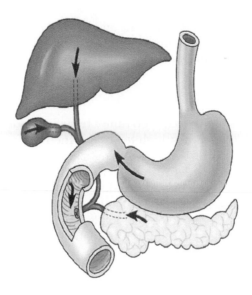

FIGURE 3.22
Effect of the pH of an organ on interaction between chitosan and oil micelles.

methanol (2:1). Radioactivity was determined in aliquots from duplicate samples by liquid scintillation counting. Cholesterol absorption efficiency was determined for each 24 h period, and the two values for each rat were averaged.

Lipid analysis: Blood samples were collected in heparinized tubes and the plasma was separated by centrifugation (experiments 1–3). In experiment 4, blood serum was collected. Liver was removed immediately after the rats were killed, rinsed, and weighed. Plasma and liver lipids were extracted and analyzed for cholesterol and triglyceride. Feces were lyophilized and pulverized. Gas–liquid chromatographic analyses of fecal, neutral, and

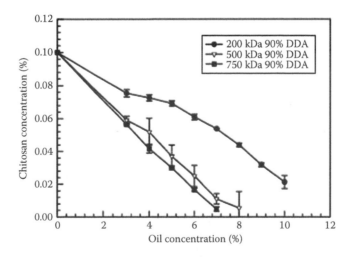

FIGURE 3.23
Effect of MW on interaction between chitosan and oil micelles.

acidic steroids were performed. 5α-Cholestane and 5β-cholanic acid were used as an internal calibration standard. Serum lipoprotein fractions were separated by sequential ultracentrifugation in the 40.3 rotor of a Beckman ultracentrifuge.

3.4.4 Antitumor

Anticancer drugs are almost nonselective on tumor tissue and normal cells and pose widespread problems such as low efficacy, high toxicity, difficult-to-control metastasis, and so on. Therefore, the anticancer drug delivery system has become the focus of research in the field of pharmacy. The targeted delivery system and sustained-release and controlled-release delivery systems have been proved to reduce the adverse effects of antitumor drugs effectively, improving clinical efficacy and patient medication compliance. Chitosan, as an anticancer drug carrier, can be made of microballs, microcapsules, nanoparticles, water, gels, implants, polymer micelles, and other formulations to achieve the role of targeting and sustained release *in vivo*.

3.4.4.1 Antitumor Activity of an LMWC

The functions of chitosan have been shown to be dependent not only on chemical structure but also on molecular size. In medicine and food industry applications, native polysaccharide is limited by its high MW, which results in its low solubility in acid-free aqueous media. Some chitosan applications require a low-molecular-weight (LMW) chitosan, which has high solubility in acid-free water and low viscosity. To be effectively absorbed in the human body, it should be converted to LMWC. LMWC is known to have biological activities such as antitumor activity [174–177], immuno-enhancing effects [174,178,179], enhancing protective effects against infection with certain pathogens in mice [180], antifungal activity, and antimicrobial activity [181].

LMWC can be prepared by enzymatic and chemical degradation of the chitosan polymer chain. Various acids have always been used for hydrolysis of chitosan to obtain LMWCs, but it seemed to be difficult to obtain water-soluble COS with a higher polymerization degree. In particular, the downstream procedure is tedious. Many oxidizing agents have also been used for the degradations, but most of them are toxic reagents such as chrome compounds, which are not desirable for application in medicine. The enzymic process of LMWC preparation seems to be generally preferable to chemical reactions, because the course under gentle conditions and product distribution can be controlled more readily, in spite of the faster rate of chemical reaction. The enzymatic method also minimizes alteration in the chemical nature of the product. However, the high cost of specific enzymes such as chitosanase and chitinase inhibits their use in industrial scale.

Recently, several hydrolytic enzymes, such as lysozyme, cellulase, papain, and pectinases, were found to catalyze the cleavage of glycosidic linkage in chitosan [182–185]. In an article on the enzymic preparation of water-soluble chitosan and its antitumor activity, cheap, commercially available hemicellulase was used to prepare water-soluble LMWC [186]. The method is suitable for scale-up manufacture of LMWC.

Preparation of samples by enzymatic hydrolysis: Crude hemicellulase solution was from Yufeng Company (Wuhan, China). Crude enzyme solution obtained was the fraction of culture supernatants that passed out of 100 kDa membrane but did not pass out of 5 kDa membrane. Further purified chitosan was obtained by the following procedure: Solid ammonium sulfate was added to the enzyme solution to 80% saturation; the solid enzyme was collected by centrifugation and redissolved in water. The solution was then loaded onto the Sephadex G25 column and deionized water was used as the eluent. The eluate was monitored for protein by measuring the absorbance at 280 nm. The first active fraction was collected as the purified hemicellulase solution.

Chitosan (200 g) was completely dissolved in 4000 mL of 2% acetic acid. After 3 h, the solution was neutralized to pH 5.5 and left overnight. The solution in the reaction vessel was placed in a water bath at 50°C, and 20 mL of enzyme solution (9.8 wt%) was added in order to initiate reaction. When 0.2 mL of the mixture was taken out and mixed with 5 mL of 4% NaOH solution and no precipitate was produced, the reaction mixture was cooled. After centrifugation, the supernatant was processed according to the following methods, to gain HCOS-B, MCOS-B, and LCOS-B samples (*cf.* Table 3.4).

Assays of antitumor activities: Antitumor effects on Sarcoma-180 (S-180) were observed in normal Kunming mice or adult BALB/c mice. The test was performed at a dose of 0.2 mL ($\sim$1.0 × 10^7 mL^{-1}) implanted subcutaneously at the right groin, and then observing the effect on the growth of the tumor in ascite form. After 24 h of tumor implantation, the test samples dissolved in physiological saline were provided once a day by intraperitoneal (i.p.) injection or by oral administration (p.o.) for 10 days, whereas 0.9% saline was provided for the control group. The animals were sacrificed, and the tumors were dissected and weighed. The tumor growth inhibition ratio was calculated by using the formula

$$\text{Inhibition rate (\%)} = \frac{100 \times (C - T)}{C}$$

where C is the average tumor weight of the control group and T is the tumor weight of the treated sample group. The spleen index was calculated by using the formula

$$\text{Spleen index} = \frac{\text{Spleen weight}}{\text{Final body weight}} \times 100$$

The maximum inhibition rate of UCOS-B reaches 64%. However, BCOS-B shows a lower activity than UCOS-B, indicating that boiling to remove enzyme modified the structure of COSs caused by side reactions such as the Maillard reaction. UCOS-B with free amine has a higher inhibitory rate than the acetate of the separated three fractions HCOS-A, MCOS-A, and LCOS-A, suggesting that the free amine group might be an important factor for the antitumor activity of chitosan.

TABLE 3.4

Plasma Pharmacokinetic Variables Following Administration of DTX (i.v.) and LMWC-DTX (p.o.) in Normal Mice

Variable	LMWC-DTX (p.o)		DTX (i.v.)	
	5 mg/kg	10 mg/kg	5 mg/kg	10 mg/kg
C_{max} (μg/mL)	0.82	2.08	65.57	125.58
T_{max} (min)	240.00	240.00	1.00	1.00
Half-life (min)	202.20	489.60	35.40	33.00
$AUC_{0 \to \infty}$ (μg h/mL)	29.02	43.20	4.69	11.34

The sample LCOS containing more molecules with lower COSs showed lower activity. This may have been due to the high content of pentamers or smallers, which are known to have no activity [187]. The sample UCOSAc from acetylation of UCOS-B also showed high antitumor activity, but it has a different optimum dose from UCOS-B. Nevertheless, a part of UCOSAc had poor water solubility.

It is interesting that the oral administration of water-soluble chitosan was effective in decreasing the weight of tumor, because lentinan was reported to have no antitumor effects by p.o. [188]. Water-soluble chitosan with small size also had a lower antitumor effect. The experiment shows that there were no significant differences in the spleen weights. Ftorafur as the positive group had a high antitumor effect and a strong side effect.

Many polysaccharides are shown to exhibit growth-inhibitory effects against solid-type tumors in experimental animals. The antitumor activity of polysaccharide seems to depend not only on chemical structure but also on molecule size [189]. For example, schizophyllan exhibits most activity within the range of 100–200 kDa, and no activity below 10 kDa. COSs and their N-acetylated analogs, which are soluble in basic physiological environment, might be good candidates for biological activity. Hexa-N-acetylchitohexaose and chito-hexaose were reported to be growth inhibitory against S-180 and MM-46 solid tumors transplanted into mice when given by i.v. administration [190]. The hexaoses were also growth inhibitory to Meth-A solid tumor transplanted in mice, but the lower homologs of the hexaoses were unable to exhibit the same effect [191]. Although the mechanisms of the antitumor activity of hexa-N-acetylchitohexaose and chitohexaose were different, they can be assumed to be acceleration of the production of and response to IL-1 and IL-2 for maturation of splenic T-lymphocytes to killer T-cells [187]. Seo et al. [192] demonstrated that water-soluble chitosan oligomers could activate murine peritoneal macrophases for tumor cell killing in the presence of IFN-γ. The amino groups as base groups might contribute a lot to the antitumor effect of chitosan.

3.4.4.2 Antitumor Activity of Chitosan Nanoparticles

The unique character of nanoparticles for their small size and quantum size effect could make chitosan nanoparticles exhibit biological activities [193]. Chitosan nanoparticles with small particle size and enhanced zeta potential have been prepared and characterized in previous reports [193–194], and their *in vitro* cytotoxic effects against various human tumor cell lines have also been studied. It was shown that chitosan nanoparticles with small particle size and positive surface charge could exhibit higher antitumor activity than other chitosan derivatives, and the physiochemical properties of nanoparticles such as particle size and zeta potential could have a significant effect on their efficacy [195]. The antitumor mechanism of chitosan nanoparticles was related to its membrane-disrupting and apoptosis-inducing activities [196].

To evaluate the *in vivo* antitumor activity of chitosan nanoparticles with different particle sizes, against the mouse tumor model, S-180 tumor and mouse hepatoma H22 (H22) with chitosan and cisplatin (cDDP) were used as reference drugs, and 0.9% saline solution was used as the blank control. Drugs were administered from the fifth day after establishing the mouse model, when the volume of subcutaneous tumor in mice grew by about 3 mm^3. Chitosan nanoparticles with different doses and different particle sizes were administered once daily by i.v. injection, i.p. injection, and p.o., respectively, for seven consecutive days. The results showed that chitosan nanoparticles exhibited very impressive antitumor efficacy *in vivo* against S-180 and H22, higher than the chitosan group. Chitosan nanoparticles elicited dose-dependent tumor-weight inhibitions (TWIs); the efficacy at a dose of 2.5 mg/kg achieved

53% and 59% against S-180 and H22, respectively, by At the same dose of 0.5 mg/kg by, chitosan nanoparticles showed much higher efficacy than the chitosan group. TWI against S-180 and H22 reached 43% and 52%, respectively, while that of the chitosan group was just about 30%. cDDP as a positive control drug exhibited higher antitumor efficacy than chitosan nanoparticles. However, cisplatin also showed great side effects compared with chitosan and nanoparticles. Chitosan nanoparticles resulted in only a small decrease in body weight of the mice relative to the saline control, which indicated weak side effects. On the contrary, cDDP led to a significant loss in body weight of mice. In the saline control group, 6 out of 12 and 7 out of 12 mice, separately in S-180 and H22 mouse models, died due to the transfer of tumor on the seventh day; cDDP also had a lethal toxicity of 4 out of 12 and 3 out of 12 mice, respectively, while in chitosan and nanoparticles groups, no lethal toxicity occurred for the inhibition of tumor growth. The histopathological slices from the liver and kidney tissues were also examined by a microscope. No pathological changes due to the administration of nanoparticles were seen, which also indicated weak side effects of chitosan nanoparticles.

For the S-180-bearing mouse model, at the same dose, the efficacy of chitosan nanoparticles (40 nm) by oral administration (p.o.), i.p. injection, and i.v. injection was 43%, 40%, and 49%, respectively. For the H22-bearing mouse model, the TWI of chitosan nanoparticles by the three administration routes was 52%, 51%, and 54%, respectively. The results showed that chitosan nanoparticles exhibit effective antitumor activities using different administration routes.

3.4.4.3 Chitosan Colloidal Drug Carrier Systems for Antitumor Activity

The oral route for colloidal drug carrier systems remains the most convenient and popular way of administration [197]. However, many anticancer drugs by oral administration are not bioavailable and adsorbable/interactive in the GI tract, because the drugs could be eliminated from the first-pass extraction by the cytochrome P450-dependent metabolic processes and the overexpression of the plasma membrane transporter P-glycoprotein (P-gp) in the physiological systems involved (intestine, liver, etc.) [198]. Application of nanoparticles with size small enough to improve adhesion and absorption to the intestinal cells and to escape from the recognition of P-gp may provide better solutions for oral administration (p.o.) of anticancer drugs. It is currently accepted that nanoparticles are taken up by the M-cells of PPs and the isolated follicles of GALT and also via the enterocytes [199]. Recently, positively charged colloidal particles were shown to be able to increase the electrostatic interaction between particles and negatively charged mucin on the mucosal surface, thus improving their bioavailability and reducing their side effects. Chitosan nanoparticles exhibited positive charge and small particle size, which is responsible for their *in vivo* efficacy.

Conventional colloidal carriers are rapidly removed from the bloodstream by the reticuloendothelial system (RES), which is a part of the mononuclear phagocyte system (MPS) after i.v. administration [200]. Nanoparticulate systems have been used to improve the blood circulating time and tumor-targeting efficacy of vincristine [201], because the tumor vascular permeability allows the penetration of particles up to 400 nm in diameter [202]. Therefore, the antitumor efficacy of chitosan nanoparticles administered by i.v. injection is probably attributed to their small particle size.

Particle size has been proved to be an important feature related to obtaining optimal *in vitro* efficacy of chitosan nanoparticles. Particle size also has a crucial impact on the *in vivo* fate of a particulate drug delivery system [203]. Decreasing particles size can increase the surface-to-volume ratio and specific surface area, which could increase the dissolution and thus increase the bioavailability of poorly water-soluble molecules [204]. The smaller-sized particles seem to have more efficient interfacial interaction with the cell membrane as compared to larger-sized particles due to the endocytosis of small-sized particles. Small-sized particles can improve the efficacy of particle-based oral drug delivery systems [205]. The use of particle size reduction to increase the oral bioavailability of drugs has been recognized [206].

Nanoparticles can prolong the blood half-life of drugs and increase efficacy by i.v. injection [207]. If particles between 30 and 100 nm are intravenously applied, the liver eliminates larger particles faster from the bloodstream compared to smaller particles. Thus, the larger the particles, the shorter their plasma half-life period [208]. As a result, with increasing particle size, the efficacy of chitosan nanoparticles administered by IV injection decreased significantly. The TWI of chitosan nanoparticles (40 nm) against S-180 and H22 was 49% and 54%, respectively [209].

Measurements of mucoadhesiveness using small intestinal brush border membrane (BBM) surfaces: Surface plasma resonance (SPR; BIAcoreX, GE Healthcare, UK) analysis was used to estimate the intestinal adhesion of LMWC and LMWC–Docetaxel (DTX). Ileal BBM vesicles from the small intestines of SD rats (180–200 g, fasted overnight) were prepared by the previously reported method (Ca²⁺ precipitation method) [210,211]. The size distributions of BBM vesicles were observed using electronic light scattering (ELS8000, Otsuka Electronics, Osaka, Japan). Ileal BBM vesicles were immobilized on an L1 sensor chip. For binding measurements, LMWC and LMWC–DTX (Figure 3.24) (each 1 and 2 mM) were dissolved in running buffer (10 mM HEPES and 150 mM NaCl, pH 7.4) and injected for 5 min at a flow rate of 2 L/min [212,213].

The solubility of DTX in water was measured to be approximately 67 μg/mL, whereas that of LMWC–DTX was approximately 1.4 mg/mL of DTX equivalent. As expected, the solubility of DTX was increased by approximately 200-fold after conjugation with LMWC. This improved water solubility enables elimination of Tween 80-based formulation, so that saline can be used to dissolve LMWC–DTX. Moreover, the parent DTX is released from the

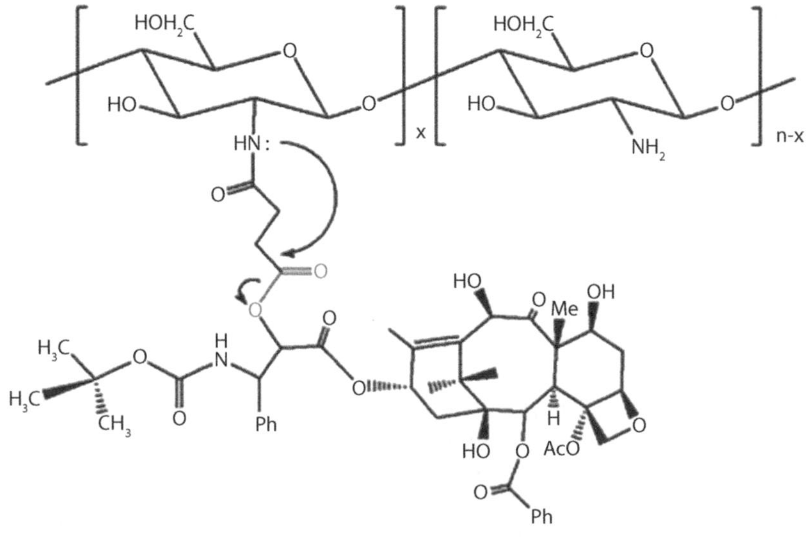

FIGURE 3.24
Scheme of the complex of LMWC–DTX.

conjugate via cleavage of the succinate linker under physiological conditions [214]. However, there is slight activity loss by two- or threefold observed with the conjugated form.

It is well known that chitosan is mucoadhesive. To examine the mucoadhesive properties of LMWC and LMWC–DTX, SPR analysis was carried out using small intestinal BBM vesicle-coated SPR chip. Figure 3.25 shows the binding response of each LMWC and the conjugate onto the BBM vesicle-coated chip surfaces. LMWC–DTX groups (1 and 2 mM LMWC equivalent) exhibited rapidly increasing response signals of ~3.4- and ~5.6-fold compared to LMWC groups (1 and 2 mM) and slow dissociation from BBM vesicles-coated surfaces. This result suggests clearly that LMWC–DTX retains the mucoadhesiveness of parent LMWC. It is speculated that the larger mucoadhesiveness of the conjugate may be attributed to the increased hydrophobicity, resulting in enhanced interactions with the intestinal epithelial layers.

Pharmacokinetic parameters after oral administration of LMWC–DTX were derived and compared with those of DTX administered intravenously (formulated in Tween 80/ethanol/saline: an identical formulation to commercial Taxotere). DTX was detectable in plasma up to 72 h for LMWC–DTX (p.o.), whereas DTX was undetectable beyond 6 h for DTX (i.v.), suggesting that DTX is released from LMWC–DTX conjugate in a sustained manner over a long period of time. The relevant pharmacokinetic parameters, including C_{max}, T_{max}, $t_{1/2}$, and $AUC_{0-\infty}$, are listed in Table 3.5. Whereas DTX (i.v.) showed a very short plasma half-life of $t_{1/2}$ =0.6 h with a rapid decrease in plasma concentration, LMWC–DTX groups (5 and 10 mg DTX 276 equivalent/kg, p.o.) exhibited significantly delayed $t_{1/2}$ values of 3.4 and 8.2 h. In addition, C_{max} of the conjugate (p.o.) was larger than that of DTX (i.v.) (2.1 ± 0.27 versus 0.82 ± 0.1).

The oral bioavailability obtained from LMWC–DTX is the highest among others reported in the literature to date. This unprecedented high absorption may be attributed to the known ability of LMWC to be mucoadhesive and to open a tight junction of intestinal epithelial layers. Furthermore, LMWC–DTX conjugates may also be able to bypass both the P-gp efflux system (displayed on intestinal epithelial cells) and cytochrome P450-mediated drug metabolism (hepatic clearance), as demonstrated in the report on oral delivery of

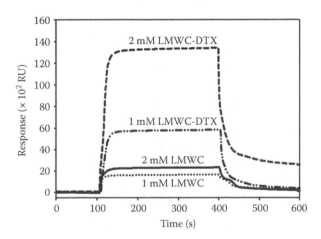

FIGURE 3.25
SPR response curve for binding of LMWC and LMWC–DTX to ileal BBM surfaces. Ileal BBM vesicles were coated onto an L1 sensor chip, after which LMWC and LMWC–DTX (each 1 and 2 mM) were injected at a flow rate of 2 L/min.

TABLE 3.5

Cytotoxicities of COS-SA, DOX HCl Solution, and DOX-COS-SA Against
MCF-7 Cells, and MCF-7/Adr Cells.

| | $IC_{50}\ n = 3(\mu g\ mL^{-1} \pm SD)$ | | |
Material	MCF- 7 Cells	MCF- 7/Adr Cells	Reversal Power
COS-SA	223.7 ± 24.8	254.1 ± 18.0	—
DOX · HCl	0.11 ± 0.02	33.7 ± 13.7	—
DOX-COS-SA-3	1.27 ± 0.12	3.26 ± 0.36	10.5
DOX-COS-SA-6	2.22 ± 0.36	5.20 ± 0.38	6.5
DOX-COS-SA-10	4.54 ± 0.35	7.70 ± 0.90	4.4

Note: Reversal power was calculated from the equation of value of drug solution against
drug resistance cells; value of drug solution against drug sensitive cells; value of
DOX-COS-SA against drug resistance cells.

paclitaxel in the form of conjugates with LMWC [215]. DTX (i.v.) (10 mg/kg) showed a
marked weight loss, indicating severe toxicity. In contrast, neither high nor low doses of
the LMWC–DTX conjugate group exhibited body weight change when compared to the
saline control group, suggesting much lower toxicity. The LMWC–DTX conjugate (p.o.) is
comparably effective in inhibiting tumor growth but is much less toxic compared to the
same dose of DTX (i.v.). The much reduced toxicity may be due to the gradual or sustained
release of DTX from the LMWC–DTX conjugate into the bloodstream after oral administration. The LMWC-based conjugate system may be used as a promising oral delivery
platform for sparingly soluble chemical drugs.

3.4.4.4 Self-Assembly Chitosan Derivatives for Antitumor Activity

Colloidal systems have found numerous applications as promising delivery vehicles for
drugs, proteins, antigens, and genes due to their low toxic side effects and enhanced therapeutic effects. Polymeric self-assembly systems (SAs) represent one type of colloidal system that has been widely investigated in terms of micellar behavior in both biotechnology
and pharmaceutics. Precise control of size and structure is a critical design parameter of
micellar systems for drug delivery applications. To control the size of an SA, chitosan was
depolymerized with sodium nitrite, and hydrophobically modified with deoxycholic acid
to form the SA in aqueous media (Figure 3.26) [216]. The size of the SA could be varied from
130 to 300 nm in diameter.

Because of the chain rigidity of chitosan, the SA was suggested to have a cylindrical
bamboo-like structure, which could form only a very poor spherical form in a bird's nest-
like structure. In the test of the potential application of the SA as a gene delivery carrier, a
significant enhancement of transfection efficiency by the SA was observed against
COS-1 cells (up to a factor of 10). This approach to control the size and structure of the
chitosan-derived SA may find a wide range of applications in gene delivery as well as in
general drug delivery applications. Lee et al. reported the delivery of adriamycin (ADR)
using the SA of the deoxycholic acid-modified chitosan [217]. Deoxycholic acid was covalently conjugated to chitosan via an hydrochloride[N-ethyl-N-(3-dimethylaminopropyl)]
carbodiimidehydrochloride (EDC)-mediated reaction to generate SA nanoparticles. ADR
was physically trapped inside the SA and slow release of ADR was thereby achieved.

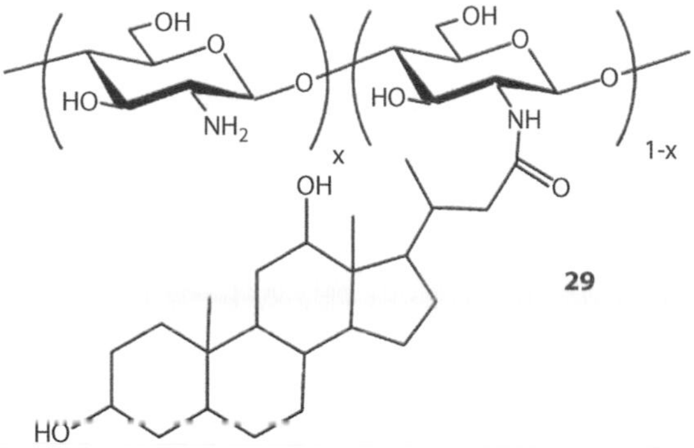

FIGURE 3.26
Deoxycholic acid-modified chitosan. (Adapted from Kim, Y. H., Gihm, S. H., and Park, C. R. 2001. *Bioconj Chem* 12: 932–938.)

Polymeric micelles can evade scavenging by the MPS because of their hydrophilic surface and generally small size (10–100 nm) [218]. As a result of the "enhanced permeability and retention (EPR) effect," the polymeric micelles largely accumulate in tumor tissue [219]. The pH of tumor tissue is mildly acidic compared with that of healthy tissue. Linkers that respond to pH changes are mainly used for small drug conjugation, such as *N-cis*-aconityl acid [220], hydrazone linkage [221], and so on. The ideal polymer–drug conjugate should be stable in blood circulation and in healthy tissues at pH 7.2, but hydrolytically degradable and releasing small drug in the mildly acidic environment of target tumor cells (pH 5–6). The conjugate of DOX attached via the hydrazone bond to *N*-(2-hydroxypropyl) methacrylamide (HPMA) copolymer showed a much higher antitumor activity *in vivo* than the free drug [221].

Drug resistance and multidrug resistance (MDR) to current chemotherapeutic agents account for the failure of human cancer chemotherapy. MDR can be the result of a variety of mechanisms that have not been unveiled completely [222]. One of the main causes of MDR is linked to the overexpression of P-gp in tumors. P-gp belongs to the ATP-binding cassette (ABC) superfamily of transporters [223], which acts as an energy-dependent drug efflux pump. P-gp expression impairs the response to chemotherapy, and the expression levels increase as tumors become drug resistant [224]. Many agents have been investigated to reverse P-gp-mediated MDR. Researchers have proposed that several polymer micelles can overcome drug resistance. The micelles were assumed to reduce the ATP production in MDR cells, while sensitive cells had no noticeable change in ATP production [225]. HPMA copolymers containing doxorubicin could overcome MDR in human acute lymphoblastic T-cells, leukemia cell lines, and mouse leukemia cell lines [226].

MCF-7 and MCF-7/Adr cells were seeded at a density of 10^5 cells/μL plate and grown for 24 h. Certain amounts (drug content was 5 μg/mL) of DOX · HCl and DOX–COS–SA were added, and the cells were further incubated for 4 and 8 h, respectively. After washing the cells with PBS three times, cellular uptake was observed by fluorescence microscopy. *In vitro* antitumor activities of DOX–COS–SA were evaluated for the determination of cytotoxicities of DOX–COS–SA using MCF-7 and MCF-7/Adr as model tumor cells, and DOX HCl solution as a control. Using the MTT method, the 50% cellular growth inhibitions (IC_{50}) for DOX HCl solution, COS–SA micelles, and DOX–COS–SA micelles with different drug loadings against MCF-7 and MCF-7/Adr were determined, and are shown in Table 3.5. The variation of cell viability with the drug concentration of DOX HCl solution

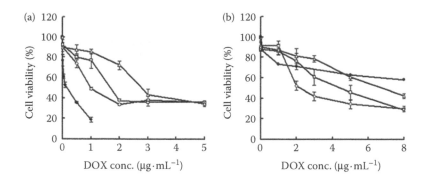

FIGURE 3.27
Cytotoxicity of DOX-COS-SA and DOX HCl solution toward MCF-7 (a) and MCF-7/Adr (b). For both cells, (◇) DOX-COS-SA-3, (○) DOX-COS-SA-6, (△) DOX-COS-SA, and (◆) DOX HCl solution. Data represent the mean standard deviation ($n = 3$). (Adapted from Hu, F. Q. et al. 2009. *Biomaterials* 30: 1–9.)

and the DOX–COS values of COS–SA in MCF–SA micelles are shown in Figure 3.27. The IC_{50} values for COS–SA in MCF-7a and MCF-7/Adr cells were determined as about 250 μg/mL, indicating that the present micelles showed low cytotoxicity against cultured cells. It can be seen that for both MCF-7 and MCF/Adr cells, the IC_{50} value of DOX–COS–SA is related to the DOX content in DOX–COS–SA. The results indicated that the higher the drug content, the lower the cytotoxicity. For MCF-7/Adr cells, the IC_{50} value of DOX HCl was above 300-fold higher than in sensitive cells. This means that MCF-7/Adr cells were DOX HCl resistant. Compared to the DOX HCl solution, DOX–COS–SA with different DOX contents did not show lower cytotoxicity in drug-sensitive MCF-7 cells. However, the IC_{50} value of DOX–COS–SA against MCF-7/Adr cells was only slightly higher than that of DOX–COS–SA against MCF-7 drug-sensitive cells and was much lower than that of DOX HCl solution in MCF-7/Adr cells. The results meant that DOX–COS–SA micelles could reverse the drug resistance of MCF-7/Adr cells. The reversal power of DOX–COS–SA against MCF-7/Adr cells was about 4–10.

ADR and DOX–CSO–SA-10 treatments effectively suppressed tumor growth; for example, 5 days after i.v. injection, tumor volumes of nude mice treated with ADR and DOX–CSO–SA-10 were significantly smaller than those treated with saline and blank COS–SA micelle solution ($p < 0.05$); after 10 days, $p < 0.001$. There were no significant differences between the tumor volumes treated with saline and blank COS–SA ($p > 0.05$). After 10 days, the tumor volumes treated with ADR (total DOX dosage was 7 mg/kg) were significantly smaller than those treated with DOX–COS–SA (total DOX dosage was 7 mg/kg), but were significantly bigger than those treated with DOX–COS–SA-10 (total DOX dosage was 14 mg/kg) ($p < 0.05$). However, after 20 days, there were no significant differences ($p > 0.05$). But for the tumor volumes treated with DOX–COS–SA-10 (total DOX dosage was 7 mg/kg) and DOX–COS–SA-10 (total DOX dosage was 14 mg/kg), there were evident significant differences ($p < 0.05$). The doses of these five groups were within the safe range. However, the injection of ADR with 2 mg/kg body weight for 7 days consecutively led to the death of nude mice (only 1 survived on the 15th day). This means that DOX–COS–SA was safer than ADR. The tumor inhibition rate of ADR (total DOX dosage was 7 mg/kg; the total drug dose was 64.33 ± 7.01%; DOX–COS–SA-10 with 7 mg/kg was 63.89 ± 7.64%; and DOX–COS–SA-10 with 14 mg/kg total drug dose was 80.70 ± 2.55%. All the tumor inhibition values were larger than 60%, which was considered to be effective treatment.

The carboxymethyl chitosan (CMC) value is one of the important characteristics for polymeric micelles as a drug delivery carrier. A low CMC value means that the copolymer can form micelles under highly diluted conditions. DOX conjugation can improve the hydrophobicity of CSO–SA, which caused the decrease in CMC value for DOX–CSO–SA. After DOX conjugation, the micellar size was bigger in comparison with CSO–SA, which might be caused by the increased DOX content in the micelles. The reduction of amino groups after DOX conjugation led to lower zeta potential of DOX–CSO–SA. The zeta potential of these micelles was still larger than 30 mV in deionized water, which means that the micelles were stable in colloidal dispersion.

The *cis*-aconityl linkage was introduced as a pH-sensitive linkage for release of DOX in a macromolecule drug. The elevation of pH results in decreased liberation of the drug from all the DOX–CSO–SA conjugates with different drug contents. The faster drug release from DOX–CSO–SA under weak acid conditions might be favorable for targeting the delivery of antitumor drugs [228], because of the lower pH of tumor tissue. The varied drug release behavior among DOX–CSO–SA with different drug contents might relate to the varied micellar size of DOX–CSO–SA. The micellar size is a key factor affecting the surface area in contact with the dissolution medium. Moreover, the larger the area in contact with the medium, the faster the drug release from the micelles.

Various lines of evidence strongly support the fact that expression of ABC transporters on the cell membrane, such as P-gp, is associated with drug resistance in cancer. P-gp functions as an energy-dependent efflux pump to remove cytotoxic agents from drug-resistant cells. The DOX uptakes of DOX–CSO–SA micelles were increased with incubation time in both MCF-7 and MCF-7/Adr cells. DOX–CSO–SA micelles may enter the cells via endocytosis, which is not a P-gp-dependent pathway.

Nano-sized polymeric carriers have been extensively applied, because they enhanced the drug's solubility and stability *in vivo* by encapsulating the hydrophobic camptothecin (CPT) into nano-sized drug carriers, wherein CPT is encapsulated into hydrophobic cores and the drug carriers are covered with hydrophilic and biocompatible polymer shells [229,230]. Furthermore, nano-sized polymeric carrier-encapsulated CPTs have exhibited a prolonged circulation time *in vivo* by avoiding the RES, and the prolonged circulation time of polymeric carriers allows the encapsulated CPT to extravasate and accumulate into tumor tissue, wherein a disorganized vasculature and defective vascular architecture develop, which is called an enhanced permeability and retention (EPR) effect in tumor tissue [231,232]. Therefore, this passive targeting of CPT-encapsulated nano-sized polymeric carriers to solid tumors has enhanced the drug's therapeutic efficacy and potentially decreased severe toxic effects.

Preparation of CPT-encapsulated and nano-sized carriers: 100 mg of aglycol chitosan 5β-cholanic acid (HGC) conjugate (Figure 3.28) was mixed in 5 mL of DMSO and CPT solutions (10, 20, and 30 mg in 2 mL of DMSO). The solution was vigorously stirred for 12 h at room temperature and dialyzed for 2 days in distilled water by using a dialysis tube with an MW cutoff of 12,000–14,000 (Spectrum, Rancho Dominquez, CA). After dialysis for 2 days, the solution was centrifuged at 10,000 *g* for 30 min to remove free CPT. The supernatant was filtered with 0.8 μm of syringe filter and lyophilized to give a white powder.

Physicochemical properties of CPT-encapsulated HGC: The critical aggregation of concentration value of HGC nanoparticles was 0.047 mg/mL, which was lower than those of LMW surfactants (e.g., 2.3 mg/mL for sodium dodecyl sulfate in water). Thus, HGC nanoparticles could maintain their nanoscale particle structure at the diluted concentration in the body. As HGC nanoparticles possess hydrophobic inner cores, the nanoparticles are stable and may encapsulate hydrophobic drugs. Because CPT is water insoluble, CPT is easily encapsulated into HGC nanoparticles by the dialysis method. Thus, we assumed that HGC

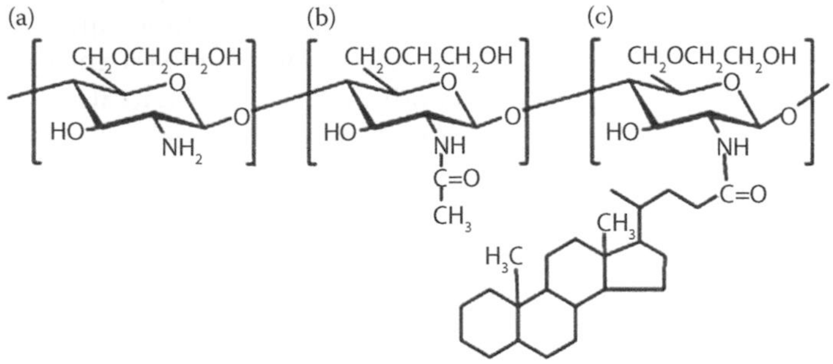

Hydrophobically modified glycol chitosan conjugate (HGC)

FIGURE 3.28
Chemical structure of HGC nanoparticles prepared by chemical coupling of hydrophilic glycol chitosan with hydrophobic 5β-cholanic acids. (Adapted from Maeda, H. et al. 2000. *J control Release* 65: 271–284.)

nanoparticles might protect the active lactone ring of CPT against hydrolysis under physiological conditions, due to the encapsulation of CPT into the hydrophobic cores in HGC nanoparticles. The freshly prepared HGC and CPT-10 wt%–HGC nanoparticles were well dispersed in aqueous conditions and the particle sizes were about 254 and 288 nm, respectively, which are confirmed by DLS measurements. Transmission electron microscopy (TEM) images also revealed that HGC and CPT-10 wt%–HGC nanoparticles were almost spherical in shape. Also, CPT–HGC nanoparticles were well dispersed and their particle sizes were maintained up to 2 weeks at 37°C in PBS, indicating thermodynamical stability in aqueous media. The loading efficiency of CPT was above 80% when the drug was present at less than 10 wt% of nanoparticles, whereas a marked decrease in the loading efficiency (to less than 45%) was seen when the drug was present at 20 wt%.

Protection of the CPT lactone ring from hydrolysis: The proportions of CPT in the lactone ring and carboxylate forms are critical in predicting tumor response to CPT because the lactone form has much higher antitumor efficacy compared to the carboxylate form. The protection effect of CPT–HGC nanoparticles on the CPT lactone ring form against hydrolysis under physiological conditions (PBS, pH 7.4, 37°C) using reversed-phase high-performance liquid chromatography (HPLC) was evaluated. As shown in Figure 3.29a, free CPT dissolved in PBS exhibited significant lactone ring opening due to rapid hydrolysis. The carboxylate form and the lactone ring form of CPT were detected at 8.7 and 11.5 min, respectively, in analytical HPLC spectra. Only 39% of CPT remained in the lactone ring form after incubation in PBS for 6 h, indicating that the unprotected CPT lactone ring was rapidly converted into the inactive carboxylate by hydrolysis. On the other hand, about 89% of the lactone ring was preserved after 6 h incubation in PBS when CPT was incorporated into HGC nanoparticles (Figures 3.29b and c). This implies that the many inner cores of HGC nanoparticles efficiently protected the lactone form of CPT from hydrolysis.

In vivo tumor-targeting characteristics of CPT–HGC nanoparticles: To estimate the *in vivo* characteristics of CPT–HGC nanoparticles, HGC nanoparticles were labeled with the near-infra-red (NIR) fluorophore, Cy 5.5 (exciting wavelength = 675 nm, emission wavelength = 695 nm), which yields a strong fluorescence signal *in vivo*. To estimate *in vivo* tumor targeting of CPT–HGC nanoparticles, 10 wt% of CPT was encapsulated into Cy 5.5-labeled HGC nanoparticles. The freshly prepared Cy 5.5-labeled CPT–HGC nanoparticles had the same physicochemical characteristics (particle size, *in vitro* stability, morphological shape, and drug-loading efficiency) as unlabeled CPT–HGC nanoparticles, whereas they presented a strong NIR fluorescence signal. After the i.v. injection of Cy

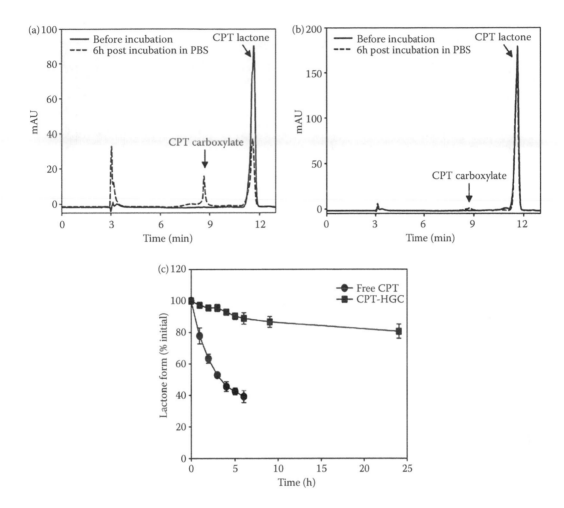

FIGURE 3.29

Protection effect of CPT-10 wt%–HGC nanoparticles on the lactone ring of CPT against hydrolysis over time under physiological conditions (pH 7.4, 37°C). Reversed-phase HPLC chromatograms of (a) CPT and (b) CPT-10 wt%–HGC nanoparticles before and after incubation for 6 h under physiological conditions (PBS, pH 7.4, 37°C). (b) Kinetic valuation of the rat of lactone ring opening for free CPT and CPT-10 wt%–HGC nanoparticles evaluated by reversed-phase HPLC under physiological conditions (PBS, pH 7.4, 37°C).

5.5-labeled CPT–HGC nanoparticles with 10 mg/kg of CPT, the time-dependent excretion profile, tumor accumulation, and tissue distribution of Cy 5.5-labeled CPT–HGC nanoparticles in tumor-bearing mice were evaluated using the Explore Optix system and the Kodak Image Station 4000 MM. First, the time-dependent excretion profile of CPT–HGC nanoparticles was clearly visualized by monitoring real-time NIR fluorescence signals in the whole body (Figure 3.30a). After the i.v. injection of Cy 5.5-labeled CPT–HGC nanoparticles, the NIR fluorescence intensity immediately increased in the whole body, due to the rapid circulation of Cy 5.5-labeled CPT–HGC nanoparticles. However, the NIR fluorescence signal in the whole body decreased as time elapsed, which was indicative of excretion by renal clearance. It is deduced that nano-sized drug carriers in the blood might be dissociated and biodegraded *in vivo* and then excreted by renal clearance. Importantly, CPT–HGC nanoparticles displayed strong fluorescence signals in tumor regions, compared to the whole body (Figure 3.30b and c). Furthermore, *ex vivo* fluorescence images

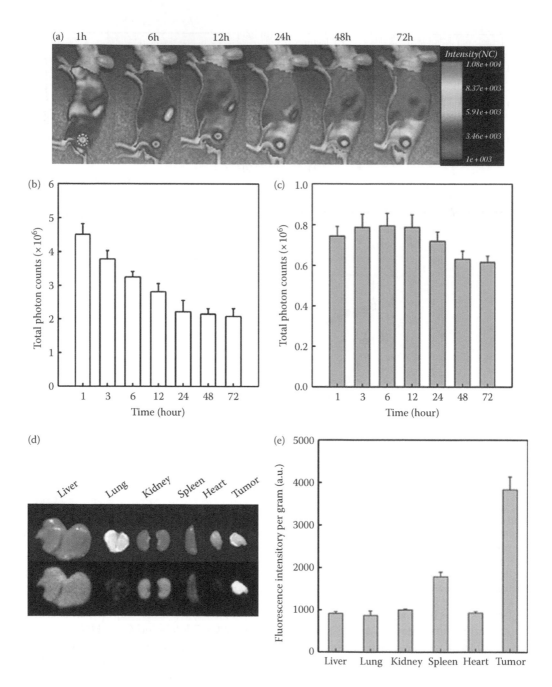

FIGURE 3.30
(a) *In vivo* NIR fluorescence images of the time-dependent excretion profile and real-time tumor-targeting characteristics of CPT-10 wt%–HGC nanoparticles in tumor-bearing mice. The tumor locations are specified with an arrow. Quantification of the *in vivo* tumor-targeting characteristics of CPT-10 wt%–HGC nanoparticles. The NIR fluorescence intensities of (b) whole body and (c) tumor tissues are shown as a function of time postadministration. (d) Representative *ex vivo* NIR fluorescence images of dissected organs and tumor of mice bearing MDA-MB231 human breast tumors, sacrificed 3 days after i.v. injection of Cy 5.5-labeled CPT-10 wt%–HGC nanoparticles. (e) Quantification of the *ex vivo* tumor-targeting characteristics of Cy 5.5-labeled CPT-10 wt%–HGC nanoparticles.

showing higher fluorescence intensity in tumors than in other major organs (Figure 3.30d) at 3 days after i.v. administration indicate that CPT–HGC nanoparticles are preferentially accumulated in tumor tissue rather than in normal organs. The highest NIR fluorescence intensity was observed in tumor tissue and the NIR fluorescence intensity was 23 times higher than those of other organs (Figure 3.30e).

The enhanced therapeutic potencies of nanoparticles are mainly due to passive targeting to tumor sites, based on the EPR effect, which is attributed to high vascularization and enhanced permeability of tumor blood vessels combined with limited lymphatic clearance of macromolecules from the tumor environment [234,235]. Nanoparticles should retain drugs while circulating, thereby preventing premature drug release before the nanoparticles accumulate in the tumor. To increase therapeutic efficacy, nanoparticle design must allow for drug release, and therefore subsequent increases in drug concentration, in tumor tissues. In addition, drug delivery in nanoparticles substantially reduces adverse side effects by virtue of the relatively low doses of drugs (compared to free drug doses) required [236,237].

3.4.4.5 Chitosan Hydrogels for Antitumors

The formation of hydrogels from polymers using noncovalent cross-linking is a useful method of preparing hydrogels for drug delivery. These gels are likely to be biocompatible as gel formation does not require the use of organic solvents or chemical reactions, which may be potentially deleterious to the drug load. Such physically cross-linked chitosan-based gels are formed by exploiting either hydrogen bonding or hydrophobic attractions. Hwang et al. [238] and Martin et al. [239] have focused on the use of pendant hydrophobic groups to achieve noncovalent cross-linking. Palmitoylglycol chitosan (GCP, Figure 3.31) hydrogel has been evaluated as an erodible controlled release system for the delivery of hydrophilic macromolecules. Fluorescein isothiocyanate (FITC)-dextran, and/or amphiphilic derivatives Gelucire 50/13 and vitamin E [D-α-tocopherol poly(ethyleneglycol)succinate] were used as model macromolecules. Hydration and erosion were governed by the hydrophobicity of the gel and the presence of amphiphilic additives. The controlled release of FITC-dextran was governed by the hydrophobicity of the gel. In a subsequent study, GCP hydrogel was evaluated for buccal delivery of the hydrophobic drug denbufylline [240]. The buccal route has been advocated as a possible means for administration of drugs that undergo extensive hepatic first-pass metabolism or that are susceptible to degradation in the GI tract.

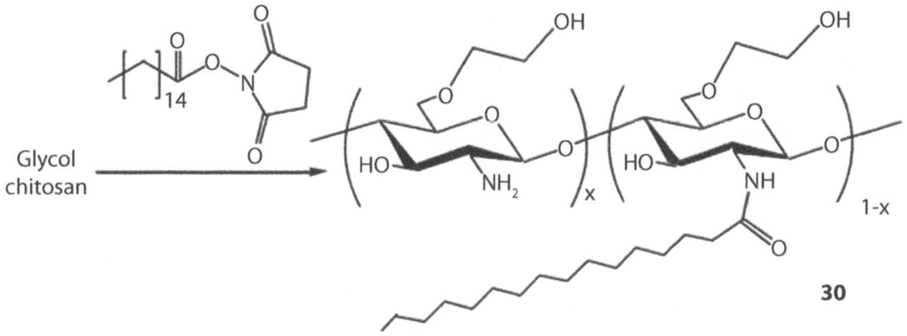

FIGURE 3.31
Scheme of the synthesis of palmitoyl glycol chitosan.

When FGF-2 was added to hydrogels, most of the FGF-2 molecules retained in the hydrogels remained biologically active, and were gradually released on biodegradation of the hydrogels *in vivo* [241,242]. The study showed that the controlled release of biologically active FGF-2 molecules from FGF-2-incorporated chitosan hydrogels caused induction of angiogenesis, and collateral circulation possibly occurred in healing-impaired diabetic (db/db) mice and in the ischemic limbs of rats. The controlled release of paclitaxel from photocross-linkable chitosan hydrogel *in vitro* has been described and its antiangiogenesis and antitumor effects *in vivo* were shown to support the possible use of chitosan hydrogel incorporating paclitaxel as a regional delivery for tumor treatment [243]. Thus, photocross-linkable chitosan hydrogel and injectable chitosan/IO_4^- heparin hydrogel are excellent carriers for controlled release of drug reagents such as FGF-2 and paclitaxel. To prepare a chitosan hydrogel incorporating paclitaxel, 1 mL of Taxol containing paclitaxel (6 mg/mL) in a vehicle composed of Cremophor EL and ethanol at a 50:50 (v/v) ratio was mixed into 1 mL of 40 mg/mL Az–CH–LA aqueous solution (at a final concentration of 20 mg/mL Az–CH–LA) using a vortex. While about 35–40% of both paclitaxel and vehicle were released from the photocross-linked hydrogel within 1 day, the releases were observed over a period of 4 days with a half-release time of 45 h [243].

Paclitaxel is a potent inhibitor of angiogenesis, cell migration, and collagenase production in addition to its antiproliferative effect on tumor cells. Chitosan hydrogel incorporating paclitaxel was found to inhibit the growth of Lewis lung cancer cells (3LL), human umbilical vein endothelial cells (HUVECs), and human dermal microvascular endothelial cells (HMVECs) with half-cell growth-inhibition concentrations of 15, 15, and 1 ng/mL, respectively. Washing chitosan hydrogels incorporating paclitaxel with the culture medium for longer than 15 days resulted in loss of the ability to inhibit cell growth except in the case of HMVECs. HMVEC growth was inhibited in the presence of the washed chitosan hydrogel incorporating paclitaxel for longer than 21 days. On the other hand, the chitosan hydrogel incorporating paclitaxel had a significantly lower inhibitory effect on fibroblast (human dermal fibroblast) growth than 3LL, HUVECs, and HMVECs.

A measurable tumor volume (about 100 mm) was formed at 12 days after subcutaneous implantation of 3LL cells. UV-laser irradiation for 30 s was able to convert the injected viscous Az–CH–LA aqueous solution (0.2 mL) into the same insoluble hydrogel through insertion of an optical crystal fiber connected to a He-Cd laser. As shown in Figure 3.32 [244], administration of paclitaxel alone and chitosan hydrogel alone reduced subcutaneous induced tumor growth of 3LL cells to various extents over 7 days. The chitosan hydrogel incorporating paclitaxel more strongly inhibited tumor growth to less than 5% of the control group value ($p < 0.0001$ versus control) than paclitaxel alone or chitosan hydrogel alone. The inhibitory effect on tumor growth of the chitosan hydrogel incorporating paclitaxel lasted for 14 days and subsequently the tumor in most mice grew again. However, a second application of the chitosan hydrogel incorporating paclitaxel 10 days after the first application had an additional antitumor effect.

To evaluate the antiangiogenesis effect of chitosan hydrogel incorporating paclitaxel, immunohistochemical staining of murine CD34 was carried out in 3LL cells treated with chitosan hydrogel incorporating paclitaxel, chitosan hydrogel alone, paclitaxel alone, and untreated control tumors. On day 8, in paclitaxel-treated and control mice, many CD34-positive stained vessels were diffusely located and clearly formed tube-like structures were found in the tumor. On the other hand, CD34-positive vessels were significantly fewer in the tumors treated with chitosan hydrogel incorporating paclitaxel. As shown in Figure 3.33, chitosan hydrogel incorporating paclitaxel significantly reduced the number of CD34-positive vessels compared with other treatments, suggesting that chitosan

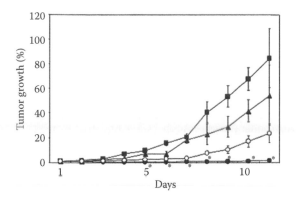

FIGURE 3.32

Inhibitory effect of paclitaxel-incorporated chitosan hydrogel on lewis lung cancer cell (3LL)-tumor growth. Tumor cells were implanted into the dorsal subcutis of mice. After tumors reached a measurable size (about 100 mm³), 200 mL of paclitaxel-incorporated chitosan hydrogel was administered beneath the tumor. Data were compared with the average tumor volume of the phosphate-buffered saline (PBS)-treated group on day 12 defined as 100%. Solid circles, paclitaxel and chitosan hydrogel; open circles, chitosan hydrogel alone; triangles, paclitaxel alone; squares, saline (control). *$P < 0.05$, paclitaxel and chitosan hydrogel versus the other three groups. (Adapted from Obara, K. 2005. *J control Release* 110: 79–89.)

hydrogel incorporating paclitaxel significantly inhibited angiogenesis in tumors. Application of chitosan hydrogel alone showed an intermediate effect of antiangiogenesis. It is thus proposed that chitosan hydrogel incorporating paclitaxel may be a promising new biomaterial to strongly inhibit vascularization and tumor growth.

It should also be noted that application of the chitosan hydrogel alone significantly inhibited tumor growth, although the inhibitory activity was lower than for the chitosan hydrogel incorporating paclitaxel. Chitosan has shown a growth-inhibition effect on tumor cells [245] and inhibition of tumor-induced angiogenesis and tumor metastasis [246]. Chitosan directly inhibits tumor cell proliferation by inducing apoptosis [247].

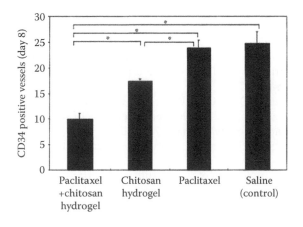

FIGURE 3.33

Effect of paclitaxel-incorporated chitosan hydrogel on 3LL-tumor vascularization. Vascularization of the 3LL tumor, evaluated immunohistochemically with antimurine CD34, markedly decreased in paclitaxel-incorporated chitosan hydrogel-treated 3LL tumors and chitosan hydrogel-treated 3LL tumors when compared with paclitaxel-treated and PBS-treated 3LL tumors. *$p < 0.05$.

3.5 Conclusions

Chitosan can be dissolved in the digestive tract under acidic conditions, combines bile acid with its ion-exchanging function, and excretes the combined bile acid outside the body; consequently, it decreases the cholesterol pool in the body. Chitosan, a deacetylated derivative of chitin, is a positively charged polymer carrier. The cell adhesion and potential uptake of chitosan particles are also most favorable due to their attraction to negatively charged cell membranes, an attractive feature for the treatment of solid tumors. Moreover, chitosan has shown favorable biocompatibility as well as the ability to increase cell membrane permeability both *in vitro* and *in vivo*. Chitosan can also be degraded by lysozymes in the body.

References

142. Suh, J. K. and Matthew, H. W. 2000. Application of chitosan-based polysaccharide biomaterials in cartilage tissue engineering: A review. *Biomaterials* 21: 2589–2598.
143. Usami, Y., Okamoto, Y., Takayama, T., Shigemasa, Y., and Minami, S. 1998. Chitin and chitosan stimulate canine polymorphonuclear cells to release leukotriene B4 and prostaglandin E2. *J Biomed Mater Res* 42: 517–522.
144. Peluso, G., Petillo, O., Ranieri, M., Santin, M., Ambrosis, L., Calabro, D., Avallone, B., and Balsamo, G. 1994. Chitosan-mediated stimulation of macrophage function. *Biomaterials* 15: 1215–1220.
145. Mori, T., Okumura, M., Matsura, M., Ueno, K., TOkura, S., Okamoto, Y., Minami, S., and Fujinaga, T. 1997. Efects of chitin and its derivates on the proliferation and cytokine production of broblasts *in vitro*. *Biomaterials* 18: 947–951.
146. Pae, H. O., Seo, W. G., Kim, N. Y., Oh, G, S., Kim, G. E., Kim, Y. H., Kwak, H. J., Yun, Y. G., Jun, C. D., and Chung, H. T. 2001. Induction of granulocytic differentiation in acute promyelocytic leukemia cells (HL-60) by water-soluble chitosan oligomer. *Leukemia Res* 25: 339–346.
147. Yoon, H. J., Moon, M. E., Park, H. S., Im, S. Y., and Kim, Y. H. 2007. Chitosanoligosaccharide (COS) inhibits LPS-induced inflammatory effects in RAW264.7 macrophage cells. *Biochem Biophy Res Comm* 358: 954–959.
148. Berthold, A., Cremer, K., and Kreuter, J. 1996. Preparation and characterization of chitosan microspheres as drug carrier for prednisolone sodium phosphate as model for anti-inflammatory drugs. *J Control Release* 39: 17–25.
149. Kofuji, K., Akamine, H., Qian, C. J., Watanabe, K., Togan, Y., Nishimura, M., Sugiyama, I., Murata, Y., and Kawashima, S. 2004. Therapeutic efficacy of sustained drug release from chitosan gel on local inflammation. *Int J Pharm* 272: 65–78.
150. Hara, N. and Okabe, S. 1985. Effects of gefarnate on acute gastric lesions in rats. *Folia Pharmacol Jpn* 85: 443–446.
151. Koji, K. 1992. Clinical application of chitin artificial skin (Beschitin W). In: Brine, C. J., Sanford, P. A., Zikakis, J. P., eds. *Advances in Chitin and Chitosan*. London: Elsevier, Advances in chitin and chitosan. pp. 9–15.
152. Ueno, H., Yamada, H., Tanaka, I., Kaba, N., Matsuura, M., Okumura, M., Kadosawa, T., and Fujinaga, T. 1999. Accelerating effects of chitosan for healing at early phase of experimental open wound in dogs. *Biomaterials* 20: 1407–1414.
153. VandeVord. P. J., Matthew, H. W., DeSilva, S. P., Mayton, L., Wu, B., and Wooley, P. H. 2002. Evaluation of the biocompatibility of a chitosan scaffold in mice. *J Biomed Mater Res* 59: 585–590.

154. Azad, A. K., Sermsintham, N., Chandrkrachang, S., and Stevens, W. F. 2004. Chitosan membrane as a wound-healing dressing: Characterization and clinical application. *J Biomed Mater Res B-Appl Biomater* 69B: 216–222.
155. Guo, X. B., Xie, Y., Zhou, N. J., and Chen, J. 2007. Effect of chitosan on the quality of gastric ulcer healing: An experimental study. *Chin J Gastroenterol* 12: 148–152.
156. Ito, M., Ban, A., and Ishihara, M. 2000. Anti-ulcer effects of chitin and chitosan, healthy foods, in rats. *Jpn J Pharmacol* 82: 218–225.
157. Lyder, C. H. 2003. Pressure ulcer prevention and management. *JAMA* 289: 223–226.
158. Phillips, T. J. 1994. Chronic cutaneous ulcers: etiology and epidemiology. *J Invest Dermatol* 102: 38S–41S.
159. Centers for Disease Control and Prevention (CDC). 2003. History of foot ulcer among persons with diabetes-United States, 2000–2002. *MMWR Morb Mortal Wkly Rep* 52: 1098–1102.
160. Azad, A. K., Sermsintham, N., Chandrkrachang, S., and Stevens, W. F. 2004. Chitosan membrane as a wound-healing dressing: characterization and clinical application. *J Biomed Mater Res B Appl Biomater* 69: 216–222.
161. Prudden, J. F., Nishihara, and G., Baker, L. 1957. The acceleration of wound healing with cartilage. I. *Surg Gynecol Obstet* 105: 283–286.
162. Muzzarelli, R. A., Mattioli-Belmonte, M., Pugnaloni, A., and Biagini, G. 1999. Biochemistry, histology and clinical uses of chitins and chitosans in wound healing. *EXS* 187: 251–264.
163. Ueno, H., Yamada, H., Tanaka, I., Kaba, N., Matsuura, M., Okumura, M., Kadosawa, T., and Fujinaga, T. 1999. Accelerating effects of chitosan for healing at early phase of experimental open wound in dogs. *Biomaterials* 20: 1407–1414.
164. Obara, K., Ishihara, M., Ishizuka, T., Fujita, M., Ozeki, Y., Maehara, Saito, Y., Yura, H., Matsui, T., Hattori, H., Kikuchi, M., and Kurita, A. 2003. Photocross-linkable chitosan hydrogel containing fibroblast growth factor-2 stimulates wound healing in healing-impaired db/db mice. *Biomaterials* 24: 3437–3444.
165. Park, C. J., Clark, S. G., Lichtensteiger, C. A., Jamison, R. D., and Johnson, A. J. 2009. Accelerated wound closure of pressure ulcers in aged mice by chitosan scaffolds with and without bFGF. *Acta Biomater* 5: 1926–1936.
166. Kanauchi, O., Deuchi, K., Imasato, Y., Shizukuishi, M., and Kobayashi, E. 1995. Mechanism for the inhibition of fat digestion by chitosan and for the synergistic effect of ascorbate. *Biosci Biotechnol Biochem* 59: 786–790.
167. Jameela, S. R., Misra, A., and Jayakrishnan, A. 1994. Cross-linked chitosan microspheres as carriers for prolonged delivery of macromolecular drugs. *J Biomater Sci Polym Edn* 6: 621–632.
168. Maezake, Y., Tsuji, K., and Nakagawa, Y. 1993. Hypocholesterolemic effect of chitosan in adult males. *Biosci Biotechnol Biochem* 57: 1439–1444.
169. Muzzarelli, R. A. A. 1997. Human enzymatic activities related to the therapeutical administration of chitin derivatives. *Cell Mol Life Sci* 53: 131–140.
170. Remunan-Lopez, C., Portero, A., Vila-Jato, J. L., and Alonso, M. J. 1998. Design and evaluation of chitosan/ethylcellulose mucoadhesive bilayered devices for buccal drug delivery. *J Control Release* 55: 143–152.
171. Tanaka, Y., Tanioka, S., Tanaka, M., Tanigawa, T., Kitamura, Y., Minami S, Okamoto, Y., Miyashita, M., and Nanno, M. 1997. Effects of chitin and chitosan particles on BALB/c mice by oral and parenteral administration. *Biomaterials* 18: 591–595.
172. Sugano, M., Watanabe, S., Kishi, A., Izume, M., and Ohtakara, A. 1988. Hypocholesterolemic action of chitosans with different viscosity in rats. *Lipids* 23: 187–191.
173. Tokoro, A., Tatewaki, N., Suzuki, K., Mikami, T., Suzuki, S., and Suzuki, M. 1988. Growth-inhibitory effect of hexa N-acetylchitohexaose and chitohexaose against Meth-A solid tumor. *Chem Pharm Bull* 36: 784–790.
174. Nishimura, S., Nishi, N., Tokura, S., Nishimura, K., and Azuma, I. 1986. Bioactive chitin derivatives. Activation of mouse-peritoneal macrophages by O-(carboxymethyl) chitins. *Carbohydr Res* 146: 251–258.

175. Tsukada, K., Matsumoto, T., Aizawa, K., Tokoro, A., Naruse, R. S., Suzuki, S., and Suzuki, M. 1990. Antimetastatic and growth-inhibitory effects of N-acetylchitohexaose in mice bearing Lewis lung carcinoma. *Jpn J Cancer Res* 81: 259–265.

176. Seo, W. G., Pae, H. O., Kim, N. Y., Oh, G. S., Park, I. S., Kim, Y. H., Kim, Y. M., Lee, Y. H., Jun, C. D., and Chung, H. T. 2000. Synergistic cooperation between water-soluble chitosan oligomers and interferon-γ for induction of nitric oxide synthesis and tumoricidal activity in murine peritoneal macrophages. *Cancer Lett* 159: 189–195.

177. Suzuki, K., Mikami, T., Okawa, Y., Tokoro, A., Suzuki, S., and Suzuki, M. 1986. Antitumor effect of hexa-N-acetylchitohexaose and chitohexaose. *Carbohydr Res* 151: 403–408.

178. Kobayashi, M., Watanabe, T., Suzuki, S., and Suzuki, M. 1990. Effect of N-acetyl-chitohexaose against Candida albicans infection of tumor-bearing mice. *Microbiol Immunol* 34: 413–426.

179. Tokoro, A., Suzuki, K., Matsumoto, T., Mikami, T., Suzuki, S., and Suzuki, M. 1988. Chemotactic response of human neutrophils to N-acetyl chitohexaose *in vitro*. *Microbiol Immunol* 132: 387–395.

180. Tokoro, A., Kobayashi, M., Tatewaki, N., Suzuki, K., and Okawa, Y. 1989. Protective effect of N-acetyl chitohexaose on Listeria monocytogenes infection in mice. *Microbiol Immunol* 33: 357–367.

181. Shahidi, F., Arachchi, J. K. V., and Jeon, Y. J. 1999. Food applications of chitin and chitosans. *Trends Food Sci Technol* 10: 37–51.

182. Yalpani, M., and Pantaleone, D. 1994. An examination of the unusual susceptibilities of aminoglycans to enzymatic hydrolysis. *Carbohydr Res* 256: 159–175.

183. Pantaleone, D., Yalpani, M., and Scollar, M. 1992. Unusual susceptibility of chitosan to enzymic hydrolysis. *Carbohydr Res* 237: 325–332.

184. Muzzarelli, R. A. A., Xia, W., Tomasetti, M., and Ilari, P. 1996. Depolymerization of chitosan and substituted chitosans with the aid of wheat germ lipase preparation. *Enzyme Microbiol Technol* 17: 541–545.

185. Shin-ya, Y., Lee, M. Y., Hinode, H., and Kajiuchi, T. 2001.Effects of N-acetylation degree on N-acetylated chitosan hydrolysis with commercially available and modified pectinases. *Biochem Eng J* 7: 85–88.

186. Qin, C. Q., Du, Y. M., Xiao, L., Li, Z., and Gao, X. H. 2002. Enzymic preparation of water-soluble chitosan and their antitumor activity. *Int J Biol Macromol* 31: 111–117.

187. Tokoro, A., Tatewaki, N., Suzuki, K., Mikami, T., Suzuki, S., and Suzuki, M. 1988. Growth-inhibitory effect of hexa-N-acetylchitohexaose and chitohexaose against Meth-A solid tumor. *Chem Pharm Bull* 36: 784–790.

188. Lu, R., Yoshida, T., Nakashima, H., Premanathan, M., Aragaki, R., Mimura, T., Kaneko, Y., Yamamoto, N., Miyakoshi, T., and Uryu, T. 2000. Specific biological activities of Chinese lacquer polysaccharides. *Carbohydr Polym* 43: 47–54.

189. Calazans, G. M. T., Lima, R. C., Franca, F. P., and Lopes, C. E. 2000. Molecular weight and anti-tumour activity of *Zymomonas mobilis levans*. *Int J Biol Macromol* 27: 245–247.

190. Suzuki, K., Mikami, T., Okawa, Y., Tokoro, A., Suzuki, S., and Suzuki, M. 1986. Antitumor effect of hexa-N-acetylchitohexaose and chitohexaose. *Carbohydr Res* 151: 403–408.

191. Seo, W. G., Pae, H. O., Kim, N. Y., Oh, G. S., Park, I. S., Kim, Y. H., Kim, Y. M., Lee, Y. H., Jun, C. D., and Chung, H. T. 2000. Synergistic cooperation between water-soluble chitosan oligomers and interferon-γ for induction of nitric oxide synthesis and tumoricidal activity in murine peritoneal macrophages. *Cancer Lett* 159: 189–195.

192. Muzzarelli, R. A. A. 1977. *Chitin*. Oxford: Pergamon Press.

193. Qi, L., Xu, Z., Jiang, X., Hu, C., and Zou, X. 2004. Preparation and antibacterial activity of chitosan nanoparticles. *Carbohydr Res* 339: 2693–2700.

194. Qi, L. and Xu, Z. 2004. Lead sorption from aqueous solutions on chitosan nanoparticles. *Colloids Surf A* 251: 183–190.

195. Wang, Y., Guan, L. F., Jia, S. J., Tseng, B., Drewe, J., and Cai, S. X. 2005. Dipeptidyl aspartyl fluoromethylketones as potent caspase inhibitors: peptidomimetic replacement of the P2 α-amino acid by a α-hydroxy acid. *Bioorg Med Chem Lett* 15: 1397–1383.

196. Qi, L. F., Xu, Z. R., Li, Y., Jiang, X., and Han, X. Y. 2005. *In vitro* effects of chitosan nanoparticles on proliferation of human gastric carcinoma cell line MGC803 cells. *World J Gastroentero* 11: 5136–5141.

197. Tobio, M., Sanchez, A., Vila, A., Soriano, I., Evora, C., Vila-Jato, J. L., and Alonso, M. J. 2000. The role of PEG on the stability in digestive fluids and *in vivo* fate of PEG-PLA nanoparticles following oral administration. *Colloid Surf B* 18: 315–323.

198. Feng, S. S. and Chien, S. 2003. Chemotherapeutic engineering: Application and further development of chemical engineering principles for chemotherapy of cancer and other diseases. *Chem Eng Sci* 58: 4087–4114.

199. Florence, A. T. 1997. The oral absorption of micro and nanoparticles: Neither exceptional nor unusua. *Pharm Res* 14: 259–266.

200. Marianne, R., Dagmar, F., and Thomas, K. 1998. Surface-modified biodegradable albumin nano- and microspheres. II: Effect of surface charges on *in vitro* phagocytosis and biodistribution in rats. *Eur J Pharm Biopharm* 46: 255–263.

201. Wang, J., Kozo, T., Tsuneji, N., and Yoshie, M. 2003. Pharmacokinetics and antitumor effects of vincristine carried by microemulsions composed of PEG-lipid, oleic acid, vitamin E and cholesterol. *Int J Pharm* 251: 13–21.

202. Fan, F., Marc, D., Dai, F., Michael, L., David, A. B., Torchilin, V. P., and Jain, R. K. 1995. Vascular permeability in a human tumor xenograft:molecular size dependence and cutoff size. *Cancer Res* 55: 3752–3756.

203. Moghimi, S. M., Hunter, A. C., and Murray, J. C. 2001. Long-circulating and target-specific nanoparticles: Theory to practice. *Pharmacol Rev* 53: 283–318.

204. Kondo, N., Iwao, T., Kikuchi, M., Shu, H., Yamanouchi, K., Yokoyama, K., Ohyama, K., and Ogyu, S. 1993. Pharmacokinetics of a micronized, poorly water-soluble drug, HO-221, in experimental animals. *Biol Pharm Bull* 16: 796–800.

205. Kreuter, J. 1991. Peroral administration of nanoparticles. *Adv Drug Deliv Rev* 7: 71–86.

206. Gary, G. L. and Kenneth, C. C. 1995. Particle size reduction for improvement of oral bioavailability of hydrophobic drugs: I. Absolute oral bioavailability of nanocrystalline danazol in beagle dogs. *Int J Pharm* 125: 91–97.

207. Williams, J., Lansdown, R., Sweitzer, R., Romanowski, M., LaBell, R., Ramaswami, R., and Unger, E. 2003. Nanoparticle drug delivery system for intravenous delivery of topoisomerase inhibitors. *J Control Release* 91: 167–172.

208. Chouly, C., Pouliquen, D., Lucet, I., Jeune, J. J., and Jallet, P. 1996. Development of superparamagnetic nanoparticles for MRI: Effect of particle size, charge and surface nature on biodistribution. *J Microencapsulation* 13: 245–255.

209. Qi, L. F. and Xu, Z. R. 2006. *In vivo* antitumor activity of chitosan nanoparticles. *Bioorg Med Chem Lett* 16: 4243–4245.

210. Prabhu, R. and Balasubramanian, K. A. 2001. A novel method of preparation of small intestinal CTE brush border membrane vesicles by polyethylene glycol precipitation. *Anal Biochem* 289: 157–161.

211. Kessler, M., Acuto, O., Storelli, C., Murer, H., Ller, M. M., and Semenza, G. 1978. A moded procedure for the rapid preparation of efficiently transporting vesicles from small intestinal brush border membranes: their use in investigating some properties of D-glucose and choline transport systems. *Biochim Biophy Acta* 506: 136–154.

212. Cho, S., Park, J. H., Yu, J., Lee, Y., Byun, Y., Chung, H. C., Kwon, I. C., and Jeong, S. Y. 2004. Preparation and characterization of reconstructed small intestinal brush border membranes for surface plasm on resonance analysis. *Pharm Res* 21: 55–60.

213. Kim, K., Cho, S., Park, J. H., Byun, Y., Chung, H., Kwon, I. C., and Jeong, S. Y. 2004. Surface plasmon resonance studies of the direct interaction between a drug/intestinal brush border membrane. *Pharm Res* 21: 1233–1239.

214. Lee, E., Kim, H. J., Lee, I. H., and Jon, S. Y. 2009. *In vivo* antitumor effects of chitosan-conjugated docetaxel after oral administration. *J Control Release* 140: 79–85.

215. Lee, E., Lee, J., Lee, I. H., Yu, M., Kim, H., Chae, S. Y., and Jon, S. 2008. Conjugated chitosan as a novel plat form for oral delivery of paclitaxel. *J Med Chem* 51: 6442–6449.
216. Kim, Y. H., Gihm, S. H., and Park, C. R. 2001. Structural characteristics of size-controlled self-aggregates of deoxycholic acid-modified chitosan and their application as a DNA delivery carrier. *Bioconj Chem* 12: 932–938.
217. Lee, K. Y., Kim, J. H., Kwon, L. C., and Jeong, S. Y. 2000. Self-aggregates of deoxycholic acid-modified chitosan as a novel carrier of adriamycin. *Colloid Polym Sci* 2278: 1216–1219.
218. Gaucher, G., Dufresne, M. H., Sant, V. P., Kang, N., Maysinger, D., and Leroux, J. C. 2005. Block copolymer micelles: preparation, characterization and application in drug delivery. *J Control Release* 109: 169–188.
219. Omelyaneko, V., Kopeckova, P., Gentry, C., and Kopecek, J. 1998. Targetable HPMA copolymer adriamycin conjugates. Recognition, internalization, and subcellular fate. *J Control Release* 53: 25–37.
220. Park, J. H., Kwon, S., Lee, M., Chung, H., Kim, J. H., Kim, Y. S., Park, R. W., Kim, I. S., Seo, S. B., Kwon, I. C., and Jeong, S. Y. 2006. Self-assembled nanoparticles based on glycolchitosan bearing hydrophobic moieties as carriers for doxorubicin: *in vivo* biodistribution and anti-tumor activity. *Biomaterials* 27: 119–126.
221. Chytil, P., Etrych, T., Konak, C., Sirova, M., Mrkvan, T., and Rihova, B. 2006. Properties of HPMA copolymer-doxorubicin conjugates with pH-controlled activation: effect of polymer chain modification. *J Control Release* 115: 26–36.
222. Teodori, E., Dei, S., Scapecchi, S., and Gualtieri, F. 2002. The medicinal chemistry of multi drug resistance (MDR) reversing drugs. *IL Farmaco* 57: 385–415.
223. Tijerina, M., Fowers, K. D., Kopeckova, P., and Kopecek, J. 2000. Chronic exposure of human ovarian carcinoma cells to free or HPMA copolymer-bound mesochlorin does not induce P-glycoprotein-mediated multi drug resistance. *Biomaterials* 21: 2203–2210.
224. Gottesman, M. M., Fojo, T., and Bates, S. E. 2002. Multi drug resistance in cancer: Role of ATP-dependent transporters. *Nat Rev Cancer* 2: 48–58.
225. Kabanov, A. V., Batrakova, E. V., and Alakhov, V. Y. 2002. Pluronic block copolymers for overcoming drug resistance in cancer. *Adv Drug Deliv Rev* 54: 759–779.
226. Stastny, M., Strohalm, J., Plocova, D., Ulbrich, K., and Rihova, B. 1999. A possibility to overcome P-glycoprotein (PGP)-mediated multi drug resistance by antibody-targeted drugs conjugated to *N*-(2-hydroxypropyl)methacrylamide (HPMA) copolymer carrier. *Eur J Cancer* 35: 459–66.
227. Hu, F. Q., Liu, L. N., Du, Y. Z., and Yuan, H. 2009. Synthesis and antitumor activity of doxorubicin conjugated stearic acid-g-chitosan oligosaccharide polymeric micelles. *Biomaterials* 30: 1–9.
228. Prabaharan, M., Grailer, J. J., Pilla, S., Steeber, D. A., and Gong, S. 2009. Folate-conjugated amphiphilic hyperbranched block copolymers based on Boltorn H40, poly-(L-lactide) and poly (ethyleneglycol) for tumor-targeted drug delivery. *Biomaterials* 30: 3009–3019.
229. Kawano, K., Watanabe, M., Yamamoto, T., Yokoyama, M., Opanasopit, P., Okano, T., and Maitani, Y. 2006. Enhanced antitumor effect of camptothecin loaded in long-circulating polymeric micelles. *J Control Release* 112: 329–332.
230. Watanabe, M., Kawano, K., Yokoyama, M., Opanasopit, P., Okano, T., and Maitani, Y. 2006. Preparation of camptothecin-loaded polymeric micelles and evaluation of their incorporation and circulation stability. *Int J Pharm* 308: 183–189.
231. Matsumura, Y. and Maeda, H. 1986. A new concept for macromolecular therapeutics in cancer chemotherapy: Mechanism of tumoritropic accumulation of proteins and antitumor agent smancs. *Cancer Res* 46: 6387–6392.
232. Maeda, H., Wu J., Sawa, T., Matsumura, Y., and Hori, K. 2000. Tumor vascular permeability and the EPR effect in macromolecular therapeutics: A review. *J Control Release* 65: 271–284.
233. Min, K. H., Park, K., Kim, Y. S., Bae, S. M., Lee, S., Jo, H. G., Park, R. W., Kim, I. S., and Jeong, S. Y. 2008. Hydrophobically modified glycol chitosan nanoparticles-encapsulated camptothecin enhance the drug stability and tumor targeting in cancer therapy. *J Control Release* 27: 208–218.

234. Hsiang, Y. H. and Liu, L. F. 1988. Identification of mammalian topoisomerase I as an intracellular target of the anticancer drug camptothecin. *Cancer Res* 48: 1722–1726.
235. Garcia-Carbonero, R. and Supko, J. G. 2002. Current perspectives on the clinical experience, pharmacology, and continued development of the camptothecins. *Clin Cancer Res* 8: 641–661.
236. Oberlies, N. H. and Kroll, D. J. 2004. Camptothecin and taxol: historic achievements in natural products research. *J Nat Prod* 67: 129–135.
237. Sriram, D., Yogeeswari, P., Thirumurugan, R., and Bal, T. R. 2005. Camptothecin and its analogues: a review on their chemotherapeutic potential. *Nat Prod Res* 19: 398–412.
238. Hwang, H. Y., Kim, I. S., Kwon, I. C., and Kim, Y. H. 2008. Tumor target ability and antitumor effect of docetaxel-loaded hydrophobically modified glycol chitosan nanoparticles. *J Control Release* 128: 23–31.
239. Martin, L., Wilson, C. G., Koosha, F., Tetley, L., Gray, A. I., Senel, S., and Uchegbu, I. F. 2006. The release of model macromolecules may be controlled by the hydrophobicity of palmitoyl glycol chitosan hydrogels. *J Control Release* 80: 87–100.
240. Martin, L., Wilson, C. G., Koosha, F., and Uchegbu, I. F. 2003. Sustained buccal delivery of the hydrophobic drug denbufylline using physical cross-linked palimitoylglycolchitosan hydrogels. *Eur J Pharm Biopharm* 55: 35–45.
241. Fujita, M., Ishihara, M., Shimizu, M., Obara, K., Ishizuka, T., Saito, Y., Yara, H., Morimoto, Y., Takase, B., Matsui, T., Kikuchi, M., and Maehara, T. 2004. Vascularization *in vivo* caused by the controlled release of fibroblast growth factor-2 from an injectable chitosan/non-anticoagulant heparin hydrogel. *Biomaterials* 25: 699–706.
242. Ishihara, M., Obara, K., Ishizuka, T., Fujita, M., Sato, M., Masuoka, K., Saito, Y., Yura, H., Matsui, T., Hattori, H., Kikuchi, M., and Kurita, A. 2003. Controlled release of fibroblast growth factors and heparin from photocross-linked chitosan hydrogels and subsequent effect on *in vivo* vascularization. *J Biomed Mater Res* 64A: 551–559.
243. Obara, K., Ishihara, M., Ozeki, Y., Ishizuka, T., Hayashi, T., Nakamura, S., Saito, Y., Yura, H., Matsui, T., Hattori, H., Takase, B., and Maehara, T. 2005. Controlled release of paclitaxel from photocross-linked chitosan hydrogels and its subsequent effect on subcutaneous tumor growth in mice. *J Control Release* 110: 79–89.
244. Ishihara, M., Nakamura, S., Masuoka, K., Takase, B., Morimoto, Y., and Maehara, T. 2006. Chitosan hydrogel as a drug delivery carrier to control angiogenesis. *J Artif Organs* 9: 8–16.
245. Carreno-Gomez, B. and Duncan, R. 1997. Evaluation of the biological properties of soluble chitosan and chitosan microspheres. *Int J Pharm* 148: 231–240.
246. Murata, J., Saiki, I., Makabe, T., Tsuta, Y., Tokura, S., and Azuma, I. 1991. Inhibition of tumor-induced angiogenesis by sulfated chitin derivative. *Cancer Res* 51: 22–26.
247. Murata, J., Saiki, I., Nishimura, S., Nishi, N., Tokura, S., and Azuma, I. 1989. Inhibitory effect of chitin heparinoids on the lung metastasis of B16-B16 melanoma. *Jpn J Cancer Res* 80: 866–872.

4

Formation of Chitosan-Based Hydrogels Network

Yuji Yin and Junjie Li

CONTENTS

4.1 Complex Tissue from Simple Molecules

The tissues of the human body contain significant extracellular space, into which extracellular matrix (ECM) molecules are secreted by the cells to form a complex hydrogel network. The ECM provides mechanical support for tissues, organizes cells into specific tissues, and controls cell behavior. In other words, ECM is a dynamic structure that provides structural and anchoring support to the cells to improve tissue architecture. It also contributes to signaling, directing cell fate and function through cell–matrix interactions. In addition, the ECM is constantly remodeled by cells during development, homeostasis, and wound healing by balancing its synthesis and degradation by a variety of enzymes.

4.1.1 ECM Component Cross-Linking

Generally, the natural ECM is mainly composed of two classes of macromolecules: polysaccharide chains of the class called glycosaminoglycans (GAGs), which are usually found covalently linked to protein in the form of proteoglycans (PGs), and fibrous proteins, including collagens, elastin, fibronectin, and laminin, which have both structural and adhesive functions. The PG molecules form highly hydrated gels, in which the assembled fibrous proteins are embedded and interact with cells through mechanical as well as chemical signals [1,2].

The ECM proteins include structural fibrous proteins such as collagen and elastin and cell-adhesive proteins such as fibrolectin and laminin. Collagen, the most abundant protein in mammals, provides tensile strength to the ECM, while other proteins, such as elastin, give the ECM its elasticity. Collagen comes in many different types. Type I collagen is the most common fibrillar collagen found in skin, bone, and tendons, and type II collagen possesses a similar fibrillar structure that provides tensile strength to the cartilage. Cells bind to the ECM mainly through adhesive proteins such as laminin and fibronectin. Laminin, which has a cross-shaped trimer structure containing a, b, and g chains, is the major adhesive protein in basal lamina with binding sites for cell membrane receptors and type IV collagen, heparan sulfate proteoglycan (HSPG), and entacin. Fibronectin, evolutionarily related to fibrinogen, is another important adhesive protein in the ECM. Fibrinogen is a V-shaped dimmer with several binding domains for mediating the connection between the ECM and cell membrane, and binds a variety of proteins such as collagen and fibrin, as well as cell-surface receptors such as integrins [3].

ECM proteins are embedded in highly negatively charged, polysaccharide-rich, gelatinous ground substances, called glycans, including GAGs and PGs. GAGs are linear polymers of repeated disaccharide derivative with two types: nonsulfated, such as hyaluronic acid (HA), and sulfated, such as chondroitin, dermatan, heparin, and keratin sulfates. Sulfated GAGs can assemble on serine-rich proteins to form PGs, such as aggrecan and HSPG. Both GAGs and PGs swell in the aqueous spaces between protein fibrils to form hydrogel, taking compressive stresses, limiting tissue collapse under pressure. Glycans also allow tissues to diffuse nutrients and provide the reservoir for signaling molecules such as growth factors (GFs) [4].

4.1.2 Performance of Cross-Linking Network

As mentioned above, ECM components undergo self-assembly as well as cell-directed assembly to form complex 3D organized hydrogel networks. Cell receptors bind both soluble and tethered signaling cues from the ECM environment. In turn, these receptor–ligand interactions trigger complex cascades of intracellular enzymatic reactions that regulate gene and protein expression, and define the fate of a cell in a tissue. Simultaneously, cells send out signals to actively construct and degrade their microenvironment. Thus, the ECM acts not only as a simple space filler and a mechanical scaffold for the cells, but also as a bioactive and dynamic environment that mediates cellular functions. Generally, the natural ECM has three basic biofunctions, including cell adhesion, proteolytic degradation, and GF binding. Cell attachment to the ECM is an obvious prerequisite for a number of important cell function processes, such as cell proliferation and cell migration. The ECM provides cell adhesive domains for binding cell surface receptors. There are various cell surface receptors, among which are integrins, selectins, CD44, and syndecan. Integrins are the major family responsible for cell attachment to the ECM; they bind to specific domains present in ECM proteins such as fibronectin, laminin, and collagen. Through binding to these functional cell-binding domains, integrins play central roles in tissue development, organization, and maintenance, by providing anchorage and triggering signals that direct cell function, cell cycle progression, and expression of differentiated phenotypes. The proteolytic degradation of the natural ECM is an essential feature of a variety of biological processes, such as cell migration, tissue repair, and remolding. Most ECM proteins, including collagen, fibrin, fibronectin, and laminin, have specific cleavage sites for degradation by enzymes, such as matrix metalloproteinases, plasmin, and elastase [3,4].

Moreover, GAGs play a critical role in assembling protein–protein complexes such as GF-receptor or enzyme-inhibitor on the cell surface and in the ECM that are directly involved in initiating cell signaling events or inhibiting biochemical pathways. Furthermore, extracellular GAGs can potentially sequester proteins and enzymes and present them to the appropriate site for activation (*cf.* Figure 4.1). Thus for a given high-affinity GAG–protein interaction, the positioning of the protein-binding oligosaccharide motifs along the GAG chain determines whether an active signaling complex is assembled on the cell surface and/or an inactive complex is sequestered in the matrix. It should be noted that high-affinity GAG–protein interactions are not the only biologically significant interactions. GAGs have been shown to play important roles in maintaining morphogen gradients across a cell or tissue, which have been implicated in developmental processes. Maintaining a gradient in the concentration of GFs or morphogens would involve graded affinities between different GAG sequences with the given protein. Thus, the nature of GAG–protein interactions coupled with their sequence diversity enables GAGs to "fine-tune" or what can be viewed as an "analog modulation" of the activity of proteins [5].

On the other hand, hydrogels are comprised of cross-linked polymer networks that have a high number of hydrophilic groups or domains. These networks have a high affinity for water, but are prevented from dissolving due to the chemical or physical bonds formed between the polymer chains. Water penetrates these networks causing swelling, giving the hydrogel its form. Fully swollen hydrogels have some physical properties common to living tissues, including a soft and rubbery consistency, and low interfacial tension with water or biological fluids. The elastic nature of fully swollen or hydrated hydrogels has been found to minimize irritation to the surrounding tissues after implantation. The low interfacial tension between the hydrogel surface and body fluid minimizes protein adsorption and cell adhesion, which reduces the chances of a negative immune reaction. Because the hydrogel's physiochemistry is similar to the native ECM, hydrogels can serve as dual-propose devices, acting as a supporting material for cells during tissue regeneration as well as delivering a drug payload [2,6,7].

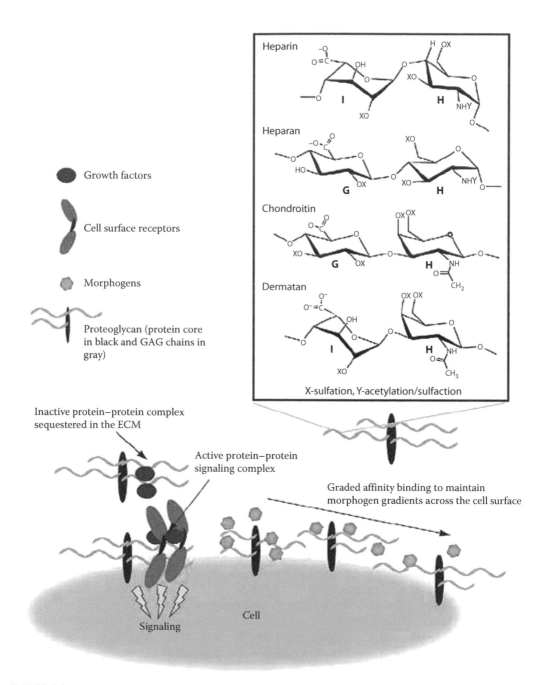

FIGURE 4.1
Structure and biological roles of GAGs. (From Raman, R., Sasisekharan, V., and Salisekharan, R. 2005. *Chem. Biol.* 12: 267–277. With permission.)

A variety of natural and synthetic polymers have been used to fabricate hydrogels. Poly(ethylene glycol) (PEG) and its derivatives, poly(vinyl alcohol) (PVA) and poly(hydroxylethyl methacrylate), have all been used to form hydrogels with variable mechanical strengths and biological responses. Natural polymers, such as polysaccharides and proteins, have also been used as the structural material in hydrogels. This is largely due to the interest in the intrinsic properties of these polymers including biocompatibility, low toxicity, and susceptibility to enzymatic degradation. Among these polymers, polysaccharides do not suffer some of the disadvantages of other naturally derived materials, such as immunogenicity and the potential risk of transmitting animal-originated pathogens. One such polysaccharide is chitosan. These attractive natural polysaccharides share the advantages of other natural polymers (lysozomal degradation, etc.), but do not induce an immune response [8].

Chitosan hydrogels have been prepared with a variety of different shapes, geometries, and formulations that include liquid gels, powders, beads, films, tablets, capsules, microspheres, microparticles, sponges (porous scaffolds), nanofibrils, textile fibers, and inorganic composites. In each preparation chitosan is either physically associated or chemically cross-linked to form the hydrogel [6].

4.2 Chitosan-Based Network

In cross-linked chitosan (cr-CS), polymeric chains are interconnected by cross-linkers, leading to the formation of a 3D network. A cross-linking network of chitosan can be formed by complexation with another polymer, generally ionic, or by aggregation after chitosan grafting [9]. Chitosan-based biomaterials can form hybrid polymer networks (HPNs) or semi- or full-interpenetrating polymer networks (semi- or full-IPNs) through the cross-linking reaction [10]. In these cross-linking systems, covalent bonds are the main interactions to form the networks, but other interactions cannot be excluded. Indeed, there are secondary interactions including hydrogen bridges and hydrophobic interactions. In general, the network structures include polyelectrolyte complex (PEC) networks and covalent cross-linking and ionic cross-linking networks (*cf.* Figure 4.2). These chitosan networks could modulate the swelling behaviors, mechanical properties, and some bioactive functions. Desirable chitosan-based network biomaterials need special interaction with or mimicry of ECM components, GFs, or cell-surface receptors. Chitosan is similar to GAGs in structure, but it is absent *in vivo*. Therefore, the hybrid networks are formed via introducing some bioactive molecule or polysaccharide. The chitosan-based network structure is an efficient method for simulating the cell growth microenvironment [11].

4.2.1 Complex Cross-Linking Network

Chitosan is a copolymer of glocosamine and N-acetyl-dD-glycoamine linked together by $\beta(1-4)$ glycoside bonds. Due to its unique cationic nature, chitosan is able to form the PEC with negatively charged polyanions, for example, proteins and GAGs. Chitosan-based PECs (CS-PECs) are generally obtained through the reaction of chitosan and polyanions. In general, the CS-PEC films' formation may be schematically classified into three main stages: (1) primary complex formation; (2) formation process within intracomplexes; and (3) intercomplex aggregations. Since chitosan has a rigid, stereo-regular structure containing bulky pyranose rings, the formation of PEC can induce a conformational change of the other polyelectrolyte if the latter has a nonrigid structure [12]. Various different characteristics of CS-PECs can be obtained by changing the chemical characteristics of the polymers' components, such as the M_W, flexibility, functional group

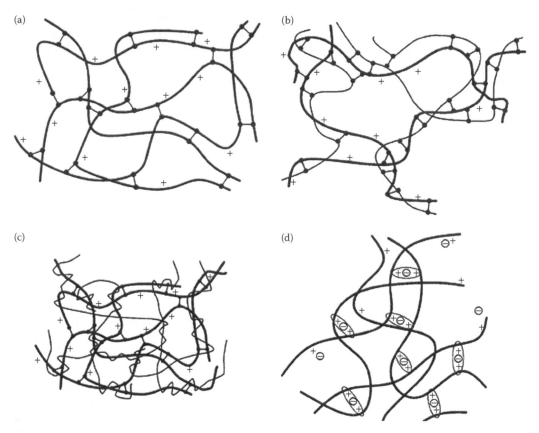

FIGURE 4.2
Structure of chitosan hydrogels formed by (a) chitosan cross-linked with itself; (b) HPN; (c) semi-interpenetrating network; and (d) ionic cross-linking of chitosan. (From Bergera, J. et al. 2004. *Eur J Pharm Biopharm* 57: 19–34. With permission.)

structure, charge density, hydrophilicity/hydrophobicity balance, stereo-regularity, and compatibility, as well as the reaction conditions, for example, the pH, ionic strength, concentration, mixing ratio, and temperature [13]. The properties of PECs are mainly determined by the degree of interaction among individual polymers. PECs depend essentially on the polymers' global charge density and this determines their relative composition in the PEC. The lower the charge density of the polymer, the higher the polymer proportion in the PEC, since more polymeric chains are required to react with other polymers. A PEC can be formed via two ionizable polymers with opposite charges individually. This means that PEC formation reaction can only occur at pH values in the vicinity of the pK_a interval of the two polyelectrolytes. The concomitant release of corresponding counterions is the main driving force of the reaction because it corresponds to an increase in entropy of the system. Other interactions may be involved in the formation of PEC structures, such as hydrogen bonding, hydrophobic interaction, or van der Waals interactions. PECs can be prepared in various forms such as film, hydrogel, microcapsule, or scaffold.

Cell attachment, morphology, and proliferation are influenced by physicochemical properties of the CS-PECs surface. The surface chemical composition of PECs is important in cell events because the cell could directly recognize the PECs and adheres to them without the aid of protein. For example, rat osteoblasts directly recognize the CS-PECs (which are composed of phosphate and carboxymethylated chitin as a polyanion and chitosan as a polycation) and adhere to them without the aid of fibronectin [14]. CS-PECs containing carboxymethyl groups as anionic sites cause the human periodontal ligament fibroblast (HPLF) to aggregate and promote differentiation because the carboxymethyl groups offer similar conditions as *in vivo* to HPLF. On the contrary, PECs containing sulfate groups cause HPLF to form a spreading morphology and proliferate well [15,16]. A higher adhesion number of cells on the chitosan/chondroitin sulfate surface are better than that on pure chitosan films [17]. This is explained by taking into account that complex formation removes the individual charges of the polymers and the chemical structure of chitosan, which is necessary for cell recognition changes.

Above all, the diversity of the structure and preparation method of CS-PEC results in a change of the physicochemical and bioactive functions. Here, some typical CS-PECs and their characteristics will be introduced.

4.2.1.1 Chitosan–Gelatin PECs

Gelatin is a partial denaturalization derivative of collagen. Its electrical nature can be changed by the collagen processing method. The alkaline process through hydrolysis of amide groups of collagen yields gelatin with a high density of carboxyl groups, which makes the gelatin negatively charged, reducing the isoelectric point (p*I*) to 5.0. Gelatin presumably retains informational signals, for example, the Arg–Gly–Asp sequence. These informational signals could improve chondrocytes attachment [18]. A PEC film can be formed via the electrostatic interaction between chitosan and gelatin. There occurs strong interaction between gelatin and chitosan in aqueous medium, which is enough to form PECs *in situ*. And the chitosan/gelatin PECs is only yielded at pH values higher than 4.7 and below pH 6.2 [19]. The strong interactions between chitosan and gelatin replace the macromolecular chain–water interactions. Therefore, the bound water content of chitosan/gelatin PECs decrease slightly when compared to chitosan. The free water content of chitosan films increases when blended with gelatin, which indicates that the structure of chitosan films is more rigid and compact than that of a composite film. The chitosan/gelatin PEC reaches the optimum interactive ratio when the content of gelatin is about 60% [20,21].

Gelatin moieties provide biocompatibility. The cell cycle analysis is carried out to assess the proliferation of L929 rat fibroblasts on chitosan/gelatin PEC films in comparison with that on chitosan films. It is found that blending chitosan and gelatin can induce cells to enter the cell cycle and to begin to proliferate. Chitosan/gelatin PECs can promote cell proliferation and inhibit cell apoptosis. This effect may be attributed to the decline in positive charge density of chitosan that may benefit cell migration [22]. A chitosan/gelatin PEC scaffold is fabricated by freezing and lyophilizing methods. Autologous chondrocytes from pigs' auricular cartilage are seeded onto the scaffold, and elastic cartilages have been successfully engineered at porcine abdomen subcutaneous tissue [23]. Moreover, chondrocyte proliferation is more distinct in chitosan–gelatin–DNA PEC scaffolds [24]. These studies indicate that the chitosan/gelatin PECs can be used as a suitable scaffold for tissue engineering.

4.2.1.2 Chitosan–Alginate PECs

Chitosan–alginate PECs are prepared by mixing aqueous solutions of chitosan and alginate. At a given pH, the composition of the PEC shifts to a lower alginate content as the degree of N-acetylation of chitosan increases. For a given chitosan sample, the higher the pH, the lower the alginate content of the PEC [25]. And the ratio of chitosan to alginate is independent of the M_W of chitosan and the composition of alginate used [26,27].

In order to fabricate homogeneous chitosan–alginate PECs films, chitosan and alginate solutions are mixed under controlled conditions to yield fine coacervates that are isolated from the reacting pot and resuspended in dilute $CaCl_2$ solutions prior to casting and drying. This method has the advantage of using an aqueous system, which is stable to storage at ambient conditions, to produce water-insoluble homogeneous membranes [28]. Increasing the $CaCl_2$ concentration does not affect membrane thickness, but improves the respective mechanical properties [29]. The mechanical strength decreases with increasing the content of chitosan in the PECs, which is due to the inhibition of chelation of calcium ions with alginate chains at high concentrations of chitosan. The pH value is another factor influencing the mechanical strength of chitosan–alginate PECs. Sankalia et al. [30] found that chitosan–alginate PECs, which are formed when a chitosan solution with pH 2 and an alginate solution with pH 6.5 are mixed, show excellent mechanical strength. The maximum interaction between the amino and carboxyl groups takes place under this condition and results in a compact film. Iwasaki et al. [31] and Tamura et al. [32] found that the chitosan–alginate scaffolds are stable regardless of the pH value of the solution. That can be attributed to (1) the interaction of amine groups on chitosan with carboxyl groups on alginate, which prevents the protonation of amino groups on chitosan, and (2) the carboxyl groups on alginate that buffer the solution and slow down the degradation of chitosan [33].

Chitosan–alginate PECs show good compatibility *in vitro* with the mouse/human fibroblasts, osteoblasts, and chondrocytes [34]. The chondrocytes on chitosan tend to form a monolayer, a possible marker of chondrocyte dedifferentiation and fibroblastic phenotype [35,36]. In contrast, the chondrocytes on chitosan–alginate PECs materials form much larger cell clusters. And cell proliferation on chitosan–alginate scaffolds is found to be faster than that on a pure chitosan scaffold [37]. In addition, chitosan–alginate PECs have the advantage of not destroying the drug structure loaded. This characteristic is especially suitable for the encapsulation of biological products with low stability, such as peptides, proteins, vaccines, and so on [38]. The chitosan–alginate PECs are also an effective controlled release carrier for nerve growth factor [39].

4.2.1.3 Chitosan/HA PECs

Chitosan/HA PECs are prepared by mixing the chitosan solution and the HA solution below the pK_a value of chitosan (6.5). Denuziere et al. [40] have reported that a PEC composed of HA and chitosan can be formed below the pK_a of HA because the ionic interaction between the polyions competes with the protonation of HA. The chitosan/HA PECs are most stable at pH values around neutrality, and are more labile in acidic than under basic conditions [41]. At the initial ionic state of polyions dissolved in formic acid, the amino groups of chitosan interact with formic acid and the carboxyl groups of HA existing in a protonated form. As the pH of the solution increases, protonated carboxyl groups competed with the precomplexed amine groups of chitosan with formic acid to form an ionic linkage between HA and chitosan [42].

The swelling degree of chitosan/HA PEC films ranges between 250% and 325% and changes in relation to the chitosan content of the network. An increase in the chitosan fraction of the films leads to an increase in the equilibrium swelling ratio [43]. This behavior may be due not only to the ratio of chitosan and the HA complexation of the network, but also to the chitosan content having a large number of water-binding sites [44]. Moreover, the swelling ratio also increases with increasing temperature [45]. The stiffness and hardness decrease with increasing the weight ratio of HA because of the soft mechanical properties of HA [46].

HA interacts with proteins such as CD44 and fibrinogen, and has an important role in many natural processes such as cell motility, cell adhesion, and wound healing. Chondrocyte adhesivity and proliferation and the synthesis of aggrecan are significantly higher in the chitosan/HA groups than in the pure chitosan group [47]. Cai and coworkers [48] found that the chitosan/HA/collagen complex film possesses promising coagulation capability, cell compatibility, and antibacteria property.

4.2.1.4 Chitosan/Heparin PECs

Chitosan/heparin PEC microparticles are prepared by one-shot addition or dropwise titration using chitosan as the starting solution. In the pH range of 1.2–6.5, ionized chitosan and heparin are able to form PECs, which result in a matrix structure with a spherical shape. Outside this pH range, the nanoparticles become unstable and break apart (as shown in Figure 4.3). This is because that at pH 7.0, chitosan is deprotonated, causing the collapse of the nanoparticles. These observations suggest that nanoparticles with pH-responsive characteristics (that are stable at pH 1.2–2.5 (simulating gastric acid)) are capable of protecting drugs from destruction by gastric acids [49]. A low pH value of the chitosan solution, a high chitosan M_W and a high chitosan concentration and heparin concentration all contributed to the large heparin/chitosan nanoparticles size [50]. And under conditions

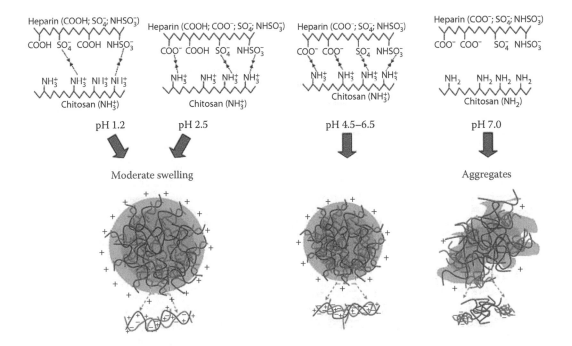

FIGURE 4.3
Schematic illustrations of the physical structures of chitosan/heparin nanoparticles in specific pH environments. (From Lin, Y. H. et al. 2009. *Biomaterials* 30: 3332–3342. With permission.)

close to a charge mixing ratio of 1, the size of chitosan/heparin nanoparticles tends to aggregate [51]. Chitosan/heparin microspheres are prepared using the water-in-oil emulsification solvent evaporation technique. The stirring speed has a particularly strong influence on the microsphere size, and microsphere size decreases as the stirring speed increases [52,53]. Chitosan/heparin PEC microparticles are excellent drug or protein release carriers.

The chitosan/heparin PEC films or scaffolds are widely used in tissue engineering. Kratz et al. [54] found that the chitosan/heparin PEC can stimulate wound healing in human skin. Moreover, the chitosan/heparin complex networks are supposed to exist as a network to create an appropriate environment for the regeneration of hepatocytes, as well as to induce growth angiogenesis for the regeneration of livers. They are potential candidates for liver tissue engineering. For example, the collagen–chitosan–heparin [55] and alginate–galactosylated chitosan/heparin [56] scaffolds, which are similar to the liver ECM, play important roles in the regulation of the morphological appearance of , hepatocytes.

4.2.1.5 Chitosan–DNA PECs

Chitosan–DNA PECs microparticles are prepared using a complex coacervation process under defined conditions. The size of the complexes is of crucial importance for cellular uptake. Small-sized complexes have the advantage of entering the cells through endocytosis and/or pinocytosis. Illum et al. [57] synthesized chitosan/DNA nanoparticles ranging from 20 to 500 nm. The chitosan/DNA PECs show excellent stability, and chitosan microparticles protect DNA during the storage time in freeze-dried form and also from nuclease degradation in the medium [58].

Incorporating positive-charged arginine (Arg) moieties into chitosan may increase the charge strength and charge density of nanoparticles and enhance the electrostatic interaction between nanoparticles and the cell membrane. Therefore, the cell uptake mediated by Arg-chitosan/DNA complexes is improved compared with chitosan/DNA complexes. The luciferase expression of Arg-chitosan is about 100-fold compared with the expression levels mediated by chitosan for HeLa cells [59]. The zeta potential of Arg-chitosan/DNA is about 0.23–12.5 mV, which increases with an increase of the nitrogen/phosphor (N/P) ratio [60]. Chitosan/DNA PEC nanoparticles administered in the anterior tibialis mice muscles reveal a high signal corresponding to β-gal gene expression within 48 h. In contrast, the administration of naked or DNA/Lipofectamine in the anterior tibialis muscle does not reveal any β-gal gene expression. From these preliminary data, the chitosan/DNA nanoparticles have the potential ability to transfect muscle cells *in vivo* and lead to protein synthesis [61].

4.2.2 Ionic Cross-Linking Network

Because chitosan is a weak polybase with thousands of positive charges, anions with sufficient charge numbers are effective in the ionic cross-linking of chitosan through electrostatic interactions. The processes of ionic cross-linking attract much attention because of the simplicity, the relatively mild preparation condition procedural, and avoidance of possible toxicity of the reagents commonly used for chemical cross-linking [62]. Many multivalent anions and metal ions are available as cross-linkers to form the chitosan cross-linking network. The properties of ionically cross-linked chitosan network are influenced by interactions between the multivalent ions cross-linkers and chitosan. Since the interactions between chitosan and ion cross-linkers depend on the molecular structure of the ions [63], these interactions can be modulated via adjusting the charge density of cross-linkers and the pH value of solutions [64,65].

A phosphate anion, such as triphosphate (TPP), hexametaphosphate (HMP), and poly-phosphate (PP), is usually used as a cross-linker for chitosan (*cf.* Figure 4.4) [66]. The ionic cross-linking density of the chitosan–TPP network or the interpolymer linkage of chito-san–PP network can be adjusted by transferring the pH value of the cross-linking agent from the basic to the acidic condition [67]. Chitosan solutions containing >20 wt% glycerol phosphate become a gel at 37°C and maintain this form for 28 days *in vitro* and *in vivo* [68]. The mechanical strength of this system formed under the acid condition decreases com-pared with that of the system formed under the basic condition. This can be attributed to the tightening of the gel network by increased shrinking of this system [69].

The swelling is lower in the sodium tripolyphosphate (STPP)-anion-cross-linked chito-san microspheres in comparison with the microspheres prepared with the sodium hexametaphosphate (SHMP) anion cross-linker. This is due to the stronger electrostatic interactions of SHMP-anion-cross-linked chitosan in comparison with STPP-anion-cross-linked chitosan [66]. The SHMP anions show strong electrostatic interactions with ion-ized chitosan, which provide sufficient opportunities to control the drug release pattern of centchroman and to make it in a much better way than reported with other phosphate cross-linkers [70].

The formation of a chitosan–glycerophosphate thermosetting gel mainly depends on the hydrogen bonding, ionic interaction, and chitosan–chitosan hydrophobic interactions. This system play an important role in successfully delivering biologically active GFs *in vivo* as well as being an encapsulating matrix for living chondrocytes for tissue-engineering appli-cations [71]. Hoyland and coworkers [72] investigated human mesenchymal stem cells (hMSCs) differentiated to nucleus pulposus (NP)-like cells in temperature-sensitive chitosan–glycerophosphate hydrogels. Here, cells can be mixed at room temperature prior to sol–gel transition and give a homogeneous cell distribution. hMSCs cultured in gels for 4 weeks in standard media express a chondrocytes phenotype. While the chondrocytic marker gene expression profile of MSCs is similar to both NP cells and articular chondro-cytes, the MSCs synthesized and deposited ECM proteins within the gel in ratios that match NP cells more closely than articular chondrocytes. Moreover, chitosan–glycerophosphate hydrogels aid chondrogenic differentiation of MSCs and inhibit osteogenic differentiation

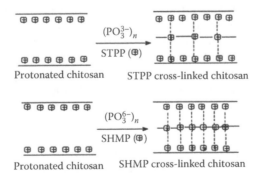

FIGURE 4.4
Formation chitosan cross-linking network via ionic cross-link using a phosphate anion. (From Gupta, K. C., and Jabrail, F. H. 2007. *J Appl Polym Sci* 104: 1942–1956. With permission.)

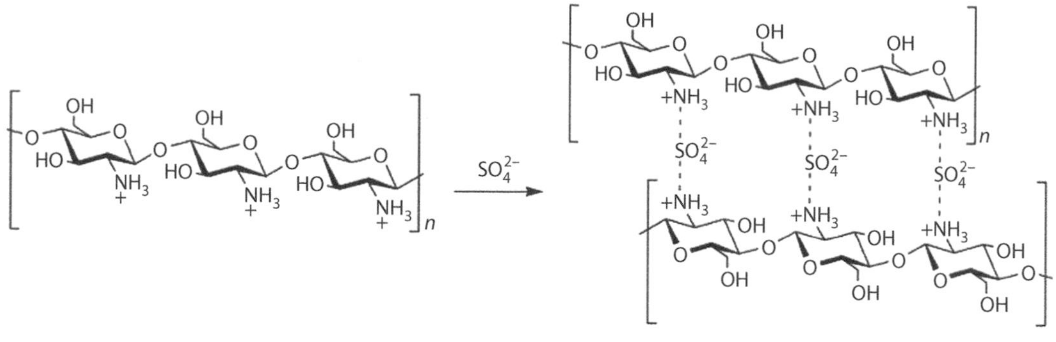

FIGURE 4.5
Ionic cross-linking of the chitosan using H_2SO_4. (From Cui, Z. et al. 2008. *Carbohydr Polym* 73: 111–116. With permission.)

and cell hypertrophy without exogenous factors. Many researchers have studied the sulfuric acid-cross-linked chitosan network. Firstly, H_2SO_4 protonates chitosan amine groups, and then the SO_4^{2-} anions slowly interact with chitosan NH_3^+ groups to form ionic bridges among the polymer chains (*cf.* Figure 4.5) [73]. After cross-linking, the surface topography becomes more homogenous and relatively flat, and the change of nanotopology can affect the surface wettability and surface reactions, for example, capillary reaction, and so on [74].

4.2.3 Covalent Cross-Linking Network

Compared with PEC networks, the functions of covalent cross-linking networks are easier to be controlled because their formation and application are not limited by pH value. However, a high cross-linking density may produce some side effects. For example, Picart et al. [75] found that chitosan/HA films cross-linked by a high 1-ethyl-3-(3-dimethylaminopropyl) carbodiimide (EDC) concentration lead to a pronounced inflammatory response *in vivo* and also to the formation of fibres. Therefore, a moderate cross-linking seems to be of greater interest in terms of biodegradability and application. One could control the cross-linking density through many ways: (1) changing the number or activity of cross-linked sites; (2) adjusting the cross-linked agent concentration; as the initiator concentration increases, the chain length between cross-links decreases and leads to stiff; (3) using different cross-linking agent types; the cross-linking degree of chitosan-based biomaterials cross-linked using EDC is lower compared with that using dialdehyde agents [76]; and (4) using different cross-linking methods (surface cross-linking or bulk cross-link). Covalent cross-linking treatments have been used to modulate the physical properties and biofunctions of chitosan-based biomaterials. Usually, the hydrophilicity–hydrophobicity, swelling behavior, biodegradation performance, mechanical properties, and biocompatibilities of cr-CS have a good relationship with the network structure as is illuminated in the following.

1. *Hydrophilicity–hydrophobicity*: The hydrophilicity of chitosan comes from the hydrophilic groups as –OH and $-NH_2$ of the chitosan chain. The reaction of a dialdehyde cross-linker with primary amino groups results in the formation of Schiff bases. Therefore, the decline in the $-NH_2$ group content enables the enhancement of the hydrophobicity of the chitosan network. The hydrophilic cross-linking agent

is also expected to improve the hydrophilicity of the cross-link network. For example, the chitosan network cross-linked by sulfosuccinic acid maintains the hydrophilic performance [77].

2. *Swelling behaviors*: In general, the swelling process of cr-CS-based biomaterials includes two stages: physical movement along free volume cavities of the network and the formation of bond water with hydrophilic groups of the covalent cross-linking network [78]. The swelling performance could be controlled by the following factors: first, the concentration of the chitosan acetic solution during the formation of the network is an important factor; the equilibrium degree of swelling increases as the concentration decreases. It can be explained that the intermolecular cross-linking reaction with the cross-linker decreases in the dilute solution, but the intramolecular cross-linking increases. Second, the cross-linking density also influences the swelling behaviors; the swelling degrees are suppressed with increasing cross-linking density. For example, the degree of swelling of chitosan fiber decreases as the concentration of cross-linker increases [79]. Third, the type and amount of other compounds in the cross-linking system are not ignored factors. For example, the swelling degree of the chitosan–polyether-cross-linked network decreases with increasing the polyether amount, which is due to the intensification of hydrogen bonding between chitosan and polyether [80–84].

3. *Degradation performance*: The degradation rate of cr-CS-based biomaterials is much lower than that of noncross-linked composites [85]. The cross-linked network may have a high stereohindrance for the penetration of lysozyme and the steric effects of the cross-linked chain among chitosan molecules, and it prevents lysozyme from binding to the chitosan substrate. In general, with increasing the cross-linking density, the degradation rate decreases. Actually, the decrease of the mobility of the chitosan chain can result in a low rate of solvent expulsion, and thus a low rate of mass loss too [86]. Compared with bulk cross-linking, after surface cross-linking there are fewer cross-linking agents left in the modified materials. Meanwhile, surface cr-CS-based biomaterials show a lower initial degradation rate because the constructed matrix begins to degrade from the cross-linking surfaces, but the degradation rate increases with the time because of lower cross-linking extent inside the matrix [87].

4. *Mechanical properties:* Cross-linking can enhance the mechanical properties of the chitosan-based biomaterials without impacting on the biocompatibility. One can modulate the mechanical performance via controlling the cross-linking density or the type and counts of other compounds in the composites systems. Du and coworkers [88] found that the proper cross-linking density is able to improve the mechanical properties of chitosan network films. For chitosan-based biomaterials scaffold fabricated through thermally induced phase separation and freeze-drying technology, the freezing temperature and concentration of acetic acid are also an important factor to influence the mechanical performance [89]. Most cells can sense biomaterials' intrinsic mechanical environment and the substrate or scaffold rigidity/stiffness can also serve as an intrinsic mechanical stimulus. Stiffer surfaces could promote the cell proliferation and the preservation of morphology. For example, about 90% of the chondrocyte cells on uncross-linked chitosan films have a spherical morphology and nebulous, punctate actin, while they are flattened with stress fibers and 40–50% of cells have a flattened morphology on the cr-CS films [90–92].

The biocompatibility of the chitosan network is the final evaluation index and it is a comprehensive effect of the above physical–chemical properties. Above all, different chemical structures and properties of the network result from different cross-linkers and cross-linking mechanisms. Cross-linkers are molecules with at least two reactive functional groups that allow the formation of bridges among polymeric chains. To date, the most commonly used cross-linkers with chitosan-based biomaterials are dialdehydes (such as glyoxal and in particular glutaraldehyde (GA), genipin, diepoxide, EDC, etc.). The details of the cross-linking mechanism and properties of the chitosan-based cross-linking network will be provided below.

4.2.3.1 Dialdehyde-Cross-Linked CS

GA is a commonly used cross-linker for chitosan and the cross-linking mechanism is shown in Figure 4.6 [93]. The chitosan-based biomaterial networks cross-linked by GA have many advantages. In fact, the easiness of synthesis, the speed of reaction, the mild experimental conditions (room temperature, pH around 4.5), and the acceptable biocompatibility of the reactants make these networks particularly promising for the synthesis of biomaterials *in situ* [94,95]. The reaction between amino groups of chitosan and GA is highly unlikely to proceed homogeneously, and the absolute stoichiometry of the reaction cannot be determined by the [–CHO]/[–NH$_2$] values. The amount of adsorbed proteins on the GA-cross-linked chitosan (GCCS) surface decreases because the positive-charged amino groups of chitosan are cross-linked by the GA. However, there are some aldehyde groups on the surface of GCCS that may bind proteins via their amino groups by the formation of azomethine bonds [96]. The mechanical performance of chitosan films or fibers can be improved by using GA as a cross-linking agent [97]. Chitosan cross-linked by GA and spacer group glycine has been reported by Gupta and Kumar [98]. The cross-linking network can be hydrolyzed in an acidic medium due to a higher swelling degree than at basic pH. These preliminary results suggest the possibility to obtain a desired pH-sensitive drug delivery system using GCCS as a carrier.

A chitosan film is formed by solution casting and then cross-linked by immersion in a GA aqueous solution. The residual aldehyde groups are blocked with a glycine solution. Neutralizing and washing until the film pH returns to the physiological range, primary rat heptocytes are seeded on the film. Hepatocytes sparsely adhere to the chitosan film in culture media. Results indicate that chitosan is a poor substrate for hepatocytes' attachment. However, it is suitable for sustaining hepatocytic functions [99].

On the other hand, GA is neurotoxic, and glyoxal is mutagenic. Therefore, even if products are purified before administration, the presence of free unreacted dialdehydes in the products cannot be completely excluded.

4.2.3.2 Genipin-Cross-Linked Chitosan

Genipin is a natural cross-linking reagent which has recently been used as a cross-linking agent for chitosan and proteins containing residues with primary amine groups. It is not cytotoxic *in vitro* [100] and is biocompatible after injection in rats [101]. The cross-linking mechanism consists of two reactions, involving different sites on the genipin molecule (as shown in Figure 4.7) [102,103]. The first step is the nucleophilic attack of amino group of the genipin C-3 carbon atom from a primary amine group to form an intermediate aldehyde group. The newly formed secondary amine reacts with the aldehyde group to form a heterocyclic compound. The step that follows is a nucleophilic substitution reaction that

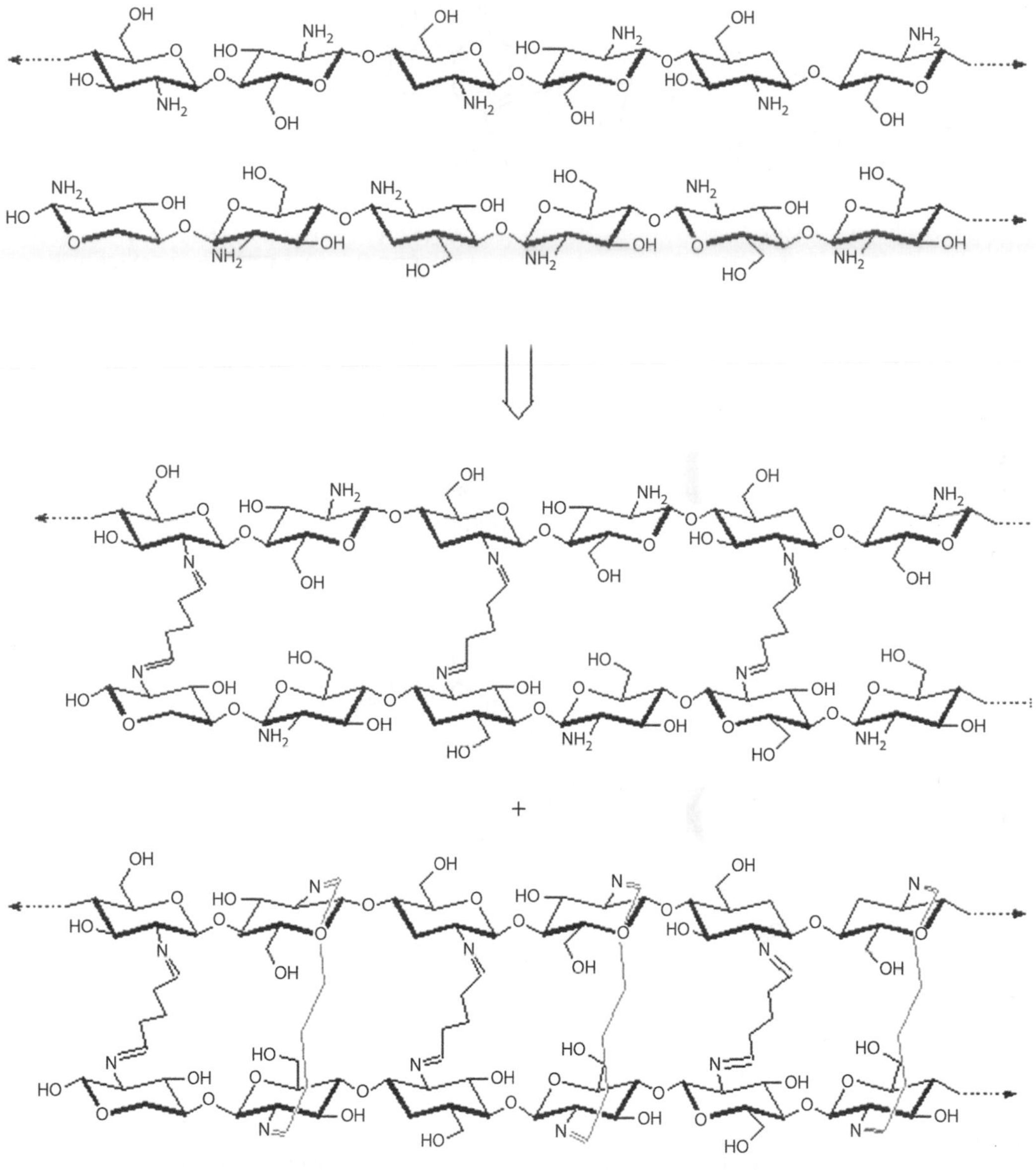

FIGURE 4.6
Sketch map of chitosan cross-linked by GA. (From Webster, A., Halling, M. D., and Grant, D. M. 2007. *Carbohydr Res* 342: 1189–1201. With permission.)

involves the replacement of the ester group on the G molecule by a secondary amide linkage. The reaction is complicated by the oxygen radical-induced polymerization of genipin that occurs once the heterocyclic compound has formed. The environmental pH condition plays an important role in influencing the cross-linking reactions for the preparation of genipin-cross-linked chitosan. Figure 4.8 shows the conformation of the network segments of the genipin-cross-linked chitosan network consisting of short cross-linking units of cyclic bridges and long cross-linking units of polymerized genipin [104].

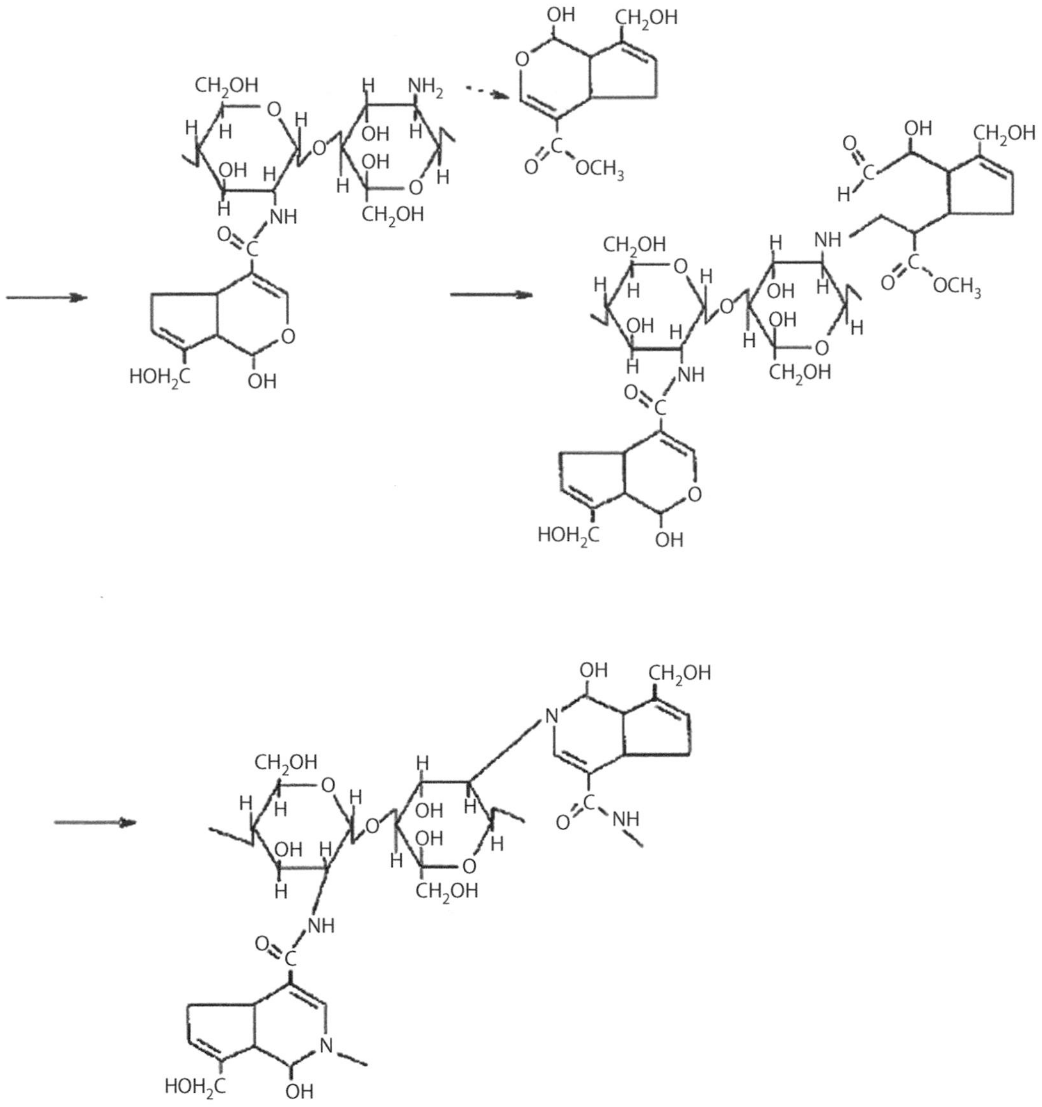

FIGURE 4.7
Reaction mechanism for the synthesis of genipin-cross-linked chitosan network. (From Mi, F. L., Sung, H. W., and Shyu, S. S. 2000. *J Polym Sci A-Polym Chem* 38: 2804–2814. With permission.)

Genipin-cross-linking-produced chitosan networks are insoluble in acidic and alkaline solutions but are able to swell in these aqueous media. The swelling characteristics of the films exhibit sensitivity to the environmental pH and temperature [105], whereas at pH 1.0 and pH 13.0, the swelling ratio increase to 315% and 240%, respectively, while at pH 7 the swelling ratio is about 62%. The increase of swelling of the cross-linked hydrogel at pH lower than 3 and higher than 11 may be ascribed to the hydrolysis of amide linkage in the cr-CS network by acid or alkaline and the regeneration of carboxyl acid and amine groups in networks. The swelling behavior is dictated by their polyelectrolyte nature. An increase in swelling is observed below the pK_a of the chitosan amine groups as they become

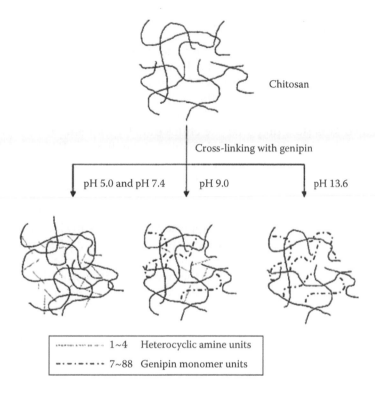

Chitosan

Cross-linking with genipin

pH 5.0 and pH 7.4   pH 9.0   pH 13.6

1~4   Heterocyclic amine units
7~88   Genipin monomer units

FIGURE 4.8
Conformations of the network segments of genipin-cross-linked chitosan gels consisting of short cross-linking units of cyclic bridges and long cross-linking units of polymerized genipin. (From Mi, F. L., Shyu, S. S., and Peng, C. K. 2005. *J Polym Sci B-Polym Chem* 43: 1985–2000. With permission.)

protonated. Genipin cross-linkers may form wasted cross-links as well as polymerize, leading to cross-links formed from not just one genipin molecule but various dimers, trimers, oligomers, and possibly polymers of genipin [106].

The degradation rate of the genipin-cross-linked chitosan network is much lower than the GA-cross-linked counterparts, because the genipin-cross-linked network may have a higher stereohindrance for the penetration of lysozyme than the GA-cross-linked network due to the bulky heterocyclic structure of genipin [101].

4.2.3.3 Diisocyanate-Cross-Linked Chitosan

Welsh and Price [107] prepared a water-soluble, blocked diisocyanate as a cross-linking agent for chitosan network formation. With increased pH or temperature, the adduct readily reacts with amines of chitosan, forming a urea linkage, at a rate much greater than that characteristic of competing reactions with alcohols or water. The cross-linker could tolerate high levels of hydration to achieve greater reaction efficiency and alternative applications, such as hydrogels. With greater control over cross-linking efficiency, material properties (such as physical, mechanical, and biological) of diisocyanate-cross-linked chitosan can be tailored to a given application [108].

4.2.3.4 Diepoxide-Cross-Linked Chitosan

A diepoxide-based bifunctional linker is used to cross-link the chitosan chains via the reactive amino groups on the chitosan backbone. The schematic representation of the cross-linking method is shown in Figure 4.9. The cross-linking chitosan network film with 1,4-butanediol diglycidyl ether increases the hydrophilicity of the surface and shows excellent cytocompatibility for chondrocyte cells [90].

Inoue and coworkers [109] prepared the chitosan network using the diepoxy-PEG as a cross-linker (*cf.* Figure 4.10). The swelling behavior of the diepoxy-PEG-cross-linked chitosan is found to rely greatly on the M_W of PEG in diepoxy-PEGs and weight percentage of the diepoxy-PEGs. The higher the diepoxy-PEG weight percentage, the lower the equilibrium swelling ratio for certain diepoxy-PEG. And the higher the M_W of PEG in diepoxy-PEG, the higher the equilibrium swelling ratio for the same weight percentage of the diepoxy-PEGs. Kulkarni et al. [110] have reported that cross-linking chitosan by PEG is accomplished by a novel yet simple method using formaldehyde. The free amino groups of chitosan, when treated with formaldehyde form intermediates of Schiff's bases ($-N=CH_2$), readily undergo addition with the hydroxyl groups of PEGs [111]. Moreover, these cross-linking networks show a significant swelling ratio in both the simulated

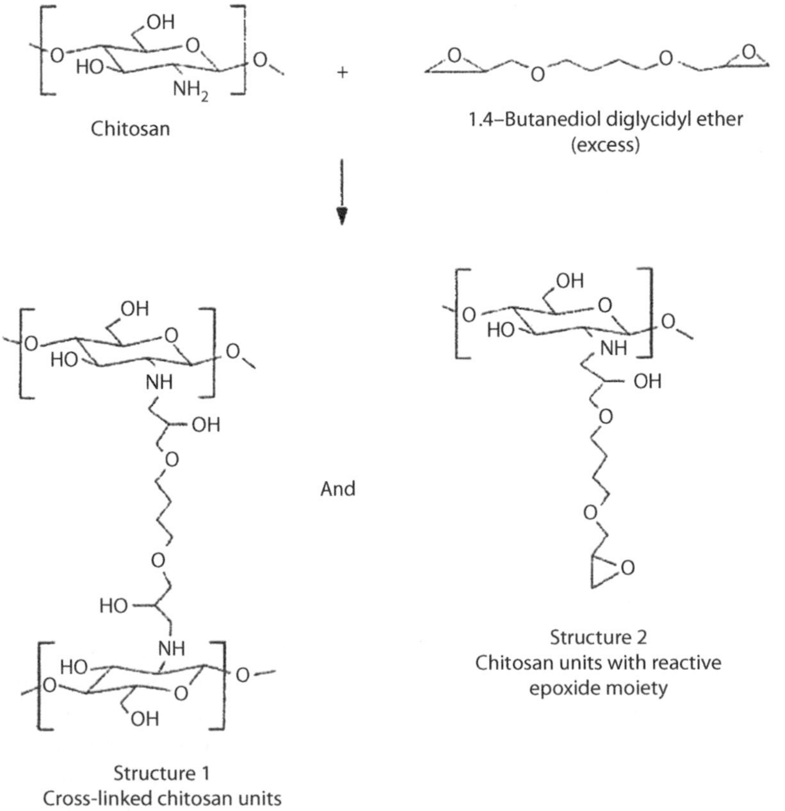

FIGURE 4.9
Schematic represenation of the strategy for cross-linking with bifunctional epoxides. (From Subramanian, A. and Lin, H. Y. 2005. *J Biomed Mater Res* 75A: 742–753. With permission.)

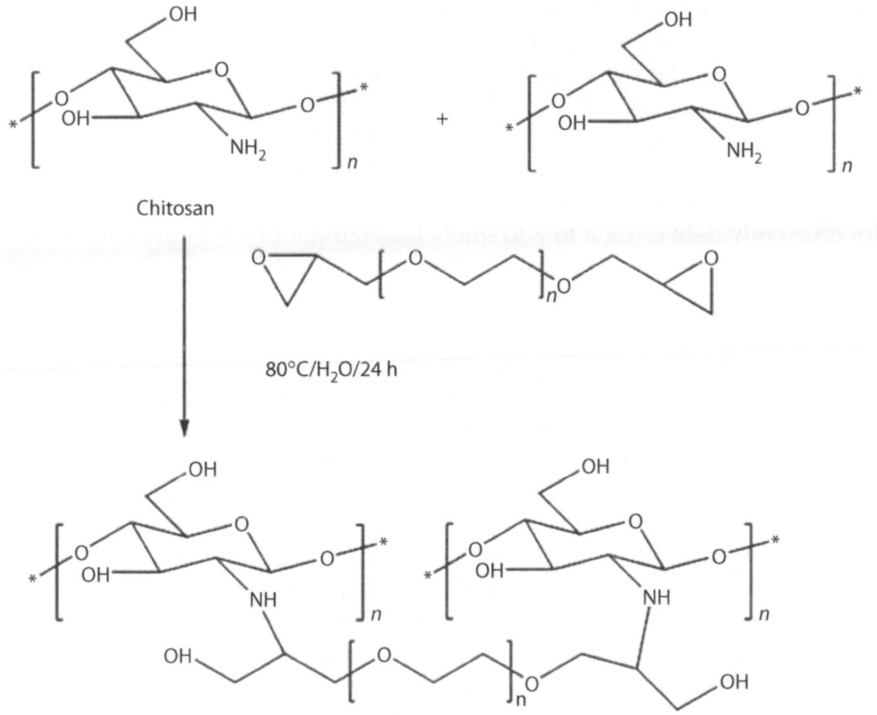

FIGURE 4.10

Reaction of cross-linked PEG hydrogel. (From Kiuchi, H., Kai, W. H., and Inoue, Y. 2008. *J Appl Polym Sci* 107: 3823–3380. With permission.)

stomach and intestinal solutions, which can be a better biomaterial than chitosan in the development of orally sustained drug delivery devices.

4.3 Multiple Component Network

4.3.1 Hybrid Cross-Linking Network

4.3.1.1 Chitosan/Protein Cross-Linking Network

4.3.1.1.1 Chitosan/Collagen Hybrid Cross-Linking Network

As a tissue-engineering scaffold, chitosan/collagen hybrid cross-linking networks show several advantages, including uniform and porous ultrastructure, less water absorption, small interval porosity, and high resistance to collagenase digestion. Incorporation of collagen into a chitosan matrix tends to increase the pore size and density and improve the structural homogeneity, which is due to the improvement of the structural stability of the matrices by chitosan in the chitosan/collagen cocross-linking network. The large number of amino groups on the chains of chitosan functions as a cross-linking bridge to increase overall matrix integrity by reinforcing the structure and cross-linking efficiency of GA in the scaffolds [112,113]. Gao and coworkers [114] found that the GA treatment has an influence on the morphology of the chitosan/collagen network scaffold. After cross-linking, the interconnected 3D porous structure of the scaffolds is retained. However, the mean pore size increased from ca. 100 μm (the uncross-linked) to >200 μm (the uncross-linked). At the same time, more sheet-like structures appear together with condensed walls.

The chitosan/collagen networks cross-linked by GA show excellent biocompatibility not only *in vitro* but also *in vivo* [114–116]. Therefore, it is widely used in tissue engineering, especially for skin tissue engineering and it is also used as a new wound-dressing material for damaged tissue recovery in various organs. The system has been explored to optimize the matrix for efficiently delivering it to and stably localizing it in the target tissues of fibroblast growth factor (FGF) [117]. The chitosan/collagen cross-linking nanofiber network is prepared by adding the synthetic polymer poly(ethylene oxide) (PEO), because collagen and chitosan cannot form nanofibers during electrospinning due to their larger net charges. The water sorption ability of the nanofiber network decreases after cross-linking [116]. Tsai et al. [118] found that chitosan/collagen network scaffolds with glutamic acid molecules as cross-linking bridges can enhance the tensile strength and improve cytocompatibility with skin fibroblasts, because the glutamic acid molecules to form cross-linking bridges might cause the chitosan/collagen-glutamic acid surface to absorb more serum proteins in the culture medium. The *N,O*-(carboxymethyl) chitosan/collagen cross-linking networks are more efficient in accelerating wound healing, because the *N,O*-(carboxymethyl) chitosan is able to stimulate the migration of fibroblasts, and the migration is significantly enhanced by *N,O*-(carboxymethyl) chitosan in a concentration-dependent manner [119]. In order to reduce the cell contraction and improve the initial cell distribution in chitosan/collagen scaffold, Tan and coworkers [120] developed a perfusion seeding system for dermal fibroblasts seeding onto collagen/chitosan sponges. High seeding efficiencies with uniform cell distributions are achieved by the perfusion seeding method, which further facilitates cell proliferation.

Combining the chitosan-cross-linked network with collagen is also able to improve the biological stability and strength of collagen to satisfy the demand of applications in bone tissue engineering. The incorporation of chitosan into a collagen scaffold increases the mechanical strength of the scaffold and reduces the biodegradation rate against collagenase [121,122]. Osteoblasts show higher levels of markers of osteoblastic differentiation at a mature stage, osteocalcin and calcium, in the chitosan/collagen network than chitosan. There are several possible reasons for this: first, osteoblasts have a specific affinity for collagen fibers; second, the stimulating effect of collagen matrix is further enhanced by the three-dimensional structure of the scaffolds; and third, chitosan improves the internal porous structure of a chitosan/collagen composite [123].

Collagen also greatly influences hepatocype growth and stability of mRNA for the expression of liver-specific function. Therefore, chitosan/collagen cross-linking network films are capable of maintaining both the attachment and function for hepatocutes [99].

4.3.1.1.2 Chitosan/Gelatin Hybrid Cross-Link Network

Chitosan/gelatin cross-linking networks are attractive for their applications in controlled release devices and tissue engineering. These networks are prepared using many cross-linkers, such as TPP, GA, genipin, EDC, and so on. In general, for chitosan/gelatin cross-linking networks, the mechanical properties improved with increasing cross-linking density. On the other hand, an increase in cross-linking density will induce a decrease in swelling and pH sensitivity. Thus, there is a practical trade-off between mechanical integrity and pH sensitivity, and both of these qualities are affected by the amount of chitosan, gelatin, and cross-linker as well as the pH at which curing is performed [124]. Chitosan/gelatin-cross-linked networks have a higher degradation rate and more loss of material than chitosan-cross-linked networks. Mechanical properties are affected by the addition of gelatin although there is no clear trend [125]. The chitosan/gelatin cross-linking network has excellent cytocompatibility [126]. For example, the cross-linked network containing 80 wt% gelatin well supports neuroblastoma cell adhesion and proliferation, which results in optimal candidates for future trials in the field of peripheral nerve regeneration [127]. In addition, it is more efficient in inducing fibrin formation and vascularization at the implant–host interface. However, the inflammatory reactions for the gelatin/chitosan network gel are significantly stronger than those for the gelatin gel [128].

Chitosan/gelatin network scaffolds are developed via their PEC formation, freeze-drying, and postcross-linking with GA. The average pore sizes of chitosan/gelatin scaffolds can be controlled within the range of 30–100 μm, and pore size can be modulated via prefreezing temperatures. Li and coworkers [129] have reported a novel method to fabricate chitosan/gelatin network scaffolds according to multilevel internal architectures via solid free form fabrication, microreplication, and lyophilization techniques. The porosity, pore size, and morphology can be easily controlled. The compression modulus of chitosan/gelatin scaffolds can be controlled within the range of 10–100 kPa [130,131]. Yao and coworkers [132] prepared the bilayer chitosan/gelatin scaffold via contacting with −56°C lyophilizing plate directly and then lyophilized. First, fibroblasts are seeded in the loose layer of the bilayer scaffold. The cell/scaffold constructs are cultured for 4 weeks. Afterward, keratinocytes were cocultured on the thick layer of fibroblast locating scaffolds, where cells proliferate well for 7 days. The results revealed that the chitosan/gelatin scaffold with multilevel internal architectures has the potential for being used in artificial skin [133].

Chitosan/gelatin microspheres can be prepared by the water-in-oil emulsion method and postcross-linking with GA. The human recombinant basic FGF (bFGF) is loaded within the microspheres by adsorption in its PBS solution. Incorporation of bFGF microspheres into the chitosan/gelatin scaffold significantly augmented the proliferation and glycosaminoglycan synthesis of human fibroblasts [134].

4.3.1.2 Chitosan/GAG Cross-Linking Network

GAGs can be cross-linked on the chitosan scaffold. The efficiency of GAG cross-linking is limited by the amounts of available amine groups on the scaffold for cross-linkage [135]. Different cross-linkers and cocross-linkers are used, such as GA, EDC, *N*-hydroxysuccinimide (NHS) and 2-morpholinoethane (MES), and Ca^{2+}, according to different GAGs.

4.3.1.2.1 Chitosan/Chondroitin Sulfate Cross-Linking Network

The tensile strength of chitosan/chondroitin sulfate, which was prepared via immobilizing chondroitin sulfate on the chitosan nonwoven scaffold using GA as a cross-linker, increases to over 200% of that of chitosan, but the elongation of chitosan/chondroitin sulfate decreased to less than 20% of that of chitosan. A possible reason is that the immobilization of chondroitin sulfate can also cause the fibers to bind with each other [136]. Chen et al. [137] augmented the GAGs (chondroitin-4-sulfate (CSA), chondroitin-6-sulfate, dermatan sulfate (DS), and heparin) onto chitosan films via cross-linking using EDC/NHS. The results suggested that the chitosan/GAG network (containing low CSA levels) leads to the maintenance of proper chondrocyte phenotype, as judged by the chondrocyte-like morphology, modest cell expansion, higher GAG and collagen production, and proper cartilage marker gene expression. The pore morphology and size agree with those of other chitosan-only scaffolds and exceed 70–120 μm, which is sufficient for uniform cell penetration and migration and improves GAG and collagen production [138].

The cross-linking of the chitosan/chondroitin sulfate composite ECMs with GA and EDC/NHS shows no obvious change in the morphology of 3D porous scaffolds. However, the cross-linking of the chitosan/chondroitin sulfate composite with Ca^{2+} produces a significant change in its porous structure. The Ca^{2+}-cross-linked chitosan/chondroitin sulfate composite ECMs have smaller pore size than GA- and EDC/NHS-cross-linked counterparts [139]. GA cross-links at the C-2 amine of glucosamine units in chitosan via imide bonds formation. However, the functional groups on chondroitin sulfate are not easy to react with GA. This suggests that the cross-linking of the chitosan/chondroitin sulfate complex with GA may produce a composite structure like semi-interpentrated networks, whereas EDC/NHS cross-linking results in the formation of amide bonds between carboxylic acid groups on chondroitin sulfate and amine groups on chitosan. Chondroitin sulfate will become cross-linked with the chitosan macromolecular chain, which is to form real chitosan/chondroitin sulfate interpenetrated networks. Calcium ions coordinated by oxygen atoms on carboxylate and sulfate groups on chondroitin sulfate are at short distances to form cross-linked networks. The chitosan/chondroitin sulfate networks show different swelling behavior due to the different cross-linked structure. The swelling ratios of the Ca^{2+}-cross-linked chitosan/chondroitin sulfate network are significantly lower than those of the GA-cross-linked ones. And different cross-linking types have different effects on the adsorption of bFGF (*cf.* Figure 4.11) [140]. In addition, the release rate of these GFs can be controlled by varying the composition of chondroitin sulfate in the sponge or initial loading content. For example, Lee and coworkers [141] found that the release rate of platelet-derived growth factor BB (PDGF-BB) increases with decreasing the chondroitin sulfate content of the system. And chitosan/chondroitin sulfate can improve the migration and proliferation of osteoblasts as compared with the chitosan scaffold alone. Furthermore, the release of PDGF-BB from the chitosan/chondroitin sulfate network scaffold significantly enhances osteoblast proliferation.

Chitosan can provide initial attachment and spreading of osteoblasts preferentially over the fibroblast [142]. Gelatin is derived from type I collagen, which plays a central role in the new bone formation from progenitors cells [143]. Moreover, chondroitin sulfate, which is the main GAG in bone, in association with collagen fibers, promotes *in vitro* mineralization[144]. Based on the advantages of these, a 3D chitosan/gelatin/chondroitin sulfate porous scaffold was cross-linked with EDC. A rat MSC scaffold was cultured with the osteogenic medium. The results demonstrated that the 3D structure provides a good environment for the osteogenic process and enhances cellular proliferation [145].

4.3.1.2.2 Chitosan/HA Network

HA is a major component of the PGs in the cartilage. Chitosan/gelatin/HA hybrid cross-linked networks were prepared via cross-linking with EDC/NHS and MES (*cf.* Figure 4.12). For studying the biocompatibility of these films, the cell cycle and apoptosis of L929 cells were evaluated. The results show that incorporated HA shortens the adaptation period of cells on the film surface, and then cells enter the normal cell cycle quickly. Moreover, the added HA would not trigger necrosis; it inhibited cell apoptosis on chitosan/gelatin films [146]. The concentration of HA in the chitosan/gelatin/HA-cross-linked network has an influence on the physical and mechanical properties and cytocompatibility of the network film. It is only the HA concentration in the range of 0.01–0.1% that benefits the ternary film [147].

A two-layer chitosan/gelatin/HA scaffold cross-linked with EDC has been constructed using the freeze-drying method. The asymmetric scaffold with different pore size layers is used for coculturing human fibroblasts and keratinocytes. The scaffold provides a

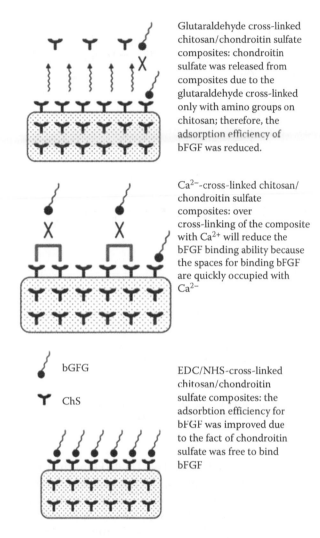

Glutaraldehyde cross-linked chitosan/chondroitin sulfate composites: chondroitin sulfate was released from composites due to the glutaraldehyde cross-linked only with amino groups on chitosan; therefore, the adsorption efficiency of bFGF was reduced.

Ca^{2-}-cross-linked chitosan/chondroitin sulfate composites: over cross-linking of the composite with Ca^{2+} will reduce the bFGF binding ability because the spaces for binding bFGF are quickly occupied with Ca^{2-}

bGFG

ChS

EDC/NHS-cross-linked chitosan/chondroitin sulfate composites: the adsorbtion efficiency for bFGF was improved due to the fact of chondroitin sulfate was free to bind bFGF

FIGURE 4.11

Schematic comparisons of bFGF-binding modes between the EDC/NHS-, GA-, and Ca^{2+}-cross-linked chitosan/ composites. (From Mi, F. L. et al. 2006. *J Biomed Mater Res* 76A: 1–15. With permission.)

stable and biocompatible microenviroment for the adhesion, proliferation, and differentiation of fibroblast and keratinocytes. The fibroblasts proliferation in the chitosan/ gelatin/HA scaffolds is significantly higher than that in the chitosan/gelatin scaffolds after 7 days. The results show that the scaffold has the potential to develop functional artificial skin [148].

4.3.1.2.3 Chitosan/Heparin Network

Heparin is a GAG used mainly as an anticoagulant or for the prevention of venous thrombosis and pulmonary embolism in patients undergoing surgery. Heparin and its related polysaccharides also play important roles in the regulation of blood vessel growth and regression. Three-dimensional, macroporous chitosan/heparin composite scaffolds are prepared by an interpolyelectrolyte and cross-linked using EDC/NHS or GA. The scaffolds

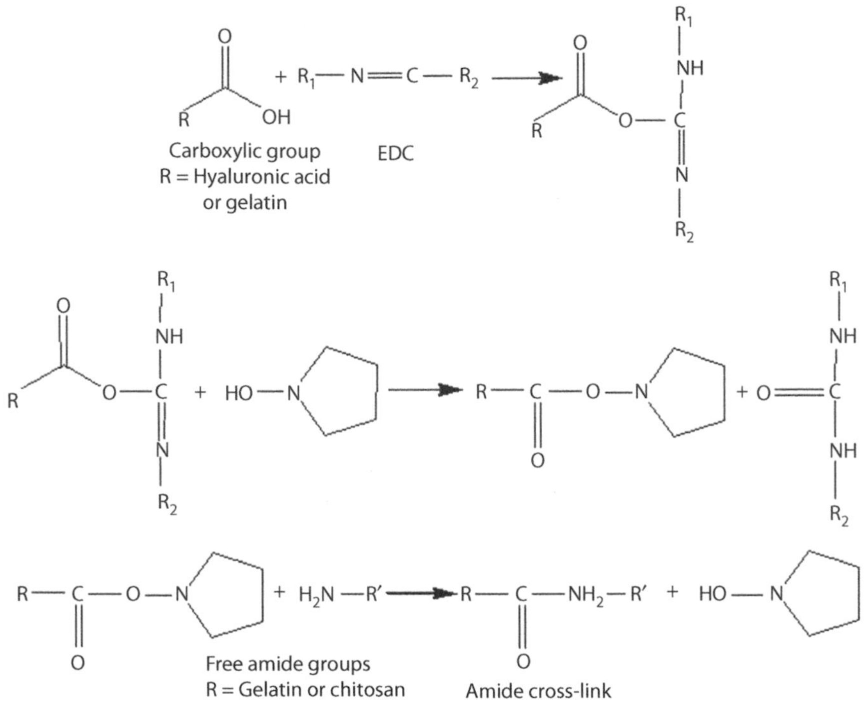

FIGURE 4.12
Mechanism of covalent attachment of HA to gelatin and chitosan using EDC and NHS. R_1=-CH$_2$-CH$_3$, R_2=-(CH$_2$)$_3$-NH$^+$-(CH$_3$)$_2$C$_1$. (From Liu, H. F. et al. 2004. *Biomaterials* 25: 3523–3530. With permission.)

show excellent cytocompatibility for fibroblast [149]. Heparin-functionalized chitosan-based scaffolds are formed via immobilizing the heparin on the chitosan-based network using a special cross-linker. In general, carbodiimide is used because of the existence of carboxylic acid groups in heparin molecules. Heparin can be immobilized on the chitosan/collagen films using the EDC/morpholinoethane sulfonic acid (MES) cross-linker system. The addition of heparin to the EDC cross-linking solution allows the remaining amino groups of collagen or chitosan to react with the carboxylic acid groups of heparin. The tensile strength and Young's modulus of the chitosan/collagen/heparin network decrease with the addition of heparin. With the introduction of heparin, more carboxyl groups are provided to take part in the cross-linking reaction with the amino groups. Most of the heparin molecules may not infiltrate into the inner part of the collagen/chitosan films and cross-linking may happen only on the surface of the films. Thus incorporation of heparin only on the surface of collagen/chitosan films can invoke adverse effects on the mechanical strength of the films. However, the mechanical strength of the collagen/chitosan/heparin film is enough to withstand the forces incurred during cell culture [150].

Mi and coworkers [151] conjugated heparin into chitosan–alginate PEC scaffolds using EDC. In the conjugation process, carboxylic acid groups of heparin are preactivated using EDC/NHS, followed by reaction of the activated heparin with the amine groups on chitosan (*cf.* Figure 4.13). bFGF is incorporated into these scaffolds through bioaffinity with heparin. The release rate can be controlled by controlling the immobilized heparin concentration and the released bFGF from the scaffold retains its biological activity.

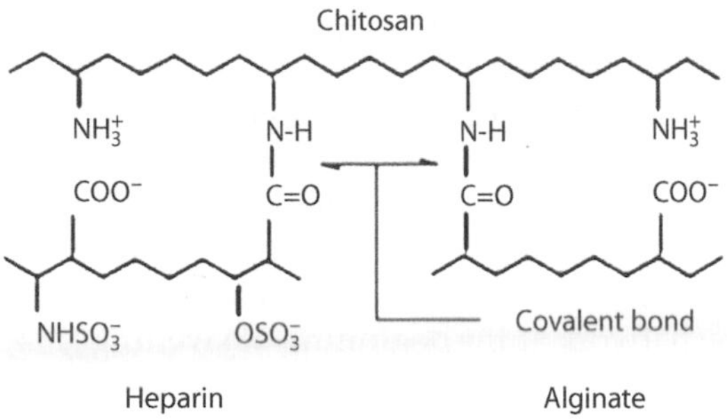

FIGURE 4.13
Heparin-functionalized chitosan–alginate PEC. (From Ho, Y. C. et al. 2009. *Int J Pharm* 376: 69–75. With permission.)

Chondrocytes seeded in the chitosan–alginate–heparin–bFGF actually show significant higher viability. bFGF is a primary promoter of cell proliferation, which stimulates the proliferation and migration of chondrocytes. Moreover, heparin can recognize and bind bFGF via the bioaffinity interaction, and coupling of heparin onto the scaffold is beneficial for the stable conjugation of bFGF under mild conditions. This may in turn help in preserving the bioactivity of the cell growth factor [152].

4.3.2 Interpenetrating Network

Entangled polymer networks can be further strengthened by interlacing secondary polymers within the cross-linked networks. Here, a cross-linked chitosan network is allowed to swell in an aqueous solution of polymer monomers. These monomers are then polymerized, forming a physically entangled polymer mesh called an interpenetrating polymer network (IPN). There are also semi-IPNs, where only one of the polymer networks is cross-linked, while the second polymer remains in its linear state. If the second polymer is also cross-linked, a full-IPN is formed. There are several chitosan-based semi-IPNs and full-IPNs. This technique allows for the specific selection of polymers that can complement the deficiencies of one another. Although the cross-linking density, hydrogel porosity, and gel stiffness can be adjusted in IPN-based hydrogels according to the target application, they have difficulty encapsulating a wide variety of therapeutic agents, especially sensitive biomolecules. In addition, IPN preparation requires the use of toxic agents to initiate or catalyze the polymerization or to catalyze the cross-linking. Complete removal of these materials from the hydrogel is challenging, making the clinical application problematic [6].

4.3.2.1 Semi-IPNs

The states of water in hydrogels and their relative amounts exert a considerable effect on the permeability and selectivity of hydrogel membranes. The activity of biological systems, such as proteins and enzymes, depends on how the water molecules associate with these biopolymers. Cross-linked chitosan–polyether semi-interpenetrating polymer network (cr-CS–PE semi-IPN) was synthesized and the state and mobility of water in cr-CS–PE semi-IPN were investigated using differential scanning calorimetry (DSC) and nuclear magnetic resonance (NMR), respectively. The results indicate that the states and mobility of water in the semi-IPN hydrogels vary with the change in water content, which is also responsible for the alteration of free volume and the diffusion coefficient [153]. A comparative study of the swelling behavior of cr-CS and its semi-IPN with poly(oxy-propylene glycol) (cr-CS/PE semi-IPN) was also carried out by using DSC, NMR, and positron annihilation lifetime spectroscopy. The results reveal that cr-CS/PE semi-IPN-containing hydrophobic moieties have more free volume for water at definite water content and restricts its mobility less, and the water clusters coexist with water molecules hydrogen-bonded to the network at the beginning of swelling [154].

The swelling and mechanical performance of a chitosan/PEO semi-IPN and a reference chitosan gel were evaluated and compared by Agnely and coworkers [155]. From the swelling study it was concluded that the semi-IPN has a promising potential because of its higher pH-dependent swelling properties, which could allow a pH-controlled release of drug in oral administration. The DSC measurements indicate that the semi-IPN contained 6% more bound water than the reference gel, probably due to the presence of the hydrophilic PEO chains. As regards the mechanical properties, which are a key parameter for the potential use of the system as an implant, the presence of the PEO physical network enlarges the elastic character for the semi-IPN compared to the chitosan reference gel.

Shyu and coworkers [156] found a route via polymer blend and cross-linking/grafting modification to obtain novel biomaterials by interpenetrating a natural polymer modified polysaccharide, 6-O-carboxymethylchitosan (6-OCC) with various waterborne polyurethane (WPU) chains. Semi-IPN membranes are prepared by cross-linking/grafting the 6-OCC/WPU composites with GA or with ethylene glycol diglycidyl ether. The results reveal that the miscibility of a 6-OCC/WPU composite membrane is increased after being converted into a semi-IPN membrane, and the antibacterial capability and thrombo resistance of the WPUs are significantly improved via the formation of the semi-IPN membranes. The results of this work suggest that the 6-OCC/WPU semi-IPN membranes may be used as a biomaterial for blood-contracting devices.

For tissue-engineering applications, it is expected that the homogeneous blending of a hydrophilic polymer with the hydrophobic polycaprolactone (PCL) chains improves water diffusion to the proximities of PCL chains, thus accelerating their hydrolytic degradation. PCL and chitosan (CHT) are immiscible polymers. Apparently homogeneous cosolutions are obtained mixing PCL solution in pure acetic acid with chitosan solutions in 1 M acetic acid for CHT/PCL weight ratios up to 30:70. Then, a PCL/CHT semi-IPN is prepared by simultaneous precipitation and CHT cross-linking with tripolyphosphate. High-porosity PCL/CHT scaffolds with open pore structure and good interconnectivity are also obtained. Mechanical properties evaluated by dynamic-mechanical analysis decrease as porosity increases. The physical interactions between functional groups of CHT and carbonyl groups of PCL are assessed by FTIR, the shifting of the main relaxation of PCL toward high temperatures as the fraction of CHT increases as well as the evolution of the thermal properties of the system [157].

To overcome the fast dissolution of Poloxamer (P) gels, improve swelling properties and sustain the release of 5-FU for longer, P gels with an interpenetrating chitosan network (CS network) that is cross-linked by GA, P-CS/GA gels were developed by Chung et al. [158]. The results indicated that the swelling ratios of all P-CS/GA gels are markedly superior to those of nonswelling P and P-CS gels. *In vitro* releases of 5-FU from P-CS/GA gels have significantly lower initial burst release and last much longer than those from gels without a CS network. The release of drugs from gels with an interpenetrating CS network can be modeled by Fickian diffusion; the characteristic constant k of drug–gel systems decrease with increasing the GA concentrations in the P-CS/GA gels and increasing the viscosities of the P, P-CS, and P-CS/GA solutions.

The multifunctional chitosan–poly(methacrylic acid)–CdSe (chitosan–PMAA–CdSe) hybrid nanogels are prepared in an aqueous solution via *in situ* immobilization of CdSe quantum dots (CdseQDs) into the chitosan–PMAA semi-IPN nanogels, which should display the properties and functions from each building block, as schematically depicted in Figure 4.14. The template chitosan–PMAA nanogel is formed either by noncovalent physical associations, such as secondary forces and physical entanglements, or by covalent cross-linkages. The covalently cross-linked nanogels are very stable in both structure and composition upon pH variation; the hybrid nanogels based on the physical associations exhibited a significant change in structure and composition in response to a pH increase to physiological conditions. The covalently cross-linked hybrid nanogels exhibit excellent structural stability as well as reversible physical property change in response to a pH variation cross the physiological condition, which can successfully integrate the optical pH-sensing and cellular imaging ability, regulated drug delivery, and low-cytotoxicity into a single nano-object. In contrast, the physically associated hybrid nanogels would not be an ideal candidate for biosensing and drug delivery. It is important to achieve progress in the development of multifunctional bionanomaterials by incorporation of functional building blocks into a single individual nanoparticle [159].

The limited solubility of chitosan in water and common organic solvents has inhibited extensive studies and utilization of chitosan. So modifications of chitosan with polymers have been widely investigated to tune its properties to fulfill some requirements for specific applications. These are carried out either by physical blending, chemical grafting, or cross-linking. For example, PEG/polydimethylsiloxane (PEG/PDMS) block copolymer, prepared by a condensation reaction between PEG diacid and PDMS diol, is incorporated into chitosan in order that good water swellability and wettability of chitosan were retained due to hydrophilic PEG blocks, whereas PDMS block in the copolymers functioned as a toughening modifier [160,161]. However, some macroscopic phase separation between the copolymer and chitosan is still observed when a high percentage of the copolymer was applied due to the absence of chemical bonding between these two phases. Therefore, PDMS/PEG–chitosan semi-IPNs were prepared, where PDMS and PEG were selected to represent hydrophobic and hydrophilic polymers, respectively, to investigate their effect on the properties of chitosan hydrogels. They are interpenetrated and locked in place in the chitosan structure, so that up to 20 wt% PDMS/PEG with high Mn (8000 g/mol) can be

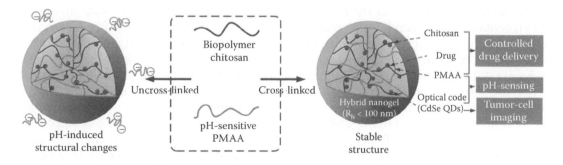

FIGURE 4.14
Schematic representation of the concept for designing multifunctional chitosan–PMAA–CdSe hybrid nanogel and its potential applications in the biomedical field. (From Wu, W. et al. 2010. *Biomaterials* 31: 8371–8381. With permission.)

incorporated. Without the formation of semi-IPN structure, hydrophobic PDMS with high Mn and high content tends to macrophase separate from chitosan continuous phase. PDMS and PEG in the chitosan semi-IPNs generally promote water swelling ability and water vapor permeability of the modified chitosan films. It is hypothesized that PEG enhanced these properties due to its hydrophilic characteristics, while in the case of PDMS–chitosan semi-IPNs, this is attributed to the formation of PDMS microphase, allowing the materials to have more polymer–air interfaces and more contact with water. Addition of PDMS/PEG to chitosan semi-IPNs slightly enhances their thermal stability and surface hydrophobicity, while their tensile properties are sacrificed [162].

4.3.2.2 Full-IPNs

Fang and coworkers [163] reported a kind of full-IPN chitosan/poly(*N*-isopropylacrylamide) (CS/PNIPAM) hydrogel that is formed by chemical combination of methylene bis-acrylamide-cross-linked PNIPAM network with a formaldehyde (HCHO)-crosslinked chitosan network. It is demonstrated that the properties of the hydrogels, including the extractability of PNIPAM within it, the phase transition behavior, the swelling dynamics in aqueous phase, the swelling behavior in ethanol/water mixtures, and even the microstructure, are quite different from those of the semi-IPN CS/PNIPAM hydrogels, in which PNIPAM is simply embedded. Like the semi-IPN CS/PNIPAM hydrogels, however, the full-IPN hydrogel is also temperature sensitive; that is, the hydrogel is transparent below 30°C, but opaque above that temperature. It is expected that this hydrogel may find some uses in separation science and in the design and preparation of new soft machines.

PVA has hydrophilic groups, which are employed in biomedical applications because of its easy preparation, excellent chemical resistance and physical properties and because it is biocompatible. Full-IPN hydrogels based on PVA and chitosan were prepared by using UV irradiation and the swelling ratio, free water content and bound water content of the IPN hydrogels were measured by Kim et al. [164]. All hydrogels swell rapidly and reach equilibrium within 1 h. The swelling ratio and free water contents increase with increasing molar ratio of hydrophilic groups of chitosan in IPNs. The PVA/chitosan IPN hydrogels exhibit swelling change in response to external stimuli such as pH and temperature, and can be useful as a novel modulation system in the biomedical field.

Considering that conventional nonporous hydrogels swell slowly and exhibit low loading capacities, which restrict their use in effective drug delivery, superporous hydrogel (SPH) containing poly(acrylic acid-co-acrylamide)/carboxymethyl chitosan (P(AA-co-AM)/O-CMC) IPNs (SPH-IPNs) are synthesized to enhance the mechanical strength, *in vitro* muco-adhesive force, and loading capacity of SPHs. The swelling ratios of SPH-IPNs decrease with increasing the O-CMC content, the GA amount, and the cross-linking time. After the introduction of the full-IPN structure, mechanical properties, *in vitro* mucoadhesive force and loading capacities of the SPH-IPNs are significantly improved and can be modulated by varying the O-CMC content. The SPH-IPNs will also be biocompatible considering the biocompatibility of both P(AA-co-AM) and O-CMC. Such characteristics suggest that the SPH-IPN may be an advantageous candidate for the mucosal drug delivery system, especially for effective peroral delivery of peptide and protein drugs [165].

SPH-IPN is also evaluated as the oral delivery vehicle for insulin, emphasizing the effect of polymer integrity on insulin absorption mechanisms. Compared to powdered SPH-IPN (P-SPH-IPN), integral SPH-IPN (I-SPH-IPN) has a higher swelling ratio, a stronger water retention capacity, and lower *in vitro* as well as *in vivo* release rates, which is beneficial for its application as an oral delivery vehicle. Although I-SPH-IPN and P-SPH-IPN have comparable *in vitro* enzymatic inhibition capacities due to their similar chemical compositions, I-SPH-IPN possesses notable superiority to P-SPH-IPN in *in vivo* enzymatic inhibition, permeation enhancing effect, and intestinal retention as a result of its preferable physical integrity that exerted stronger mechanical pressures to the intestinal epithelia. Therefore, oral delivery of I-SPH-IPN induces significant insulin absorption and hypoglycemic effect, while P-SPH-IPN proves ineffective. In the oral acute and subacute toxicity assessments, minimal cumulative toxicity indicates good tolerance of the SPH-IPN. The SPH-IPN is an effective and safe carrier for oral delivery of protein drugs, where polymer integrity plays an important role in effective drug absorption. This work concerning polymer integrity-related absorption mechanisms can help in formulating strategies to improve the oral bioavailability of protein drugs using expandable formulations as delivery vehicles, such as films and hydrogels [166].

4.4 Composite Network

It has been proved that chitosan can potentiate the differentiation of osteoprogenitors cells and may facilitate the formation of bones [167,168]. However, the mechanical properties of chitosan do not satisfy the requirements of bone tissue repair. Thus, the chitosan/calcium phosphate (chitosan/CaP) composites (especially chitosan/hydroxyapatite (HAp) composites) are developed in order to improve the mechanical properties. Moreover, the chitosan/CaP composites can imitate the components and structures of natural bone and can improve the bioactivity and bone bonding ability. The adhesive and flexible properties of chitosan make it bind the CaP particles together and prevent the migration of CaP particulate into the surrounding tissue upon postimplantation. Besides, smoothness of the composites may not damage or harm any soft tissues. In general, the chitosan/CaP composites can be formed via blending of chitosan and CaP or mineralization of the chitosan matrix.

4.4.1 Blending Composites

Incorporation of calcium phosphate salt, such as β-tricalcium phosphate (β-TCP), calcium phosphate, and HAp, into the chitosan matrix can improve the biocompatibility and hard tissue integration and assists in tailoring degradation and resorption kinetics. Chitosan/CaP composites are made by a simple mixing-and-heating method with the aim of improving the properties of chitosan. The conventional method for fabricating the chitosan/CaP composite is as follows: CaP powder is mixed with chitosan in an acetic acid solution, and then the mixture is impressed into a mold, and finally it is freeze-dried to make a scaffold composite. The major advantages of this approach are simplicity and low cost [168,169]. These chitosan/CaP composites can be used as bone tissue-engineering scaffolds and drug controlled release carriers.

4.4.1.1 Chitosan/β-TCP Composite System

With the β-TCP powder as a filler to reinforce the microstructure of the chitosan scaffolds, both the compressive modulus and the yield strength are greatly improved. And the compressive strength increases with increasing the β-TCP content [170]. When β-TCP is introduced into chitosan scaffolds, not only physical incorporation of the secondary phases into the chitosan matrix occurs, but also chemical reactions among the chitosan and β-TCP might take place. That is because of the high surface charge density of chitosan and the ability of chitosan to form ionic complexes. The β-TCP powders are dispersed homogeneously on the surfaces of the solid walls of the pores; β-TCP powders are expected to slowly dissolve in physiological media and increase the concentrations of the Ca and P ions [171].

The chitosan/β-TCP scaffold supports the proliferation of osteoblast cells as well as their differentiation as indicated by high ALPase activities and deposition of mineralized matrices by cells. Small bone-like spicules are observed as early as 14 days. The chitosan/β-TCP scaffolds can be used as a matrix to grow osteoblast in a 3D structure for transplantation into a site for bone regeneration *in vivo* [172,173]. Moreover, chitosan/β-TCP composites are developed as bone substitutes and tissue-engineering scaffolds with a releasing function for some drug or GF with osteogenic effect. Zhang and Zhang [174] reported that the initial burst of antibiotic gentamicin-sulfate release in chitosan/β-TCP is greatly reduced, and the release rate in the second stage after the initial burst is higher and steadier than that of pure chitosan scaffold. However, the release rate of transforming growth factor-β (β-TGF) in chitosan/β-TCP composites is higher than that in chitosan at the initial stage. And the concentration of released β-TGF from the chitosan/β-TCP microgranules for 28 days is sufficient to induce a biological effect. The initial burst release can be beneficial to the early healing and regenerative effect, and the following continuous release can help osteoblasts proliferate [175,176].

4.4.1.2 Chitosan/HAp Composite System

In the chitosan/HAp composite system, the chitosan network not only serves as a matrix to the HAp particles but also provides an anchoring site for HAp particles in the structure. There are multiple interactions between chitosan and HAp. For example, HAp may interact with the plentiful amino and hydroxyl groups of chitosan by the formation of hydrogen bonds [177]. Ca^{2+} ions, which appear on the terminal surface of HAp crystals, have a coordination number of 7 and are strictly held in the composite through coordination with the $-NH_2$ of chitosan. Wilson and Hull [178] prepared the nano-HAp–chitosan composites via surface modification of nanophase HAp with chitosan. Chitosan exhibits strong adsorption interactions with HAp, which enhance colloid stability for the processing of chitosan/HAp nanocomposites and cause an increase in specific surface areas. However, the hybrid composite seems to be dissociated possibly due to the degradation of the chitosan [179].

The addition of nHAp to pure chitosan leads to a decrease in the degree of water absorption. However, the water retention ability of chitosan scaffolds and chitosan/HAp is similar with only small differences. The compression modulus of hydrated scaffolds significantly increases on the incorporation of nHAp and increases with increasing nHAp content in the scaffold, which can be attributed to the strong interaction between chitosan and HAp. Favorable biological responses of preosteoblast (MC 3T3-E1) on nanocomposite scaffolds include improved cell adhesion, higher proliferation, and well spreading morphology in relation to pure chitosan scaffold [180].

Oliveira et al. [181] prepared the chitosan/HAp bilayer scaffold; the bilayered scaffolds exhibit excellent physicochemical properties, which appear to make them a suitable candidate to be used as a supportive structure for cell functions. Moreover, the *in vitro* cell culture studies demonstrate that both HAp and chitosan layers provide an adequate 3D support for the attachment, proliferation, and differentiation of MSCs into osteoblasts and chondrocytes, respectively. The chitosan/HAp scaffolds show promising biological behavior and may therefore find applications in bone tissue engineering and osteochondral defects.

A biomimetic HAp/chitosan/gelatin network composite scaffold is developed through phase separation of HAp powder suspension in an acid aqueous solution of chitosan–gelatin and GA under freeze-drying conditions. The pore size of scaffolds ranges from several microns to ca. 500 µm, and the porosity can be adjusted by changing the solid content of the original component ratio. Typical data of porosity is 90% and the pore size is ca. 300–500 µm. Rat caldaria osteoblasts seeding onto the scaffold exhibit excellent bioactivity and can facilitate bone formation [182,183]. And this scaffold leads to enhancement of ECM proteins and calcium, which favors the adhesion and osteogenic differentiation of MSCs [184].

4.4.2 Mineralization Composites

Bone tissue is extremely strong and dense, which makes it well suited for providing load-bearing support and protection to the body. It is mainly composed of mineral of HAp set onto collagen fiber. Bone is characterized by hierarchical organization. Here, the mineral structure is incorporated into the ECM, where a network of collagen fiber-holding cells together serves as a template for biomineralization [185]. HAp crystal is sedimented *in situ* on a chitosan-based matrix in order to mimic the structure of bone. Coprecipitation and surface coating are the main approaches to prepare chitosan–HAp mineralization composites.

4.4.2.1 Mineralization through Coprecipitation

Chitosan can also serve as a template for mineralization due to its special functional groups, such as $-NH_2$ and C=O. The process of chitosan mineralization in the case when a stepwise coprecipitation approach is used is shown in Figure 4.15 [186]. Small HAp crystallites are able to align along the chitosan molecule upon aggregation through the interaction between the calcium ions on the HAp surface and the amino groups of the chitosan molecule. In other words, the self-assembly phenomenon for the *c*-axis of HAp nanocrystals parallel to the chitosan molecules can be described by the formation of HAp nucleation centers on the amino groups in chitosan, resulting in the subsequent crystal growth of HAp nanocrystals [187].

Porous Hap–chitosan–alginate composite scaffolds are fabricated by *in situ* coprecipitation methods; eventually, the pore structure is locally collapsed and appears to be agglomerated. The size of HAp crystals can be controlled via changing the contents of chitosan in the chitosan–alginate complex. A higher amount of chitosan leads to a smaller average crystallite size of HAp [188]. In general, the average size of HAp crystals formed via mineralization is ca. 15–100 nm and the crystallinity is lower when compared with those formed in solution. The maximum compressive strength of the HAp/chitosan composite is about 120 MPa corresponding to the 30:70 chitosan/HAp composite, while the compressive strength of 20:70 chitosan/HAp composites is ca. 100 MPa. This may be caused by chemical and mechanical interlocking between HAp and chitosan that accounts for the efficient stress transfer in the composite system. Besides, the interactions such as hydrogen bonding and chelation between the two phases also contribute to the good mechanical properties of the chitosan/HAp composite [189].

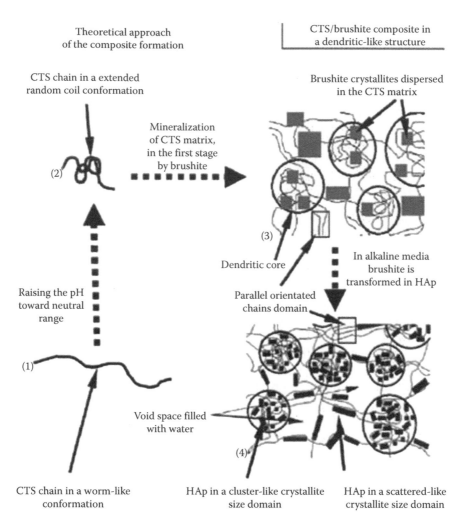

FIGURE 4.15
Main stages in the formation of the chitosan/HAp (CTS/HAp) composite structure. (From Rusu, V. M. et al. 2005. *Biomaterials* 26: 5414–5426. With permission.)

The resorbability of nano-HAp can be increased by the addition of chitosan. Possible reasons for this are the following: first, the presence of chitosan macromolecules can further stimulate the release of calcium ions from the composite matrix; second, the low crystallinity also improves the resorbability [190]. Mineralization of the alginate–chitosan core-shell capsules is used for the encapsulation and release of a range of human cell types (e.g., human bone marrow cells, articular cartilage progenitor cells, and adipocytes) and GF (e.g., recombinant human morphogenetic protein-2 (rh-BMP-2)). The factor can be delivered to mouse C1C12 promyoblast cells [191].

4.4.2.2 Mineralization through Surface Coating

The apatite coating on chitosan/gelatin films can be formed via the biomimetic process in SBF or Ca/P buffer solution. The properties of apatite coating could be controlled by (1) charged density of chitosan–gelatin network films; (2) intensities of interactions among the corresponding ionic groups and/or polar groups; and (3) accessibility of these corresponding groups [192]. The surface properties of chitosan/gelatin could control the nucleation and growth of HAp crystals (*cf.* Figure 4.16). The average size of nHA crystals decreases with increasing gel content and increases with increasing calcium and phosphate concentrations. The DD of the chitosan and the concentration of SBF have significant effects on the microstructure and crystallinity of biomimetically deposited calcium phosphate coatings. The crystallinity of coatings on the chitosans with higher DD is better because chitosans with higher DD are also most hydrophilic. This can have an effect on the nucleation and growth of calcium phosphate crystals [193]. It is found that osteoblasts proliferate to a greater extent on amorphous carbonated CaP than on more crystalline CaP [194]. Therefore, one can modulate the osteoblast behavior by changing the properties of the template.

Incorporating nano-HAp crystallines into chitosan can accelerate the biomineralization process and influence the topography because the nano-HAp particles can act as nucleation sites [195]. The biomineralization behavior of *N*-methylene phosphochitosan scaffolds is superior to that of the chitosan scaffold in Ca^{2+} and HPO_4^{2-} solutions or the SBF solution due to the exiting of PO_4^{3-} in the template [196]. For the same reason, stronger interactions between the carboxyl group and Ca^{2+}, the incorporation of gelatin into chitosan also accelerates the formation of nano-HAp coating through repeated deposition in PO_4^{3-} and Ca^{2+} ion solutions. The size of nanocrystals can be adjusted by changing the ratio of chitosan and gelatin, concentrations of PO_4^{3-} and Ca^{2+}, and the reaction temperature [192]. The surface topography can be modulated by the deposition times [197]. The nano-HAp coating chitosan-based biomaterials is a suitable substrate for osteoblast-like cell distribution, attachment, and migration. And it also accelerates osteoblastic differentiation at an early stage, and promotes ECM formation in comparison with chitosan [198,199]. In addition, it can also inhibit the proliferation of cancer cells [200].

4.5 Self-Assembly Network

There are very complex and diverse self-assembled structures from building units (amino acid, carbohydrate, and lipids) in a living system. The key point lies in the chemical structure of these units that should carry all the information to direct their self-assembly process [201]. Self-assembly is the spontaneous formation of ordered structures and is an important nanotechnology tool that may be utilized for spatially orienting macromolecules with nanoscale precision. Self-assembly is a "bottom-up" approach in which smaller building block molecules associate with each other in a coordinated fashion to form larger, more complex supramolecules. The organization of these building blocks into supramolecules is governed by molecular recognition due to noncovalent interactions such as hydrogen bonding, as well as electrostatic and hydrophobic interactions [3]. Commonly used chitosan self-assembly methods include self-assembled nanoparticles and self-assembled multilayers.

4.5.1 Self-Assembly Nanoparticles

The self-assembly nanoparticles can be employed to control the drug release behaviors and it is also an effective method for controlling the spatial organization of cells [202].

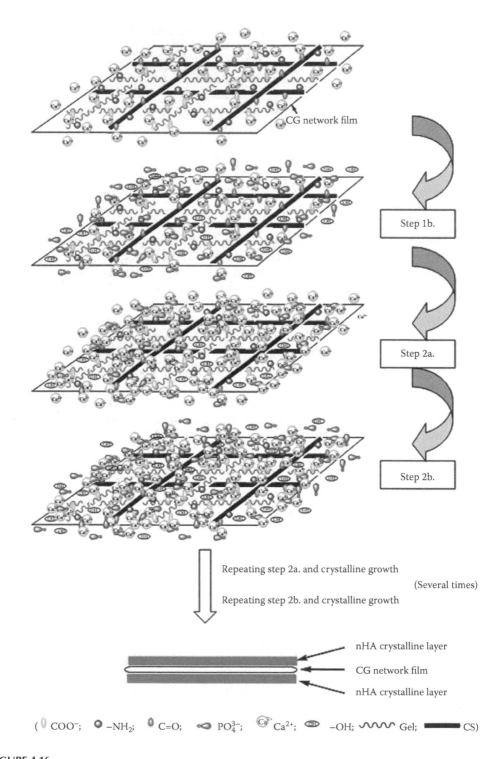

FIGURE 4.16
Schematic representation of the mechanism of nHA crystalline formation *in situ* on the surface of CG network films. (From Li, J. J. et al. 2007. *Biomaterials* 8: 781–790. With permission.)

Amphiphilic chitosan-based biomaterials are developed by conjugating hydrophobic groups and/or hydrophilic groups into chitosan molecules. Amphiphilic chitosan can form nanosized self-assembly particles with a hydrophobic core and a hydrophilic shell due to the intra- and/or intermolecular interactions of hydrophobic segments in the aqueous media. The hydrophobic microdomains are formed by the association of hydrophobic groups. Chitosan backbones coil to form the hydrophilic shells outside these hydrophobic microdomains. Furthermore, inter- and/or intramolecular hydrogen bondings among tightly packed chitosan backbones will promote the self-assembly of hydrophobically modified polysaccharides (*cf.* Figure 4.17) [203]. These self-assemblies have potential applications in biotechnology and medicine due to their unique supramolecular structures.

Grafting an amphiphilic biblock copolymer on chitosan molecules can also endow the chitosan with amphiphilicity. Amphiphilic N-phthaloylchitosan-grafted mPEG (PLC-g-mPEG) is a good model to fulfill the conditions for colloidal phenomena where the nanospheres are induced. The stability of the appearance of the milky solution is enhanced in protic solvents where hydrogen bonds are accomplished. And the nanosize can be controlled by the length of the mPEG chain. mPEG with M_n = 5 kDa gives spheres with sizes about 80–100 nm, whereas mPEG with M_n = 550 Da provides spheres with an average size of 400–500 nm [204,205]. The favorable conditions for the guest molecules to incorporate into chitosan nanosphere are high hydrophobicity of the guest itself and positive charge. An effective guest incorporation is achieved by dispersing the PLC-g-mPEG nanosphere in a guest–isopropanol solution, or so-called the heterogeneous system (*cf.* Figure 4.18) [206,207].

PLC-g-mPEG forms a core-shell micellar structure after dialysis of the polymer solutions in dimethyl sulfoxide or dimethylformamide (DMF) against water. Camptothecin (CPT) can load into the inner core of the micelles by the dialysis method with high stability and with a sustained release against PBS buffer, pH 7.4. Phthaloylchitosan units of the hydrophobic chain of the polymers and drug contents are important factors for the incorporation

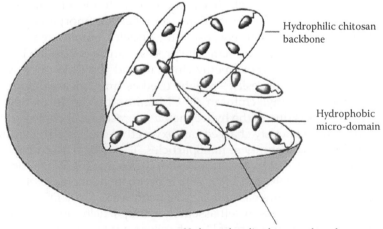

Hydrophilic chitosan backbone

Hydrophobic micro-domain

Hydrogen bonding between the polar groups

FIGURE 4.17
Schematic representation of amphiphilic chitosan self-assembly nanoparticles. (From Wang, Y. S. et al. 2007. *Eur Polym J* 43: 43–51. With permission.)

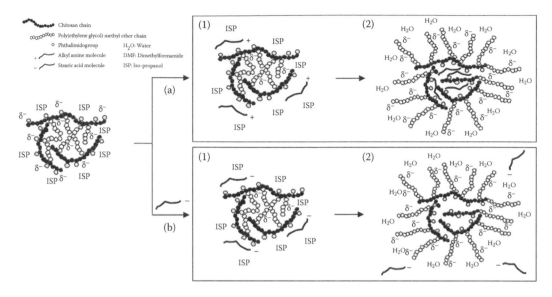

FIGURE 4.18
Formation mechanisms of *N*-phthaloylchitosan grafted mPEG nanoparticles via the heterogeneous system. (From Opanasopit, P. et al. 2007. *Colloid Surf B* 60: 117–124; Yoksan, R. and Chirachanchai, S. 2008. *Bioorg Med Chem* 16: 2687–2696. With permission.)

efficiency and stability of drug-loaded micelles. And the DD of chitosan is a key factor in controlling the yield, stability of the drug-loaded micelles, and drug release behavior. As the DD increases, the stability of CPT-loaded micelles increases, and a sustained release is obtained at high DD [207]. Furthermore, the internalization of the drug in the micelles notably hinders the hydrolytic opening of the lactone ring in the physiological environment (PBS buffer, pH 7.4) and in human serum albumin (HSA) [206,208].

N-Phthaloyl-carboxymethylchitosan with suitable balance of the attractive and repulsive forces could self-organize in a selective and repulsive to form the multilamellar vesicles derivative. It could be self-assembled to form various morphologies of crew-cut aggregates including vesicles, vesicle encapsulating vesicles, onion-like vesicles, and large compound micelles in the mixture system. The process can be controlled by adjusting the concentration of *N*-phthaloyl-carboxymethylchitosan and the ratio of *N*, *N*-DMF in the mixture solution [209]. The nanovesicles may be used as time release devices. For cholesterol-modified *O*-carboxymethyl chitosan (*O*-CM-chitosan), the formation of the self-aggregated nanoparticles is due to the hydrophobic interactions of cholesterol moieties in aqueous media, and the negatively charged carboxymethyl groups also play an important role in the morphology and stability of nanoparticles. The critical assembly concentration of *O*-CM-chitosan conjugates decreases from 0.03 to 0.006 mg/mL when the DS of cholesterol moiety increases from 6.9% to 12.5%. This is because the increase of hydrophobicity makes *O*-CM-chitosan molecules easier to aggregate in water [210]. DS also influences the interaction between *O*-CM-chitosan self-assembly nanoparticles and bovine serum albumin (BSA). The higher-order structure of BSA changes on interaction with *O*-CM-chitosan self-assembly nanoparticles and its stability against a denaturant such as urea remarkably improves [211]. The hydrophobic anticancer drug, paclitaxel (PTX), can spontaneously transfer from the aqueous medium into the hydrophobic cores of *O*-CM-chitosan (with DS

6.9%) self-assembled nanoparticles due to the driving force of hydrophobic interaction. These nanovesicles can be used to modify the biodistribution of PTX *in vivo*, which is advantageous for enhancing the therapeutic index and reducing the toxicity of PTX [212].

Yao and coworkers [213] prepared the pH-sensitive chitosan/ovalbumin nanogels through self-assembly; in the system chitosan chains are supposed to be partly trapped in the nanogel core upon heating because of the electrostatic attraction between chitosan and ovalbumin, and the rest of the chitosan chains form the shell of the nanogels. The nanogels do not change the size distribution after long-time storage and do not dissociate in the pH range of 2–10.5. The dispersibility, size, and hydrophobicity/hydrophilicity of the nanogel are pH dependent. The nanogels are good candidates for cosmetic and pharmaceutical applications. They can absorb positively charged drugs at alkaline pH through electrostatic attractions and release them at acidic pH, where nanogels also carry positive charges. The nanogels can absorb molecules with low polarity at acidic pH, where the core of the nanogels is relatively hydrophobic, and release them at neutral pH, where the nanogels are more hydrophilic.

4.5.2 Self-Assembly Multilayer

The electrostatic layer-by-layer (LBL) self-assembly is based on the attraction between positively and negatively charged molecules, which seem to be a good choice as a driving force for the multilayer's buildup [214]. Compared with the classic chemical immobilization method, the LBL technique has the least demand for chemical bonds. The multilayers built by the LBL method afford a more stable coating than those prepared by physical adsorption because of the electrostatic attractions between layer and layer and between layer and substrate. One important feature of this method is the adsorption at every step of the polyanion/polycation assembly, which results in recharging of the outermost layer during the film fabrication process. The overcompensating adsorption, more than equal charge, allows for charge reversal on the surface. It has two important consequences: first, repulsion of equally charged molecules and thus self-regulation of the adsorption and restriction to a single layer, and second, the ability of an oppositely charged molecule to be adsorbed in a second step on top of the first one [214]. The LBL self-assembly of polyanions and chitosan into multilayered coatings is a versatile, inexpensive yet efficient technique to "build" a biologically active surface. Electrostatic LBL assembly can be used to prepare the nanoscale bioactive coating on chitosan-based biomaterials [215]. Chitosan LBL self-assembly multilayer films open many new opportunities for us to achieve the ideal model surface whose properties are controllable [216]. The polyelectrolyte multilayer (PEM) deposition has also become a well-established methodology for clinical applications that require biomaterials with finely engineered surfaces, such as implant materials, stents, prostheses, and artificial organs. In these systems, the PEM mediates the cellular responses upon the device implantation, controls processes such as inflammation and tissue regeneration, and modulates the adhesion, migration, and proliferation of cells. The chemical composition, surface topography, and rheological characteristics of PEMs control their functions and their interactions in the biological milieu.

4.5.2.1 Chitosan/Protein Self-Assembly

As is known to all, collagen fibrillogenesis *in vivo* is a complex process that includes intracellular and extracellular compartments. Collagen molecules undergo fibril assembly in the extracellular zone and the assembly process is regulated by fibroblasts, which also determines the proper architecture and components of the matrices. Collagen molecules self-assembly *in vitro* is strongly affected by the microenvironment in which the cells are cultured. When the collagen solution and chitosan solution are mixed, and the temperature of the mixture is raised to 37°C, the collagen self-assembly fibers are formed. And the average diameter of chitosan/collagen assembly fibers is larger than that for collagen alone. The electrostatic forces between chitosan and collagen molecules play important roles in fibril self-assembly [217].

Collagen/sulfated chitosan self-assembly multilayers are prepared on the surface of Ti. The electrostatic attraction between NH_3^+ groups of collagen and SO_3^- groups of sulfated chitosan is the main driving force leading to LBL assembly. The coated surface topography changes from rough to mirror-like smoothness. The collagen/sulfated chitosan multilayers show excellent anticoagulation properties *in vitro*. As for the structure of the multilayers, every two layers partly overlap each other; even if the outermost layer is sulfated chitosan, some groups of collagen will still be exposed. It is expected that the collagen component of the multilayer will promote endothelial cell adhesion and growth on the surface [218].

Chitosan/gelatin PEM self-assembly films can be formed via the electrostatic interaction. Due to the difference in chemical nature and M_W between chitosan and gelatin molecules, PEM films express different surface topographic structures. The size and conformation of chitosan molecules cannot change significantly during the drying process, which is because chitosan molecules are rigid and possess high intrinsic stiffness due to abundant intramolecular hydrogen bonds [219]. Moreover, gelatin molecules are flexible and their molecular conformation tends to change remarkably. Therefore, the surface with chitosan as the outmost coating layer shows no characteristic morphology and structure, in sharp contrast to the tree-like structure for the surface with gelatin as the outermost coating layer. The same outermost layer has similar surface morphology and structure irrespective of the deposition cycle. Gelatin as the terminating layer in polyelectrolyte multilayer films is biocompatible and nontoxic for surface engineering [220].

Chitosan is uniquely positioned to emerge as an important platform for biofunctionalized fiber assemblies because this aminopolysaccharide can form fibers and can participate in simple protein assembly mechanisms. Shi et al. [221] have reported that the histidine-tagged proteins can assemble on the chitosan fiber via nickel-mediated (*cf.* Figure 4.19). Nickel-mediated protein G binding to chitosan enables the subsequent assembly of antibodies to the fibers and the assembly behaviors could be controlled.

4.5.2.2 Chitosan/Polysaccharide Self-Assembly

The LBL approach can be used to prepare thin PEM films according to a predesigned architecture with a precise thickness control. When the surface charges of PEM and bioactive substances, for example, peptide, are opposite, PEM could act as "sponge" to load the bioactive substance into the films. The chitosan/polysaccharide PEM can be used as the drug delivery carrier, biosensor, and scaffold for tissue engineering.

4.5.2.2.1 Chitosan/Hyaluronic Acid PEM

The chitosan/HA multilayer films can be used in the surface modification of cardiovascular devices, intraocular implants, tissue engineering scaffolds, and drug delivery systems. Chitosan/HA multilayer film is formed on the positively charged substrate surface through

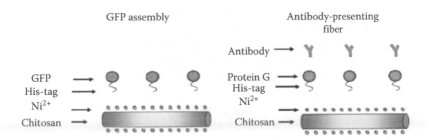

FIGURE 4.19
Assembly process of histidine-tagged protein on chitosan fibers. (From Shi, X. W. et al. 2008. *Biomacromolecules* 9: 1417–1423.)

aminolysis using low-M_W polyethyleneimine. The M_W of chitosan is an important factor in building the PEM films. The film buildup process is more rapid for low-M_W chitosan, because the high-M_W chitosans are difficult to distinguish within experimental errors even if the increase is slightly steeper for the low-M_W chitosan [222]. In addition, the M_W of chitosan has only a marginal effect on the stability of the films [223].

The chitosan/HA multilayer films exhibited a more homogeneous feature and a nicer miscibility at nanometer scale and had a lower roughness than pure chitosan films [224]. The surface morphologies of HA- and chitosan-terminated films may therefore show some fine structural differences. Deposition of the second layer of HA and chitosan already results in the surface being densely covered with larger spheres. And islands grow in size and lose their spherical shape as the multilayer buildup is continued to five bilayers. The film thickness in the exponential growth phase depends on the M_W of the nondiffusing species HA and the diffusing species chitosan; the higher the M_W of the polysaccharides, the thicker the multilayer for a given number of deposited bilayers [225]. The contact angle of chitosan/HA PEMs coated on the NiTi metal surface decreases with increasing the layer number. The contact angle reaches about 30° upon deposition of seven single layers and remains constant upon further polyelectrolyte layer deposition [226]. It is found that at least four bilayers are necessary to mask the substrate with respect to the properties of the multilayer water interface [227].

One can modulate the viscoelasticity and hydrophilicity of chitosan/HA multilayers via the construction of ternary films consisting of chitosan/HA and phosphorylcholine-modified chitosan/HA (PC-CS/HA) bilayers or varying the degree of PC grafting onto chitosan. PC-CS/HA PEMs are rougher and thicker than chitosan/HA films. In addition, the incorporation of PC can modify the pK_a of the chitosan, thus the coatings become more stable in neutral and basic media. The high water content of HA/PC-CS films reflects the known ability of the phosphorylcholine group to undergo hydrogen bond interactions with water molecules [228].

Chitosan/HA PEMs are rapidly degraded by both lysozyme and R-amylase. The cross-linking chitosan/HA PEMs, which are prepared through immersion of the chitosan/HA PEMs in an EDC-NHS solution, are much more resistant to all enzymatic degradation due to the existence of amide and ester bonds [229].

Tabrizian and coworkers [230] demonstrated the possibility of self-assembling paclitaxel-loaded PEMs using a hyaluronan ester prodrug of PTX by combining the prodrug approach and the LBL technique. One could easily envisage, with this strategy, designing PEMs with multiple drugs and/or with complex release behaviors based on appropriate chemical design of the prodrugs. It is Lu and Hu [231] loaded positively charged myoglobin (Mb) in the interior of PEM films of chitosan/HA. The electrostatic interaction may be the main driving force for Mb to be loaded into multilayer films. However, other interactions, such as the hydrophobic force and hydrogen bonding, cannot be ruled out completely.

The chitosan/HA-cross-linked multilayer coating exhibits nonadherence to NIH-3T3 fibroblasts, but this nonadherence is not due to the cytotoxic effect. These chitosan/HA PEM surfaces appear to be promising as a potential new noninteractive coating for invasive medical devices (e.g., catheters) and are also useful for the culture of naturally nonadherent cells (e.g., chondrocytes) [232]. Osteoblast adhesion onto the Ti surface, which is modified using chitosan/HA PEMs, is inhibited due to the presence of the HA chains. However, the immobilization of RGD (Arg-Gly-Asp) on the surface of such functionalized substrates tries to counteract this adverse effect. The immobilized RGD has a profound beneficial influence on osteoblast adhesion and proliferation, and retains high antibacterial efficacy [233]. The chitosan/HA PEM can also be constructed on damaged and healthy aortic porcine arteries using a perfusion chamber matching closely the conditions achievable *in vivo*. Strong adhesion of the coating onto the artery is ensured by depositing the first chitosan layer, a polycation exhibiting excellent bioadhesive properties toward negatively charged surfaces such as those presented by damaged arteries. The multilayer has an effective protective effect against platelet adhesion onto damaged arteries. Moreover, this effect can be improved when the l-arginine are introduced into multilayers [234].

4.5.2.2.2 Chitosan–Alginate PEM

Both chitosan and alginate are weak polyelectrolytes, and thus their charge density can be easily tuned by pH. The chitosan–alginate assembly systems are commonly developed as a complex planar membrane and microcapsule (*cf.* Figure 4.20) [235,236]. Their multilayer films are formed by the LBL method. There are small globules on the surface of chitosan–alginate PEM. In addition, with increasing the assembly pH, the size of the globules becomes larger and larger. Different assembly pH values induce a change of the conformation of the chitosan molecules. When the assembly pH of alginate is 3, the assembled structure is relatively homogeneous, which means that the alginate molecules are adsorbed homogeneously on the surface. At higher assembly pH values, chitosan develops a loopier and globular conformation, weakens the electrostatic repelling, and induces the aggregation of chitosan molecules. Thus, chitosan assembly with alginate molecules produces a more globular complex (*cf.* Figure 4.20).

The multilayer films can load antibody with pI 6.0–6.5 on the active site of the negatively charged multilayer film surface. Its loading capacity decreases with increasing assembly pH of alginate [235]. Shen and coworkers [237] employed mercaptoacetic acid (MAA) to form a self-assembled monolayer (SAM) on the gold electrode surface of the quartz–crystal microbalance (QCM), which resulted in a negatively charged surface through the formulation of the MAA-SAM layer. The HSA antibodies were coupled to alginate via activation with EDC-NHS, which prepared the negatively charged alginate-HSA antibodies. The immobilization of the antibodies on QCM is achieved with a positively charged chitosan layer used as the double-sided linker to attach the negatively charged alginate-HSA antibodies to the negatively charged MAA–SAM layer (*cf.* Figure 4.21). The aforementioned immobilization methodology was applied as a piezoelectric immunosensor for detecting HSA in human serum.

Chitosan–alginate assembly nanotubes are prepared by the LBL assembly technique by depositing chitosan and alginate onto the inner pores of a polycarbonate template alternately [238]. Their nanotubes form after the removal of the template. The thickness of the

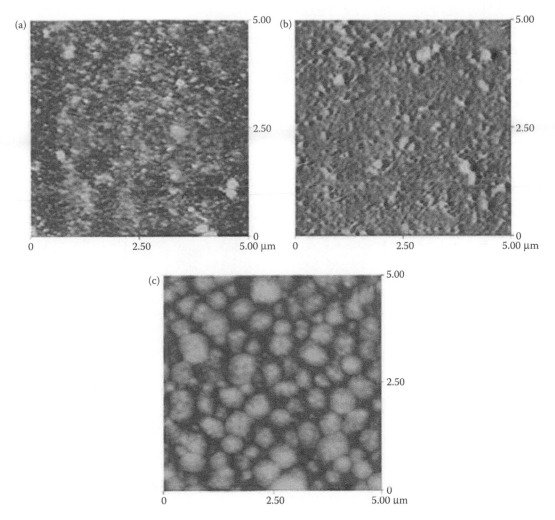

FIGURE 4.20
AFM images acquired in the phosphate–citrate buffer (pH 5.0). The number of layers of all these chitosan–alginate multilayer films is six. The assembly pH of chitosan of all these multilayer films is 3.0. The assembly pH of alginate is (a) 3.0, (b) 4.0, and (c) 5.0. The Z range (maximum height) is (a) 30 nm, (b) 100 nm, and (c) 400 nm. (From Yuan, W. Y. et al. 2007. *Langmuir* 23: 13046–13052. With permission.)

nanotube wall can be controlled by changing the assembled layers. The nanotubes are internalized into the HeLa cells and localized in the cell cytoplasm.

Core-shell chitosan–alginate nanoparticles can be formed on liposomes via LBL assembly. Low-M_W chitosan favors the creation of smaller chitosan–alginate nanoparticles, as compared to high-M_W chitosan [239]. The mean particle size decreases when chitosan was absorbed on a previously adsorbed alginate layer. This behavior might be explained by the ability of the shorter polymer chains of alginate to easily diffuse between the longer polymer chains of chitosan due to the strong ionic electrostatic interactions and complexation of the polymers forming a denser network. These core-shell assembly nanoparticles not only possess a high loading capacity that can be altered by the number of polyelectrolyte layers, but also provide sustained release of the entrapped protein for extended periods of

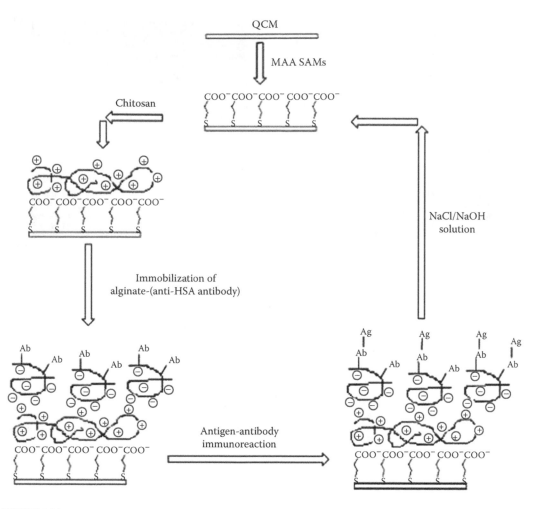

FIGURE 4.21
Schematic diagram of the immunoassay procedures. (From Deng, T. et al. 2005. *Anal Chim Acta* 532: 137–144. With permission.)

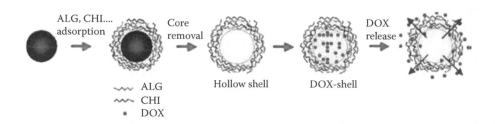

FIGURE 4.22
Schematic illustration of the procedure for the loading and release of doxorubicin (DOX) in the LBL self-assembled chitosan–alginate shells. (From Tao, X. et al. 2007. *Int J Pharm* 336: 376–381. With permission.)

time [240]. LBL assembly chitosan–alginate microshells are also effective drug release carriers. The forming process of the microshell that uses the melamine formaldehyde as the core and the loading-releasing behaviors for anticancer drugs are illustrated in Figure 4.22 [241]. The constructed microshells display an intact spherical shape with an inner hollow and shells [242]. The microshells are stable and can retain spherical shape structure intact for a period of at least 1 month due to the interaction between the $-NH_2$ groups of chitosan and $-COOH$ groups of alginate. The release rate of encapsulated drug from chitosan–alginate microshells decreases with increasing the number of assembly layers. Increasing the deposition temperature can increase the thickness and perfection of the chitosan–alginate multilayer assembly film and provide an efficient method for controlling the release rate [243]. Cross-linking neighboring layers will be an effective method for protecting the multilayer film made by LBL assembly from enzymatic erosion and for prolonging the release of the encapsulated drug [244]. The EDC cross-linking can improve the alginate–chitosan films' resistance to pepsin erosion more effectively than GA cross-linking. The reason is that the EDC joins chitosan and alginate macromolecules together over the multilayer film, thus producing a more compact alginate–chitosan multilayer film with lower mobility. When chitosan is partially degraded, the chitosan residues are still linked to the alginate chains, which will enhance the film stability. GA cross-linking only occurs among chitosan macromolecules, which contributes little towards the film stability [245].

References

1. Zhang, X., Reagan, M. R., and Kaplan, D. L. 2009. Electrospun silk biomaterial scaffolds for regenerative medicine. *Adv Drug Deliv Rev* 61: 988–1006.
2. Geckil, H., Xu, F., Zhang, X., Moon, S. J., and Demirci, U. 2010. Engineering hydrogels as extracellular matrix mimics. *Nanomedicine* 5: 469–484.
3. Shekaran, A. and Garcia, A. J. 2011. Nanoscale engineering of extracellular matrix-mimetic bioadhesive surfaces and implants for tissue engineering. *Biochim Biophys Acta* 1810: 350–360.
4. Zhu, J. 2010. Bioactive modification of poly(ethylene glycol) hydrogels for tissue engineering. *Biomaterials* 31: 4639–4656.
5. Raman, R., Sasisekharan, V., and Salisekharan, R. 2005. Structural insights into biological roles of protein–glycosaminoglycan interactions. *Chem Biol* 12: 267–277.
6. Bhattarai, N., Gunn, J., and Zhang, M. 2010. Chitosan-based hydrogels for controlled, localized drug delivery. *Adv Drug Deliv Rev* 62: 83–99.
7. Malafaya, P. B., Silva, G. A., and Reis, R. L. 2007. Natural–origin polymers as carriers and scaffolds for biomolecules and cell delivery in tissue engineering applications. *Adv Drug Deliv Rev* 59: 207–233.
8. Wang, C., Varshney, R. R., and Wang, D. 2010. Therapeutic cell delivery and fate control in hydrogels and hydrogel hybrids. *Adv Drug Deliv Rev* 62: 699–710.
9. Prashanth, K. V. H. and Tharanathan, R. N. 2006. Cross-linked chitosan—preparation and characterization. *Carbohydr Res* 341: 169–173.
10. Tsai, H. S. and Wang, Y. 2008. Properties of hydrophilic chitosan network membranes by introducing binary cross-link agents. *Polym Bull* 60: 103–113.
11. Bergera, J., Reista, M., Mayera, J. M., Feltb, O., Peppasc, N. A., and Gurny, R. 2004. Structure and interactions in covalently and ionically cross linked chitosan hydrogels for biomedical applications. *Eur J Pharm Biopharm* 57: 19–34.
12. Yao, K. D., Tu, H. L., Chang, F., Zhang, J. W., and Liu, J. 1997. pH sensitivity of the swelling of a chitosan–pectin polyelectrolyte complex. *Angew Makromol Chem* 245: 63–72.

13. Dumitriu, S. and Chornet, E. 1998. Inclusion and release of proteins from polysaccharide-based polyion complexes. *Adv Drug Deliv Rev* 31: 223–246.
14. Harnano, T., Chiba, D., Nakatsuka, K., Nagahata, M., Teramoto, A., Kondo, Y., Hachimori, A., and Abe, K. 2002. Evaluation of a polyelectrolyte complex (PEC) composed of chitin derivatives and chitosan, which promotes the rat calvarial osteoblast differentiation. *Polym Adv Technol* 13: 46–53.
15. Hamano, T., Teramoto, A., Iizuka, E., and Abe, K. 1998. Effects of polyelectrolyte complex (PEC) on human pedodontal ligament fibroblast (HPLF) function. I. Three-dimensional structure of HPLF cultured on PEC. *J Biomed Mater Res* 41: 257–269.
16. Denuziere, A., Ferrier, D., Damour, O., and Domard, A. 1998. Chitosan–chondroitin sulfate and chitosan-hyaluronate polyelectrolyte complexes: Biological properties. *Biomaterials* 19: 1275–1285.
17. Peniche, C., Fernadez, M., Rodriguez, G., Parra, J., Jimenez, J., Lopez, B. A., Gomez, D., and San, R. J. 2007. Cell supports of chitosan/hyaluronic acid and chondroitin sulphate systems. Morphology and biological behaviour. *J Mater Sci Mater Med* 18: 1719–1726.
18. Solchaga, L. A., Yoo, J. U., Lundberg, M., Dennis, J. E., Huibregtse, B. A., Goldberg, V. M., and Caplan, A. L. 2000. Hyaluronan-based polymers in the treatment of osteochondral defects. *J Orthop Res* 18: 773–780.
19. Yin, Y. J., Li, Z., Sun, Y., and Yao, K. 2005. A preliminary study on chitosan/gelatin polyelectrolyte complex formation. *J Mater Sci* 40: 4649–4652.
20. Cheng, M., Deng, J., Yang, F., Gong, Y., Zhao, N., and Zhang, X. 2003. Study on physical properties and nerve cell affinity of composite films from chitosan and gelatin solutions. *Biomaterials* 24: 2871–2880.
21. Yin, Y., Yao, K., Cheng, G., and Ma, J. 1999. Properties of polyelectrolyte complex films of chitosan and gelatin. *Polym Int* 48: 429–432.
22. Mao, J., Cui, Y., Wang, X., Sun, Y., Yin, Y., Zhao, H., and Yao, K. 2004. A preliminary study on chitosan and gelatin polyelectrolyte complex cytocompatibility by cell cycle and apoptosis analysis. *Biomaterials* 25: 3973–3981.
23. Xia, W., Liu, W., Cui, L., Liu, Y., Zhong W., Liu D., Wu, J., Chua, K., and Cao, Y. 2004. Tissue engineering of cartilage with the use of chitosan–gelatin complex scaffolds. *J Biomed Mater Res Part B: Appl Biomater* 71B: 373–380.
24. Guo, T., Zhao, J., Chang, J., Ding, Z., Hong, H., Chen, J., and Zhang, J. 2006. Porous chitosan–gelatin scaffold containing plasmid DNA encoding transforming growth factor-beta 1 for chondrocytes proliferation. *Biomaterials* 27: 1095–1103.
25. Lee, K. Y., Park, W. H., and Ha, W. S. 1997. Polyelectrolyte complexes of sodium alginate with chitosan or its derivatives for microcapsules. *J Appl Polym Sci* 63: 425–432.
26. Becheran, M. L., Peniche, C., and Arguelles-Monal, W. 2004. Study of the interpolyelectrolyte reaction between chitosan and alginate: Influence of alginate composition and chitosan molecular weight. *Int J Biol Macromol* 34: 127–133.
27. Abreu, F. O. M. S., Bianchini, C., Forte, M. M. C., and Kist, T. B. L. 2008. Influence of the composition and preparation method on the morphology and swelling behavior of alginate–chitosan hydrogels. *Carbohydr Polym* 74: 283–289.
28. Wang, L. H., Khor, E., and Lim, L. Y. 2001. Chitosan–alginate–CaCl$_2$ system for membrane coat application. *J Pharm Sci* 90: 1134–1142.
29. Wang, L. H., Khor, E., Wee, A., and Lim, L. Y. 2002. Chitosan–alginate PEC membrane as a wound dressing: Assessment of incisional wound healing. *J Biomed Mater Res* 63: 610–618.
30. Sankalia, M. G., Mashru, R. C., Sankalia, J. M., and Sutariya, V. B. 2007. Reversed chitosan–alginate polyelectrolyte complex for stability improvement of alpha-amylase: Optimization and physicochemical characterization. *Eur J Pharm Biopharm* 65: 215–232.
31. Iwasaki, N., Yamane, S. T., Majima, T., Kasahara, Y., Minami, A., and Harada, K. 2004. Feasibility of polysaccharide hybrid materials for scaffolds in cartilage tissue engineering: Evaluation of chondrocyte adhesion to polyion complex fibers prepared from alginate and chitosan. *Biomacromolecules* 5: 828–833.

32. Tamura, H., Tsuruta, Y., and Tokura, S. 2002. Preparation of chitosan-coated alginate filament. *Mater Sci Eng C* 20: 143–147.
33. Li, Z. S., Ramay, H. R., Hauch, K. D., Xiao, D. M., and Zhang, M. Q. 2005. Chitosan–alginate hybrid scaffolds for bone tissue engineering. *Biomaterials* 26: 3919–3928.
34. Yan, X. L., Khor, E., and Lim, L. Y. 2001. Chitosan–alginate films prepared with chitosan of different molecular weights. *J Biomed Mater Res* 58: 358–365.
35. Nettles, D. L., Elder, S. H., and Gilbert, J. A. 2002. Potential use of chitosan as a cell scaffold material for cartilage tissue engineering. *Tissue Eng* 8: 1009–1016.
36. de Haart, M., Marijnissen, W., van Osch, G., and Verhaar, J. A. N. 1999. Optimization of chondrocyte expansion in culture—Effect of TGF beta-2, bFGF and L-ascorbic acid on bovine articular chondrocytes. *Acta Orthop Scand* 70: 55–61.
37. Li, Z. S. and Zhang, M. Q. 2005. Chitosan–alginate as scaffolding material for cartilage tissue engineering. *J Biomed Mater Res* 75A: 485–493.
38. Li, S., Wang, X. T., Zhang, X. B., Yang, R. J., Zhang, H. Z., and Zhu, L. Z. 2002. Studies on alginate–chitosan microcapsules and renal arterial embolization in rabbits. *J Control Release* 84: 87–98.
39. Kim, S. J., Lee, K. J., and Kim, S. I. 2004. Swelling behavior of polyelectrolyte complex hydrogels composed of chitosan and hyaluronic acid. *J Appl Polym Sci* 93: 1097–1101.
40. Denuziere, A., Ferrier, D., and Domard, A. 1996. Chitosan–chondroitin sulfate and chitosan–hyaluronate polyelectrolyte complexes. *Physico-chemical aspects Carbohydr Polym* 29: 317–323.
41. Kim, S. J., Yoon, S. G., Lee, K. B., Park, Y. D., and Kim, S. I. 2003. Electrical sensitive behavior of a polyelectrolyte complex composed of chitosan/hyaluronic acid. *Solid State Ion* 164: 199–204.
42. Son, T. I., Park, S. H., Kang, H. S., Son, Y. S., Kim, C. H., and Jang, E. C. 2005. Preparation of human epidermal growth factor/low-molecular-weight chitosan conjugates and their effect on the proliferation of human dermal fibroblast *in vitro*. *J Ind Eng Chem* 11: 34–41.
43. Kim, S. J., Lee, K. J., and Kim, S. I. 2004. Swelling behavior of polyelectrolyte complex hydrogels composed of chitosan and hyaluronic acid. *J Appl Polym Sci* 93: 1097–1101.
44. Lee, S. J., Kim, S. S., and Lee, Y. M. 2000. Interpenetrating polymer network hydrogels based on poly(ethylene glycol) macromer and chitosan. *Carbohydr Polym* 41: 197–205.
45. Kim, S. J., Shin, S. R., Lee, K. B., Park, Y. D., and Kim, S. I. 2004. Synthesis and characteristics of polyelectrolyte complexes composed of chitosan and hyaluronic acid. *J Appl Polym Sci* 91: 2908–2913.
46. Lee, S. B., Lee, Y. M., Song, K. W., and Park, M. H. 2003. Preparation and properties of polyelectrolyte complex sponges composed of hyaluronic acid and chitosan and their biological behaviors. *J Appl Polym Sci* 90: 925–932.
47. Yamanea, S., Iwasaki, N., Majima, T., Funakoshi, T., Masuko, T., Haradac, K., Minami, A., Monde, K., and Nishimura, S. 2005. Feasibility of chitosan-based hyaluronic acid hybrid biomaterial for a novel scaffold in cartilage tissue engineering. *Biomaterials* 26: 611–619.
48. Wu, Y. Z., Hu, Y., Cai, J. Y., Ma, S. Y., and Wang, X. P. 2008. Coagulation property of hyaluronic acid–collagen/chitosan complex film. *J Mater Sci: Mater Med* 19: 3621–3629.
49. Lin, Y. H., Chang, C. H., Wu, Y. S., Hsu, Y. M., Chiou, S. F., and Chen, Y. J. 2009. Development of pH-responsive chitosan/heparin nanoparticles for stomach-specific anti-*Helicobacter pylori* therapy. *Biomaterials* 30: 3332–3342.
50. Liu, Z. H., Jiao, Y. P., Liu, F. N., and Zhang, Z. Y. 2007. Heparin/chitosan nanoparticle carriers prepared by polyelectrolyte complexation. *J Biomed Mater Res Part A* 83A: 806–812.
51. Boddohi, S., Moore, N., Johnson, P. A., and Kipper, M. J. 2009. Polysaccharide-based polyelectrolyte complex nanoparticles from chitosan, heparin, and hyaluronan, *Biomacromolecules* 10: 1402–1409.
52. He, Q., Ao, Q., Wang, A. J., Gong, Y. D., Zhao, N. M., and Zhang, X. F. 2007. *In vitro* cytotoxicity and protein drug release properties of chitosan/heparin microspheres. *Tsinghua Sci Technol* 12: 361–365.

53. Andersson, M. and Löfroth, J. E. 2003. Small particles of a heparin/chitosan complex prepared from a pharmaceutically acceptable microemulsion, Small particles of a heparin/chitosan complex prepared from a pharmaceutically acceptable microemulsion. *Int J Pharm* 257: 305–309.

54. Kratz, G., Arnander, C., Swedenborg, J., Back, M., Falk, C., Gouda, I., and Larm, O. 1997. Heparin–chitosan complexes stimulate wound healing in human skin. *Scand J Plast Reconstr Surg Hand Surg* 31: 119–123.

55. Wang, X. H., Yan, Y. N., Liu, F., Xiong, Z., Wu, R., Zhang, R. J., and Lu, Q. P. 2005. Preparation and characterization of a collagen/chitosan/heparin matrix for an implantable bioartificial liver. *J Biomater Sci Polymer Edn* 16: 1063–1080.

56. Seo, S. J., Choi, Y. J., Akaike, T., Higuchi, A., and Cho, C. S. 2006. Alginate–galactosylated chitosan–heparin scaffold as a new synthetic extracellular matrix for hepatocytes. *Tissue Eng* 12: 33–44.

57. Illum, L., Jabbal, G. I., Hinchcliffe, M., Fisher, A. N., and Davis, S. S. 2001. Chitosan as a novel nasal delivery system for vaccines. *Adv Drug Deliv Rev* 51: 81–96.

58. Guliyeva, U., Oner, F., Ozsoy, S., and Haziroglu, R. 2006. Chitosan microparticles containing plasmid DNA as potential oral gene delivery system. *Eur J Pharm Biopharm* 62: 17–25.

59. Zhu, D. W., Zhang, H. L., Bai, J. G., Liu, W. G., Leng, X. G., and Song, C. X. 2007. Enhancement of transfection efficiency for HeLa cells via incorporating arginine moiety into chitosan. *Chinese Sci Bull* 52: 3207–3215.

60. Gao, Y., Xu, Z. H., Chen, S. W., Gu, W. W., Chen, L. L., and Li, Y. P. 2008. Arginine-chitosan/DNA self-assemble nanoparticles for gene delivery: *In vitro* characteristics and transfection efficiency. *Int J Pharm* 359: 241–246.

61. Mansouri, S., Lavigne, P., Corsi, K., Benderdour, M., Beaumont, E., and Fernandes, J. C. 2004. Chitosan–DNA nanoparticles as non-viral vectors in gene therapy: Strategies to improve transfection efficacy. *Eur J Pharm Biopharm* 57: 1–8.

62. Prabaharan, M. and Mano, J. F. 2005. Chitosan-based particles as controlled drug delivery systems. *Drug Deliv* 12: 41–57.

63. Shu, X. Z. and Zhu, K. J. 2002. The influence of multivalent phosphate structure on the properties of ionically cross-linked chitosan films for controlled drug release. *Eur J Pharm Biopharm* 54: 235–243.

64. Aksungur, P., Sungur, A., Unal, S., Iskit, A. B., Squier, C. A., and Senel, S. 2004. Chitosan delivery systems for the treatment of oral mucositis: *In vitro* and *in vivo* studies. *J Control Release* 98: 269–279.

65. Aral, C. and Akbuga, J. 1998. Alternative approach to the preparation of chitosan beads. *Int J Pharm* 168: 9–15.

66. Gupta, K. C. and Jabrail, F. H. 2007. Controlled-release formulations for hydroxy urea and rifampicin using polyphosphate-anion-cross-linked chitosan microspheres. *J Appl Polym Sci* 104: 1942–1956.

67. Mi, F. L., Shyu, S. S., Wong, T. B., Jang, S. F., Lee, S. T., and Lu, K. T. 1999. Chitosan–polyelectrolyte complexation for the preparation of gel beads and controlled release of anticancer drug. II. Effect of pH-dependent ionic cross-linking or interpolymer complex using tripolyphosphate or polyphosphate as reagent. *J Appl Polym Sci* 74: 1093–1107.

68. Cho, M. H., Kim, K. S., Ahn, H. H., Kim, M. S., Kim, S. H., and Khang, G. 2008. Chitosan gel as an *in situ*-forming scaffold for rat bone marrow mesenchymal stem cells *in vivo*. *Tissue Eng Part A* 14: 1099–1108.

69. Rayment, P. and Butler, M. F. 2008. Investigation of ionically cross-linked chitosan and chitosan-bovine serum albumin beads for novel gastrointestinal functionality. *J Appl Polym Sci* 108: 2876–2885.

70. Gupta, K. C. and Jabrail, F. H. 2006. Preparation and characterization of sodium hexameta phosphate cross-linked chitosan microspheres for controlled and sustained delivery of centchroman. *Int J Biol Macromol* 38: 272–283.

71. Chenite, A., Chaput, C., Wang, D., Combes, C., Buschmann, M. D., and Hoemann, C. D. 2000. Novel injectable neutral solutions of chitosan form biodegradable gels *in situ*. *Biomaterials* 21: 2155–2161.

72. Richardson, S. M., Hughes, N., Hunt, J. A., Freemont, A. J., and Hoyland, J. A. 2008. Human mesenchymal stem cell differentiation to NP-like cells in chitosan–glycerophosphate hydrogels. *Biomaterials* 29: 85–93.

73. Cui, Z., Xiang, Y., Si, J. J., Yang, M., Zhang, Q., and Zhang, T. 2008. Ionic interactions between sulfuric acid and chitosan membranes. *Carbohydr Polym* 73: 111–116.

74. Karakecili, A. G., Satriano, C., Gumusdereliioglu, M., and Marletta, G. 2007. Surface characteristics of ionically cross-linked chitosan membranes. *J Appl Polym Sci* 106: 3884–3888.

75. Picart, C., Schneider, A., Etienne, O., Mutterer, J., Schaaf, P., and Egles, C. 2005. Controlled degradability of polysaccharide multilayer films *in vitro* and *in vivo*. *Adv Funct Mater* 15: 1771–1780.

76. Hofmann, T. 2001. In *Chemistry and Physiology of Selected Food Colorants*. Ames, J. M. and Hofmann, T., eds., pp. 135–151. Washington DC: American Chemical Society.

77. Tsai, H. S. and Wang, Y. Z. 2008. Properties of hydrophilic chitosan network membranes by introducing binary cross-link agents. *Polym Bull* 60: 103–113.

78. Cheng, G. X., Liu, J., Zhao, R. Z., Yao, K. D., Sun, P. C., and Men, A. J. 1998. Studies on dynamic behavior of water in cross-linked chitosan hydrogel. *J Appl Polym Sci* 67: 983–988.

79. Lee, S. H., Park, S. Y., and Choi, J. H. 2004. Fiber formation and physical properties of chitosan fiber cross-linked by epichlorohydrin in a wet spinning system: The effect of the concentration of the cross-linking agent epichlorohydrin. *J Appl Polym Sci* 92: 2054–2062.

80. Yao, K. D., Peng, T., Goosen, M. F. A., Min, J. M., and He, Y. Y. 1993. pH-sensitivity of hydrogels based on complex forming chitosan: Polyether interpenetrating polymer network. *J Appl Polym Sci* 48: 343–354.

81. Yao, K. D., Liu, J., Zhao, R. Z., Wang, W. H., and Wei, L. 1998. Dynamic water absorption characteristics of chitosan-based hydrogels—An investigation by positron annihilation lifetime spectroscopy. *Angew Makromol Chem* 255: 71–75.

82. Yao, K. D., Liu, J., Cheng, G. X., Zhao, R. Z., Wang, W. H., and Wei, L. 1998. The dynamic swelling behaviour of chitosan-based hydrogels. *Polym Int* 45: 191–194.

83. Cuan, Y. L., Shao, L., and Yao, K. D. 1996. A study on correlation between water state and swelling kinetics of chitosan-based hydrogels. *J Appl Polym Sci* 61: 2325–2335.

84. Goycoolea, F. M., Heras, A., Aranaz, I., Galed, G., Fernandez-Valle, M. E., and Arguelles Monal, W. 2003. Effect of chemical cross-linking on the swelling and shrinking properties of thermal and pH-responsive chitosan hydrogels. *Macromol Biosci* 3: 612–619.

85. Cao, W. L., Cheng, M. Y., Ao, Q., Gong, Y. D., Zhao, N. M., and Zhang, X. F. 2005. Physical, mechanical and degradation properties, and Schwann cell affinity of cross-linked chitosan films. *J Biomater Sci Polym Edn* 16: 791–807.

86. Yu, L. M. Y., Kazazian, K., and Shoichet, M. S. 2007. Peptide surface modification of methacrylamide chitosan for neural tissue engineering applications. *J Biomed Mater Res* 82A: 243–255.

87. Lu, G. Y., Kong, L. J., Sheng, B. Y., Wang, G., Gong, Y. D., and Zhang, X. F. 2007. Degradation of covalently cross-linked carboxymethyl chitosan and its potential application for peripheral nerve regeneration. *Eur Polym J* 43: 3807–3818.

88. Tang, R. P., Du, Y. M., and Fan, L. H. 2003. Dialdehyde starch-cross-linked chitosan films and their antimicrobial effects. *J Polym Sci B-Polym Phys* 41: 993–997.

89. Hsieh, C. Y., Tsai, S. P., Ho, M. H., Wang, D. M., Liu, C. E., and Hsieh, C. H. 2007. Analysis of freeze-gelation and cross-linking processes for preparing porous chitosan scaffolds. *Carbohydr Polym* 67: 124–132.

90. Subramanian, A. and Lin, H. Y. 2005. Cross-linked chitosan: Its physical properties and the effects of matrix stiffness on chondrocyte cell morphology and proliferation. *J Biomed Mater Res* 75A: 742–753.

91. Discher, D. E., Janmey, P., and Wang, Y. L. 2005. Tissue cells feel and respond to the stiffness of their substrate. *Science* 310: 1139–1143.

92. Georges, P. C. and Janmey, P. A. 2005. Cell type-specific response to growth on soft materials. *J Appl Physiol* 98: 1547–1553.
93. Webster, A., Halling, M. D., and Grant, D. M. 2007. Metal complexation of chitosan and its glutaraldehyde cross-linked derivative. *Carbohydr Res* 342: 1189–1201.
94. Agarwal, R. and Gupta, M. N. 1995. Evaluation of gluteraldehyde-modified chitosan as a matrix for hydrophobic interaction chromatography. *Anal Chim Acta* 313: 253–357.
95. Crescenzi, V., Francescangeli, A., Taglienti, A., Capitani, D., and Mannina, L. 2003. Synthesis and partial characterization of hydrogels obtained via glutaraldehyde cross-linking of acety-lated chitosan and of hyaluronan derivatives. *Biomacromolecules* 4: 1045–1054.
96. Gong, H. P., Zhong, Y. H., Li, J. C., Gong, Y. D., Zhao, N. M., and Zhang, X. F. 2000. Studies on nerve cell affinity of chitosan-derived materials. *J Biomed Mater Res* 52: 285–295.
97. Knaul, J. Z., Hudson, S. M., and Creber, K. A. M. 1999. Cross-linking of chitosan fibers with dialdehydes: Proposal of a new reaction mechanism. *J Polym Sci B-Polym Phys* 37: 1079–1094.
98. Gupta, K. C. and Kumar, M. N. V. R. 2000. Drug release behavior of beads and microgranules of chitosan. *Biomaterials* 21: 1115–1119.
99. Li, K. G., Qu, X. J., Wang, Y., Tang, Y. F., Qin, D. J., and Wang, Y. J. 2005. Improved performance of primary rat hepatocytes on blended natural polymers. *J Biomed Mater Res* 75A: 268–274.
100. Sung, H. W., Huang, R. N., Huang, L. L. H., and Tsai, C. C. 1999. *In vitro* evaluation of cytotoxic-ity of a naturally occurring cross-linking reagent for biological tissue fixation. *J Biomater Sci Polym Edn* 10: 63–78.
101. Mi, F. L., Tan, Y. C., Liang, H. F., and Sung, H. W. 2002. *In vivo* biocompatibility and degradabil-ity of a novel injectable-chitosan-based implant. *Biomaterials* 23: 181–191.
102. Mi, F. L., Sung, H. W., and Shyu, S. S. 2000. Synthesis and characterization of a novel chitosan-based network prepared using naturally occurring cross-linker. *J Polym Sci A-Polym Chem* 38: 2804–2814.
103. Butler, M. F., Ng, Y. F., and Pudney, P. D. A. 2003. Mechanism and kinetics of the cross-linking reaction between biopolymers containing primary amine groups and genipin. *J Polym Sci B-Polym Chem* 41: 3941–3953.
104. Mi, F. L., Shyu, S. S., and Peng, C. K. 2005. Characterization of ring-opening polymerization of genipin and pH-dependent cross-linking reactions between chitosan and genipin. *J Polym Sci B-Polym Chem* 43: 1985–2000.
105. Jin, J., Song, M., and Hourston, D. J. 2004. Novel chitosan-based films cross-linked by genipin with improved physical properties. *Biomacromolecules* 5: 162–168.
106. Butler, M. F., Clark, A. H., and Adams, S. 2006. Swelling and mechanical properties of biopoly-mer hydrogels containing chitosan and bovine serum albumin. *Biomacromolecules* 7: 2961–2970.
107. Welsh, E. R. and Price, R. R. 2003. Chitosan cross-linking with a water-soluble, blocked diiso-cyanate. 2. Solvates and hydrogels. *Biomacromolecules* 4: 1357–1361.
108. Lin-Gibson, S., Walls, H. J., Kennedy, S. B., and Welsh, E. R. 2003. Reaction kinetics and gel properties of blocked diisocyinate cross-linked chitosan hydrogels. *Carbohydr Polym* 54: 193–199.
109. Kiuchi, H., Kai, W. H., and Inoue, Y. 2008. Preparation and characterization of poly(ethylene glycol) cross-linked chitosan films. *J Appl Polym Sci* 107: 3823–3380.
110. Kulkarni, A. R., Hukkeri, V. I., Sung, H. W., and Liang, H. F. 2005. A novel method for the syn-thesis of the PEG-cross-linked chitosan with a pH-independent swelling behavior. *Macromol Biosci* 5: 925–928.
111. Benson, M. T. 2003. Density functional investigation of melamine-formaldehyde cross-linking agents. 1. Partially substituted melamine. *Ind Eng Chem Res* 42: 4147–4155.
112. Ma, J. B., Wang, H. J., He, B. L., and Chen, J. T. 2001. A preliminary *in vitro* study on the fabrica-tion and tissue engineering applications of a novel chitosan bilayer material as a scaffold of human neofetaf dermal fibroblasts. *Biomaterials* 22: 331–336.

113. Tan, W., Krishnaraj, R., and Desai, T. A. 2001. Evaluation of nanostructured composite collagen–chitosan matrices for tissue engineering. *Tissue Eng* 7: 203–210.
114. Ma, L., Gao, C. Y., Mao, Z. W., Zhou, J., Shen, J. C., and Hu, X. Q. 2003. Collagen/chitosan porous scaffolds with improved biostability for skin tissue engineering. *Biomaterials* 24: 4833–4841.
115. Wu, X. M., Black, L., Santacana-Laffitte, G., and Patrick, C. W. 2007. Preparation and assessment of glutaraldehyde-cross-linked collagen–chitosan hydrogels for adipose tissue engineering. *J Biomed Mater Res* 81A: 59–65.
116. Chen, J. P., Chang, G. Y., and Chen, J. K. 2008. Electrospun collagen/chitosan nanofibrous membrane as wound dressing. *Colloid Surf A* 313: 183–188.
117. Wang, W., Lin, S. Q., Xiao, Y. C., Huang, Y. D., Tan, Y., and Cai, L. 2008. Acceleration of diabetic wound healing with chitosan-cross-linked collagen sponge containing recombinant human acidic fibroblast growth factor in healing-impaired STZ diabetic rats. *Life Sci* 82: 190–204.
118. Tsai, S. P., Hsieh, C. Y., Hsieh, C. Y., Wang, D. M., Huang, L. L. H., and Lai. J. Y. 2007. Preparation and cell compatibility evaluation of chitosan/collagen composite scaffolds using amino acids as cross-linking bridges. *J Appl Polym Sci* 105: 1774–1785.
119. Chen, R. N., Wang, G. M., Chen, C. H., Ho, H. O., and Sheu, M. T. 2006. Development of N,O-(carboxymethyl)chitosan/collagen matrixes as a wound dressing. *Biomacromolecules* 7: 1058–1064.
120. Ding, C. M., Zhou, Y., He, Y. N., and Tan, W. S. 2008. Perfusion seeding of collagen-chitosan sponges for dermal tissue engineering. *Process Biochem* 43: 287–296.
121. Lee, S. B., Kim, Y. H., Chong, M. S., and Lee, Y. M. 2004. Preparation and characteristics of hybrid scaffolds composed of beta-chitin and collagen. *Biomaterials* 25: 2309–2317.
122. Taravel, M. N. and Domard, A. 1993. Relation between the physicochemical characteristics of collagen and its interactions with chitosan: I. *Biomaterials* 14: 930–938.
123. Arpornmaeklong, P., Suwatwirote, N., Pripatnanot, P., and Oungbho, K. 2007. Growth and differentiation of mouse osteoblasts on chitosan-collagen sponges. *International J Oral Maxillofac Surg* 36: 328–337.
124. Mao, J. S., Kondu, S., Ji, H. F., and McShane, M. J. 2006. Study of the near-neutral pH-sensitivity of chitosan/gelatin hydrogels by turbidimetry and microcantilever deflection. *Biotechnol Bioeng* 95: 333–341.
125. Huang, Y., Onyeri, S., Siewe, M., Moshfeghian, A., and Madihally, S. V. 2005. *In vitro* characterization of chitosan–gelatin scaffolds for tissue engineering. *Biomaterials* 26: 7616–7627.
126. Kim, S., Nimni, M. E., Yang, Z., and Han, B. 2005. Chitosan/gelatin-based films cross-linked by proanthocyanidin. *J Biomed Mater Res Part B: Appl Biomater* 75B: 442–450.
127. Chiono, V., Pulieri, E., Vozzi, G., Ciardelli, G., Ahluwalia, A., and Giusti, P. 2008. Genipin-cross-linked chitosan/gelatin blends for biomedical applications. *J Mater Sci Mater Med* 19: 889–898.
128. Wang, X. H., Yu, X., Yan, Y. N., and Zhang, R. J. 2008. Liver tissue responses to gelatin and gelatin/chitosan gels. *J Biomed Mater Res* 87A: 62–68.
129. He, J. K., Li, D. C., Liu, Y. X., Yao, B., Lu, B. H., and Lian, Q. 2007. Fabrication and characterization of chitosan/gelatin porous scaffolds with predefined internal microstructures. *Polymer* 48: 4578–4588.
130. Jameela, S. R., Lakshmi, S., James, N. R., and Jayakrishnan, A. 2002. Preparation and evaluation of photocross-linkable chitosan as a drug delivery matrix. *J Appl Polym Sci* 86: 1873–1877.
131. Shen, F., Cui, Y. L., Yang, L. F., Yao, K. D., Dong, X. H., and Jia, W. Y. 2000. A study on the fabrication of porous chitosan/gelatin network scaffold for tissue engineering. *Polym Int* 49: 1596–1599.
132. Mao, J. S., Zhao, L. G., Yin, Y. J., and Yao, K. D. 2003. Structure and properties of bilayer chitosan–gelatin scaffolds. *Biomaterials* 24: 1067–1074.
133. Mao, J. S., Zhao, L. G., Yao, K. D., Shang, Q. X., Yang, G. H., and Cao, Y. L. 2003. Study of novel chitosan–gelatin artificial skin *in vitro*. *J Biomed Mater Res* 64A: 301–308.

134. Liu, H. F., Fan, H. B., Cui, Y. L., Chen, Y. P., Yao, K. D., and Goh, J. C. H. 2007. Effects of the controlled-released basic fibroblast growth factor from chitosan–gelatin microspheres on human fibroblasts cultured on a chitosan–gelatin scaffold. *Biomacromolecules* 8: 1446–1455.

135. Chen, Y. L., Lee, H. P., Chan, H. Y., Sung, L. Y., Chen, H. C., and Hu, Y. C. 2007. Composite chondroitin-6-sulfate/dermatan sulfate/chitosan scaffolds for cartilage tissue engineering. *Biomaterials* 28: 2294–2305.

136. Jou, C. H., Chen, W. C., Yang, M. C., Hwang, M. C., Chou, W. L., and Lin, S. M. 2008. *In vitro* biocompatibility of three-dimensional chitosan scaffolds immobilized with chondroitin-6-sulfate. *Polym Adv Technol* 19: 377–384.

137. Chen, Y. L., Chen, H. C., Lee, H. P., Chan, H. Y., and Hu, Y. C. 2006. Rational development of GAG-augmented chitosan membranes by fractional factorial design methodology. *Biomaterials* 27: 2222–2232.

138. Griffon, D. J., Sedighi, M. R., Schaeffer, D. V., Eurell, J. A., and Johnson, A. L. 2006. Chitosan scaffolds: Interconnective pore size and cartilage engineering. *Acta Biomater* 2: 313–320.

139. Peng, C. K., Yu, S. H., Mi, F. L., and Shyu, S. S. 2006. Polysaccharide-based artificial extracellular matrix: Preparation and characterization of three-dimensional, macroporous chitosan and chondroitin sulfate composite scaffolds. *J Appl Polym Sci* 99: 2091–2100.

140. Mi, F. L., Shyu, S. S., Peng, C. K., Wu, Y. B., Sung, H. W., and Wang, P. S. 2006. Fabrication of chondroitin sulfate–chitosan composite artificial extracellular matrix for stabilization of fibroblast growth factor. *J Biomed Mater Res* 76A: 1–15.

141. Park, Y. J., Lee, Y. M., Lee, J. Y., Seol, Y. J., Chung, C. P., and Lee, S. J. 2000. Controlled release of platelet-derived growth factor-BB from chondroitin sulfate–chitosan sponge for guided bone regeneration. *J Control Release* 67: 385–394.

142. Fakhry, A., Schneider, G. B., Zaharias, R., and Senel, S. 2004. Chitosan supports the initial attachment and spreading of osteoblasts preferentially over fibroblasts. *Biomaterials* 25: 2075–2079.

143. Yang, X. B. B., Bhatnagar, R. S., Li, S., and Oreffo, R. O. C. 2004. Biomimetic collagen scaffolds for human bone cell growth and differentiation. *Tissue Eng* 10: 1148–1159.

144. Bouvier, M., Couble, M. L., Hartmann, D. J., Gauthier, J. P., and Magloire, H. 1990. Ultrastructural and immunocytochemical study of bone-derived cells cultured in three-dimensional matrices: influence of chondroitin-4 sulfate on mineralization. *Differentiation; Res biological diversity* 45: 128–137.

145. Machado, C. B., Ventura, J. M. G., Lemos, A. F., Ferreira, J. M. F., Leite, M. F., and Goes, A. M. 2007. 3D chitosan–gelatin–chondroitin porous scaffold improves osteogenic differentiation of mesenchymal stem cells. *Biomed Mater* 2: 124–131.

146. Mao, J. S., Wang, X. H., Cui, Y. L., and Yao, K. D. 2003. Effects of hyaluronic acid–chitosan–gelatin complex on the apoptosis and cell cycle of L929 cells. *Chinese Sci Bull* 48: 1807–1810.

147. Liu, H. F., Yin, Y. J., Yao, K. D., Ma, D. R., Cui, L., and Cao, Y. L. 2004. Influence of the concentrations of hyaluronic acid on the properties and biocompatibility of Cs-Gel-HA membranes. *Biomaterials* 25: 3523–3530.

148. Liu, H. F., Yin, Y. J., and Yao, K. D. 2007. Construction of chitosan–gelatin-hyaluronic acid artificial skin *in vitro*. *J Biomater Appl* 21: 413–430.

149. Yu, S. H., Wu, Y. B., Mi, F. L., and Shyu, S. S. 2008. Polysaccharide-based artificial extracellular matrix: Preparation and characterization of three-dimensional, macroporous chitosan, and heparin composite Scaffold. *J Appl Polym Sci* 109: 3639–3644.

150. Yu, X., Bichtelen, A., Wang, X. H., Yan, Y. N., Lin, F., Xiong, Z., Wu, R., Zhang, R. J., and Lu, Q. P. 2005. Collagen/chitosan/heparin complex with improved biocompatibility for hepatic tissue engineering. *J Bioact Compat Polym* 20: 15–28.

151. Ho, Y. C., Mi, F. L., Sung, H. W., and Kuo, P. L. 2009. Heparin-functionalized chitosan–alginate scaffolds for controlled release of growth factor. *Int J Pharm* 376: 69–75.

152. Tan, H. P., Gong, Y. H., Lao, L. H., Mao, Z. W., and Gao, C. Y. 2007. Gelatin/chitosan/hyaluronan ternary complex scaffold containing basic fibroblast growth factor for cartilage tissue engineering. *J Mater Sci Mater Med* 18: 1961–1968.

153. Yao, K. D., Liu, W. G., and Liu, J. 1999. The unique characteristics of water in chitosan–polyether semi-IPN hydrogel. *J Appl Polym Sci* 71: 449–453.
154. Yao, K. D., Liu, J., Cheng, G. X., Zhao, R. Z., Wang, W. H., and Wei, L. 1998. The dynamic swelling behaviour of chitosan-based hydrogels. *Polym. Int.* 45, 191–194.
155. Khalid, M. N., Agnely, F., Yagoubi, N., Grossiord, J. L., and Couarraze, G. 2002. Water state characterization, swelling behavior, thermal and mechanical properties of chitosan based networks. *Eur J Pharm Sci* 15: 425–432.
156. Yu, S. H., Mi, F. L., Shyu, S. S., Tsai, C. H., Peng, C. K., and Lai, J. Y. 2006. Miscibility, mechanical characteristic and platelet adhesion of 6-*O*-carboxymethylchitosan/polyurethane semi-IPN membranes. *J Membrane Sci* 276: 68–80.
157. Cruz, D. M. G., Coutinho, D. F., Mano, J. F., Ribelles, J. L. G., and Sanchez, M. S. 2009. Physical interactions in macroporous scaffolds based on poly(3-caprolactone)/chitosan semi-interpenetrating polymer networks. *Polymer* 50: 2058–2064.
158. Chung, T. W., Lin, S. Y., Liu, D. Z., Tyan, Y. C., and Yang, J. S. 2009. Sustained release of 5-FU from Poloxamer gels interpenetrated by cross-linking chitosan network. *Int J Pharm* 382: 39–44.
159. Wu, W., Shen, J., Banerjee, P., and Zhou, S. 2010. Chitosan-based responsive hybrid nanogels for integration of optical pH-sensing, tumor cell imaging and controlled drug delivery. *Biomaterials* 31: 8371–8381.
160. Rutnakornpituk, M. and Ngamdee, P. 2006. Surface and mechanical properties of microporous membranes of poly(ethyleneglycol)-polydimethylsiloxane copolymer/chitosan. *Polymer* 47: 7909–7917.
161. Rutnakornpituk, M., Ngamdee, P., and Phinyocheep, P. 2005. Preparation and properties of polydimethylsiloxane-modified chitosan. *Carbohydr Polym* 63: 229–237.
162. Rodkate, N., Wichai, U., Boontha, B., and Rutnakornpituk, M. 2010. Semi-interpenetrating polymer network hydrogels between polydimethylsiloxane/polyethylene glycol and chitosan. *Carbohydr Polym* 81: 617–625.
163. Wang, M. Z., Fang, Y., and Hu, D. D. 2001. Preparation and properties of chitosan-poly(*N*-isopropylacrylamide) full-IPN hydrogels. *React. Funct. Polym.* 48: 215–221.
164. Kim, S. J., Park, S. J., and Kim, S. I. 2003. Swelling behavior of interpenetrating polymer network hydrogels composed of poly(vinyl alcohol) and chitosan. *React Funct Polym* 55: 53–59.
165. Yin, L., Fei, L., Cui, F., Tang, C., and Yin, C. 2007. Superporous hydrogels containing poly(acrylic acid-co-acrylamide)/O-carboxymethyl chitosan interpenetrating polymer networks. *Biomaterials* 28: 1258–1266.
166. Yin, L., Ding, J., Zhang, J., He, C., Tang, C., and Yin, C. 2010. Polymer integrity related absorption mechanism of superporous hydrogel containing interpenetrating polymer networks for oral delivery of insulin. *Biomaterials* 31: 3347–3356.
167. Klokkevold, P. R., Vandemark, L., Kenney, E. B., and Bernard, G. W. 1996. Osteogenesis enhanced by chitosan (poly-*N*-acetyl glucosaminoglycan) *in vitro*. *J Periodontol* 67: 1170–1175.
168. Mukherjee, D. P., Tunkle, A. S., Roberts, R. A., Clavenna, A., Rogers, S., and Smith, D. 2003. An animal evaluation of a paste of chitosan glutamate and hydroxyapatite as a synthetic bone graft material. *J Biomed Mater Res Part B: Appl Biomater* 67B: 603–609.
169. Ding, S. J. 2006. Preparation and properties of chitosan/calcium phosphate composites for bone repair. *Dent Mater J* 25: 706–712.
170. Yin, Y. J., Ye, F., Cui, J. F., Zhang, F. J., Li, X. L., and Yao, K. D. 2003. Preparation and characterization of macroporous chitosan-gelatin/β-tricalcium phosphate composite scaffolds for bone tissue engineering. *J Biomed Mater Res Part A* 67A: 844–855.
171. Zhang, Y. and Zhang, M. Q. 2001. Synthesis and characterization of macroporous chitosan/calcium phosphate composite scaffolds for tissue engineering. *J Biomed Mater Res* 55: 304–312.
172. Lee, Y. M., Park, Y. J., Lee, S. J., Ku, Y., Han, S. B., and Choi, S. M. 2000. Klokkevold PR. chung CP. Tissue engineered bone formation using chitosan.tricalciun phosphate sponges. *J Periodontal* 71: 410–417.

173. Kuo, S. M., Chang, S. J., Niu, G. C. C., Lan, C. W., Cheng, W. T., and Yang, C. Z. 2009. Guided tissue regeneration with use of β-TCP/chitosan composite membrane. *J Appl Polym Sci* 112: 3127–3134.

174. Zhang, Y. and Zhang, M. Q. 2002. Calcium phosphate/chitosan composite scaffolds for controlled *in vitro* antibiotic drug release. *J Biomed Mater Res* 62: 378–386.

175. Lee, J. Y., Seol, Y. J., Kim, K. H., Lee, Y. M., Park, Y. J., Rhyu, I. C., Chung, C. P., and Lee, S. J. 2004. Transforming growth factor (TGF)-β1 releasing tricalcium phosphate/chitosan microgranules as bone substitutes. *Pharm Res* 21: 1790–1796.

176. Lee, Y. M., Park, Y. J., Lee, S. J., Ku, Y., Han, S. S., Klokkevold, P. R., and Chung, C. P. 2000. The bone regenerative effect of platelet-derived growth factor-BB delivered with a chitosan/tricalcium phosphate sponge carrier. *J periodontal* 71: 418–424.

177. Kikuchi, M., Ikoma, T., Itoh, S., Matsumoto, H. N., Koyama, Y., and Takakuda, K. 2004. Biomimetic synthesis of bone-like nanocomposites using the self-organization mechanism of hydroxyapatite and collagen. *Composites Sci Technol* 64: 819–825.

178. Wilson, O. C. and Hull, J. R. 2008. Surface modification of nanophase hydroxyapatite with chitosan. *Mater Sci Eng C* 28: 434–437.

179. Ding, S. J. 2007. Biodegradation behavior of chitosan/calcium phosphate composites. *J Non-Cryst Soli* 353: 2367–2373.

180. Thein-Han, W. W. and Misra, R. D. K. 2009. Biomimetic chitosan-nanohydroxyapatite composite scaffolds for bone tissue engineering. *Acta Biomater* 5: 1182–1197.

181. Oliveira, J. M., Rodrigues, M. T., Silva, S. S., Malafaya, P. B., Gomes, M. E., and Viegas, C. A. 2006. Novel hydroxyapatite/chitosan bilayered scaffold for osteochondral tissue-engineering applications: Scaffold design and its performance when seeded with goat bone marrow stromal cells. *Biomaterials* 27: 6123–6137.

182. Yin, Y. J., Zhao, F., Song, X. F., Yao, K. D., Lu, W. W., and Leong, J. C. 2000. Preparation and characterization of hydroxyapatite/chitosan–gelatin network composite. *J Appl Polym Sci* 77: 2929–2938.

183. Zhao, F., Yin, Y. J., Lu, W. W., Leong, J. C., Zhang, W. J., and Zhang, J. Y. 2002. Preparation and histological evaluation of biomimetic three-dimensional hydroxyapatite/chitosan–gelatin network composite scaffolds. *Biomaterials* 23: 3227–3234.

184. Zhao, F., Grayson, W. L., Ma, T., Bunnell, B., and Lu, W. W. 2006. Effects of hydroxyapatite in 3-D chitosan–gelatin polymer network on human mesenchymal stem cell construct development. *Biomaterials* 27: 1859–1867.

185. Subburaman, K., Pernodet, N., Kwak, S. Y., DiMasi, E., Ge, S., and Zaitsev, V. 2006. Templated biomineralization on self-assembled protein fibers. *Proc Nat ACAD Sci USA* 103: 14672–14677.

186. Rusu, V. M., Ng, C. H., Wilke, M., Tiersch, B., Fratzl, P., and Peter, M. G. 2005. Size-controlled hydroxyapatite nanoparticles as self-organized organic–inorganic composite materials. *Biomaterials* 26: 5414–5426.

187. Yamaguchi, I., Tokuchi, K., Fukuzaki, H., Koyama, Y., Takakuda, K., and Monma, H. 2001. Preparation and microstructure analysis of chitosan/hydroxyapatite nanocomposites. *J Biomed Mater Res* 55: 20–27.

188. Jin, H. H., Lee, C. H., Lee, W. K., Lee, J. K., Park, H. C., and Yoon, S. Y. 2008. *In-situ* formation of the hydroxyapatite/chitosan–alginate composite scaffolds. *Mater Lett* 62: 1630–1693.

189. Zhang, L., Li, Y. B., Yang, A. P., Peng, X. L., Wang, X. J., and Zhang, X. 2005. Preparation and *in vitro* investigation of chitosan/nano-hydroxyapatite composite used as bone substitute materials. *J Mater Sci Mater Med* 16: 213–219.

190. Murugan, R. and Ramakrishna, S. 2004. Bioresorbable composite bone paste using polysaccharide based nano hydroxyapatite. *Biomaterials* 25: 3829–3835.

191. Green, D. W., Leveque, I., Walsh, D., Howard, D., Yang, X. B., and Partridge, K. 2005. Biomineralized polysaccharide capsules for encapsulation, organization, and delivery of human cell types and growth factors. *Adv Funct Mater* 5: 917–923.

192. Li, J. J., Chen, Y. P., Yin, Y. J., Yao, F. L., and Yao, K. D. 2007. Modulation of nano-hydroxyapatite size via formation on chitosan–gelatin network film *in situ*. *Biomaterials* 8: 781–790.

193. Suzuki, S., Grondahl, L., Leavesley, D., and Wentrup-Byrne, E. 2005. *In vitro* bioactivity of MOEP grafted ePTFE membranes for craniofacial applications. *Biomaterials* 26: 5303–5312.

194. Chesnutt, B. M., Yuan, Y., Brahmandam, N., Yang, Y., Ong, J. L., and Haggard, W. O. 2007. Characterization of biomimetic calcium phosphate on phosphorylated chitosan films. *J Biomed Mater Res* 82A: 343–353.

195. Kong, L. J., Gao, Y., Lu, G. Y., Gong, Y. D., Zhao, N. M., and Zhang, X. F. 2006. A study on the bioactivity of chitosan/nano-hydroxyapatite composite scaffolds for bone tissue engineering. *Eur Polym J* 42: 3171–3179.

196. Yin, Y. J., Luo, X. Y., Cui, J. F., Wang, C. Y., Guo, X. M., and Yao, K. D. 2004. A study on biomineralization behavior of N-methylene phosphochitosan scaffolds. *Macromol Biosci* 4: 971–977.

197. Li, J. J., Dou, Y., Yang, J., Yin, Y. J., Zhang, H., Yao, F. L., Wang, H. B., and Yao, K. D. 2009. Surface characterization and biocompatibility of micro- and nano-hydroxyapatite/chitosan–gelatin network films. *Mater Sci Eng C* 29: 1207–1215.

198. Manjubala, I., Scheler, S., Bossert, J., and Jandt, K. D. 2006. Mineralisation of chitosan scaffolds with nano-apatite formation by double diffusion technique. *Acta Biomater* 2: 75–84.

199. Manjubala, I., Ponomarev, I., Wilke, I., and Jandt, K. D. 2008. Growth of osteoblast-like cells on biomimetic apatite-coated chitosan scaffolds. *J Biomed Mater Res Part B: Appl Biomater* 84B: 7–16.

200. Li, J. J., Yin, Y. J., Yao, F. L., Zhang, L. L., and Yao, K. D. 2008. Effect of nano- and micro-hydroxyapatite/chitosan–gelatin network film on human gastric cancer cells. *Mater Lett* 62: 3220–3223.

201. Rodriguez-Hernandez, J., Checot, F., Gnanou, Y., and Lecommandoux, S. 2005. Toward "smart" nano-objects by self-assembly of block copolymers in solution. *Prog Polym Sci* 30: 691–724.

202. Kumar, G., Wang, Y. C., Co, C., and Ho, C. C. 2003. Spatially controlled cell engineering on biomaterials using polyelectrolytes. *Langmuir* 19: 10550–10556.

203. Wang, Y. S., Liu, L. R., Jiang, Q., and Zhang, Q. Q. 2007. Self-aggregated nanoparticles of cholesterol-modified chitosan conjugate as a novel carrier of epirubicin. *Eur Polym J* 43: 43–51.

204. Yoksan, R., Matsusaki, M., Akashi, M., and Chirachanchai, S. 2004. Controlled hydrophobic/hydrophilic chitosan: Colloidal phenomena and nanosphere formation. *Colloid Polym Sci* 282: 337–342.

205. Yoksan, R., Akashi, M., Hiwatari, K., and Chirachanchai, S. 2003. Controlled hydrophobic/hydrophilicity of chitosan for spheres without specific processing technique. *Biopolymers* 69: 386–390.

206. Opanasopit, P., Ngawhirunpat, T., Rojanarata, T., Choochottiros, C., and Chirachanchai, S. 2007. Camptothecin-incorporating N-phthaloylchitosan-g-mPEG self-assembly micellar system: Effect of degree of deacetylation. *Colloid Surf B* 60: 117–124.

207. Yoksan, R. and Chirachanchai, S. 2008. Amphiphilic chitosan nanosphere: Studies on formation, toxicity, and guest molecule incorporation. *Bioorg Med Chem* 16: 2687–2696.

208. Opanasopit, P., Ngawhirunpat, T., Chaidedgumjorn, A., Rojanarata, T., Apirakaramwong, A., and Phongying, S. 2006. Incorporation of camptothecin into N-phthaloyl chitosan-g-mPEG self-assembly micellar system. *Eur J Pharm Biopharm* 64: 269–276.

209. Peng, X. H. and Zhang, L. N. 2007. Formation and morphologies of novel self-assembled micelles from chitosan derivatives. *Langmuir* 23: 10493–10498.

210. Wang, Y. S., Liu, L. R., Weng, J., and Zhang, Q. Q. 2007. Preparation and characterization of self-aggregated nanoparticles of cholesterol-modified O-carboxymethyl chitosan conjugates. *Carbohydr Polym* 69: 597–606.

211. Wang, Y. S., Jiang, Q., Liu, L. R., and Zhang, Q. Q. 2007. The interaction between bovine serum albumin and the self-aggregated nanoparticles of cholesterol-modified O-carboxymethyl chitosan. *Polymer* 48: 4135–4142.

212. Wang, Y. S., Jiang, Q., Li, R. S., Liu, L. L., Zhang, Q. Q., and Wang, Y. M. 2008. Self-assembled nanoparticles of cholesterol-modified O-carboxymethyl chitosan as a novel carrier for paclitaxel. *Nanotechnology* 19: 145101.

213. Yu, S. Y., Hu, J. H., Pan, X. Y., Yao, P., and Jiang, M. 2006. Stable and pH-sensitive nanogels prepared by self-assembly of chitosan and ovalbumin. *Langmui* 22: 2754–2759.

214. Decher, G. 1997. Fuzzy nanoassemblies: Towards to layered polymeric multicomposites. *Science* 277: 1232–1237.
215. He, W. and Bellamkonda, R. V. 2005. Nanoscale neuro-integrative coatings for neural implants. *Biomaterials* 26: 2983–2990.
216. Esker, A. R., Mengel, C., and Wegner, G. 1998. Ultrathin films of a polyelectrolyte with layered architecture. *Science* 280: 892–895.
217. Tsai, S. W., Liu, R. L., Hsu, F. Y., and Chen, C. C. 2006. A study of the influence of polysaccharides on collagen self-assembly: Nanostructure and kinetics. *Biopolymers* 83: 381–388.
218. Li, Q. L., Huang, N., Chen, J., Wan, G., Zhao, A., and Chen, J. 2009. Anticoagulant surface modification of titanium via layer-by-layer assembly of collagen and sulfated chitosan multilayers. *J Biomed Mater Res* 89: 575–584.
219. Brugnerotto, J., Desbrieres, J., Roberts, G., and Rinaudo, M. 2001. Characterization of chitosan by steric exclusion chromatography. *Polymer* 42: 9921–9927.
220. Cai, K. Y., Rechtenbach, A., Hao, J. Y., Bossert, J., and Jandt, K. D. 2005. Polysaccharide–protein surface modification of titanium via a layer-by-layer technique: Characterization and cell behaviour aspects. *Biomaterials* 26: 5960–5971.
221. Shi, X. W., Wu, H. C., Liu, Y., Tsao, C. Y., Wang, K., and Kobatake, E. 2008. Chitosan fibers: Versatile platform for nickel-mediated protein assembly. *Biomacromolecules* 9: 1417–1423.
222. Richert, L., Lavalle, P., Payan, E., Shu, X. Z., Prestwich, G. D., and Stoltz, J. F. 2004. Layer by layer buildup of polysaccharide films: Physical chemistry and cellular adhesion aspects. *Langmuir* 20: 448–458.
223. Kujawa, P., Sanchez, J., Badia, A., and Winnik, F. M. 2006. Probing the stability of biocompatible sodium hyaluronate/chitosan nanocoatings against changes in salinity and pH. *J Nanosci Nanotechnol* 6: 1565–1574.
224. Feng, Q., Zeng, G. C., Yang, P. H., Wang, C. X., and Cai, J. Y. 2005. Self-assembly and characterization of polyelectrolyte complex films of hyaluronic acid/chitosan. *Colloid Surf A* 257–58: 85–88.
225. Kujawa, P., Moraille, P., Sanchez, J., Badia, A., and Winnik, F. M. 2005. Effect of molecular weight on the exponential growth and morphology of hyaluronan/chitosan multilayers: A surface plasmon resonance spectroscopy and atomic force microscopy investigation. *J Am Chem Soc* 127: 9224–9234.
226. Thierry, B., Winnik, F. M., Merhi, Y., Silver, J., and Tabrizian, M. 2003. Bioactive coatings of endovascular stents based on polyelectrolyte multilayers. *Biomacromolecules* 4: 1564–1571.
227. Chen, W. and McCarthy, T. J. 1997. Layer-by-layer deposition: A tool for polymer surface modification. *Macromolecules* 30: 78–86.
228. Kujawa, P., Schmauch, G., Viitala, T., Badia, A., and Winnik, F. M. 2007. Construction of viscoelastic biocompatible films via the layer-by-layer assembly of hyaluronan and phosphorylcholine-modified chitosan. *Biomacromolecules* Oct 8: 3169–3176.
229. Etienne, O., Schneider, A., Taddei, C., Richert, L., Schaaf, P., and Voegel, J. C. 2005. Degradability of polysaccharides multilayer films in the oral environment: An *in vitro* and *in vivo* study. *Biomacromolecules* 6: 726–733.
230. Thierry, B., Kujawa, P., Tkaczyk, C., Winnik, F. M., Bilodeau, L., and Tabrizian, M. 2005. Delivery platform for hydrophobic drugs: Prodrug approach combined with self-assembled multilayers. *J Am Chem Soc* 127: 1626–1627.
231. Lu, H. Y. and Hu, N. F. 2006. Loading behavior of {chitosan/hyaluronic acid}(n) layer-by-layer assembly films toward myoglobin: An electrochemical study. *J Phys Chem B* 110: 23710–23708.
232. Croll, T. I., O'Connor, A. J., Stevens, G. W., and Cooper-White, J. J. 2006. A blank slate? Layer-by-layer deposition of hyaluronic acid and chitosan onto various surfaces. *Biomacromolecules* May 7: 1610–1622.
233. Chua, P. H., Neoh, K. G., Kang, E. T., and Wang, W. 2008. Surface functionalization of titanium with hyaluronic acid/chitosan polyelectrolyte multilayers and RGD for promoting osteoblast functions and inhibiting bacterial adhesion. *Biomaterials* 29: 1412–1421.

234. Thierry, B., Winnik, F. M., Merhi, Y., and Tabrizian, M. 2003. Nanocoatings onto arteries via layer-by-layer deposition: Toward the *in vivo* repair of damaged blood vessels. *J Am Chem Soc* 125: 7494–7495.

235. Yuan, W. Y., Dong, H., Li, C. M., Cui, X. Q., Yu, L., and Lu, Z. S. 2007. pH-Controlled construction of chitosan–alginate multilayer film: Characterization and application for antibody immobilization. *Langmuir* 23: 13046–13052.

236. Maurstad, G., Morch, Y. A., Bausch, A. R., and Stokke, B. T. 2008. Polyelectrolyte layer interpenetration and swelling of alginate–chitosan multilayers studied by dual wavelength reflection interference contrast microscopy. *Carbohydr Polym* 71: 672–681.

237. Deng, T., Wang, H., Li, J. S., Shen, G. L., and Yu, R. Q. 2005. A novel biosensing interfacial design based on the assembled multilayers of the oppositely charged polyelectrolytes. *Anal Chim Acta* 532: 137–144.

238. Yang, Y., He, Q., Duan, L., Cui, Y., and Li, J. B. 2007. Assembled alginate–chitosan nanotubes for biological application. *Biomaterials* 28: 3083–3090.

239. Douglas, K. L., and Tabrizian, M. 2005. Effect of experimental parameters on the formation of alginate–chitosan nanoparticles and evaluation of their potential application as DNA carrier. *J Biomater Sci Polym Edn* 16: 43–56.

240. Haidar, Z. S., Hamdy, R. C., and Tabrizian, M. 2008. Protein release kinetics for core-shell hybrid nanoparticles based on the layer-by-layer assembly of alginate and chitosan on liposomes. *Biomaterials* 29: 1207–1215.

241. Tao, X, Chen, H., Sun, X. J., Chen, H. F., and Roa, W. H. 2007. Formulation and cytotoxicity of doxorubicin loaded in self-assembled bio-polyelectrolyte microshells. *Int J Pharm* 336: 376–381.

242. Tao, X., Sun, X. J., Su, J. M., Chen, J. F., and Roa, W. 2006. Natural microshells of alginate–chitosan: Unexpected stability and permeability. *Polymer* 47: 6167–6171.

243. Ye, S. Q., Wang, C. Y., Liu, X. X., and Tong, Z. 2005. Deposition temperature effect on release rate of indomethacin microcrystals from microcapsules of layer-by-layer assembled chitosan and alginate multilayer films. *J Control Release* 106: 319–328.

244. Ye, S. Q., Wang, C. Y., Liu, X. X., Tong, Z., Ren, B., and Zeng, F. 2006. New loading process and release properties of insulin from polysaccharide microcapsules fabricated through layer-by-layer assembly. *J Control Release* 112: 79–87.

245. Wang, C. Y., Ye, S. Q., Dai, L., Liu, X. X., and Tong, Z. 2007. Enhanced resistance of polyelectrolyte multilayer microcapsules to pepsin erosion and release properties of encapsulated indomethacin. *Biomacromolecules* 8: 1739–1744.

5

Environment–Stimuli Response of Chitosan-Based Hydrogels

Junjie Li and Fanglian Yao

CONTENTS

5.1 Introduction

Hydrogels can exhibit dramatic changes in their swelling behaviors, network structure, permeability, or mechanical strength in response to different stimuli (such as temperature, pH, ionic strength, chemicals, and fields), both internal and external to the body [1]. Chitosan-based hydrogels are "smart" or "intelligent" in the sense that they can perceive the prevailing stimuli and respond by showing changes in their physical or chemical behavior. Moreover, some systems have been developed to combine two or more stimuli–response mechanisms into one polymer system. For example, pH-sensitive chitosan-based hydrogels may also respond to temperature. These stimuli-responsive properties of chitosan-based hydrogels have been widely investigated and explored for the biomedical field, especially for drug-controlled release.

5.2 pH Response

The presence of amino groups in chitosan (pK_a = 6.2–6.5) results in pH-sensitive character. The pH sensitivity of a chitosan-based hydrogel is a change in volume of the hydrogel in response to pH changes in the surrounding medium, caused by the presence of weakly acidic or basic character. One characteristic phenomenon of pH-sensitive hydrogels is the dynamic swelling corresponding to different pH values of the surrounding medium. The swelling takes place because of ionization by acid or base transfer from the surrounding bulk solution. The acid or base character of the bulk solution causes the gels to swell or shrink [2]. Various methods have been employed for elucidating the swelling behavior of pH-sensitive chitosan-based hydrogels; they include weighing of hydrogel slabs, calculating the volume change by measuring the diameter of hydrogel discs, and spectroscopic and microelectro-mechanical methods.

The mechanism of water transport could be diffusion, convection, or both during the swelling process. Water and solute molecules travel within the gel by the osmotic pressure gradient (due to the water concentration gradient) between the inside and outside of the hydrogels. From the structural point of view, all pH-sensitive hydrogels have either acidic or basic groups; these groups can ionize and develop fixed charges on the polymer network, which results in electrostatic repulsive forces, responsible for pH-dependent swelling/shrinkage of the hydrogels. For cationic chitosan-based hydrogels, amino groups are protonated below the pK_a of chitosan, leading to swelling of the hydrogel at a pH below the chitosan pK_a because of a large osmotic swelling force due to the presence of ions (*cf.* Figure 5.1). Small changes in pH (especially in the vicinity of pK_a) can result in significant changes in the mesh size of the chitosan hydrogel networks [3]. Considering that the pK_a of chitosan is ~6.5, at pH > pK_a, chitosan is found to form dissociated precipitates rather than a massive hydrogel because the aggregation of chitosan polymers occurred too rapidly and locally [4]. Recently, the pH-sensitive chitosan-based hydrogels are prepared via chemical modification or composites with other compounds. Different chitosan-based hydrogel networks have specific pH responses. The swelling and pH responsiveness can

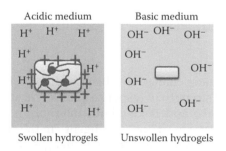

FIGURE 5.1
The pH-responsive swelling of chitosan-based hydrogels.

be adjusted by the components and the connection mode of each component. In general, two cross-linking methods have been developed for preparing chitosan-based hydrogels: physical or chemical cross-linking.

5.2.1 Physical Cross-Linking of Chitosan-Based Hydrogels

5.2.1.1 Chitosan-Derivative-Based Hydrogels

It is a very effective method to obtain pH-sensitive hydrogels via grafting some special chemical function group or polymer on chitosan chains. Poly(α-hydroxy acids) can generate acidic degradation products at the implanted site, which evokes an undesirable tissue reaction [5]. The acid by-product may lead to local disturbance due to poor vascularization in the surrounding tissue. Chitosan may be combined with acid-producing biodegradable polymers, so that local toxicity due to the acid by-products can be alleviated. Physically cross-linked chitosan-g-poly(α-hydroxy acids) hydrogels have been carried out by direct grafting of α-hydroxy acids onto chitosan in the absence of catalysts. The structure of the graft copolymers can change according to the pH value of the environment because there are unreacted amino groups of chitosan in chitosan-g-poly(α-hydroxy acids) acid copolymers, which would be protonated in acid solutions. In the acidic condition, the acid can be attached to the hydrogels, as shown in Figure 5.2. The swelling process of hydrogels contains the protonation of amino groups by the acid in the low pH value (pH $< pK_b$) by the ionic bonds; therefore, the chitosan-g-poly(α-hydroxy acids) hydrogels are able to imbibe a lot of water and swell quickly. However, the swelling ability of the hydrogels becomes unchanged when the pH value is higher than pK_b [6]. Moreover, the pH-sensitive behaviors could be modulated via adjusting the side groups and degree of substitution. However, the side groups and degree of substitution have less effect on sample swelling above pK_b. For example, Albertsson and coworkers [7] found that chitosan-g-poly(lactic acid) hydrogels appear to have higher water uptake values than chitosan-g-poly(glycolic acid) hydrogels at pH 2.2, but they have similar water uptake at pH 7.4. Yao et al. [8,9] obtained the cytocompatible poly(chitosan-g-L-lactic acid) through grafting oligo(L-lactic acid) onto the amino groups on chitosan without a catalyst. These graft copolymers have a higher strength than chitosan and the swelling behaviors are influenced by pH (as shown in Figure 5.3). When pH < 2, with increasing buffer pH, the concentration of charged ionic groups in the films increases. The swelling of the samples will increase due to enhancement of the osmotic pressure and charge repulsion. At higher pH, the degree of ionization is reduced due to deprotonation of the amino units of chitosan and the swelling of the films decreases. In addition, the hydrophobic side-chain aggregation and hydrogen bonds

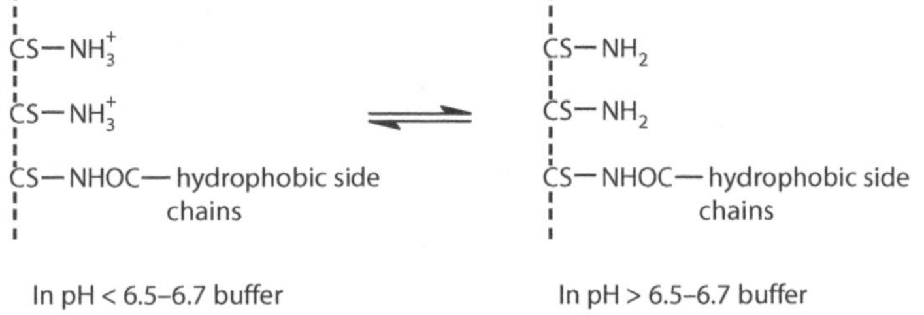

FIGURE 5.2
Structure change of the chitosan graft copolymer in acidic and alkaline buffers.

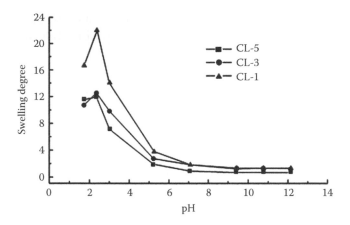

FIGURE 5.3
Effect of the LA/CS feed ratio and pH value on the equilibrium water uptake of the CL films (CL-1, CL-3, and CL-5 indicate that the lactic acid/chitosan ratio = 0.5, 2.0, and 4.0 w/w, respectively).

in the copolymers are much stronger, which will also lead to lower swelling ability of the hydrogels.

Hydrophobically modified chitosan can form hydrogels via a change in the environmental pH. The balance between charge repulsion and hydrophobic interaction on hydrophobically modified chitosan chains is sensitive to the environmental pH. For example, N-palmitoyl chitosan (NPCS) solution flows almost like a liquid at large shear rates due to the shear-thinning effect when pH < 6.5; when pH is raised from 6.5 to 7.0, NPCS solution shows a drastic increase in G' by about an order of magnitude and the material is in the form of hydrogel, as shown in Figure 5.4 [10]. That means that NPCS solution can transform into hydrogels within a narrow pH range (pH 6.5–7.0).

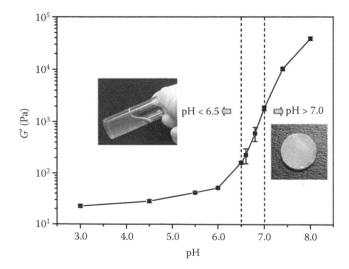

FIGURE 5.4
Elastic modulus (G') of aqueous NPCS (originally at a concentration of 1% w/v) measured at a constant frequency of 0.1 Hz as a function of pH ($n = 5$).

Amphiphilic chitosan-based hydrogels are developed by conjugating hydrophobic groups and/or hydrophilic groups into chitosan molecules. Amphiphilic chitosan can aggregate into nano micelles or particles, and these micelles or particles have special pH sensitivity because their formation and dissociation depend on the pH of the environment. The rationale for designing pH-sensitive nanoparticles was based on either the protonation or deprotonation of amino groups of chitosan. In general, the structure of micelles or particles is loose when pH < pK_a (chitosan) and becomes compact when pH > pK_a (chitosan) [11]. For example, when the pH is ~4, chains of the pH-sensitive graft copolymer, poly[(2-dimethylamino)ethyl methacrylate]-graft-chitosan (PDMAEMA-g-chitosan), extend because chitosan and dimethylamino ethyl methacrylate (DMAEMA) segments are almost fully protonated. When pH values are in the vicinity of the pK_a of chitosan, amino groups of chitosan are deprotonated and their hydrophobicity increases, resulting in the formation of micelles with chitosan core and the partially deprotonated DMAEMA segments as the shell. When pH > 7, both DMAEMA and chitosan segments are deprotonated, and double-layered hard spheres are formed, as shown in Figure 5.5 [12].

5.2.1.2 Chitosan–Polyanion Polymer Polyelectrolyte Complex

Chitosan–polyanion polymer polyelectrolyte complex (CS-PEC) hydrogels are generally obtained either by the reaction of chitosan or polyanions. CS-PEC forming reaction can only occur when the pH values are between the pK_a of chitosan and $pK_{a'}$ of polyanion polymer. That is to say, pH can control the formation and dissociation of CS-PECs. Therefore, most properties of CS-PEC hydrogels depend on the pH of the environment. In general, CS-PECs show the lowest swelling degree in the range of $pK_{a'}$ < pH < pK_a due to the strong interactions between chitosan and polyanion polymer. However, CS-PECs swell obviously at pH < $pK_{a'}$ and/or pH > pK_a. Pectin is an acidic polysaccharide that has repeating units of α (1, 4)-L-rhamnose units. A polyelectrolyte complex is formatted from anionic pectin and cationic chitosan. The PEC swells obviously at pH < 3 and pH > 8, and does not swell in the range of 3 < pH < 8. Moreover, its degree of swelling in an acidic medium is much more than that in an alkaline medium. The swelling of the PEC correlates with its composition and is also affected by the degree of deacetylation (DD) and the methoxy level of pectin [13]. Yoshizawa et al. [14,15] found that the chitosan/polyalkyleneoxide–maleic acid copolymer (CS/PAOMA) PEC films swell at low pH and shrink at pH between 4.8 and 6.5, and the swelling increases after pH 6.5. These swelling behaviors can be attributed to the electrostatic interaction between the protonation of amino groups in chitosan and the ionization of carboxyl groups in PAOMA. The pK_a of chitosan is 6.5 and the pK_a of PAOMA is 4.8. In different pH media, corresponding groups (e.g., NH_3^+ and COO^-) play different roles between intermolecules.

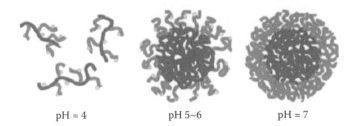

pH = 4   pH 5~6   pH = 7

FIGURE 5.5
Schematic representation of the microstructure of PDMAEMA-g-chitosan copolymer at different pH values.

5.2.2 Chemical Cross-Linking of Chitosan-Based Hydrogels

Chemical cross-linking is an effective method for preparing pH-sensitive chitosan-based hydrogels. The amino groups of the glucosamine residue within chitosan chains can serve as cross-linking sites, for example, by reacting with glutaraldehyde, glyoxa, proanthocyanidin, genipin, and so on, to form cross-linking between linear chitosan chains that leads to gel formation. But the pH-sensitivity of pure chitosan cross-linking hydrogels does not satisfy the application. First, amphoteric cross-linking hydrogels can be formed via introducing some negative groups into chitosan in order to modulate the pH-sensitive capability. In addition, a chitosan-based heterocyclic polymer network (HPN) could be formed via the addition of other polymers and cross-linked. In this system, chitosan and polymer are cross-linked by co-cross-linkers and form a covalent network, as shown in Figure 5.6a. On the other hand, when other polymer chains interpenetrate and interact with chitosan via hydrogen bonds or physical interactions, the chitosan-based semi-interpenetrating polymer network (semi-IPN) is formed (*cf.* Figure 5.6b). The HPN and semi-IPN technique can be used to improve the properties of chitosan-based gels. Moreover, their pH sensitivity could be modulated via adjusting the composition and cross-linking degree.

5.2.2.1 Amphoteric Cross-Linking Hydrogels

The density of –NH$_2$ of chitosan has a very important role in the pH sensitivity of chitosan-based hydrogels. Therefore, an effective method for modulating pH sensitivity is by changing the density of –NH$_2$ of a chitosan network. Introducing negative groups into chitosan chains could improve the swelling degree of chitosan-based hydrogels in neutral and basic media. For example, the swelling degree of carboxymethyl chitosan hydrogels is higher

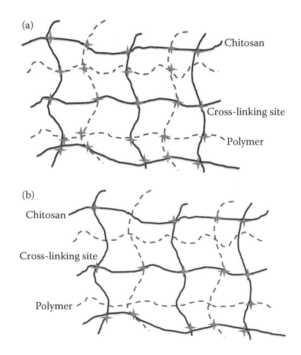

FIGURE 5.6
Schematic representation of (a) chitosan-based HPN hydrogels and (b) semi-IPN hydrogels.

than that of chitosan hydrogels [16]. When pH is equal to isoelectric point (p*I*) of chitosan-based amphoteric cross-linking hydrogels, the numbers of $-NH_2$ and negative groups are equal and ionic interactions between opposite charges result in the lowest swelling degree. When pH > p*I*, a larger concentration of negative groups inside the hydrogels are ionized, which results in an osmotic pressure and makes the amphoteric cross-linking hydrogels swell, and the swelling degree increases with increasing pH. When pH < 7, the dissociation of carboxyl groups is inhibited and $-NH_2$ is protonated. When pH < p*I*, the dominant ionic groups of amphoteric cross-linking hydrogels are $-NH_3^+$, and the swelling increases with decreasing pH. The effect of substitution degree (SD) on swelling degree is somewhat "complex." The swelling degree is almost unchanged when pH = p*I*. When pH < p*I*, the swelling degree of amphoteric cross-linking hydrogels increases with decreasing SD. However, when pH > p*I*, the opposite phenomenon can be observed. For example, the higher the SD value that *N*-(2-carboxybenzyl) chitosan cross-linking hydrogels (CBCSG) possess, the bigger the swelling degree it exhibits in the pH range 7.4–9.0. In the pH range 1.0–5.0, the result is contrary to the above-mentioned results (*cf.* Figure 5.7) [17]. Yang et al. [18] found that poly(acrylic acid)-modified chitosan-based cross-linked hydrogels exhibit similar swelling behaviors.

5.2.2.2 Chitosan-Based Semi-IPN Hydrogels

At low pH, the swelling process of the chitosan-based semi-IPN involves the protonation of amino groups in the gels and relaxation. The equilibrium swelling degree of semi-IPN hydrogels increases and the semi-IPN becomes more pH sensitive with decreasing cross-linking degree. However, at high pH, where there are no protonation and hydrogen bonding association, there is almost no effect of cross-linking degree on the equilibrium degree of swelling and pH sensitivity. In addition, with decreasing chitosan content in the semi-IPN, the semi-IPN becomes less pH sensitive.

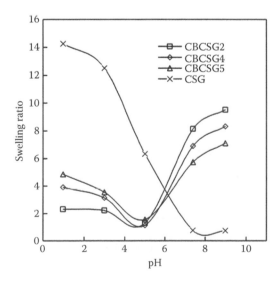

FIGURE 5.7

Swelling characteristics of the CBCSG with different SD values in different buffer solutions for 24 h. SD: CBCSG2 (2.62 mmol/g), CBCSG4 (2.10 mmol/g), CBCSG5 (1.64 mmol/g), and CSG2 (0).

Cross-linked chitosan/poly(oxypropylene glycol) semi-IPN hydrogels based on the complex formed by physical and chemical cross-linking, for example, imine bonds and interactions between macromolecular chains including hydrogen bonding, display pH sensitivity. The rate of swelling is highly pH dependent and can be divided into three parts (*cf.* Figure 5.8) [19]: (1) When pH > 6, the swelling degree of the semi-IPN is very limited, because the inherent hydrophobicity of the hydrogels dominates. The content of bonding water is very low, almost approaching zero [20]. (2) When pH ranges from 2 to 4.84, the semi-IPN rapidly swells due to the protonation of amino groups. (3) When pH = 1, the swelling and swelling rate of the semi-IPN is prior to that in other pHs because of the highest protonation degree of amino groups in the gels. In acid medium, the composition of the swelling medium has a complex effect on the state of the water in the hydrogel (*cf.* Figure 5.9). Moreover, the swelling behaviors are also relative to the composition of semi-IPN hydrogels. Compared with pure chitosan cross-linking hydrogels, the semi-IPN has a lower sorption rate and exhibits low swelling degree because poly(oxypropylene glycol) provides cross-linking in the semi-IPN. Meanwhile, the swelling reversibility of pure chitosan hydrogels is low when its medium pH changes interval, but the semi-IPN can maintain excellent swelling reversibility (*cf.* Figure 5.10) [21]. That is to say, poly(oxypropylene glycol) within the semi-IPN not only enhances the flexibility of the semi-IPN, but also influences the swelling behaviors of the semi-IPN via macromolecular interactions. The poly(oxypropylene glycol)-containing hydrophobic moieties offer more free volume to water as a definite water content and restrict its mobility less; therefore, the content of bond water within the semi-IPN hydrogels is higher than that within pure cross-linking chitosan hydrogels [22].

Some hydrophilic polymers, such as poly(ethylene glycol) (PEG), poly(vinyl alcohol) (PVA), and poly(vinylpyrrolidone), are blended with chitosan to obtain pH-sensitive chitosan-based semi-IPN hydrogels. There are several types of hydrogen bonds in this semi-IPN; some are intramolecular hydrogen bonds and others are intermolecular hydrogen bonds. The hydrogels swell the most in acidic medium compared to neutral or basic

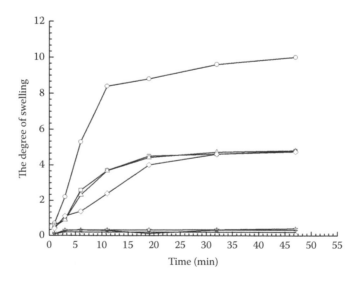

FIGURE 5.8
Swelling kinetics of chitosan/poly(oxypropylene glycol) semi-IPN in different pH solutions at 37°C and ionic strength $I = 0.1$; (O) pH = 1, ($\square$) pH = 2, (Δ) pH = 3.19, ($\lozenge$) pH = 4.84, ($\star$) pH = 6, (+) pH = 7, ($\times$) pH = 8.99, and (*) pH = 12.

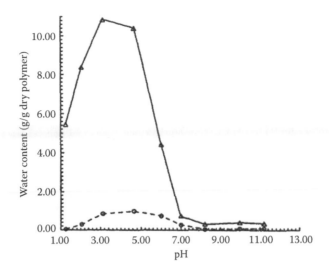

FIGURE 5.9
Water contents as a function of pH for the cross-linking chitosan/poly(oxypropylene glycol) semi-IPN hydrogels at equilibrium swollen state. Solid line: total water; dashed line: bound water.

medium and the swelling equilibrium is established faster at neutral or basic medium than at acidic medium. In addition, the different hydrogel compositions have a certain effect on the swelling performance. For example, in chitosan/PEG and chitosan/PVA semi-IPN hydrogels, the bound water decreases as the percentage of chitosan decreases because of the weaker water-binding ability of the –OH group compared to the $-NH_3$ group due to its fewer polar moieties [23].

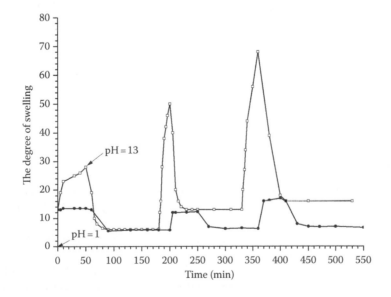

FIGURE 5.10
Degree of swelling as a function of time for chitosan/poly(oxypropylene glycol) (solid) and chitosan (blank) hydrogels after repeated changes of pH between 1 and 13.

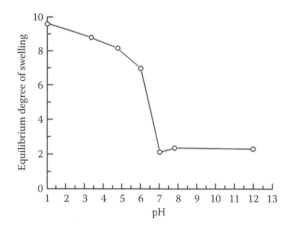

FIGURE 5.11

Swelling behavior of the chitosan–gelatin hybrid network specimen with a—CHO/–NH$_2$ molar ratio of 10 in solutions of different pH values with ionic strength $I = 0.1$ at 37°C.

5.2.2.3 Chitosan-Based HPN Hydrogels

The uncross-linked polymer of the chitosan-based semi-IPN hydrogels is always subject to diffusion in the solvent, especially in swelled condition. HPN hydrogels may overcome the problem via cocross-linking.

Gelatin is a denatured form of collagen, composed of glycine, praline, hydroxyproline, arginine, and other amino acids. The amphiphilic protein (pI = 4.96) can provide amino groups for cocross-linking with chitosan to prepare a chitosan/gelatin hybrid polymer network (HPN). The pH-sensitive swelling behavior of HPN gel is displayed in Figure 5.11 [24]. The data show that the degree of swelling declines sharply at pH 7.0; this can be explained by the fact that the hydrogen bonds within the chitosan/gelatin HPN dissociate in an acidic medium. The elastic modulus of chitosan/gelatin HPN hydrogels in basic medium is higher than that in acidic medium due to the reassociation of hydrogen bondings between networks [25]. An increase in cross-link density induced a decrease in swelling and pH sensitivity. The pH-sensitive chitosan hydrogel properties can be tuned by preparatory conditions and the inclusion of gelatin [26].

5.3 Temperature Response

It is well known that thermosensitive behaviors in a polymer solution can generally be considered as a change in intermolecular interactions in response to temperature. These polymer chains contain either moderately hydrophobic groups (if too hydrophobic, the polymer chains would not dissolve in water at all) or a mixture of hydrophilic and hydrophobic segments. When a polymer is dissolved in water, there are three types of interactions that take place: between polymer molecules, polymer and water, and between water molecules [27]. These interactions are the main drive force underlying the formation of thermosensitive hydrogels. At low temperature, water molecules are presumed to form enclosed structures that surround the polymer chains. At high temperature, water is released from polymer chains due to the high rotation energy of water, and the dewatered hydrophobic polymer segments begin to associate with each other, and hydrogels result. These polymer solutions exhibit a separation from solution and solidification above a certain temperature defined as the lower critical solution temperature (LCST). Above the LCST, they turn into a gel, becoming extremely hydrophobic and insoluble [28]. In general, as the polymer chain contains more hydrophobic constituents, LCST becomes lower. From a thermodynamic point of view, thermoreversible behavior in a polymer system can generally be regarded as a change in the driving force in response to temperature variation. From the molecular structure point of view, the thermosensitive hydrogels usually display a change in hydrophobicity or efficiency of hydrogen bonding when temperature increases.

Some chitosan-based hydrogels have thermosensitivity. As clinically applicable hydrogels, thermosensitive chitosan-based hydrogels preferably assume a liquid form below body temperature and gel readily at body temperature. In addition, their swelling behaviors could change under temperature stimuli. Chitosan possesses hydrophobic ($-CH_3$) and hydrogen bonding favoring groups ($-OH$, $-NH$, and $-C=O$). However, intermolecular interactions of pure chitosan change little under temperature stimulation due to its high hydrophobicity. It should provide a favorable environment to form a gel structure under temperature stimulation through the following mechanisms: (1) Incorporating some functional groups to reduce hydrogen bond interactions between chitosan and water by a screening effect at low temperature and to enhance the chitosan–chitosan interactions over those of chitosan–water via the hydrophobic effect at high temperature and (2) introducing some amphiphilic thermosensitive polymer containing hydrophilic and hydrophobic segments. Therefore, some functional group or polymer is introduced into the chitosan network via grafting, block or blending. These functional groups or polymers can modulate the hydrophilic–hydrophobic balance via temperature change, and endow the chitosan with thermosensitivity (*cf.* Figure 5.12) [29]. If the chitosan chains in hydrogels are not covalently cross-linked in this system, thermosensitive hydrogels can undergo sol–gel phase transitions, instead of swelling–shrinking transitions. Moreover, most of these thermosensitive chitosan-based hydrogels also have pH sensitivity due to the presence of amino groups. If the chitosan-based thermosensitive hydrogels can be turned into liquid at room temperature, undergoing gelation when in contact with physiological fluids, they will play a very important role in the applications of drug release, cell encapsulation, and tissue engineering.

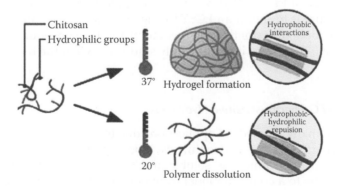

FIGURE 5.12
Schematic representation of thermoreversible networks of chitosan graft copolymer resulting in semisolid gel at body temperature and liquid below room temperature.

5.3.1 Chitosan/Polyol Thermosensitive Hydrogels

Polyol can stabilize certain compounds in aqueous solutions and promote the formation of a shield of water around some macromolecules or polymer chains [30]. Therefore, when hydroxyl composites are incorporated into a chitosan network, chitosan chains can maintain a certain stability and cannot build up a 3D network structure at low temperature because of the difficulty of creating contacts between the junction chains. However, at high temperature, water molecules have enough energy from the shackles of chitosan chains. The dewatered chitosan chains associate with each other via hydrophobic interaction. Thus, many hydroxyl groups, composites, or polymers are introduced into the chitosan network via chemical modification, grafting, or blending to obtain chitosan-based thermosensitive hydrogels.

5.3.1.1 Hydroxybutyl Chitosan Derivative Thermosensitive Hydrogels

Hydroxybutyl chitosan, a promising thermoresponsive polymer, is synthesized by conjugation of hydroxybutyl groups to the hydroxyl and amino reactive sites of chitosan. It can be easily applied as a mildly viscous solution without spatial restriction, but quickly transforms into a pliable and durable hydrogel when the temperature is increased. Moreover, this process is reversible. At temperatures below LCST, hydrogen bonds exist not only between the OH group of hydroxybutyl groups and the OH and NH_2 groups of the chitosan chains but also between the hydroxybutyl groups and water. That is to say, hydroxybutyl chitosan chains are surrounded by water molecules. When the temperature is higher than LCST, the intermolecular hydrogen-bonding interactions decrease and the energized water molecules surrounding the hydroxybutyl chitosan are removed. Hydrophobic interactions between interchains of hydroxybutyl chitosan become more and more strong, which results in hydrogel formation. Moreover, the hydrogels can transform into solution when the temperature decreases to below LCST [31].

LCST of hydroxybutyl chitosan depends on the molecular weight (MW) and SD of hydroxybutyl. The higher the MW the lower the LCST. The lower the SD the higher the LCST [32]. Gel transformation time is related to temperature. Therefore, the gel is formed in <100 s when the temperature is 25°C, which is higher than the LCST (20°C, MW 900 kDa, and SD 1.23). However, when the temperature is elevated to 37°C, gel is formed quickly in <50 s [31]. For hydroxybutyl chitosan hydrogel films, the film surface appears to be rough and is filled with small agglomerates with different heights when the temperature is higher than LCST (*cf.* Figure 5.13). The result is likely caused by the increase of hydrophobicity of the polymer chain and the subsequent dewetting of the chitosan films. The film surface is significantly smoother when the temperature is below LCST [33].

5.3.1.2 Chitosan/PEG Thermosensitive Hydrogels

PEG is also used in many biomedical applications due to its outstanding physicochemical and biological properties such as hydrophilicity, biocompatibility, and lack of toxicity. PEG solutions are known to become less soluble and precipitate at higher temperatures in aqueous solutions due to a conformational transition to a less polar form. Chitosan/PEG composite hydrogels exhibit excellent thermosensitivity. For chitosan-g-PEG, at low temperatures, chitosan chains are covered with water molecules attached by hydrogen bonds between hydrophilic groups of PEG and water molecules. Thus, direct association between

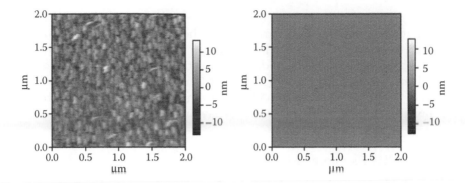

FIGURE 5.13
AFM topographic images of hydroxybutyl chitosan film immersed in pure water at 37°C (left) and 18°C (right).

polymer chains is disrupted, thereby rendering the graft polymer soluble in water. With increasing temperature, both chitosan and PEG polymer chains gradually lose the attached water molecules, the hydrophobic interactions between chitosan chains interactions start to prevail, and a gel is formed (*cf.* Figure 5.14) [34]. In addition, the physical junction zones of polymer chain segments increase and gel is formed. However, the high grafted rate of

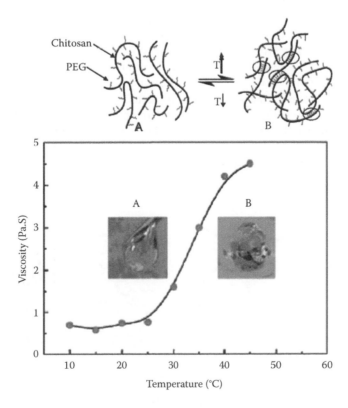

FIGURE 5.14
Schematic representation of thermoreversible hydrogel formulation of aqueous chitosan-g-PEG solution and the temperature dependence of viscosity of PEG-g-chitosan solution.

PEG would suppress hydrophobic interactions between chitosan chains, thereby resulting in a solution that does not gel at body temperature. Thermoreversible chitosan/PEG hydrogels are obtained when PEG is grafted in an amount of 45–55 wt% [35]. Similar trends were observed by Ganji and Abdekhodaie [36] for thermosensitive chitosan/PEG block copolymers. Harding and coworkers [37] found that the swelling ratio of cross-linked chitosan-g-PEG hydrogels increases with increasing temperature. And the chitosan/PEG semi-IPN also exhibits similar swelling behaviors [38].

5.3.1.3 Chitosan/PVA Thermosensitive Hydrogels

PVA, a water-soluble polyhydroxy polymer, has been frequently explored as implant material for drug delivery systems and surgical repairs because of its excellent mechanical strength, biocompatibility and nontoxicity. The formation of chitosan/PVA hydrogels could be controlled by temperature. The chitosan/PVA composites are liquid solutions at low temperature (about 4°C), but gel under physiological conditions [39]. At low temperature, it is very difficult to construct hydrogel networks using chitosan and PVA because of the difficulty of creating contacts between the junction chains. In this condition, hydrogen bonds exist not only between the OH and NH_2 groups of chitosan and the OH group of PVA but also between PVA and water due to the high hydrophilicity of PVA, which can lead to the dissolution of chitosan chains. In addition, the low temperature can also reduce the mobility of chitosan molecules, which further prevents the association of chitosan chains (*cf.* Figure 5.15a). However, the high temperature can reduce the intermolecular hydrogen-bonding interactions and accelerate the mobility of chitosan molecules. So the energized water molecules surrounding the chitosan chains are removed. The dewatered hydrophobic chitosan chains associate with each other (*cf.* Figure 5.15b) [40]. That is to say, chitosan is responsible for the hydrophobic interactions at high temperature, while PVA content is related to the hydrogen-bonding interactions at low temperature. Therefore, the proportion of PVA in the gel increases, gelation time becomes longer at 37°C, the aperture turns smaller, and hence the intensity of the gel increases. When the ratio of PVA to chitosan is greater than 10:1, chitosan/PVA would not be thermosensitive; hence, the content of PVA should be kept at a certain degree [41].

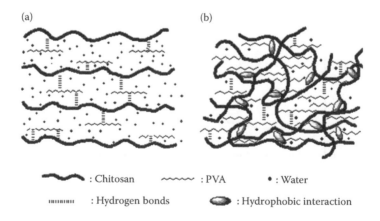

(a)   (b)

⬬⬬⬬ : Chitosan   ∿∿∿ : PVA   • : Water

⬩⬩⬩ : Hydrogen bonds   ⬭ : Hydrophobic interaction

FIGURE 5.15
Formation mechanism of chitosan/PVA gel: (a) solution at low temperature and (b) gel at high temperature.

5.3.1.4 Chitosan/Polyol Salt Thermosensitivity Hydrogels

Chitosan/glycerophosphate (chitosan/GP) hydrogel, a novel thermosensitive hydrogel first reported by Chenite et al. [42], is an important system due to its sol–gel transition at body temperature. Chitosan/GP is a physical hydrogel formed when hydrogen bonds between chitosan/GP and water become unstable at higher temperatures. As shown in Figure 5.16, this system remains liquid at room temperature and solidifies into a hydrogel as the temperature is increased to body temperature [43]. Chitosan/GP hydrogels have a heterogeneous microstructure, with large interconnected solvent-rich areas and a polymer-rich phase of agglomerates that aggregate into chains and large volume particulates (*cf.* Figure 5.17). GP plays two essential roles in the chitosan/CG system: (1) to increase the pH value of chitosan solution to the physiological range of 7.0–7.4 and to prevent immediate precipitation or gelation of chitosan solution, which is due to its mild basic character and potentially due to the attraction of phosphate moieties of GP to the remaining charged amine of chitosan, and thereby exposing the glycerol moiety to separate chitosan chains in solution and maintain its solubility at low temperature; (2) to allow for controlled hydrogel formation when an increase in temperature is imposed [44]. There are three interactions in the chitosan/GP system [45]: (1) electrostatic attraction between the amino group of chitosan and the phosphate group of glycerophosphate; (2) hydrogen bonding between chitosan chains; and (3) chitosan–chitosan hydrophobic interactions. At low temperatures, GP can promote the protective hydration of the chitosan chains; strong chitosan–water interactions protect the chitosan chains against aggregation. Chitosan adopts a compact conformation due to intramolecular hydrogen bonds, and the physical junctions that could form a gel are confined inside the coil. It is therefore a poor conformation to build up a three-dimensional (3D) structure because of the difficulty of creating contacts between the junction zones [46]. Upon heating, sheaths of water molecules are removed by the glycerol moiety, and new hydrogen bonds form between hydrophobic groups as they collapse to form separate domains. The hydrophobic associations cooperate to form junction points and chitosan molecules can unfold freely, which in turn allows the association of chitosan macromolecules. Moreover, GP is freely diffusible after gelation and is not retained in the hydrogels [47].

In general, the thermosensitivity of chitosan/GP solution can be controlled by the DD of chitosan, the MW of chitosan, the concentration of chitosan, the amount of GP, and the medium. (1) The hydrogel of chitosan/GP can rapidly form at body temperature when the DD is ca. 75.4%, whereas chitosan/GP hydrogels with other DD values form either slowly or remain unchanged. Thus, the optimal DD for chitosan/GP thermosensitive hydrogel preparation is 75.4% [48]; (2) the increase of MW is favorable for hydrogel transition and a

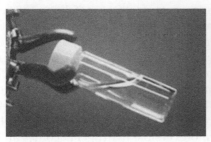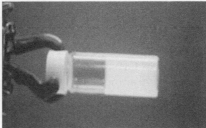

FIGURE 5.16
Chitosan/GP formulation at room temperature (left) and at 37°C (right).

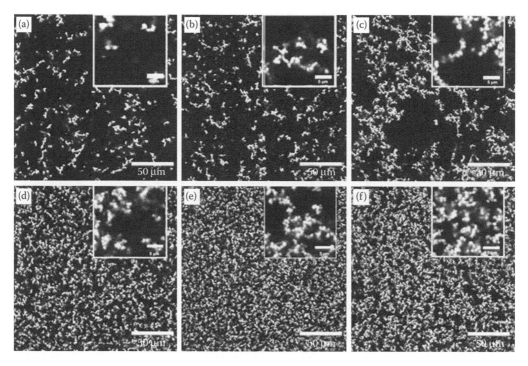

FIGURE 5.17
Microstructural images of chitosan/GP hydrogels from LSCM; inset: optically magnified 10×. Chitosan compositions: (a) 0.25 wt%/vol%, (b) 0.5 wt%/vol%, (c) 0.75 wt%/vol%, (d) 1.0 wt%/vol%, (e) 1.25 wt%/vol%, and (f) 1.5 wt%/vol%. White areas represent the polymer-rich phase; scale bars represent 50 μm, and 5 μm in the inset.

high-MW chitosan is optimal for hydrogel preparation; (3) chitosan solution with high concentration are not practically useful to obtain thermosensitive hydrogel owing to their high viscosity. In general, the concentration of chitosan solution ranges from 1.0% to 2.0% and this is beneficial for the transition hydrogels. Two lengths are found for chitosan chains in the chitosan/GP hydrogel, which are highly concentration dependent. The polymer-rich hydrophobic domains of these particles have a characteristic length of 35 nm, which decreases with increasing chitosan concentration, and the polymer-poor more hydrophilic regions have a correlation length of 12 nm, which increases with increasing chitosan concentration [49]; (4) the gel transition temperature decreases with increasing amounts of GP [50]. Moreover, if the gels returned to a liquid solution, they were called thermoreversible hydrogels, whereas those which remained as gel at low temperature were called thermoirreversible hydrogels. To some extent, chitosan/GP is a thermoreversible hydrogel, which depends on the amount of GP and chitosan in the solution. The hydrophobic interaction is reversible under temperature stimulation, but hydrogen bonds are not influenced by temperature. High amounts of GP make chitosan/GP irreversible. At high concentration of GP salt, the hydrogen bonds between chitosan chains and chitosan–water molecules predominate due to the neutralization effects of GP. Since hydrogen bonds are not temperature dependent, cooling the hydrogel does not affect the gel structure. Ganji et al. [51] found that as the GP salt concentration increases from 0.33 to 0.40 M in a solution composed of 2% w/v chitosan, a thermoreversible hydrogel becomes an irreversible hydrogel. (5) The gel transition temperature is also influenced by the medium. Chen and coworkers [52] found that the viscosity of chitosan/GP hydrogels prepared with different acids increase as follows: nitric acid < chloroacetic < hydrochloric < carboxylic acids (formic, acetic propionic, butyric, isobutyric) < lactic acid. Hydrogels prepared with carboxylic acids showed higher viscosity than inorganic acids.

However, Ma and coworkers [53] found that the chitosan/GP system does not behave appropriately as a pH-sensitive drug carrier. Its swelling degree decreases in both acidic and basic media. It showed high initial drug release in both acidic and basic conditions. At acidic medium, the amino groups in chitosan/GP hydrogel are protonated and interact with the free GP, which results in shrinkage of hydrogel. At basic medium, the ionic interaction between chitosan and GP is destroyed, which results in weight loss of the hydrogel in solution and the swelling degree decreases. Quaternized chitosan/GP hydrogels have appropriate pH sensitivity, and dissolve promptly in acidic solution, whereas they nearly kept their original state in neutral or basic conditions. However, compared to the chitosan/GP system, the thermosensitivity of quaternized chitosan/GP hydrogels decreases because quaternization decreased the crystallinity and improved the water solubility of chitosan, both of which contributed to reducing the gelation capacity. On the other hand, polymer interchain repulsion due to the high cationic charge can also hinder polymer gelation. Therefore, high SD is not beneficial for the gelation formation of the quaternized chitosan/GP system [54]. In order to overcome this disadvantage, PEG is incorporated into the quaternized chitosan/GP system. The chitosan/PEG/GP system has excellent temperature and pH sensitivity, which can be utilized for facilitating the nasal drug delivery of peptide drug [55].

5.3.2 Chitosan/Amphiphilic Polymer Thermosensitive Hydrogels

5.3.2.1 Chitosan/Pluronic Hydrogels

Triblock poly(ethylene oxide)–poly(propylene oxide)–poly(ethylene oxide), (PEO–PPO–PEO) copolymer (commercially available as Pluronic or Poloxamers) is well known to have a fast thermally reversible property. Some of them have been proved by FDA. The LCST could be controlled by the ratio of the hydrophobic PPO segment to the hydrophilic PEO segment. The more the PPO constituents, the lower the LCST. Most of the Pluronic have an LCST well above normal body temperature. Pluronic F127 is found to gel at a concentration of 20 wt% at 25°C, which is less than that of the other members of the Pluronic series. At room temperature (<25°C), the solution behaves as a mobile liquid, which is transformed into a transparent gel at body temperature [56]. Chitosan-g-Pluronic 127 (CP) also exhibits reversible thermosensitive properties at 30–35°C according to the incorporated Pluronic concentration without any treatment. The LCST of CP is lower than that of Pluronic itself at the same concentration. Sol–gel transition of CP does not occur if chitosan is over 17 wt% in the copolymer owing to the increased hydrophilic property of chitosan [57]. At low temperature, the CP copolymer is retained in the monomer state (solution phase). With increasing temperature, CP aggregates are formed by hydrophobic interaction and CP hydrogels are formed by packing of the aggregates in the aqueous solution (*cf.* Figure 5.18). The hydrophobic interactions of the PPO group and dehydrated chitosan were suggested to be the main force driving the formation of CP hydrogels [58].

5.3.2.2 Chitosan/PNIPAAm Hydrogels

Poly(*N*-isopropylacrylamide) (PNIPAAm) is a well-known member of the thermoresponsive polymer family. Its transition from a hydrophilic to a hydrophobic structure occurs

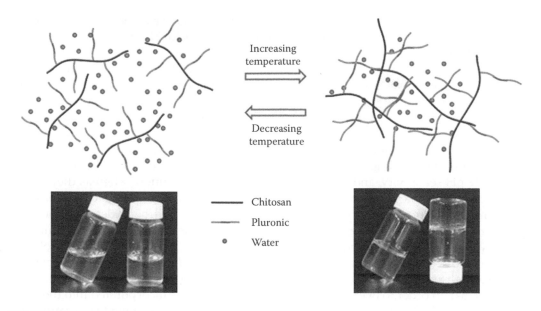

FIGURE 5.18
Hydrogel formation of the thermosensitive CP hydrogel in aqueous solution via the hydrophobic interaction of a PPO group in Pluronic and the dehydrated chitosan chain.

dramatically at what is known as the LCST. Experimentally, the LCST of PNIPAAm is in the range of 30–35°C [59]. At a temperature below its LCST, linear PNIPAAm is water soluble; however, at an LCST temperature or higher, the hydrogen bond interactions between PNIPAAm and water become weak and water would be released. PNIPAAm would undergo a coil-to-globule transition and become insoluble. PNIPAAm can be combined into chitosan-based hydrogels and endow the chitosan-based hydrogels excellent thermosensitivity. Many studies concern chitosan/PNIPAAm hydrogels.

Chitosan/PNIPAAm semi-IPN or IPN is one of the most common thermosensitive hydrogels. Lee and Chen [60] examined chitosan/PNIPAAm semi-IPN and glutaraldehyde-cross-linked IPN hydrogels and found that the swelling ratios of IPN gels are lower than those of semi-IPN gels, the reason being that the addition of cross-linked chitosan to the PNIPAAm hydrogel makes the network structure of the gel denser and more hydrophobic. The PNIPAAm/chitosan semi-IPN and IPN hydrogels de-swell more quickly at their gel transition temperatures (*cf.* Figure 5.19). Gel transition temperature for the present gels is not affected by the addition of the chitosan component in the gels. That is to say, the LCST of chitosan/PNIPAAm depends on the PNIPAAm. In the chitosan/PPNIPAAm IPN and the semi-IPN system, chitosan chains and the PNIPAAm network give a relatively independent polymer system, in which each retained its own properties [61]. For the same reason, the LCST of the carboxymethyl chitosan/PNIPAAM semi-IPN is also ca. 30–35°C. In addition, the swelling–deswelling behaviors of the carboxymethyl chitosan/PNIPAAM semi-IPN hydrogel have good reversibility, and this process may be repeated many times, with better reproduction [62]. However, incorporation of PEG can improve the LCST, because PEG would weaken the interactions between PNIPAAm and chitosan, which leave PNIPAAm more opportunity to interact with water molecules. As a result, more heat would be required to break the hydrogen bonds. In addition, the PEG-incorporated chitosan/PNIPAAm would be more hydrophilic, and such an increase in hydrophilicity in

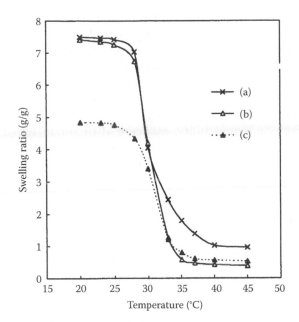

FIGURE 5.19
Equilibrium swelling ratios as a function of temperature for PNIPAAm/chitosan gels in water. (a) PNIPAAm, (b) chitosan/PNIPAAm semi-IPN, and (c) chitosan//PNIPAAm IPN.

a PNIPAAm system is well known to increase LCST [63]. During the swelling progress, there are two competitive phenomena that determine the behaviors of the gel as the temperature rises: the hydration capacity of chitosan increases, whereas that of PNIPAAm decreases as segments collapse due to the temperature-controlled conformational transition. Therefore, the temperature-dependent swelling behavior is the result of a fine balance that is influenced by both the degree of cross-linking and the chitosan to PNIPAAm ratio [64]. Chitosan/PNIPAAm IPN or semi-IPN hydrogels are prepared in acidic medium because of insolubility of chitosan in neutral and basic media, which limits the application of chitosan/PNIPAAm hydrogels to some extent. Soluble chitosan-g-PNIPAAm copolymer can overcome this disadvantage and provide a more effective method for preparing injectable hydrogels. In chitosan-g-PNIPAAm copolymer, chitosan chains could be considered as pendant chains instead of the backbone. Thus, the initial hydrophilic/hydrophobic balance of the backbone did not change. Consequently, the LCST of the resulting hydrogels nearly underwent no change [65]. Although the swelling ratios of chitosan-g-PNIPAAm copolymer hydrogels underwent a sharp decrease around LCST, the thermosensitivity is influenced by the grafting ratio and concentrations. The higher the grafting ratio of PNIPAAm, the sharper the thermosensitivity [66]. Different concentrations of the chitosan-g-PNIPAAm copolymer solution had different thermosensitivities. In general, the lower the concentration, the higher the thermosensitivity. This may stem from the fact that with increasing concentration of the copolymer, the concentration of segments also increases. As a result, the free movement of segments is restricted, and hydrophobic association between macromolecules is strengthened to a certain extent, and so gels are rapidly formed [67].

Chitosan/PNIPAAm hydrogels also have excellent pH sensitivity. For example, Lee et al. [68] found that the swelling ratio of chitosan-g-PNIPAAm hydrogels decreases with increasing pH value. That is to say, the swelling behaviors of chitosan/PNIPAAm hydrogels can be controlled by temperature and pH, which endow these hydrogels with potential applications. However, some problems remain to be addressed, such as the possibility to prepare graft-copolymers with precise MW and MW distribution in the absence of chitosan-g-PNIPAAm. And some research found that acrylamide-based polymers, in general, are not suitable for biomedical applications due to cell toxicity. The presence of unreacted monomeric residues with acrylamide-based polymers may be responsible for their toxicity. The observation that acrylamide-based polymers activate platelets when in contact with blood, along with the poorly understood metabolism of PNIPAAm and its nondegradability, makes it difficult to win FDA approval [69]. Therefore, it can be expected that in the next few years an improvement of graft copolymerization of chitosan leads to the preparation of smart polymers based on chitosan with excellent biocompatibility.

5.3.2.3 Chitosan/PNVCL Hydrogels

Poly(N-vinylcaprolactam) (PNVCL) is one of several nonionic water-soluble polymers with thermosensitivity. Compared with PNIPAAm, PNVCL is nontoxic because it does not produce small amide derivatives upon hydrolysis. Aqueous PNVCL gels undergo two heat-induced transitions: a low-temperature transition at 31.5°C, attributed to microsegregation of hydrophobic domains, and a higher-temperature transition around 37.5°C, corresponding to the gel volume collapse itself [70]. Gong and coworkers [71] grafted carboxyl-terminated poly(N-vinylcaprolactam) (PNVCL–COOH) chains onto a chitosan backbone and found that its aqueous solution shows a temperature-dependent transmittance change due to the introduction of thermosensitive PNVCL graft chains. And the LCST value of chitosan-g-PNVCL is ca. 32°C, which is the same as that for pure PNVCL-COOH (cf. Figure 5.20). Above this temperature, disruption of hydrogen bonding with water and increasing hydrophobic interaction among caprolactam groups [72]. In addition, the thermosensitivity is influenced by the pH of the medium, and the phase transmittance in acidic medium is slightly higher than that in neutral or basic medium.

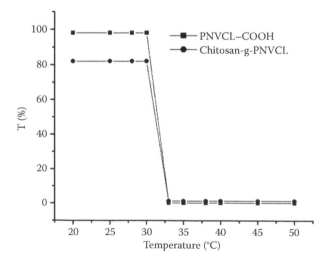

FIGURE 5.20
Optical transmittance of pure PNVCL–COOH (3% w/v) and chitosan-g-PNVCL copolymer (3% w/v) at pH 7.4.

5.4 Ionic Response

The swelling of chitosan-based hydrogels, especially for CS-PEC hydrogels, is affected by the ionic strength of the medium. Generally, the swelling capacity of chitosan-based hydrogels in salt solutions significantly decreases in comparison to that in distilled water. And the swelling degree decreases with increasing ionic concentration. The Donnan effect is considered as the main driving force for the swelling of chitosan-based gels. Therefore, with the increase of the ionic strength outside the gel, the ionic swelling pressure decreased, resulting in a decrease of swelling degree [73]. In addition, the type of salt also influences the swelling degree of chitosan-based hydrogels. For example, in comparison to the equilibrium swelling degree of chitosan/hydrolyzed polyacrylamide PEC hydrogels obtained with chloride salt solutions of the same concentration, the swelling capacity decreased with the charges of metal cations increasing ($K^+ > Mg^{2+} > Ca^{2+} > Al^{3+}$). This may be explained by the complexing ability arising from the coordination of the multivalent cations with carboxylate groups. This leads to an increase in the cross-linking density, which makes the network shrink [74]. Liu and coworkers [75] found a bit higher swelling capacity of chitosan/poly(methacrylic acid) hydrogels swollen in $CaCl_2$–HCl solution compared to those swollen in NaCl–HCl solution at the same ionic strength.

5.5 Electro-Response

Electrosensitive hydrogel is one kind of intelligent (smart) hydrogel, which can swell, shrink, or bend under electric stimulus. Sometimes, the hydrogels show swelling on one side and de-swelling on the other side, resulting in bending of the hydrogels. The deformation of a polymer hydrogel under an electric field is due to the voltage-induced motion of ions and the concomitant expansion of one side and contraction of the other. Chitosan, as a polycation polysaccharide, also have the electrosensitivity. Moreover, some cationic or anionic polymers are incorporated into the chitosan network in order to modulate the electro-responsive behaviors. In general, the electrosensitive capacity of these chitosan-based hydrogels is influenced by the following: (1) the pH value of the medium: Under electric field stimulation, chitosan/polycation hydrogels can experience greater swelling pressure on the side near the cathode than on the side near the anode and tended to bend toward the anode due to the protonation of $-NH_2$ and other cations. The blending capacity decreases in basic medium. For the same reason, amphoteric chitosan/polyanion hydrogels bend toward the anode in acidic medium. But they bend toward the cathode in basic medium, polyanions are ionized, and the amino groups remain in their original uncharged state [76] (*cf.* Figure 5.21); (2) the ionic strength of the medium: electrosensitive bending behavior does not occur in pure water because pure water is an insulating medium. Free ions of the medium are very necessary for realizing the electrosensitivity. Therefore, the ionic strength is another factor that influences the bending behavior of the hydrogels. There exists a critical ionic strength (CIS). The chitosan-based hydrogels exhibit maximal electrosensitive bending at CIS. Below CIS, the bending angle increases with increasing ionic strength. An increase in the ionic strength of a medium induces an increase in the free ions moving from the surrounding solution toward their counterelectrodes or into the chitosan-based hydrogels itself. However, above the CIS, the bending angle decreases with

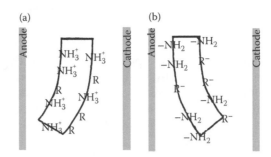

FIGURE 5.21
Bending motion of amphoteric chitosan/polyanion hydrogels in different electrolyte pH solutions. (a) Acidic medium and (b) basic medium.

increasing ionic strength, which is because a shielding effect of the polyions, by the other ions in the electrolytic solute, would occur, leading to a reduction in the electrostatic repulsion of the polyions. For example, Kim et al. [77] found that the equilibrium bending angle of the chitosan/poly(hydroxyethyl methacrylate) semi-IPN hydrogel showed an apparent peak with a 1.0 wt% aqueous NaCl solution; (3) the electric voltage: the effect of electric voltage was quite simple; that is, the higher the electric voltage applied, the higher the bending rate and the greater the equilibrium bending angle the hydrogel shows. And it exhibits a reversible bending behavior in proportion to the applied electric field. For example, the chitosan/hyaluronic acid PEC hydrogels showed a reversible bending behavior during voltage cyclic loading (*cf.* Figure 5.22) [78].

Chitosan-based electric-sensitive hydrogels could be used in drug delivery systems. Control of the "on–off" of drug release is achieved by varying the intensity of electric stimulation. And reversible behaviors endow it with potential applications in artificial muscles. However, at present, this application-based electric-sensitive chitosan-based hydrogels are still in their infancy because these hydrogels require a controllable voltage source [79].

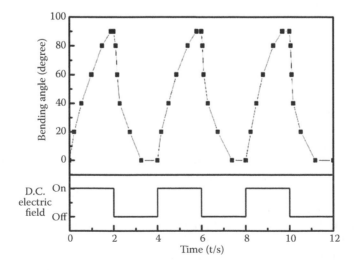

FIGURE 5.22
Reversible bending behavior of the chitosan/hyaluronic acid PEC hydrogels in a 0.8 wt% aqueous NaCl solution with changes in the applied voltage.

5.6 Summary

Stimuli-responsive chitosan-based hydrogels have been developed recently. Most chitosan-based hydrogels have dual- or multi-sensitivity. These responsive properties endow chitosan-based hydrogels with a wide range of potential biomedical applications, such as drug delivery systems and tissue engineering.

For tissue engineering, thermosensitive chitosan-based hydrogels could be used as the injectable hydrogels for cartilage or bone tissue. Artificial muscles could be prepared using electrosensitive chitosan-based hydrogels. However, low responsive rate and low mechanical strength limit their application. With an understanding of the stimuli-responsive mechanism, responsive rate controllable chitosan-based hydrogels should be designed by changing the structure and composition of the chitosan network or by changing the size of hydrogels. For example, the thermosensitive capacity could modulate the hydrophilic–hydrophobic balance. Chemical cross-linking is an effective method for improving the mechanical properties. The choice of the cross-linking agent is very critical due to toxicity of some cross-linking agents. Moreover, the responsive capacity may decrease or even disappear due to the cross-linking effect. Therefore, it is a great challenge to develop a novel chitosan-based hydrogel with rapid responsive capacity and excellent mechanical strength. With respect to drug delivery, chitosan-based hydrogels that can respond to their environments will provide new and improved methods of delivering molecules for therapeutic applications. One can select the chitosan-based hydrogels according to the type and properties of drug. In order to adapt the complexity of life system, the chitosan-based hydrogels should have gradient stimuli responsiveness.

References

1. Peppas, N. A., Hilt, J. Z., Khademhosseini, A., and Langer, R. 2006. Hydrogels in biology and medicine: From molecular principles to bionanotechnology. *Adv Mater* 18: 1345–1360.
2. Gehrke, S. H. and Cussler, E. L. 1989. Mass transfer in pH-sensitive hydrogels. *Chem Eng Sci* 44: 559–566.
3. Gupta, P., Vermani, K., and Garg, S. 2002. Hydrogels: From controlled release to pH-responsive drug delivery. *Drug Discov Today* 7: 569–579.
4. Montembault, A., Viton, C., and Domard, A. 2005. Rapidly *in situ* forming hydrophobically-modified chitosan hydrogels via pH-responsive nanostructure transformation. *Biomacromolecules* 6: 653–662.
5. Landes, C. A. and Kriener, S. 2003. Resorbable plate osteosynthesis of sagittal split osteotomies with major bone movement. *Plast Reconstr Surg* 111: 1828–1840.
6. Qu, X., Wirsen, A., and Albertsson, A. C. 1999. Structural change and swelling mechanism of pH-sensitive hydrogels based on chitosan and D, L-lactic acid. *J Appl Polym Sci* 74: 3186–3192.
7. Qu, X., Wirsen, A., and Albertsson, A. C. 2000. Novel pH-sensitive chitosan hydrogels: Swelling behavior and states of water. *Polymer* 41: 4589–4598.
8. Yao, F. L., Chen, W., Wang, H., Liu, H. F., Yao, K. D., Sun, P. C., and Hai Lin, H. 2003. A study on cytocompatible poly(chitosan-g-L-lactic acid). *Polymer* 44: 6435–6441.
9. Yao, F. L., Liu, C., Chen, W., Bai, Y., Tang, Z. Y., and Yao, K. D. 2003. Synthesis and characterization of chitosan grafted Oligo(L-lactic acid). *Macromol Biosci* 3: 653–656.

10. Chiu, Y. L., Chen, M. C., Chen, C. Y., Lee, P. W., Mi, F. L., Jeng, U. S., Chen, H. L., and Sung, H. W. 2009. Rapidly *in situ* forming hydrophobically-modified chitosan hydrogels via pH-responsive nanostructure transformation. *Soft Matter* 5: 962–965.

11. Ye, Y. Q., Feng-Liang Yang, F. L., Hu, F. Q., Du, Y. Z., Yuan, H., and He-Yong Yu, H. Y. 2008. Core-modified chitosan-based polymeric micelles for controlled release of doxorubicin. *Int J Pharm* 352: 294–301.

12. Bao, H. Q., Hu, J. H., Gan, L. H., and Li, H. 2009. Stepped association of comb-like and stimuli-responsive graft chitosan copolymer synthesized using ATRP and active ester conjugation methods. *J Polym Sci A: Polym Chem* 47: 6682–6697.

13. Yao, K. D., Tu, H. L., Chang, F., Zhang, J. W., and Liu, J. 1997. pH sensitivity of the swelling of a chitosan–pectin polyelectrolyte complex. *Angew Makromol Chem* 245: 63–72.

14. Yoshizawa, T., Shin-ya, Y., Hong, K. J., and Kajiuchi, T. 2004. pH- and thermosensitive permeation through polyelectrolyte complex films composed of chitosan and polyalkyleneoxide–maleic acid copolymer. *J Membr Sci* 241: 347–354.

15. Yoshizawa, T., Shin-ya, Y., Hong, K. J., and Kajiuchi, T. 2005. pH- and thermosensitive release behaviors from polyelectrolyte complex films composed of chitosan and PAOMA copolymer. *Eur J Pharm Biopharm* 59: 307–313.

16. Chen, S. C., Wu, Y. C., Mi, F. L., Lin, Y. H., Yu, L. C., and Sung, H. W. 2004. A novel pH-sensitive hydrogel composed of *N,O*-carboxymethyl chitosan and alginate cross-linked by genipin for protein drug delivery. *J Control Release* 96: 285–300.

17. Lin, Y. W., Chen, Q., and Luo, H. B., 2007. Preparation and characterization of *N*-(2-carboxybenzyl)chitosan as a potential pH-sensitive hydrogel for drug delivery. *Carbohyd Res* 342: 87–95.

18. Yang, L. M., Shi, L. L, Chen, J., Pei, Y., Zhu, F., and Xia, Y. B. 2005. Preparation and characterization of pH-sensitive hydrogel film of chitosan/poly(acrylic acid) copolymer. *Macromol Symp* 225: 95–102.

19. Yao, K. D., Peng, T., Feng, H. B., and He, Y. J. 1994. Swelling kinetics and release characteristic of cross-linked chitosan: Polyether polymer network (semi-IPN) hydrogels. *J Polym Sci A: Polym Chem* 32: 1213–1223.

20. Guan, Y. L., Shao. L., Liu, J., and Yao, K. D. 1996. pH effect on correlation between water state and swelling kinetics of the cross-linked chitosan/polyether semi-IPN hydrogel. *J Appl Polym Sci* 62: 1253–1258.

21. Yao, K. D., Peng, T., Goosen, M. F. A., Min, J. M., and He, Y. Y. 1993. pH-sensitivity of hydrogels based on complex forming chitosan–polyether interpenetrating polymer network. *J Appl Polym Sci* 48: 354–353.

22. Yao, K. D., Liu, J., Cheng, G. X., Zhao, R. Z., Wang, W. H., and Wei, L. 1998. The dynamic swelling behaviour of chitosan-based hydrogels. *Polym Int* 45: 191–194.

23. Wang, T. and Gunasekaran, S. 2006. State of water in chitosan–PVA hydrogel. *J Appl Polym Sci* 101: 3227–3232.

24. Yao, K. D., Yin, Y. J., Xu, M. X., and Feng, Y. 1995. Investigation of pH-sensitive drug delivery system of chitosan/gelatin hybrid polymer network. *Polym Int* 38: 77–82.

25. Yao, K. D., Liu, W. G., Lin, Z., and Qiu, X. H. 1999. *In situ* atomic force microscopy measurement of the dynamic variation in the elastic modulus of swollen chitosan/gelatin hybrid polymer network gels in media of different pH. *Polym Int* 48: 794–798.

26. Mao, J. S., Kondu, S., Ji, H. F., and McShane, M. J. 2006. Study of the near-neutral pH-sensitivity of chitosan/gelatin hydrogels by turbidimetry and microcantilever deflection. *Biotechnol Bioeng* 95: 333–341.

27. Klouda, L., Antonios G., and Mikos, A. G. 2008. Thermoresponsive hydrogels in biomedical applications. *Eur J Pharm Biopharm* 68: 34–45.

28. Carreira, A. S., Gonçalves, F. A. M. M., Mendonça, P. V., Gil, M. H., and Coelho, J. F. J. 2010. Temperature and pH responsive polymers based on chitosan: Applications and new graft copolymerization strategies based on living radical polymerization. *Carbohyd Polym* 80: 618–630.

29. Bhattarai, N., Gunn, J., and Zhang, M. Q. 2010. Chitosan-based hydrogels for controlled, localized drug delivery. *Adv Drug Deliv Rev* 62: 83–99.

30. Back, J. F., Oakenfull, D., and Smith, M. B. 1979. Increased thermal stability of proteins in the presence of sugars and polyols. *Biochemistry* 18: 5191–5196.
31. Wei, C. Z., Chun-Lin Hou, C. L., Qi-Sheng Gu, Q. S., Jiang, L. X., Zhu, B., and Sheng, A. S. 2009. A thermosensitive chitosan-based hydrogel barrier for post-operative adhesions' prevention. *Biomaterials* 30: 5534–5540.
32. Dang, J. M., Sun, D. D. N., Shin-Ya, Y., Sieber, A. N., Kostuik, J. P., and Leonga, K. W. 2006. Temperature-responsive hydroxybutyl chitosan for the culture of mesenchymal stem cells and intervertebral disk cells. *Biomaterials* 27: 406–418.
33. Chen, B. Y., Dang, J., Tan, T. L., Fang, N., Chen, W. N., Leong, K. W., and Chan, V. 2007. Dynamics of smooth muscle cell deadhesion from thermosensitive hydroxybutyl chitosan. *Biomaterials* 28: 1503–1514.
34. Bhattarai, N., Ramay, H. R., Gunn, J., Matsen, F. A., and Zhang, M. Q. 2005. PEG-grafted chitosan as an injectable thermosensitive hydrogel for sustained protein release. *J Control Release* 103: 609–624.
35. Bhattarai, N., Matsen, F. A., and Zhang, M. Q. 2005. PEG-grafted chitosan as an injectable thermoreversible hydrogel. *Macromol Biosci* 5: 107–111.
36. Ganji, F. and Abdekhodaie, M. J. 2008. Synthesis and characterization of a new thermosensitive chitosan–PEG diblock copolymer. *Carbohyd Polym* 74: 435–441.
37. El-Sherbiny, I. M., Abdel-Bary, E. M., and Harding, D. R. K. 2006. Swelling characteristics and *in vitro* drug release study with pH- and thermally sensitive hydrogels based on modified chitosan. *J Appl Polym Sci* 102: 977–985.
38. Khurma, J. R. and Nand, A. V. 2008. Temperature and pH sensitive hydrogels composed of chitosan and poly (ethylene glycol). *Polym Bullet* 59: 805–812.
39. Tang, Y. F., Du, Y. M., Li, Y., Wang, X. Y., and Hu, X. W. 2009. A thermosensitive chitosan/poly(vinyl alcohol) hydrogel containing hydroxyapatite for protein delivery. *J Biomed Mater Res* 91A: 953–963.
40. Tang, Y. F., Du, Y. M., Hu, X. W., Shi, X. W., and Kennedy, J. F. 2007. Rheological characterisation of a novel thermosensitive chitosan/poly(vinyl alcohol) blend hydrogel. *Carbohyd Polym* 67: 491–499.
41. Qi, B. W., Yu, A. X., Zhu, S. B., Chen, B., and Li, Y. 2010. The preparation and cytocompatibility of injectable thermosensitive chitosan/poly(vinyl alcohol) hydrogel. *J Huazhong Univ Sci Technol Med Sci* 30: 89–93.
42. Chenite, A., Chaput, C., Wang, D., Combes, C., Buschmann, M. D., Hoemann, C. D, Leroux, J. C., Atkinson, B. L., Binette, F., and Selmani, A. 2000. Novel injectable neutral solutions of chitosan form biodegradable gels *in situ*. *Biomaterials* 21: 2155–2161.
43. Ruel-Gariepy, E., Shive, M., Bichara, A., Berrada, M., Dorothee Le Garrec, D. L, Cheniteb, A., and Lerouxa, J. C. 2004. A thermosensitive chitosan-based hydrogel for the local delivery of paclitaxel. *Eur J Pharm Biopharm* 57: 53–63.
44. Chenite, A., Buschmann, M., Wang, D., Chaput, C., and Kandani, N. 2001. Rheological characterisation of thermogelling chitosan/glycerol–phosphate solutions. *Carbohyd Polym* 46: 39–47.
45. Ruel-Gariepya, E., Cheniteb, A., Chaput, C., Guirguisa, S., and Leroux, J. C. 2000. Characterization of thermosensitive chitosan gels for the sustained delivery of drugs. *Int J Pharm* 203: 89–98.
46. Cho, J., Heuzey, M. C., Begin, A., and Carreau, P. J. 2005. Physical gelation of chitosan in the presence of α-glycerophosphate: The effect of temperature. *Biomacromolecules* 6: 3267–3275.
47. Wang, L. M. and Stegemann, J. P. 2010. Thermogelling chitosan and collagen composite hydrogels initiated with β-glycerophosphate for bone tissue engineering. *Biomaterials* 31: 3976–3985.
48. Zhou, H. Y., Xi Guang Chen, X. G., Kong, M., Liu, C. S., Cha, D. S., and Kennedy, J. F. 2008. Effect of molecular weight and degree of chitosan deacetylation on the preparation and characteristics of chitosan thermosensitive hydrogel as a delivery system. *Carbohyd Polym* 73: 265–273.
49. Crompton, K. E., Forsythe, J. S., Horne, M. K., Finkelsteincan, D. I., and Knott, R. B. 2009. Molecular level and microstructural characterisation of thermally sensitive chitosan hydrogels. *Soft Matter* 5: 4704–4711.

50. Filion, D., Lavertu, M., and Buschmann, M. D. 2007. Ionization and solubility of chitosan solutions related to thermosensitive chitosan/glycerol–phosphate systems. *Biomacromolecules* 8: 3224–3234.
51. Ganji, F., Abdekhodaie, M. J., and Ramazani, A. 2007. Gelation time and degradation rate of chitosan-based injectable hydrogel. *J Sol–Gel Sci Technol* 42: 47–53.
52. Zhao, Q. S., Cheng, X. J., Ji, Q. X., Kang, C. Z., and Chen, X. G. 2009. Effect of organic and inorganic acids on chitosan/glycerophosphate thermosensitive hydrogel. *J Sol–Gel Sci Technol* 50: 111–118.
53. Wu, J., Su, Z. G., and Ma, G. H. 2006. A thermo- and pH-sensitive hydrogel composed of quaternized chitosan/glycerophosphate. *Int J Pharm* 315: 1–11.
54. Rossi, S., Marciello, M., Bonferoni, M. C., Ferrari, F., Sandri, G., Dacarro, C., Grisoli, P., and Caramella, C. 2010. Thermally sensitive gels based on chitosan derivatives for the treatment of oral mucositis. *Eur J Pharm Biopharm* 74: 248–254.
55. Wu, J., Wei, W., Wang, L. Y., Su, Z. G., and Ma, G. H. 2007. A thermosensitive hydrogel based on quaternized chitosan and poly (ethylene glycol) for nasal drug delivery system. *Biomaterials* 28: 2220–2232.
56. Almgren, M., Bahadur, P., Jansson, M., Li, P., Brown, W., and Bahadur, A. 1992. Static and dynamic properties of a (PEO–PPO–PEO) block copolymer in aqueous solution. *J Colloid Interface Sci* 151: 157–165.
57. Chung, H. J., Go, D. H., Bae, J. W., Jung, I. K., Joon Woo Lee, J. W., and Park, K. D. 2005. Synthesis and characterization of Pluronic grafted chitosan copolymer as a novel injectable biomaterial. *Current Appl Phys* 5: 485–488.
58. Park, K. M., Lee, S. Y., Joung, Y. K., Na, J. S., Lee, M. C., and Park, K. D. 2009. Thermosensitive chitosan–Pluronic hydrogel as an injectable cell delivery carrier for cartilage regeneration. *Acta Biomater* 5: 1956–1965.
59. Schild, H. G. 1992. Poly(N-isopropylacrylamide): Experiment, theory and application. *Prog Polym Sci* 17: 163–249.
60. Lee, W. F. and Chen, Y. J. 2001. Studies on preparation and swelling properties of the N-isopropylacrylamide/chitosan semi-IPN and IPN hydrogels. *J Appl Polym Sci* 82: 2487–2496.
61. Chen, X. C., Song, H., Fang, T., Bai, J. X., Jian Xiong, J., and Ying, H. J. 2010. Preparation, characterization, and drug-release properties of pH/temperature-responsive poly(N-isopropylacrylamide)/chitosan semi-IPN hydrogel particles. *J Appl Polym Sci* 116: 1342–1347.
62. Guo, B. L. and Gao, Q. Y. 2007. Preparation and properties of a pH/temperature-responsive carboxymethyl chitosan/poly(N-isopropylacrylamide) semi-IPN hydrogel for oral delivery of drugs. *Carbohyd Res* 342: 2416–2422.
63. Sun, G. M., Zhang, X. Z., and Chu, C. C. 2007. Formulation and characterization of chitosan-based hydrogel films having both temperature and pH sensitivity. *J Mater Sci: Mater Med* 18: 1563–1577.
64. Verestiuc, L., Ivanov, C., Barbu, E., and Tsibouklis, J. 2004. Dual-stimuli-responsive hydrogels based on poly (N-isopropylacrylamide)/chitosan semi-interpenetrating networks. *Int J Pharm* 269: 185–194.
65. Zhang, F. F., Zhong, H., Zhang, L. L., Chen, S. B., Zhao, Y. J., and Zhu, Y. L. 2009. Synthesis and characterization of thermosensitive graft copolymer of N-isopropylacrylamide with biodegradable carboxymethylchitosan. *Carbohyd Polym* 77: 785–790.
66. Don, R. M. and Chen, H. R. 2005. Synthesis and characterization of AB-cross-linked graft copolymers based on maleilated chitosan and N-isopropylacrylamide. *Carbohyd Polym* 61: 334–347.
67. Guo, B. L., Yuan, J. F., and Gao, Q. Y. 2008. Preparation and release behavior of temperature- and pH-responsive chitosan material. *Polym Int* 57: 463–468.
68. Lee, S. B., Ha, D. I., Cho, S. C., Kim, S. J., and Lee, Y. M. 2004. Temperature/pH-sensitive comb-type graft hydrogels composed of chitosan and poly (N-isopropylacrylamide). *J Appl Polym Sci* 92: 2612–2620.
69. Hatefi, A. and Amsden, B. 2002. Biodegradable injectable *in situ* forming drug delivery systems. *J Control Release* 80: 9–28.

70. Mikheeva, L. M., Grinberg, N. V., Mashkevich, A. Ya., and Grinberg, V. Ya. 1997. Microcalorimetric study of thermal cooperative transitions in poly(*N*-vinylcaprolactam) hydrogels. *Macromolecules* 30: 2693–2699.

71. Prabaharan, M., Grailer, J. J., Steeber, D. A., and Gong, S. Q. 2008. Stimuli-responsive chitosan-graft-poly (*N*-vinylcaprolactam) as a promising material for controlled hydrophobic drug delivery. *Macromol Biosci* 8: 843–851.

72. Laukkanen, A., Valtola, L., Winnik, F. M., and Tenhu, H. 2004. Formation of colloidally stable phase separated poly (*N*-vinylcaprolactam) in water: A study by dynamic light scattering, microcalorimetry, and pressure perturbation calorimetry. *Macromolecules* 37: 2268–2274.

73. Chen, L. Y., Du, Y. M., and Huang, R. H. 2003. Novel pH, ion sensitive polyampholyte gels based on carboxymethyl chitosan and gelatin. *Polym Int* 52: 56–61.

74. Cao, J., Tan, Y. B., Che, Y. J., and Ma, Q. 2010. Fabrication and properties of superabsorbent complex gel beads composed of hydrolyzed polyacrylamide and chitosan. *J Appl Polym Sci* 116: 3338–3345.

75. Chen, S. L., Liu, M. Z., Jin, S. P., and Chen, Y. 2005. Synthesis and swelling properties of pH-sensitive hydrogels based on chitosan and poly(methacrylic acid) semi-interpenetrating polymer network. *J Appl Polym Sci* 98: 1720–1726.

76. Shang, J., Shao, Z. Z., and Chen, X. 2008. Electrical behavior of a natural polyelectrolyte hydrogel: chitosan/carboxymethylcellulose hydrogel. *Biomacromolecules* 9: 1208–1213.

77. Kim, S. J., Kim, H. I., Shin, S. R., and Kim, S. I. 2004. Electrical behavior of chitosan and poly(hydroxyethyl methacrylate) hydrogel in the contact system. *J Appl Polym Sci* 92: 915–919.

78. Kim, S. J., Yoon, S. G., Lee, K. B., Park, Y. D., and Kim. S. I.. 2003. Electrical sensitive behavior of a polyelectrolyte complex composed of chitosan/hyaluronic acid. *Solid State Ion* 164: 199–204.

79. Qiu, Y. and Park, K. 2001. Environment-sensitive hydrogels for drug delivery. *Adv Drug Deliv Rev* 53: 321–339.

6

Chitosan-Based Gels for the Drug Delivery System

Jin Zhao

CONTENTS

6.1 Introduction

To date, a large number of active compounds have been discovered that serve as therapeutics for curing complex disease. Yet, very few have shown clinical success. One major challenge is the delivery of an effective dose of a given cytotoxic agent to the target site without losing its functionality, while at the same time minimizing unintended harmful side effects [1]. As is well known, during systemic administration, drugs lose functionality very soon and the blood plasma concentration of the drug can quickly drop below an effective level. Readministration is required, leading to an increase in the risk of an overdose. Another problem is that many medications such as peptide and protein, antibody, vaccine, and gene-based drugs, in general, may not be delivered using common routes because they might be susceptible to enzymatic degradation or cannot be absorbed into the systemic circulation efficiently in order to be therapeutically effective, due to molecular size and charge issues [2].

Under such circumstances, a drug delivery system (DDS) becomes an alternative technique for improving the pharmacological properties of traditional chemotherapeutics. Active therapeutics are incorporated into a polymeric network structure, and drug release profile, absorption, distribution, and elimination are modified in order to improve product efficacy and safety as well as patient convenience and compliance [3]. According to the application, the drug is released from a formulation over a period of time from a few hours to a month to several years in a controlled manner. A large variety of synthetic and natural polymers have been studied as drug carriers, such as poly(L-lactic acid) and its copolymers poly(L-glycolic acid) (PLGA), poly(ethylene glycol) (PEG) copolymers, poly(cyanoacrylates), poly(anhydrides), poly(ortho esters), polyphosphazene, poly(vinyl alcohol) (PVA), poly(vinyl pyrrolidone), poly(acrylic) acid (PAA), cellulose derivatives, hyaluronic acid derivatives, alginate, collagen, gelatin, starch, dextran, and chitosan. DDSs have capitalized on their wide-ranging hydrophobic and hydrophilic components and their polymer–polymer, polymer–drug, polymer–solvent, or polymer–physiological medium interactions [4]. Although many synthetic materials perform well for incorporating drugs and controlling sustained drug release, they may not be the most proper candidates due to their nonbiodegradability, relative hydrophobicity, and poor biocompatibility. Natural polymers such as collagen, hyaluronic acid, and chitosan have a number of advantages over synthetic polymers. For example, the need for harsh processing conditions is reduced, the material source is abundant, and production is both relatively environmentally safe and of low cost [5]. All these combined with the properties of good biocompatibility and biodegradability make natural macromolecules promising drug vehicles.

As most natural polymers are hydrophilic, they are usually in the form of hydrogel when used as drug carriers. Hydrogels are hydrated, water-insoluble polymeric networks cross-linked by water-soluble precursors [6–8]. They are able to swell and retain a significant portion of water but are not dissolved when placed in an aqueous solution [6,7]. The amount of water in the polymer matrix is at least 20% and can reach values of 99% by weight [9]. The design and preparation of hydrogels have significantly attracted the attention of the biomedical community because of their physiochemical similarity with the native extracellular matrix both compositionally and mechanically [8,10]. Unique properties such as biodegradability, tunable chemical and three-dimensional physical structure, good mechanical properties, high water content, and possible control over the swelling kinetics [11] have offered great potential for the utilization of hydrogels in drug delivery applications [12–15]. Their highly porous structure can easily be controlled by changing the density of cross-links in the gel matrix and the affinity of the hydrogels for the aqueous environment in which they are swollen. Their porosity also permits the loading of drugs into the gel vehicle and subsequent drug release at a rate dependent on the diffusion coefficient of the small molecule or macromolecule through the gel network. Indeed, the advantages of using hydrogels for drug delivery may be largely pharmacokinetic: specifically a depot formulation is created from which drugs slowly elute, maintaining a high local concentration of drugs in surrounding tissues over an extended period, although hydrogels can also be used for systemic delivery. Hydrogels are generally highly biocompatible, as reflected in their successful use in the peritoneum and other sites *in vivo*. Biocompatibility is promoted by the high water content of hydrogels and the physiochemical similarity of hydrogels to the native extracellular matrix, both compositionally (particularly in the case of carbohydrate-based hydrogels) and mechanically. Biodegradability or dissolution may be designed into hydrogels via enzymatic, hydrolytic, or environmental pathways. However, degradation is not always desirable depending on the timescale and location of the DDS. Hydrogels are also relatively deformable and can conform to the shape of the surface to which they are applied. In the latter context, the muco- or bioadhesive properties of some hydrogels can be advantageous in immobilizing them at the site of application or in applying them on surfaces that are not horizontal [10].

Moreover, hydrogels can be tailored into different shapes or geometries in terms of the requirements of the drug release profile. For example, they can be formulated into slabs, rods, nanoparticles, microspheres, membranes, sponges, films, and liquids [6,16].

Hydrogels also have several limitations. The low tensile strength of some hydrogels, when they are used in load-bearing applications, can lead to the premature dissolution or flowing away of the hydrogel from a targeted local site. The quantity and homogeneity of drug loading into hydrogels may be limited, particularly in the case of hydrophobic drugs. The high water content and large pore sizes of most hydrogels often result in relatively rapid drug release, from over a few hours to a few days. Efforts are being made to create novel hydrogel systems and improve the properties in order to solve these problems.

Among the effective drug release vehicles prepared by using natural polymer hydrogels, chitosan-based gels have received a great deal of attention because of their well-documented biocompatibility, biodegradability, low toxicity, mucoadhesivity as well as many other special properties [17]. In this chapter, we will focus on chitosan-based gels for DDS and their recent progress.

6.2 Chitosan and Chitosan Derivatives for DDS

Chitosan is a linear polysaccharide composed of randomly distributed β-(1–4)-linked D-glucosamine and *N*-acetyl-D-glucosamine units and has structural characteristics similar to glycosaminoglycans. It is generally prepared by alkaline deacetylation of chitin, which is the main component of the exoskeleton of crustaceans, such as shrimps. As chitin is the second most abundant natural biomacromolecule in nature, chitosan is easy to obtain. Chitosan shares the advantages of other natural polymers, including biocompatibility, low toxicity, and susceptibility to enzymatic degradation, but does not induce an immune response [4] and can be sterilized conveniently through many methods [18]. The primary amino groups impart special properties that make chitosan unique compared with other natural materials. Chitosan has pH-sensitive properties due to the protonation–deprotonation equilibrium of the amino groups, thus allowing the fabrication of pH-controlled release carriers that are based on chitosan [19]. Positively charged via protonation of aliphatic amines, chitosan is able to interact with negatively charged polymers, macromolecules, and polyanions on contact in an aqueous environment, which facilitates the incorporation of some macromolecule drugs [20]. Chitosan also has many other chemical and physical properties that have sparked great interest in its use as a matrix in DDS. For example, chitosan has antiulcer and antacid activities that prevent or weaken drug irritation in special delivery sites such as the stomach [21]. In addition, chitosan is mucoadhesive [22] and can adhere to mucosal surfaces. This property makes it a useful polymer for mucosal drug delivery. In view of the above-mentioned properties, chitosan is an ideal material for use as a drug vehicle and is extensively used in DDSs.

However, chitosan also has some disadvantages [20]: its low solubility at a physiological pH of 7.4 limits its use as an absorption enhancer in nasal or peroral delivery systems. Its ability to rapidly adsorb water and its higher swelling degree in aqueous environments lead to fast drug release, hardly supporting the sustained and controlled release of active agents. Chemical modification of chitosan is a powerful tool to control the interaction of polymer with drugs and to enhance load capability, improving bulk properties for the preparation of sustained drug release systems. On the other hand, chemical modification of chitosan is also extremely necessary when fabricating proper DDSs with the required release profile.

6.2.1 Functional Groups-Modified Chitosan

6.2.1.1 N-Alkylated Chitosan

Chitosan has a number of hydroxyl and amino groups along its molecular chain. These groups provide so much hydrogen bonding (H-bonding) between adjacent chains that chitosan cannot dissolve in neutral aqueous solution. This largely limits its clinical applications, for example, in the DDS. Alkylated chains were introduced into chitosan to break the strong interaction of neighboring molecules and make it soluble in a pH 7.4 environment [23]. By doing this, hydrophobic interactions are strengthened, and chitosan may become a candidate hydrophobic drug carrier for delivering drugs such as bleomycin with palmitoyl chains and taxol and vitamin B_2 (VB$_2$) with dodecyl chains [24]. Tien et al. [25] prepared N-acylated chitosan to introduce hydrophobicity for use as a matrix for drug delivery. It was found that derivatization reduced the hydration of the matrix and played a role in network stabilization by hydrophobic interactions. Acylation with longer side chains resulted in a higher degree of order and crushing strength but lower swelling. Drug dissolution kinetics showed longer release times for higher degrees of functionalization. Moreover, it was also reported that alkylated chitosan was proposed as a nonviral vector for gene transfection, because hydrophobic chains could weaken the strong interactions between primary amino groups and phosphate groups, which was reported to resist DNA unpacking within the cell to a certain degree [26]. As a result, transfection efficiency could be considerably increased by the incorporation of hydrophobic moieties.

Synthesis methods of N-alkylated chitosan have been reported by many groups. One common method is to dissolve chitosan in acetic acid and mix an aliphatic aldehyde into the solution subsequently. Through the addition of excess NaBH$_4$, the Schiff base formed is reduced and this leads to the final alkylation of chitosan [27] (*cf.* Figure 6.1). Another commonly used method was reported by Yao and coworkers [28]. Alkylated chitosans were prepared by modifying chitosan with alkyl bromide (*cf.* Figure 6.2).

6.2.1.2 Thiolated Chitosan

Thiol groups were introduced into chitosan. One motive is to enhance the mucoadhesive properties of chitosan. Thiolated chitosan has shown strong mucoadhesive properties by forming disulfide bonds with cysteine-rich domains of mucus glycoproteins, leading to an improvement in mucoadhesion of up to 140-fold that of unmodified chitosan [29]. The localization of a DDS at a given target site (i.e., nasal mucosa) was guaranteed and permeation of drugs was enhanced in this way. The study by Krauland et al. [30] showed that the bioavailability of an insulin-loaded chitosan-based vehicle via nasal administration was significantly greater for a thiolated chitosan carrier than for an unmodified

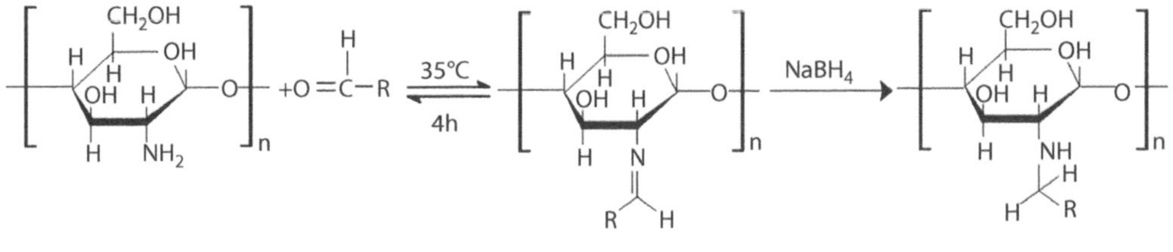

FIGURE 6.1
N-alkylated chitosan prepared via Schiff base reduction.

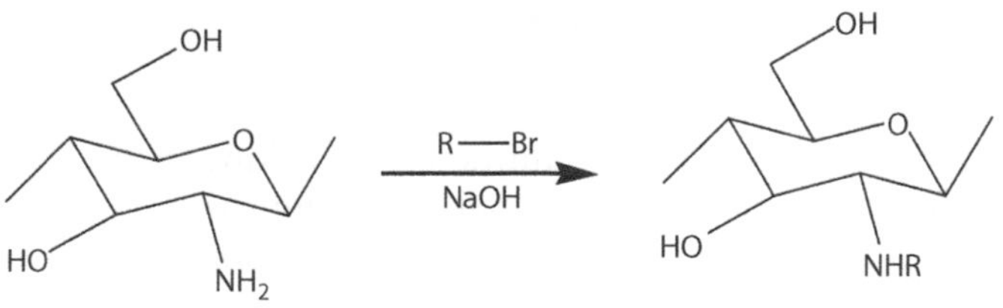

FIGURE 6.2
N-alkylated chitosan prepared with alkyl bromide.

chitosan carrier. Another important reason for the thiolation of chitosan lies in the motivation to increase the mechanical properties of the hydrogel and the introduction of *in situ* gelling features to the DDS. Hornof et al. [31] demonstrated that the elastic properties increased with increasing thiol group content. Krauland et al. showed that inter- and/or intramolecular disulfide bonds can be formed in order to obtain an *in situ* chitosan hydrogel [32]. The release of a fluorescent dextran can be controlled by the degree of this cross-linking process. Furthermore, as thiols are very active groups, they can easily interact with either acrylates or vinyl sulfones. Several kinds of *in situ* chitosan-based hydrogels for drug release can be prepared via Michael addition of the above functional groups [33,34].

Thiolated chitosan is usually synthesized by coupling chitosan with *N*-acetyl-L-cysteine via 1-ethy-3-(3-dimethylaminopropyl-carbodiimide) hydrochloride (EDAC.HCl) and 1-hydroxybenzotrizole (*cf.* Figure 6.3) [33].

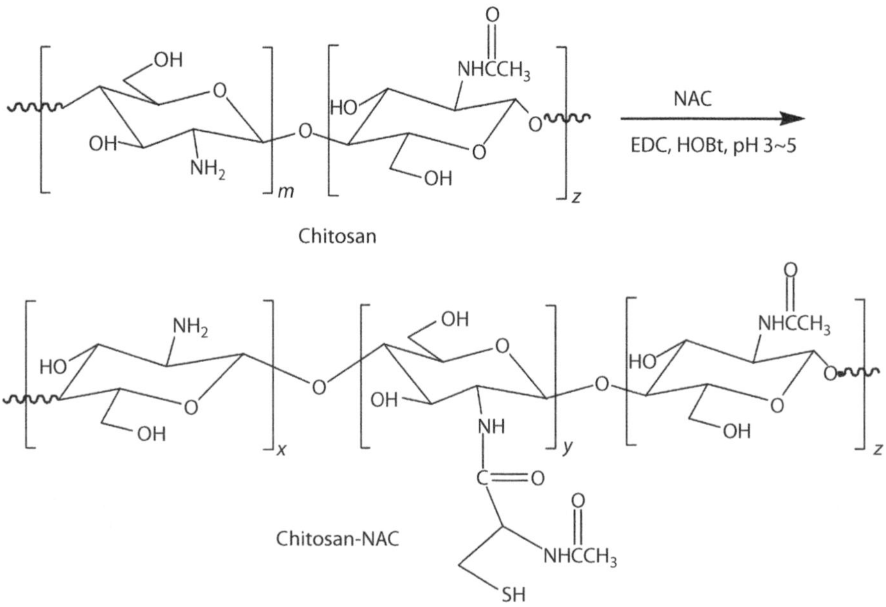

FIGURE 6.3
Synthesis of thiol-containing chitosan.

6.2.2 Polymer-Grafted Chitosan

Apart from some functional groups, polymers were also incorporated into chitosan as grafted chains to modulate the hydrophilic and hydrophobic equilibrium of hydrogel, to obtain different drug release profiles according to the practical requirements, to tailor the degradation behavior, or to create an *in situ* gelation drug vehicle.

6.2.2.1 Chitosan-g-Pluronic

Pluronic is a temperature-sensitive triblock copolymer of poly(ethylene oxide)/poly (propylene oxide)/poly(ethylene oxide) (PEO–PPO–PEO), consisting of more than 30 different nonionic surface-active agents, with ethylene oxide/propylene oxide weight ratios varying from 1:9 to 8:2. Pluronic series were liquid at room temperature or below and were found to form a gel at different elevated temperatures. Chung et al. [35] coupled chitosan and monocarboxy Pluronic using 1-ethyl-3-(3-dimethylaminopropyl)-carbodiimide (EDC) and N-hydroxysuccinimide (NHS) as coupling agents (*cf.* Figure 6.4). In this way, chitosan became soluble in physiological conditions and turned into a thermosensitive hydrogel used for DDSs with a sol–gel transition at body temperature. The most important fact was

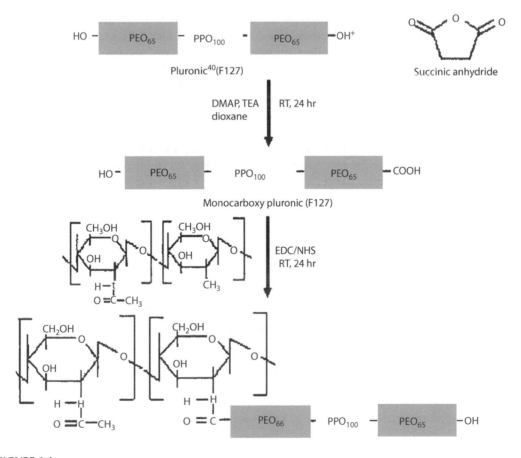

FIGURE 6.4
Schematic representation of the procedure for preparation of chitosan-Pluronic. (From Chung, H. J. et al. 2005. *Macromol Symp* 224: 275–286. With permission.)

that the hydrophobic block was introduced into chitosan, which could change the strong hydrophilicity of chitosan and improve its properties as a DDS. The decomposition of the ester linkages as well as the degradation of chitosan in the hydrogel caused the collapse of the gel, which may last for 30 days [36]. The degradation behavior can be adjusted by the ratio of ethylene oxide/propylene oxide, grafting percentage, and molecular weight of Pluronic.

6.2.2.2 Chitosan-g-PEG

Bhattarai et al. [37,38] also developed a chitosan-poly(ethylene oxide) (PEO) copolymer (chitosan-g-PEG) that was produced by chemically grafting monohydroxy PEG onto the chitosan backbone using Schiff base and sodium cyanoborohydride chemistry (*cf.* Figure 6.5). The resultant copolymer was an injectable liquid at low temperature and transformed to a semisolid hydrogel at body temperature. The hydrogel was proved to be capable of acting as a protein drug carrier by studying the release of bovine serum albumin (BSA) as a model protein [38].

6.2.2.3 Chitosan-g-Cyclodextrin [20]

Cyclodextrin has gained prominence in recent years because its hydrophobic cavity is capable of binding aromatic and other small organic molecules [20], and therefore facilitates the entrapment and controlled release of hydrophobic drugs [10]. Chitosan-g-cyclodextrin is one of the most attractive drug vehicles for delivering hydrophobic molecules. Tojima et al. [39] prepared chitosan-g-cyclodextrin via the reductive amination strategy (*cf.* Figure 6.6). Briefly, an aldehyde group was introduced into α-cyclodextrin. The aldehyde group reacted with the amine group of chitosan when mixing their solutions to form Schiff base, which was subsequently reduced using $NaBH_3CN$ as the reductive agent. A coupling reaction was also employed to prepare chitosan-g-cyclodextrin by using EDC [40]. Details of the reaction procedure are shown in Figure 6.7 [20].

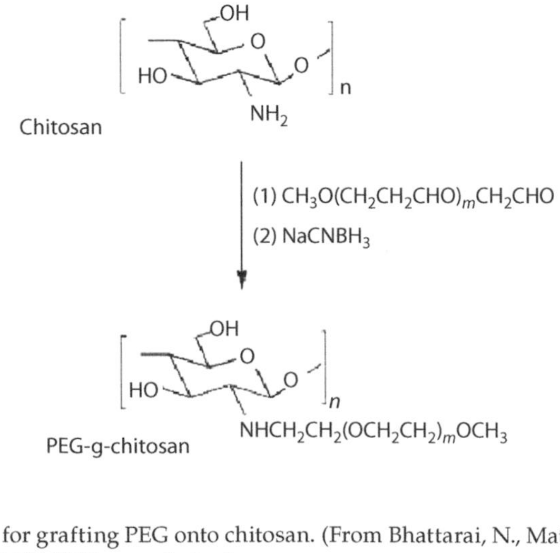

FIGURE 6.5
Chemical reaction scheme for grafting PEG onto chitosan. (From Bhattarai, N., Matsen, F. A., and Zhang, M. Q. 2005. *Macromol Biosci* 5: 107–111. With permission.)

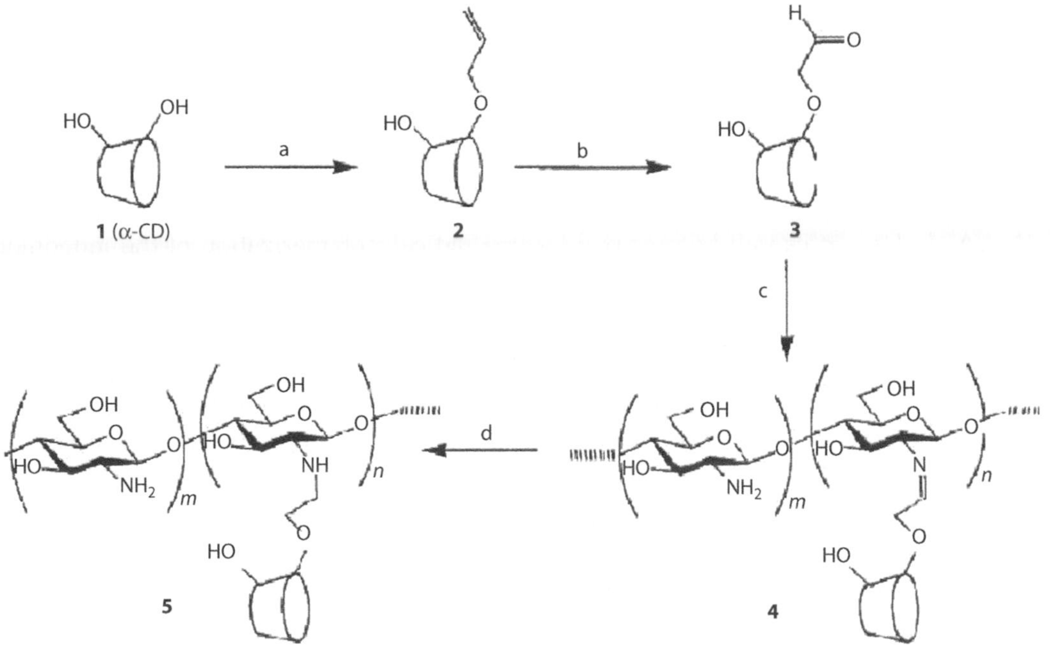

FIGURE 6.6
Preparation of chitosan-g-cyclodextrin via the reductive amination strategy. Reagent and conditions: (a) LiH–LiI, DMSO, and then allyl bromide; (b) O3 in 50% aqueous MeOH; (c) chitosan in acetate buffer (pH 4.4); and (d) NaBH$_3$CN in acetate buffer (pH 4.4). (From Tojima, T. et al. 1998. *J Polym Sci A Polym Chem* 36: 1965–1968. With permission.)

6.2.3 Graft Copolymer of Chitosan

Another way of improving chitosan performance and enlarging its potential applications is chemical modification of chitosan by grafting vinyl monomer(s) [41] and initiating the monomer's free radical polymerization.

One of the more intensively investigated monomers is *N*-isopropylacrylamide (NIPAM), whose polymer is well known to have a thermally reversible property. It has a lower critical solution temperature (LCST) of around 32°C in aqueous solution, that is, it dissolves in water below the LCST and precipitates from aqueous solution above the LCST [35].

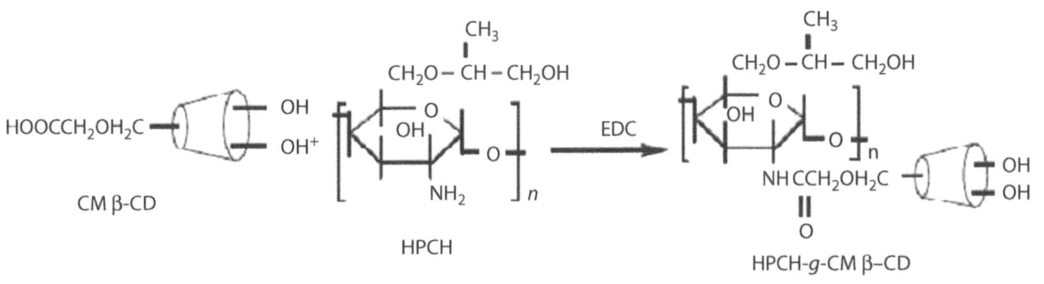

FIGURE 6.7
Preparation of chitosan-g-cyclodextrin by using EDC coupling reaction. (From Mani, P. 2008. *J Biomater Appl* 23: 5–35. With permission.)

This characteristic is an advantage in the design of DDSs. Grafting poly(N-isopropylacrylamide) (PNIPAAm) onto chitosan provided chitosan temperature-responsive properties and improved the mechanical properties of its hydrogel [41]. Chung et al. [35] prepared chitosan-g-PNIPAAm copolymer by graft polymerization of NIPAM onto chitosan using cerium ammonium nitrate as an initiator (*cf.* Figure 6.8). The efficiency and percentage of copolymerization increased as monomer concentration increased. Similar work has been done by Kim et al. [42] and Cai et al. [43]. Different chitosan graft copolymers with HEMA, AA, VA, and so on can all be prepared by free radical polymerization of the monomer using cerium ammonium nitrate as initiator [44–46]. The synthesis procedure was similar to the above reports. Drug/chitosan-based hydrogel interaction, hydrogel properties, that is, swelling behavior, and drug release profile greatly depended on the type of graft molecules and the grafting amount of these monomers. However, the greatest disadvantage of this method is that the molecular weights and the molecular weight distributions of the synthetic polymer side chain cannot be controlled as desired due to the reaction feature of free radical polymerization.

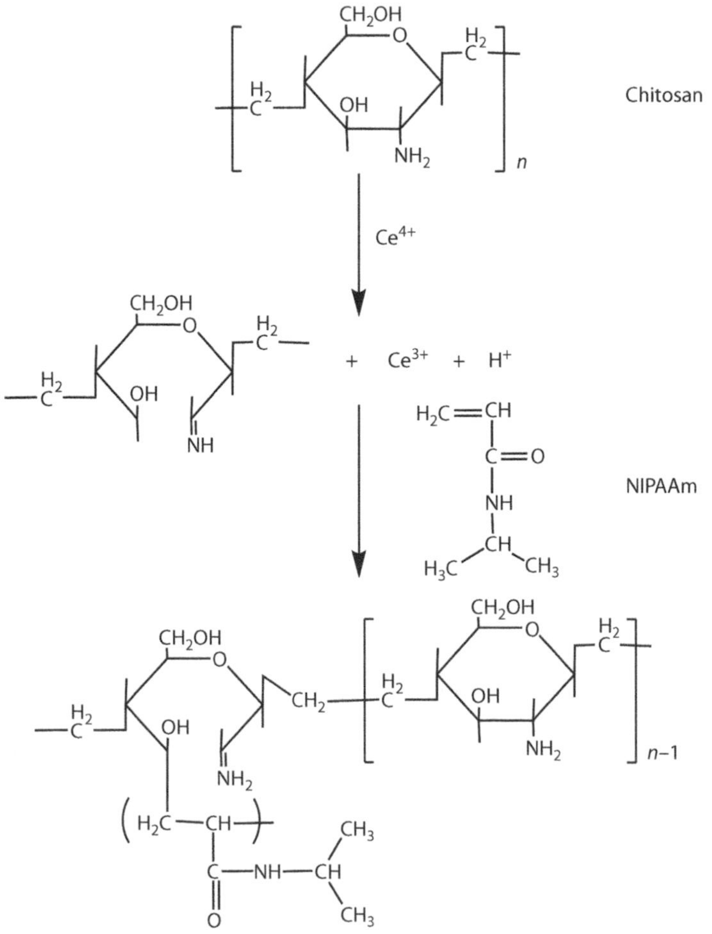

FIGURE 6.8
Schematic representation of the procedure for preparation of chitosan-g-PNIPAAm.

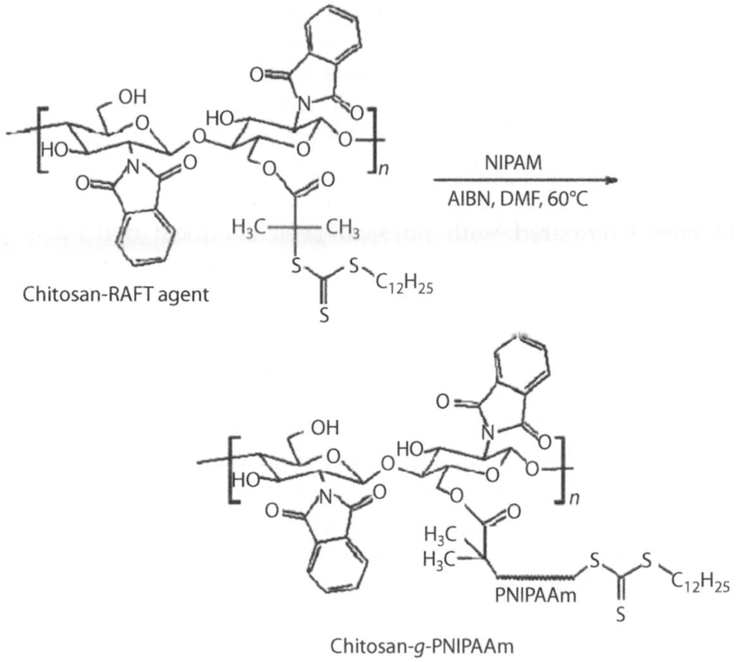

FIGURE 6.9
Schematic representation of the modifications and graft polymerization of chitosan by using the RAFT approach (From Tang, J. et al. 2008. *Int. J. Biol. Macromol.* 43: 383–389. With permission.)

Recently, controlled/living radical polymerization methods, such as atom transfer radical polymerization and reversible addition fragmentation transfer (RAFT), were employed to synthesize chitosan graft copolymers with controlled topologies and graft-controlled segments. Zhu and coworkers [47] were the first research team to successfully synthesize chitosan-g-PNIPAAm and chitosan-g-PAA using the RAFT approach (*cf.* Figure 6.9). They prepared chitosan-RAFT agents in dry dimethylformamide (DMF) by reacting N-phthaloylchitosan with S-1-dodecyl-S'-(α,α'-dimethyl-α"-acetic acid)trithiocarbonate in the presence of 1,3-dicyclohexylcarbodiimide and 4-(N, N-dimethylamino)pyridine. Both graft copolymers were carried out in dry DMF, using azobisisobutyronitrile as initiator. The results showed that PNIPAAms from the polymerization mixtures had controlled molecular weights and narrow molecular weight distributions [47]. The "well-defined" chitosan-g-PNIPAAms with thermally responsive property would enable chitosan to be used in drug delivery applications [47].

6.3 Chitosan-Based Gel Formation Principles

Irrespective of the kinds of shapes and geometries the chitosan hydrogels are in, they are formed by physical or chemical cross-links of the macromolecules [4,6,9,10], being appropriately used to give the three-dimensional structures specific mechanical and chemical characteristics. The cross-link can be formed by covalent or noncovalent interactions. Noncovalent hydrogels are called physical gels when the networks are cross-linked through molecular entanglements and secondary forces such as H-bonding, ionic force and hydrophobic association while covalently cross-linked hydrogels are called chemical gels [6]. The biggest advantage of physical hydrogels as drug vehicles is that no toxic cross-linking entities are involved during gel formation. Yet they have their limitations. These vehicles always suffer from weak mechanical strength, uncontrolled dissolution of the hydrogel, and fast release of drugs. It is also difficult to precisely control physical gel pore size, chemical functionalization, and degradation or dissolution, leading to inconsistent performance *in vivo*. Compared with physical gels, chemical hydrogels provide good mechanical strength and controllable drug release profiles but suffer from side effects [48]. A wide range of cross-linking strategies can be used, including using some cross-linking agents, polymerization, and various other chemical cross-linking techniques. The main disadvantage of this approach is that toxic reagents need to be completely removed prior to hydrogel implantation, which may be difficult to achieve without also leaching loaded drugs out of the hydrogel [10]. Another issue is that chemical hydrogels have a defined dimensionality and high elasticity, which hinder their extrusion through a needle when implanted *in vivo*. Converting the preformed gel into micro- or nanoparticles, or an *in situ* gelation system can sometimes solve the latter problem; however, potential risks of exposure to irradiation and the use of toxic cross-linkers should be deliberatively considered. Today, both physical and chemical cross-linking strategies are being pursued to achieve *in situ* gelation [10].

6.3.1 Physical Cross-Linked Hydrogels

There are three major physical interactions (i.e., charge interactions, hydrophobic associations, and H-bonding) that lead to the gelation of a chitosan solution in response to the environmental stimuli of pH, temperature, or ionic strength.

6.3.1.1 Charge Interactions

Charge interactions may occur between a polymer and a small molecule or between two polymers of opposite charge to form a hydrogel.

As for small-molecule cross-linking, chitosan, as a polycation owing to the protonation of amino groups, interacts with negatively charged molecules through an electrostatic force. Small negatively charged molecules, that is, sulfate, citrate, and tripolyphosphate (TPP), were reported to be capable of forming ionic complexes with chitosan [49,50]. The properties of their hydrogels were influenced by the degree of deacetylation and concentration of chitosan and particularly by the charge density and size of the anionic agents. In this kind of system, attention should be paid to the fact that chitosan has a pK_a of ca. 6.5 and may possess little or no charge above pH 6, limiting its ability to form ionic complexes. Therefore, anionic molecules that retain a high charge density must be chosen to ensure strong ionic interactions and to have a small enough molecular weight to freely diffuse throughout the polymer matrix and quickly form electrostatic bonds [4].

As for polymer–polymer cross-linking, chitosan, a cationic polysaccharide, has been complexed with anionic polymers, such as proteins (i.e., collagen, gelatin, and fibroin), anionic polysaccharides (i.e., pectin, carboxymethyl cellulose, and alginate), and anionic synthetic polymers (i.e., polyalkyleneoxide–maleic acid (PAOMA) copolymer), to form polyelectrolyte complexes (PECs) [51]. The properties of PECs are mainly determined by the degree of interaction between individual polymers. The latter condition depends essentially on their global charge densities and determines their relative composition in the PECs. The lower the charge density of the polymer, the higher the polymer proportion in the PECs, since more polymeric chains are required to react with the other polymers. In addition, as PECs are reported to be formed between two oppositely charged polymers, a PEC-forming reaction can only occur at pH values in the vicinity of the pK_a interval of the two polyelectrolytes. For instance, Yao and coworkers found that interaction between gelatin (pH_{iso} 4.7) and chitosan (pK_a 6.5) in the aqueous medium was enough to form PECs at a pH range from 4.7 to 6.2 [52]. Research also showed that the stability of PEC hydrogel depends on charge density, solvent, ionic strength, pH, and temperature [4].

6.3.1.2 Hydrophobic Interactions

Polymers with hydrophobic domains can cross-link in aqueous environments via reverse thermal gelation, known as "sol–gel" chemistry. That is, they are liquid at room temperature or below and form a solid-like hydrogel when the temperature increases. This special type of physical hydrogel has been studied. They are called injectable thermosensitive hydrogels and have been adapted for *in vivo* use, where they solidify *in situ* upon injection, and are attractive in DDSs due to less invasive delivery. Polymers with such gelation properties are typically moderately hydrophobic, and hydrophobic interactions between chains are proposed as the main driving force of gelation. As shown in Figure 6.10 [10], with an increase of temperature, hydrophobic domains aggregate to minimize the hydrophobic surface area contacting bulk water, reducing the amount of structured water surrounding the hydrophobic domains and maximizing solvent entropy. The temperature at which gelation occurs depends on the concentration of the polymer, the length of the hydrophobic block, and the chemical structure of the polymer: the more hydrophobic the segment, the larger the entropic cost of water structuring, the larger the driving force for hydrophobic aggregation, and the lower the gelation temperature [10].

One successful chitosan-based injectable thermosensitive system was developed by Chenite et al. [53,54] utilizing chitosan and polyol salts. In their study, glycerophosphate (GP), a polyol-phosphate salt, was added to an aqueous chitosan solution where it neutralized the ammonium groups of chitosan and permitted chitosan solutions with pH values of 7 without precipitation. Gelation by increasing temperature was believed to be mainly caused by the increased hydrophobic association between the chitosan chains at elevated temperatures [53,54]. The temperature of gelation in this chitosan–GP system can be controlled primarily through the regulation of solution pH [55]. If desired, gelation at human body temperature can be achieved, such as a solution with a 2% chitosan concentration

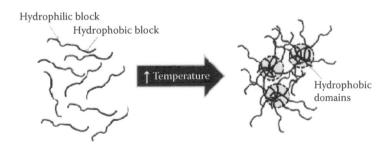

FIGURE 6.10
Mechanism of *in situ* physical gelatin driven by hydrophobic interactions. (From Hoare, T. R. and Kohane, D. S. 2008. *Polymer* 49: 1993–2007. With permission.)

and a pH of 7.2, which gels at 37°C, while slight acidification to pH 6.85 increases the gelation temperature to nearly 50°.

As mentioned in Section 1.2.2, chitosan-g-PEG prepared by Bhattarai et al. was soluble at physiological pH and exhibited injectable property, due to the graft of PEG chains. The sol–gel transition on increasing the temperature of the copolymer above 25°C was controlled by the degree of substitution of PEG on the chitosan chain, PEG molecular weight, and concentrations of the polymers [37,38]. While not fully understood, gelation mechanism involving hydrophobic interactions, hydrogen bonding, and hydrophobic associations were supposed to be the main driving force. It was believed that at low temperatures the H-bonding between PEG and water molecules dominates, while at high temperatures the hydrophobic interactions between polymer chains prevail [4,37,56]. The hydrophilic–hydrophobic transition results in gel formation [4].

Other examples of chitosan-based copolymers are chitosan-g-NIPAAm and chitosan-g-Pluronic [35,41]. PNIPAAm and Pluronic are themselves thermosensitive synthetic polymers that can form gels at elevated temperature. Their structures share the common characteristic of having both hydrophilic and hydrophobic domains. When grafted onto chitosan molecules, they convert chitosan into physically cross-linked hydrogel. The increase in strength of the hydrophobic interactions of hydrophobic groups with increasing temperature enhances the interactions between adjacent chitosan chains, leading to the formation of hydrogel. The gelation temperature primarily depends on the content ratio of chitosan and the grafted chains [57], that is, the balance between hydrophilic and hydrophobic interactions. Take chitosan-g-Pluronic for example: the gelation temperature was controlled by chitosan content, and gelation did not occur when the chitosan content was >17 wt% [35,57].

6.3.1.3 Hydrogen Bonding

By blending with some water-soluble nonionic polymers, chitosan can form hydrogels through other secondary bonding, that is, H-bonding [58–61]. This is because chitosan possesses many hydroxyl and amino groups along its molecular chain, which provides chances for chitosan to cross-link with other macromolecules having hydroxyl and amino groups (i.e., PVA and cellulose) through H-bonding [58–61]. PVA is the most commonly used polymer of this kind, since a number of –OH groups exist on the chain. The mixing of chitosan and PVA forms junction points in the form of interpolymer complexation or crystallites after a series of freezing/thawing cycles. The chain–chain interactions act as cross-linking sites of the hydrogel. In the case of chitosan–PVA polymer blends, increasing the chitosan content negatively affects the formation of PVA crystallites, leading to the formation of hydrogels with less ordered structures [4]. PVA was also grafted onto chitosan to form chitosan-g-PVA, avoiding the phase separation during mixing of component materials [59]. This polymer can form physically cross-linked hydrogel through the same mechanism.

6.3.2 Chemical Cross-Linked Hydrogel

Several chemical ways were explored to build covalent bonds to cross-link chitosan, leading to the formation of hydrogel. The mechanism of the formation of these hydrogels mainly includes Schiff base formation, Michael addition, enzyme (horseradish peroxidase—HRP)-catalyzed reaction, polymerization, and so on. Some small-molecule cross-linkers and/or functional groups conjugated to polymers are often involved in the procedure.

6.3.2.1 Schiff Base Formation

It is well known that bifunctional aldehydes, such as glutaraldehyde and phthalaldehyde, can be used to cross-link chitosan. The mechanism of this cross-linking method involves the formation of Schiff base. A Schiff base bridge is formed via reaction of the aldehyde groups with the $-NH_2$ groups of chitosan. Chitosan molecules are then bonded together in this way and engender gelation. This reaction is very fast and can improve the mechanical properties and stabilize the hydrogel. However, glutaraldehyde is cytotoxic, and even trace amounts of unreacted cross-linkers harm the body and impair the global biocompatibility of a chitosan delivery system [62]. Moreover, glutaraldehyde may react with the drug loaded and limit its therapeutic efficacy (i.e., denaturing protein drugs bioactivity). Researchers have developed some new cross-linkers that are relatively safer to make up for the drawbacks of these hydrogels.

Genipin, as a natural cross-linker, was investigated in order to cross-link chitosan due to its lower toxicity and slower degradation rate compared to the glutaraldehyde-cross-linked chitosan gels [62]. Interactions between genipin and chitosan have nothing to do with Schiff base formation but are just a nucleophilic substitution. Amide linkage was formed to cross-link the whole network. However, the exact mechanism of reaction depends on pH, which plays a role in the degree of cross-linking and in the degree of condensation of genipin in the connection. Yao and coworkers [28] synthesized a noncytotoxic cross-linker by oxidizing glucose and prepared alkylated chitosan gels cross-linked by oxidized glucose via Schiff base formation. The resultant chitosan-based hydrogel was used as a pH-sensitive carrier in delivering vitamins.

Cross-linkers for Schiff base formation used above are almost small molecules. More recently, macromolecules were modified to produce cross-linkers that are more biocompatible and less cytotoxic [63–65]. Rinaudo developed a new way to cross-link chitosan in aqueous solution in order to develop a controlled drug release system [63]. Nonionic polysaccharides were oxidized to obtain polyaldehydic derivatives capable of reacting with the free $-NH_2$ of chitosan. The Schiff base formed was reduced in the presence of a reducing agent ($NaBH_3CN$). The advantage of this reaction is that the covalent bond between chitosan and the aldehydic substrate is stable irrespective of the pH. Moreover, considering that the formation of Schiff base cross-linkage is extremely fast, usually within seconds, it does not seem an ideal mechanism to form injectable DDSs. However, since the movement flexibility of macromolecules is lower than that of the smaller molecules, the cross-linking reaction speed may decrease slightly. Weng's report showed that using oxidized dextran as the macromolecular cross-linker of chitosan, the gelation triggered by Schiff base formation happened within 1–5 min [64]. The higher the oxidation degree of dextran, the faster the gelation. This made Schiff base formation a possible mechanism for preparing injectable chitosan hydrogel for drug delivery.

6.3.2.2 Michael Addition

Chitosan hydrogels have also used Michael addition reactions [33,34,66,67] to form cross-linkages. Michael addition is a kind of reaction between thiols and either acrylates or vinyl sulfones, forming sulfide linkages. This approach is popular today for *in situ* hydrogel preparation because the reaction is highly selective versus biological amines and can be carried out under physiological conditions [66]. Moreover, its rapid reaction speed, the relative biological inertness of polymeric precursors, and relatively benign reactivity with biomolecules have sparked investigators' interest in them [4,10].

Chitosan-based hydrogel has been prepared by using acrylated chitosan with thiolated PEO. Unsaturated C=C of acrylated chitosan reacted via Michael addition with the –SH group of thiolated PEO [34]. Chitosan hydrogel can also be prepared by Michael addition of thiolated chitosan and the arylated group bearing polymer, such as PEG diacrylate, as described recently in the literature [33]. The gelation time varies from 30 min to ca. 2 h, depending on the content of free thiols in thiolated chitosan, the ratio of thiol groups to arylate groups, and temperature [33]. In addition, as mentioned in Section 1.1.2, this chitosan-based hydrogel also benefits from enhanced mucoadhesive properties, which can assist in the oral delivery of therapeutics.

Efficient design of Michael addition cross-linked hydrogels is further facilitated by the development of kinetic modeling approaches for predicting the rates of hydrogel formation and degradation and/or the release kinetics of model proteins entrapped or covalently bonded to the hydrogel network [10]. Such model approaches have considerable potential for the bottom-up design of future drug delivery vehicles.

6.3.2.3 Enzyme-Catalyzed Reaction

The enzyme-catalyzed cross-linking reaction using, for example, peroxidase is an emerging approach for the formation of *in situ* hydrogels, and many recent research works have focused on it [68–72]. The cross-linkages were formed as follows: First, a phenolic hydroxyl (Ph) group is incorporated into a polymer. Then HRP, an enzyme, was used to catalyze the oxidation of electron donors using H_2O_2, resulting in polyphenols linked at the aromatic ring by C–C and C–O coupling between Ph groups. This reaction can be carried out under mild conditions, such as under physiological environments.

Chitosan-based *in situ* hydrogels can be formed by following this mechanism. In a typical reaction, Ph groups were introduced into the chitosan through the conjugation of chitosan and 3-(p-hydroxyphenyl)propionic acid using EDC/NHS [68]. The resultant chitosan derivatives became soluble at neutral pH. Hydrogels were obtained through the HRP-catalyzed cross-linking reaction by consuming H_2O_2 in neutral aqueous solution. The gelation time of the solution was within seconds and was dependent on the extent of introduced Ph groups, temperature, and concentrations of HRP and H_2O_2. Similar routes were used by Jin et al. [69] to prepare chitosan-based *in situ* hydrogel. The gelation times reported by them varied from 10 s to 4 min with a decrease of the polymer concentration from 3 to 1 wt%. Although the enzyme-catalyzed reaction was considered as a safe principle for *in situ* hydrogel formation, the concentration of toxic H_2O_2 required to speed up gelation should be controlled below a certain value. Hence, there may be a balance between gelation time and bioactivity of the system.

6.3.2.4 Polymerization

Apart from the reaction of functional groups on the polymer, another useful principle to form hydrogel is through polymerization.

Photopolymerization to form hydrogels has attracted considerable interest in the field of tissue engineering and drug delivery. Photosensitive functional groups are incorporated into polymers, and then by adding photoinitiator, polymerization can occur on irradiation with ultraviolet (UV) light. The latter step helps to cross-link the original polymer, building up the whole hydrogel network.

A water-soluble photopolymerizable chitosan has been prepared by grafting 4-azido-benzoic acid to free amine groups of lactose-modified chitosan [73,74]. Thus, azide groups were introduced into chitosan. After UV irradiation, the azide is converted into a reactive nitrene group that binds chitosan's free amino groups, causing gelation within 60 s. The acrylate group is another common photosensitive group and is often used in photopolymerization [75,76]. Photopolymerizable chitosan derivatives have been prepared previously through methacrylation using reaction aldehyde intermediates [77]. However, this photopolymerizable chitosan derivative is only soluble at acidic pH, whereas solubility at physiological pH values is required for the synthesis of useful biocompatible hydrogels for biological applications. Thus, a useful chitosan-based photopolymerizable precursor should be solubility in aqueous solution at physiological pH. Gao et al. [76] prepared such a water-soluble (methacryloyloxy)ethyl carboxyethyl chitosan as a photopolymerizable prepolymer through Michael addition reaction between chitosan and ethylene glycol acrylate methacrylate. By blending prepolymer with D-2959 photoinitiator in solution, hydrogels were created under UV irradiation.

Ease of formation, high gelation speed, and so on make photopolymerization a promising way to obtain *in situ* forming hydrogel. However, toxicity of photoinitiator and exposure to UV irradiation may result in protein denaturation when protein drug was loaded or may do harm to neighboring cells and tissues, which should be taken into account when choosing the method.

On the other hand, as is well known, the interpenetrating network (IPN) technique can be used to improve the properties of chitosan-based gels [51,78]. A cross-linked chitosan network can be allowed to swell in an aqueous solution of polymer monomers. These monomers are then polymerized, forming a physically entangled polymer mesh called IPN. When the second polymer is linear (without being cross-linked), a semi-IPN results. When the second polymer is also cross-linked, a full-IPN is formed (*cf.* Figure 6.11). Chitosan-based IPNs can also be formed as follows: Take IPNs of PNIPAAm and chitosan for example [78]; their IPNs were prepared by free radical polymerization and cross-linking of NIPAM with bis(acrylamide) in chitosan solutions and subsequent immersion in glutaraldehyde solutions to post-cross-link the chitosan.

The IPN technique allows for the specific selection of polymers that can complement the deficiencies of one another. For instance, a hydrophilic polymer can be chosen to enhance the structural characteristics of the hydrogel, while a biocompatible polymer may limit the

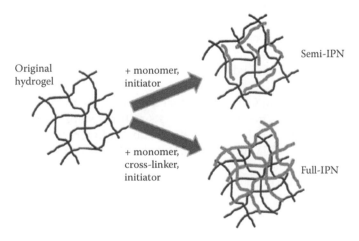

FIGURE 6.11
Formation and structure of semi- and full-IPNs. (From Hoare, T. R. and Kohane, D. S. 2008. *Polymer* 49: 1993–2007. With permission.)

immunological response. Therefore, the main advantages of IPN are that relatively dense hydrogel matrices can be produced, which feature stiffer and tougher mechanical properties, more widely controllable physical properties, and (frequently) more efficient drug loading compared to conventional hydrogels.

Although cross-linking density, hydrogel porosity, and gel stiffness can be adjusted in IPN-based hydrogels according to the target application, they have difficulty encapsulating a wide variety of therapeutic agents, especially sensitive biomolecules. In addition, IPN preparation requires the use of toxic agents to initiate or catalyze the polymerization or to catalyze the cross-linking. Complete removal of these materials from the hydrogel is challenging, making the clinical application problematic [4].

6.4 Geometries of Chitosan Gels and Their Preparation Methods

Chitosan-based gels for DDSs have been fabricated into a variety of different shapes and geometries for various administration routes such as oral, buccal, nasal, transdermal, parenteral, vaginal, cervical, intrauterine, and rectal. Different methods were used in order to obtain these shapes and geometries.

6.4.1 Scaffolds

Hydrogel can be made into bulk matrices with different shapes, that is, scaffolds, for several bioapplications, especially for tissue engineering, such as hard tissue replacement. Certain active agents or bioactive molecules (i.e., growth factors and antibiotics) can be released from these scaffolds to enhance the replacement. Scaffolds are prepared into various shapes in terms of the defects that are needed to be replaced. Chitosan is a good candidate for preparing these types of matrices [16].

Freeze-drying or lyophilization is the most popular technique to fabricate chitosan-based scaffolds [79]. Solutions of chitosan are frozen to result in phase separation. After drying in a lyophilizer, ice is removed, generating a porous material whose pore size and orientation can be controlled by variation of the freezing rate. Porous chitosan scaffolds can also be prepared using a rapid prototyping system. Chitosan matrix was endowed with special shapes and microstructure through computational modeling. Neutralization of the acetic acid by the sodium hydroxide results in a precipitate to form a gel-like chitosan structure [80].

Recently, a new supercritical CO_2 fluid-assisted process for the production of chitosan scaffolds was proposed [81]. This method consists of three steps: formation of a chitosan hydrogel by thermally induced phase separation; substitution of water with a suitable solvent; and drying of the gel using supercritical CO_2. Using this process, chitosan nanostructured networks were produced with filaments of diameters around 50 nm, without any collapse of the gel nanostructure, characterized by high porosity (>91%) and high compressive modulus (150 kPa).

6.4.2 Particles and Spheres

Hydrogels can be confined to smaller dimensions such as microparticles or microspheres. When the size of microparticles is in the submicrometer range, they are known as nanoparticles. Micro/nanoparticles or spheres may increase the life span of active constituents and control the release of bioactive agents [82]. Since their size varies from nanometers to several micrometers, micro/nanoparticles have a large surface area for multivalent bioconjugation [83] and can be used for controlled release of insoluble drugs. It is necessary to fulfill some criteria in order to design effective micro/nanoparticle DDSs [84]. The first criterion is that micro/nanoparticles should be stable enough to circulate in the bloodstream for a long time. Instability of these particles may result in burst release of therapeutics, bringing about adverse side effects. Effective ligands for certain cells should be incorporated on their surface for targeting drug release. The second criterion is that the dimension of nanoparticles should be less than 200 nm in diameter. This can facilitate cellular uptake of the nanoparticles through a receptor-mediated endocytosis (RME) to cross cell membranes as well as reduce nanoparticle uptake by the mononuclear phagocyte system, simultaneously increasing their circulation time in blood. The last criterion is the biodegradability of micro/nanoparticles. Biodegradation should not only modulate the release behaviors of drugs for a desired period of time, but also enable removal of the empty device after drug release.

There are several common methods for fabricating micro/nanoparticle DDSs.

6.4.2.1 Emulsification

Emulsification is the most popular technique to obtain micro/nanoparticles [85,86]. The general methods for emulsification include inverse (mini) emulsion, inverse microemulsion (or the reverse micelle method), and membrane emulsification [87].

Thr inverse (mini) emulsion method yields kinetically stable water-in-oil (w/o) macroemulsions at, below, or around the critical micellar concentration (CMC) of surfactants. Tween 80 as an oil-soluble surfactant is often used to implement colloidal stability of the inverse emulsion. Cyclohexane, hexane, and mineral oil are hydrophobic organic solvents commonly used for the inverse (mini) emulsion method. Micrometer-sized microparticles are often obtained by this method. Chitosan microparticles may be produced as follows: Aqueous droplets of chitosan are added via a syringe into an oil phase (mineral oil) as the suspension medium, forming a w/o emulsion. Chitosan is stably dispersed in continuous organic phase with the aid of oil-soluble surfactants. To this suspension, a chemical cross-linking agent that can react with the functional amine group of chitosan, usually a bifunctional chemical reagent such as glutaraldehyde, hexamethylene diisocyanate or ethylene glycol diglycidyl ether, is added [16]. A schematic representation of the technique is given in Figure 6.12 [16]. The chitosan microparticles obtained are washed with petroleum ether, sodium bisulfide, and acetone, respectively, to remove excess cross-linking agent and oil. The final chitosan microparticles are well-shaped, spherical particles varying in the size range of tens to hundreds of micrometers in diameter [86]. The size and size distribution of chitosan microparticles can be changed by stirring rate, concentration of chitosan, chitosan molecular weight, chitosan/solvent ratio, and extent of cross-linking.

Another emulsification method for producing micrometer-sized particles is membrane emulsification [87]. It involves the use of a membrane with a highly uniform pore size ranging from 0.1 to 18 μm. Through the membrane, an aqueous solution of biopolymers permeates under adequate pressure into an organic solvent containing oil-soluble surfactants, producing a w/o emulsion. The aqueous droplets of biopolymers are hardened by physical or chemical cross-linking, producing microparticles with a uniform-sized distribution. Chitosan-based microparticles loaded with insulin prepared via this method had diameters in the range from 4 to 15 μm.

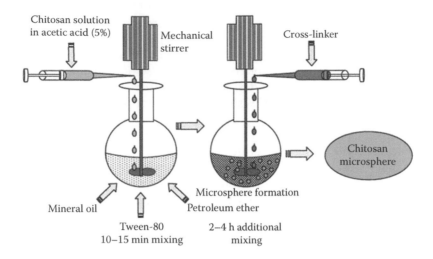

FIGURE 6.12
Schematic representation of the suspension cross-linking technique. (From Denkbas, E. B. and Ottenbrite, R. M. 2006. *J Bioact Compat Polym* 21: 351–368. With permission.)

The inverse microemulsion method has been utilized to prepare ultrafine polymeric nanoparticles with narrow size distribution [87,88]. Similar to the inverse (mini) emulsion method, this method also involves a w/o dispersion. However, it requires the addition of a large amount of oil-soluble surfactants above the critical threshold to prepare reverse micelles, producing thermodynamically stable microemulsions [84,87]. The resulting micellar droplets have nanometer-sized particles ranging from tens to hundreds of nanometers in diameter [87]. In a typical preparation [89], a lipophilic surfactant was dissolved in hexane, and then aqueous solutions of chitosan and hydrophilic drugs were added with continuous stirring to avoid any turbidity. The entire mixture solution was homogeneous and optically transparent. An additional amount of water may be added to obtain nanoparticles of larger size. To this transparent solution, a cross-linking agent (glutaraldehyde) was subsequently added with continuous stirring. It was reported that chitosan-based nanoparticles containing doxorubicin-modified dextran have a diameter of 100 nm [89].

6.4.2.2 Coacervation

In this process, the polymer is solubilized to form a solution. This is followed by the addition of a solute, which forms insoluble polymer derivative and precipitates the polymer. As for chitosan, the physicochemical property of its insolubility in an alkaline pH medium but coacervating in contact with an alkaline solution is utilized to obtain microparticles. This process avoids the use of toxic organic solvents in the other methods.

Berthold and Kreuter [90] prepared drug-loaded chitosan microspheres using sodium sulfate as a precipitant. The addition of sodium sulfate to the aqueous acid solution of chitosan containing a surfactant resulted in decreased solubility of chitosan, leading to precipitation of chitosan as a poorly soluble derivative. Microspheres were purified by centrifugation and resuspended in demineralized water. It was reported that particles produced accordingly have better acid stability than observed by other methods.

In addition, particles can also be produced by blowing chitosan solution into an alkali sodium hydroxide solution using a compressed air nozzle to form coacervate droplets [18].

Separation and purification of particles were done by filtration/centrifugation followed by successive washings with hot and cold water. The size of particles varied depending on the compressed air pressure or spray-nozzle diameter, while the drug release profile was controlled by using a cross-linking agent to harden these particles.

6.4.2.3 Aqueous Cross-Linking Gelation Method

Covalent chemical cross-linking and physical cross-linking in aqueous solution were both used for the preparation of chitosan-based submicrometer-sized particles.

Examples of the chemical cross-linking method include the use of a carbodiimide coupling reaction of chitosan with a PEG dicarboxylic acid as a water-soluble cross-linker in aqueous medium at pH 6.5 [91]. Chitosan-based nanoparticles with a diameter of 4–24 nm were formed. The average size of the particles in their swollen state was in the range of 50–120 nm. Particle size largely depended on the ratio of cross-linking and the molecular weight of chitosan [91]. Because these chitosan particles are nanosized at neutral pH, they are attractive candidates as delivery biomolecules for a variety of biomedical applications.

To avoid the possible toxicity of reagents and other undesirable effects, reversible physical cross-linking by electrostatic interaction, instead of chemical cross-linking, has been explored to prepare fine chitosan nanoparticles. In this method, chitosan, as a polycation, cross-linked with polyanion (i.e., TPP [92,93] and polyethyleneimine [94]) through electrostatic interactions. TPP is the most commonly used physical cross-linker. Recently, Csaba et al. [92] prepared chitosan/TPP nanoparticles for oligonucleotide and plasmid DNA delivery. Chitosan and TPP were separately dissolved in ultrapure water at different concentrations. Nanoparticles were formed instantaneously upon the dropwise addition of a fixed volume of TPP solution to a fixed volume of chitosan solution under magnetic stirring. Owing to the negligible toxicity of the carrier cross-linked by electrostatic interaction, these nanoparticles showed high encapsulation efficiencies for plasmid DNA and oligonucleotide. Gene expression of these particles was proved to be comparable to other efficient gene delivery systems. In addition, this research showed that chitosan/TPP nanoparticles were suitable for the simultaneous encapsulation and sustained release of other active molecules together with DNA [92].

6.4.2.4 Spray Drying Method

Spray drying is a widely used technique for preparing capsules, granules, powders, and agglomerates. This method involves the use of a spray dryer, mainly consisting of an atomizer and a drying chamber. Chitosan is first dissolved in aqueous acetic acid solution, drug is dissolved or dispersed in the solution, and then a suitable cross-linking agent is added. This solution or suspension is then atomized in a stream of hot air, which induces quick evaporation of solvent from the droplets in the drying chamber, resulting in the formation of microparticles. The obtained particles settle into a bottom collector, and are further dried in a vacuum chamber or modified in separate experiments. Various process parameters have to be controlled to obtain the desired size of particles. The size of the particles is determined by measuring nozzle size, spray flow rate, atomization speed, and extent of cross-linking [18,84].

6.4.2.5 Sieving Method

A sieving method for preparing microparticles was included in the review by Agnihotri et al. [18]. They reported their own novel method to produce chitosan microparticles [18].

In this method, chitosan was dissolved in acetic acid solution to form a thick jelly mass that was cross-linked by adding glutaraldehyde. The nonsticky cross-linked mass was passed through a sieve with a suitable mesh size to obtain microparticles. NaOH solution was used to remove unreacted excess glutaraldehyde. This method is devoid of tedious procedures, and can be scaled up easily. The average size of drug-loaded microparticles was in the range of 543–698 μm.

6.4.3 Membranes and Films

Hydrogel membranes or films have been widely used as drug carriers in the case of transdermal drug delivery. Several key properties enable the hydrogel membranes or films to be one of the ideal carriers for skin drug delivery, including flexibility and elasticity sufficient to follow the movements of the skin, enough strength to resist abrasion, high water vapor transmission rate, effective drug permeability, bioadhesion, and a good feel for the patient [95]. Chitosan has film-forming ability, bioadhesivity, antimicrobial activity, wound healing, and absorption-enhancing properties [96]. By using a proper fabrication technique, chitosan-based membranes or films with good mechanical and physical properties can be prepared, acting as an eligible drug carrier.

One of the most common techniques for the preparation of chitosan membranes or films is the solvent cast-evaporation method [97]. In a typical procedure, a clear solution of chitosan was obtained by dissolving chitosan in an aqueous solution of acetic acid. The biopolymer solution was cast onto clean glass Petri dishes, and the solvent was slowly evaporated at room temperature or in an air oven at 50–60°C. The dry chitosan films were easily separated from the glass surfaces which were then immersed into a cross-linking solution containing glutaraldehyde. PEC membranes of chitosan were also prepared by mixing with another polyanion and then casting on glass dishes to evaporate the solvent [95,98].

Recently, electrospinning techniques have increasingly been used to prepare polymer membranes with continuous nanometer-scaled fibers as novel drug vehicles [99–101]. This technique involves the use of an electrospinning setup (as shown in Figure 6.13). Chitosan is dissolved in an appropriate solvent to obtain a transparent solution. Then the solution is added into a syringe attached with a clinic-shaped metal capillary. The feeding rate of the solution was set via a syringe pump. When a high voltage is applied between the metal capillary tip and a grounded collector, the liquid droplets are charged and are subsequently

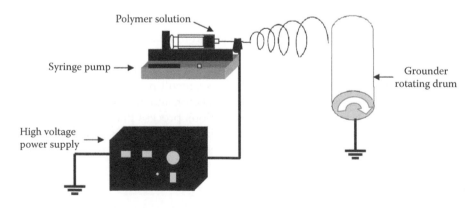

FIGURE 6.13
Schematic diagram of the electrospun scaffold experimental setup.

stretched into liquid jets, which are finally deposited on the collector as ultrafine fibrous membranes after the evaporation of solvent. The obtained membranes are further cross-linked, usually in a glutaraldehyde vapor. Since the electrospinning of chitosan itself sometimes proved to be difficult, chitosan was mixed with other synthetic or natural polymers, such as PEO, PVA, PLGA, collagen, and so on [100]. Jiang et al. [101] prepared ibuprofen-loaded chitosan-based membranes composed of PLGA and PEG-g-chitosan by electrospinning. Ibuprofen conjugated to the side chains of PEG-g-chitosan was released sustainably for more than 2 weeks from the membrane.

6.4.4 Liquids

When we say that a hydrogel is in the form of liquid, it means that the hydrogels can be formed by heating or cooling their solutions [6]. Hydrogels that undergo a sol–gel transition upon heating are always called injectable or *in situ* thermosensitive hydrogels. Today, *in situ* thermosensitive hydrogels have attracted wide attention as DDSs because of several advantages, such as the facile procedure and the minimally invasive surgical procedure [102]. Such a system enables therapeutic drugs such as cells, genes, peptides, and proteins to be simply mixed with the aqueous polymer solution at low temperatures and then form a semisolid hydrogel after injection into the body at a target site. It may also be possible to fill up a defect or target site completely with these injectable hydrogels, including bioactive molecules.

Chitosan can only be dissolved in an acid aqueous solution. However, by simply adding GP into its solution, the pH reached about 7. Thus this solution showed thermosensitive property. It remained in liquid state at room temperature, whereas it formed a hydrogel at body temperature. The preparation procedure is very simple, but one thing that needs to be paid attention to is that GP solution should be added carefully drop by drop to chitosan solution, obtaining a clear and homogeneous liquid solution [53,54]. Certain copolymers of chitosan and other synthetic polymers, for example, chitosan-g-PEG and chitosan-g-PNIPAM, exhibit thermosensitive property too. The preparation process is so simple that only dissolution of them into water is needed.

6.5 Drug Loading

Delivering a drug to the right part of the body in the correct dose and for long enough for it to have an effect can be tricky. Some drugs are highly toxic and need to be targeted specifically to avoid damaging healthy cells; others must bypass the liver or else they will be degraded; while some need to be released slowly over a long period if they are to be effective. Because of the diversity in the chemistry and size of the delivered molecules, the drug loading for controlled release in any particular hydrogel can differ widely from one application to another. The method by which the drugs are loaded directly impacts the availability of the drugs during release [4]. There are typically three methods to load drugs into the hydrogel.

6.5.1 Physical Entrapment

Loading drugs by diffusion or simple mixing is known as physical entrapment. The easiest loading method involves the diffusion process of the drugs. When a hydrogel is formed, it is allowed to immerse into a suitable drug solution [102]. The drugs slowly diffuse into the gel through the pores on the gel. When placed *in vivo*, the drug will then diffuse back out of the hydrogel into the environment. This approach is very simple and will not influence the bioactivity or therapeutic efficiency of the drugs. Small molecular drugs can diffuse readily into the hydrogel. However, for some molecules with large sizes, it is not so easy for them to migrate through the small pores of the hydrogel. In the latter case, drugs are mixed into the polymer solution before gelation begins. After cross-linking of the polymer solution, drugs are entrapped into the hydrogel as a result. This method may suffer from possible deactivation of the drugs during gelation.

Although the above methods are very easy to carry out, they have to face the same problems. The drug entrapment efficiency of these systems is not very high due to little interaction between the matrix and the drug itself. The release of loaded molecules is not well regulated. A rapid burst release is always observed during the initial hydrogel swelling in the release medium. These burst releases can lead to losses of an extremely large part of the loaded molecules, influencing the therapeutic effect of the drugs. To increase drug loading efficiency, electrostatic interactions between molecules with opposite charges are utilized to enhance the binding between drugs and hydrogels. Chitosan hydrogels are usually performed as attractive carriers for protein or gene delivery because positively charged amines (under slightly acidic conditions) allow electrostatic interaction with carboxyl acid groups on protein or with phosphate-bearing nucleic acids to form PECs [103]. Alonso and coworkers [104] prepared insulin-loaded chitosan nanoparticles based on ionic interaction between both molecules. The loading capacity was up to 55%. Similar high entrapment efficiency was also reported by others [105]. Despite this improvement, charge interactions were found to be too weak to prolong the release time [105,106]. A strong burst effect within a short time was still observed (Figure 6.14). Therefore, binding between a loaded drug and the hydrogel matrix should be enhanced further to extend the duration of drug release.

6.5.2 Covalent Incorporation

Another strategy to incorporate drugs into a hydrogel matrix is chemical covalent incorporation. Since a chemical bond is always stronger than a physical one, drugs can be incorporated more tightly and a high burst release can be avoided to some extent [107–109]. Most importantly, the release is regulated by chemical/enzymatic cleavage of the polymer–drug bond or hydrolysis of the polymer backbone [4,110]. Wu et al. [107] developed chitosan–methotrexate covalently conjugated nanoparticles as a potential delivery system for methotrexate. Methotrexate was chemically conjugated to chitosan by using glutaraldehyde as a cross-linking agent. An *in vitro* release test showed that the stable covalent bonding of chitosan and methotrexate was beneficial for providing slow release for the drug. Doxorubicin was also reported to be chemically conjugated to acrylated chitosan via an amide linkage in order to obtain sustained-release profiles [109]. Doxorubicin–chitosan conjugates significantly reduced the burst release of free doxorubicin from 90% to 10% and prolonged the release profile from 5 days to 3 weeks, compared with hydrogels without the conjugates (*cf.* Figure 6.15).

6.5.3 Composite Systems

If the retardation of drug release using cross-linked hydrogels is not sufficient to slow the release rate for long-term applications, another system may be incorporated into the

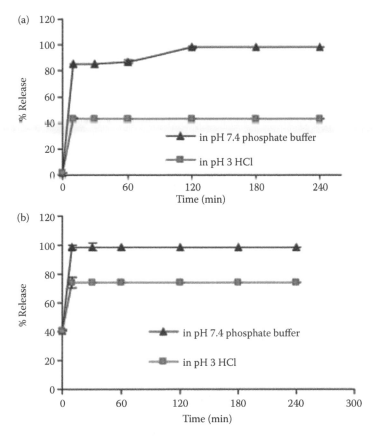

FIGURE 6.14
Release profiles of diclofenac (a) and salicylic acid (b) from washed chitosan micro/nanoparticles in different media. (From Boonsongrit, Y., Mitrevej, A., and Mueller, B. W. 2006. *Eur J Pharm Biopharm* 62: 267–274. With permission.)

hydrogel to help it achieve the goal [111–113]. Particle-based drug delivery vehicles, that is, micro/nanoparticles, have a proven capacity for long-term release. As a result, growing interest has focused on overcoming the inherent pharmacological limitations of bulk hydrogels by coformulating particulate systems into the hydrogel matrix to form composite hydrogel networks [10]. In the composite hydrogel, apart from the advantages that particles bring about, micro/nanoparticles can also be sheltered and protected by the bulk hydrogel from uncontrolled movement [114]. In typical composite systems for drug release, therapeutics can be loaded into micro/nanoparticles prior to hydrogel encapsulation [112,113]. Alternatively, particles can be designed to be charged; drugs with opposite charge are loaded via electrostatic interactions with particles in a bulk hydrogel. As reported by Tang et al. recently, a thermosensitive chitosan/PVA hydrogel containing chitosan derivative nanoparticles with different charges was prepared for delivering propranolol and diclofenac sodium. They showed that releases of the two drugs were both the fastest with pure hydrogels, indicating that the electrostatic effect between nanoparticles and drugs reduced the burst release and the addition of nanoparticles was helpful in slowing the suitable drug release (*cf.* Figure 6.16) [111].

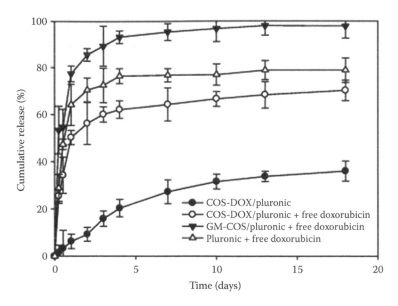

FIGURE 6.15
In vitro-release profile of doxorubicin hydrogels at 37°C. Each point is mean ± standard deviation ($n = 3$). (COS-DOX represented doxorubicin–chitosan conjugates). (From Cho, Y. I. et al. 2009. *Eur J Pharm Biopharm* 73: 59–65. With permission.)

6.5.4 Hydrophobic Drug Loading into Hydrogels

Due to their inherent hydrophilic nature, hydrogels have been effectively used to deliver hydrophilic small-molecule drugs that have high solubility in both the hydrophilic hydrogel matrix and the aqueous solvent swelling the hydrogel. However, with the development of pharmaceutics and life science, some hydrophobic drugs are becoming increasingly important clinically to cure disease and regenerate tissue. The issue of loading and delivering poorly soluble drugs proves to be a difficult challenge, because hydrophobic drugs are sparingly soluble in both the aqueous and the hydrogel phases.

Previous strategies of loading hydrophobic drugs include the multiple emulsion technique. In this method, the drug is dissolved in a suitable solvent and then emulsified in chitosan aqueous solution in order to form an oil-in-water (o/w) emulsion. Also a surfactant stabilizing the emulsion is added. This o/w emulsion can be further emulsified into liquid paraffin to obtain multiple emulsions. By using a suitable cross-linking agent, drugs are loaded into the chitosan matrix. Organic solvents may make it difficult to completely remove them. In addition, the strategies mentioned above can also be employed to improve hydrophobic drug loading into hydrogels. However, sometimes modification of the drugs and chemical reaction may lead to weakening the activity and therapeutic efficiency of the drugs. Compatibility between hydrophobic drugs and the hydrophilic network can be accomplished by introducing hydrophobic domains directly into otherwise hydrophilic hydrogel networks instead. In this way, the loading of hydrophobic drugs is improved significantly.

The most common approach for generating hydrophobic domains within the bulk hydrogel is by attaching small hydrophobic moieties to the polymer before gelation. Martin et al. [115] prepared hydrophobic pendants containing chitosan (palmitoyl glycol chitosan) hydrogels by freeze-drying an aqueous dispersion of the polymer in the presence of a hydrophobic drug denbufylline. Results showed that the sustained delivery of denbufylline

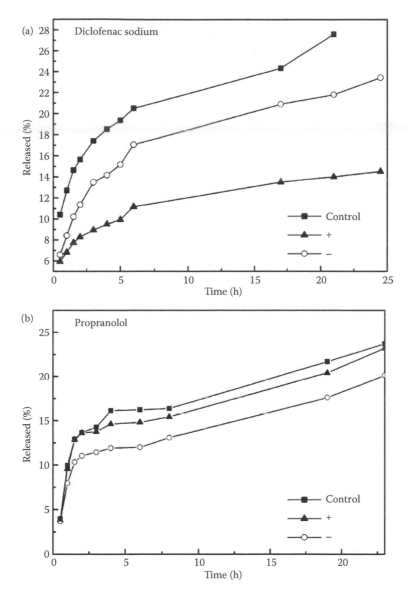

FIGURE 6.16
Drug delivery of chitosan/PVA gels with different charges drugs. *Control*: pure chitosan/PVA hydrogel; +: hydrogel with positive nanoparticles; –: hydrogel with negative nanoparticles. (From Tang, Y. F. et al. 2010. *Polym Bull* 64: 791–804. With permission.)

was achieved successfully. Apart from this, a special structure, cyclodextrin, is of interest for introducing hydrophobic domains while still maintaining the bulk hydrophilicity and swelling state of the hydrogel [10]. Cyclodextrin, as mentioned in Section 6.2.2.3, possesses a hydrophilic exterior and a hydrophobic interior cavity that is capable of binding hydrophobic molecules, and therefore provides ideal binding sites for these kinds of drugs. By grafting cyclodextrin onto chitosan, a chitosan-g-cyclodextrin is prepared [40,116]. A controlled release study suggested that *p*-nitrophenol entrapped with a chitosan-g-cyclodextrin hydrogel was released slowly and equilibrium was reached after 15 h, while chitosan hydrogel, as a control, released almost all of the *p*-nitrophenol within several hours [116]. It was suggested that a chitosan-g-cyclodextrin may serve as a promising carrier for controlled release of hydrophobic drugs.

6.6 Drug Release

6.6.1 Drug Release Mechanisms

Understanding the mechanisms and identifying the key parameters that govern drug release from hydrogels are the most important in order to accurately predict the entire release profile. Drug release behaviors from hydrogels are very different from nonhydrophilic polymers due to their hydrophilicity and high water absorbability. From various modelistic studies on the possible release mechanisms of an active agent from a hydrogel, as a function of time, focused on the rate-limiting step of the release phenomena, drug release mechanisms from hydrogels can be classified into the following: diffusion-controlled, swelling-controlled, and chemically controlled mechanisms [117].

6.6.1.1 Diffusion-Controlled Mechanism

The diffusion-controlled mechanism is the most widely applicable mechanism to describe drug release from hydrogels. Fick's law of diffusion with either constant or variable diffusion coefficients is commonly used in modeling diffusion-controlled release [118]. Diffusion-controlled hydrogel delivery systems can be either reservoirs or matrixes. Fick's first law of diffusion is usually used to describe a reservoir release system, whereas Fick's second law of diffusion is used to describe a matrix system [117]. Diffusion coefficient is an empirical parameter, usually assumed to be constant to simplify the modeling. Once the diffusion coefficient is determined, drug concentration profiles can be obtained to dictate the drug release kinetics. However, Fick's law is not available when more complex geometries or nonconstant drug diffusivities are incorporated into the model [117].

Drug diffusion out of a hydrogel matrix is primarily dependent on mesh sizes within the matrix of the gel [118]. Actually, molecule diffusion coefficient is related to hydrogel characteristics. That is, hydrogel characteristics, such as structure of the gel, polymer composition, water content, and size of the drugs, are taken into account as factors influencing the drug release profile. It was reported that typical mesh sizes for biomedical hydrogels range from 5 to 100 nm in their swollen state [4], which is much larger than the size of most small-molecule drugs. Therefore, the diffusion of small-molecule drugs is not significantly hindered in the swollen state, whereas macromolecules such as protein and peptides, due to their hydrodynamic radii, will not have a sustained release unless the structure and mesh size of the swollen hydrogels are designed appropriately to obtain the desired rates of macromolecular diffusion [118].

6.6.1.2 Swelling-Controlled Mechanisms

Another mechanism for drug delivery is swelling-controlled delivery. Hydrogels may undergo a swelling-driven phase transition from a glassy state where entrapped molecules remain immobile to a rubbery state where molecules rapidly diffuse. When diffusion of the drug is faster than hydrogel distention, swelling is considered to control the release behavior. In a swelling-controlled delivery system, the drug molecules are able to diffuse out of the rubbery phase of the polymer. Since no drug diffuses out of the glassy region of the polymer, the drug release is related to the velocity and position of the glass–rubbery interface [119]. A very important phenomenon of macromolecular relaxation takes place at the glass–rubbery interface, and significantly affects the drug release of this mechanism. Therefore, the rate of molecule release depends on the swelling rate of polymer networks.

There are many mathematical models to describe swelling-controlled release. Among them, the Korsmeyer and Peppas model is considered to be a rigorous description [120]. In this model, drug diffusion, polymer relaxation, and the "moving-boundary" conditions in which the gel expands heterogeneously as water penetrates and swells the gels are all taken into account [119,120].

6.6.1.3 Chemically Controlled Mechanisms

In addition to diffusion and swelling-controlled delivery systems, a third type of molecule release mechanism is chemically controlled delivery. It is determined by chemical reactions occurring within the gel matrix. These reactions include (1) cleavage of pendant polymer chains via hydrolytic or enzymatic degradation; (2) reversible or irreversible reactions occurring between the polymer network and releasable drug; (3) surface erosion; and (4) bulk degradation. Among these reactions, one point that needs to be clarified is that surface erosion may occur when the rate of water transport into the polymer is much lower than the rate of bond hydrolysis. However, owing to the inherently high water content of hydrogels, surface erosion only occurs in enzymatic degrading systems where the rate of transport of enzyme into the gel is lower than the rate of enzymatic degradation.

Any of the above four reactions could be the rate-determining step and will control the entire rate of drug release. Therefore, chemically controlled release can be further categorized according to the type of chemical reaction occurring during drug release. Many models are developed to describe the chemically controlled mechanism [117,119]. But under certain circumstances, diffusion should also be included in the model to accurately predict drug release.

Generally, the liberation of encapsulated or tethered drugs can occur through the degradation of pendant chains or during surface erosion or bulk degradation of the polymer backbone.

6.6.2 Drug Release Stimuli

Usually, the hydrogel-based delivery systems are classified into two major categories: (1) time-controlled systems (inert hydrogel) and (2) stimuli-induced release systems (intelligent or smart hydrogel). Stimuli-induced release systems are also called "stimuli-sensitive/responsive," "environment-sensitive/responsive," or "responsive" hydrogel systems. These smart hydrogels are developed to deliver drugs in response to a fluctuating condition in a way that desirably coincides with the physiological requirements at the right time and proper place. Despite the huge attraction toward novel DDSs based on environment-sensitive hydrogels in past and recent times, these systems have disadvantages of their own. The most considerable drawback of stimuli-sensitive hydrogels is their significantly slow response time, with the easiest way to achieve fast-acting responsiveness being to develop thinner and smaller hydrogels that, in turn, bring about fragility and loss of mechanical strength in the polymer network and the hydrogel device itself [118].

Environmental stimuli contain physical stimuli such as temperature, electricity, magnetic field, and chemical stimuli such as pH, enzyme, ions, and specific molecular recognition events. Depending on changes in the nature of the external environment, responsive hydrogels undergo drastic alterations in their structure/behavior, which facilitate drug payload release. Environmental stimuli can induce three types of hydrogel conformational changes: swelling, dissolution, or degradation [4]. Swelling of the hydrogel opens the "pores" of the polymer network, which allows for faster diffusion of entrapped molecules out of the hydrogel. Dissolution and degradation represent the physical breakup of the hydrogel. When the cross-linkages between polymer chains break, the hydrogel dissolves, subsequently allowing release of the drug. Degradation is the destruction of the polymer chains themselves (i.e., by enzymes), causing drug release. Each of these mechanisms can be executed with a number of different hydrogel preparation strategies.

6.6.2.1 pH-Sensitive Release

The pH gradient in the human gastrointestinal (GI) tract ranges from 1 to 7.5 (saliva, 5–6; stomach, 1–3; small intestine, 6.6–7.5; and colon, 6.4–7.0). When drugs are delivered via oral administration, the most preferred route, they are expected to go through different pH environments to reach the target site. The therapeutic efficiency may be affected due to exposure to harsh environmental conditions, such as extreme acidic gastric juice. Hence, pH is one of the important environmental parameters for DDSs. To achieve successful oral delivery of drugs, pH-sensitive hydrogels are commonly used to protect medicine from invalidation in harsh environments or to guarantee effective drug release within the GI tract selectively. These gels exhibit dramatic changes on pH, namely, swelling and deswelling, thus controlling drug release behavior. All the pH-sensitive polymers contain pendant acidic (e.g., carboxylic and sulfonic acids) or basic (e.g., ammonium salts) groups that either accept or release protons in response to changes in environmental pH [121].

Neutral or anionic polymers do not exhibit significant pH-sensitive behavior under acidic conditions, while the cationic chitosan is responsive at low pH [4]. As mentioned previously, chitosan exhibits pH-sensitive behavior as a weak polybase due to protonation of amine groups at low pH and deprotonation at higher pH. Moreover, it is believed that cationic hydrogels protonate and swell more when external pH is lower than the pK_a of the ionizable groups (amino groups in chitosan have a pK_a value of ca. 6.5) [122]. This characteristic leads to dissociation of H-bonding between chitosan chains, together with chain repulsion and water inside the gel, facilitating drug release at acidic medium. By cross-linking properly, chitosan hydrogels may serve as drug carriers for the delivery of some chemical drugs into the stomach where pH is 1–3. However, for the delivery of medicines to the intestine where pH is ca. 7.5, this property causes a limitation. Modified chitosan is used to prepare chitosan-based hydrogels in order to deliver certain drugs to the intestine. For example, thiolated chitosan was synthesized as a drug delivery carrier to minimize drug release in acidic sites, such as in the stomach [123]. The release amounts of indomethacin (IM) from thiolated chitosan beads were found to increase with increase in pH of the dissolution medium. The release rate of IM at pH 7.4 was shown to be higher than that at pH 1.4 due to the ionization of thiol groups and high solubility of IM in alkaline medium. The higher release rate in simulated intestinal fluid enables drug delivery to take place preferentially in the intestine, avoiding then drug leakage in the stomach.

Graft copolymers of chitosan can also be used as pH-sensitive drug release systems. Hydrogels for colon-specific drug delivery were synthesized by graft copolymerization of chitosan and acrylic acid using N,N'-methylene-bis-(acrylamide) as a cross-linker [124]. These hydrogels have good pH sensitivity due to the charge balance of the amine groups of chitosan and the carboxyl groups of acrylic acid in the graft copolymer network. The content of chitosan and the degree of cross-linking were reported to be key factors influencing the swelling kinetics. By tailoring these factors, a very low equilibrium swelling degree of the hydrogel in the range of pH 2.2–4.0 and the largest degree of swelling at pH 7.4 were observed. Moreover, a decrease of swelling degree was observed on increasing the pH to beyond 7.4. Therefore, no drug release in the stomach together with a little amount of release in the small intestine can be achieved, which enables this hydrogel to be a potential candidate for application in oral colon-specific DDSs.

An IPN or PEC of chitosan and another polymer or polyelectrolyte is also used to release drugs through the pH-sensitive mechanism [125–128]. Swelling in IPN hydrogels is moderated by the amount of hydrophobic/hydrophilic groups and the cross-linking density [125], while swelling of the PEC complexes is due to a change in the charge balance inside the hydrogel [128]. If the charge density of either polymer or polyelectrolyte is no longer sufficiently high enough to ensure complexation, then the polyelectrolyte "glue" can no longer hold the polymer chains together, leading to swelling or dissolution. By selecting polymers or polyelectrolytes based on their isoelectric points, PEC swelling and dissolution can be tailored for drug release at varying pH values [4].

6.6.2.2 pH and Temperature Dual-Sensitive Release

Chitosan hydrogels are a type of hydrogel exhibiting pH-sensitive property. Sometimes temperature-sensitive polymers are introduced into the chitosan system to obtain a pH/temperature dual-sensitive DDS. One of the most attractive features of temperature-responsive hydrogels as drug carriers is their intelligent property or autoadjustable function to external temperature changes. The combination of pH- and temperature-sensitiveness is quite useful in protecting drugs from degradation, to avoid drugs causing unwanted adverse effects, when they pass through different organs and tissues, and to deliver drugs to specific tissues [129]. For example, chitosan-coated alginate beads containing PNIPAAm are used as a controlled pH- and temperature-sensitive DDS with improved encapsulation efficiency and delayed release rate [130]. The author proposed that the LCST of the systems could be adjusted to around 37°C or even higher temperatures in future work. Such systems could be physiologically relevant, for instance, for targeted drug release of solid tumors in the intestinal tract [130]: (1) the drug administered orally can bypass the acidity of gastric fluids without liberating substantial amounts of drug and go into the intestinal fluids; (2) the tumor is subjected to local hyperthermia (typically between 37°C and 42°C), which triggers drug release.

Ma et al. [131] prepared pH- and temperature-sensitive carboxymethyl chitosan-graft-poly(N,N-diethylacrylamide) (CMCTS-g-PDEA) hydrogels as carriers of VB_2 at different pH values. It was found that VB_2 released only 10% in pH 1.2 buffer solutions and as much as 26% in pH 7.4 buffer solutions within the same time. This pH-sensitiveness was due to the formation of a large number of hydrogen bonds between the –COOH and –OH groups in CMCTS and/or the –$CONR_2$ groups in PDEA in acidic solution. Thus, from a more practical point of view, these hydrogel systems can bypass the acidity of gastric fluid without liberating substantial amounts of the loaded drug and accomplish purpose in specific drug-controlled release in the intestine. On the other hand, this hydrogel was also found to release its contents slower at 37°C than at 25°C. The temperature-sensitive phenomenon was attributed to the hydrophobic interaction of PEDA chain overwhelming the H-bonding of polymer chain with water when the temperature increased. Thus, the drug release behavior could be controlled further in this way.

PEC hydrogels can also be used as dual-sensitive carriers for ionic drugs. PEC films composed of chitosan and an anionic polymer, PAOMA copolymer, were created [132]. The drug release characteristics of this PEC in response to changes in environmental pH and temperature were studied using salicylic acid as the model drug. Both a decrease in pH from 7.2 to 3.8 and a decrease in temperature from 50°C to 25°C resulted in a corresponding decrease in the drug release rate. According to the authors, this responsiveness was because of the repulsive forces between the carboxyl groups in PAOMA and the anionic groups in model drugs at higher pH and the increase of release area caused by the phase transition of PAOMA at higher temperature.

Recently, a new method was employed to prepare smart microgels that consist of well-defined temperature-sensitive cores with pH-sensitive shells [133]. The microgels were synthesized by the aqueous graft copolymerization of NIPAM from chitosan. As a result, the cores were composed of well-defined poly(N-isopropylacrylamide) whereas the shells were composed of chitosan. Therefore, their responsiveness to pH and temperature can be manipulated individually. This unique smart hydrogel may be applicable in a further DDS for a certain purpose.

6.6.2.3 Electric-Sensitive Release

Electric-sensitive delivery systems are usually prepared from polymers containing electrosensitive moieties such as polyelectrolytes. Under the influence of an electric field, electroresponsive hydrogels generally deswell or bend, depending on the shape and orientation of the gel. The gel bends when it is parallel to the electrodes, whereas deswelling occurs when the hydrogel lies perpendicular to the electrodes [134]. The main mechanisms of drug release from the electroresponsive hydrogels include ejection of the drug solution during deswelling, diffusion, electrophoresis of charged drugs, and electro-induced gel erosion [135]. The use of chitosan gels as matrices for electrically modulated drug delivery was investigated recently [136]. In this study, release time profiles for neutral (hydrocortisone), anionic (benzoic acid), and cationic (lidocaine hydrochloride) drug molecules from chitosan gels were monitored in response to milliampere currents as a function of time. The results showed that drug release from the various formulations, involving several electrokinetic and physicochemical factors, was greater at higher milliampere current. The author stated that hydrocortisone release from the gels was probably due to the electroosmotic and diffusional forces, while the release of benzoic acid and lidocaine hydrochloride involved the additional contribution of drug polarity.

IPN hydrogels made up of PEG macromer and chitosan that exhibited electrosensitive behavior have been synthesized [137]. The electrical response of IPN hydrogels was investigated by applying electrical current to the hydrogels immersed in a NaCl solution. The extent of the bending behavior of the IPN hydrogel depends on IPN hydrogel composition and applied electric field strength. The applied voltage can increase the deformation of the hydrogels in both extent and speed. The author also proposed that the bending behavior of these swollen hydrogels under an electric field at various applied voltages could be applicable for electrically controlled drug release systems.

More recently, a nanocomposite hydrogel composed of chitosan and montmorillonite (MMT) has been prepared and the release of VB_2 under electrostimulation was studied

[138]. The drug release behavior was strongly influenced by the applied voltage and the concentration of MMT, which affected the cross-linking density of the nanohydrogels. And the release mechanism changed from a diffusion-controlled mode to a swelling-controlled mode under electrostimulation. This new class of nanohydrogels was reported to provide an interesting alternative as a long-standing electrically induced DDS with reliable drug release performance.

6.6.2.4 Enzyme-Sensitive Release

To achieve more specific release of drugs, responsiveness to enzymes that are localized to different areas of the body could be the best choice. Enzyme-controlled DDSs have been developed for colon-specific therapeutic delivery [139–141]. In an enzyme-controlled system, local enzymes produced from microflora in the human colon such as amylase, pectinase, and β-D-glucosidase break down a prodrug or a formulation containing biodegradable polymers such as pectin, guar gum, and chitosan to release the drug. Glycosidic linkages on chitosan are susceptible to glycosidic hydrolysis by microbial enzymes in the colon. Therefore, chitosan can be used as a colon-specific drug delivery vehicle.

Zhang et al. [139] prepared a multiparticulate system of chitosan hydrogel beads for colon-specific delivery of macromolecules using fluorescein isothiocyanate-labeled BSA as the model protein. The hydrogel bead was formed by polyelectrolyte complexation of chitosan with TPP. Drug release indicated that rat cecal and colonic enzymes can attack chitosan even after it has been cross-linked and its solubility reduced, resulting in a greater protein release under conditions pertaining to the colon.

In terms of chitosan-based hydrogels, an enzyme-sensitive system may, at the same time, be in response to some other stimuli, such as pH of the environment [140,141]. Nunthanid et al. [141] recently developed a colonic DDS based on a combination of time-, pH-, and enzyme-controlled systems. A combination of chitosan acetate (CSA) and hydroxypropyl methylcellulose was used as compression-coats for 5-aminosalicylic acid tablets. These chitosan-based coats were capable of retarding the release of aminosalicylic acid until the dosage forms reach the colon and there the drug was released. The delay release mechanisms during the lag time were time- and pH-controlled by the swelling gel erosion of both polymers in the acidic medium and the less solubility at high pH of CSA, respectively. The solubility of CSA at low pH facilitates drug release, while the degradation of CSA by the enzyme in the colon plays an important role in the release of the drug and helps accelerate drug release in the colon.

6.6.2.5 Glucose-Sensitive Release

In addition to the commonly used stimuli described above, other stimuli have also been used for making environment-sensitive hydrogels in order to deliver certain kinds of drugs. For example, an insulin delivery system usually requires a glucose-sensing ability to trigger the release of necessary amounts of insulin. A glucose-sensitive *in situ* gelling system based on chitosan for pulsatile delivery of insulin was developed by Kashyap et al. [142]. Glucose oxidase, an enzyme that can specifically interact with glucose and sense its levels, together with insulin, was added into a chitosan-GP solution that can form hydrogels at body temperature. These gels were found to release the entrapped insulin in a pulsatile manner in response to changes in physiological glucose concentrations. The release mechanism of this glucose-sensitive system may be as follows: Glucose oxidase immobilized in pH-sensitive chitosan hydrogels can sense glucose levels and convert glucose to gluconic acid in the presence of oxygen. The formation of the acid results in a decrease in pH; this triggers swelling in pH-sensitive chitosan hydrogels, thereby causing changes in its pore size and consequently facilitating the release of insulin by the diffusion-mediated process [142].

Recently, Manna et al. fabricated a multilayer thin film of PVA–borate and chitosan. This film was glucose sensitive and its disintegration was observed in the presence of glucose. The mechanism of glucose-triggered multilayer membrane degradation was discussed by the author. In the presence of glucose, borax molecules prefer to complex with glucose rather than PVA hydroxyl groups and thus the physically cross-linked gel loses its gelation behavior. As a result, glucose disintegrates the physically cross-linked PVA–borate complex, as shown in Figures 6.17 [143]. The glucose-triggered release of an anticancer drug, doxorubicin, from the multilayer thin film was also studied, as it is well known that cancer cells possess high concentrations of glucose. The results showed that at higher concentrations of glucose, complete disassembly of the multilayer thin film occurred and this caused the release of the drug. Therefore, this chitosan-based thin film can be utilized to target anticancer therapeutics release in cancer cells.

6.6.3 Targeted Drug Release

Drugs can be released from a hydrogel over a period of time in a controlled manner. The process could be a time-controlled one or an environmental stimuli-triggered one as mentioned above. However, in order to achieve a more specific or a more accurate administration, targeted release systems appear. These systems protect the specific drug until it reaches the desired location (e.g., a tumor or a specific organ) where the drug is released in a controlled way. This strategy could revolutionize the delivery of drugs and has the potential not only to reduce the amount of drug required to obtain effective therapy, but also to virtually eliminate nonspecific side effects.

Targeted drug delivery can be used to treat many diseases, such as cardiovascular diseases and diabetes. However, the most important application of targeted drug delivery is to treat cancerous tumors.

A targeted DDS is comprised of three components: a therapeutic agent, a targeting moiety, and a carrier system [144]. The environmental stimuli mentioned above can also be used as signals (targeting moiety) for targeting application. One can find an example of a pH-sensitive chitosan-based hydrogel used as a colon-specific DDS in Section 6.6.2.1. Such a DDS is known as a kind of physical targeted DDS. Apart from this, there are still two kinds of targeted drug delivery: active targeted drug delivery, such as some antibody medications; and passive targeted drug delivery, such as the enhanced permeability and retention (EPR) effect.

6.6.3.1 Passive Targeting: EPR Effect

Passive targeting is based on the EPR effect of the vasculature surrounding tumors, which can lead to the selective accumulation of macromolecular drugs in tumor tissues [145]. This specific passive accumulation of macromolecules was attributed to defective tumor vasculature with disorganized endothelium at the tumor site and a poor lymphatic drainage system. Researchers have taken advantage of this characteristic to deliver various drugs by encapsulating them within nanoparticles or conjugating them with polymers. Today, it is evident that long circulating macromolecules and nanosized particulates accumulate passively at the tumors due to the EPR effect [144].

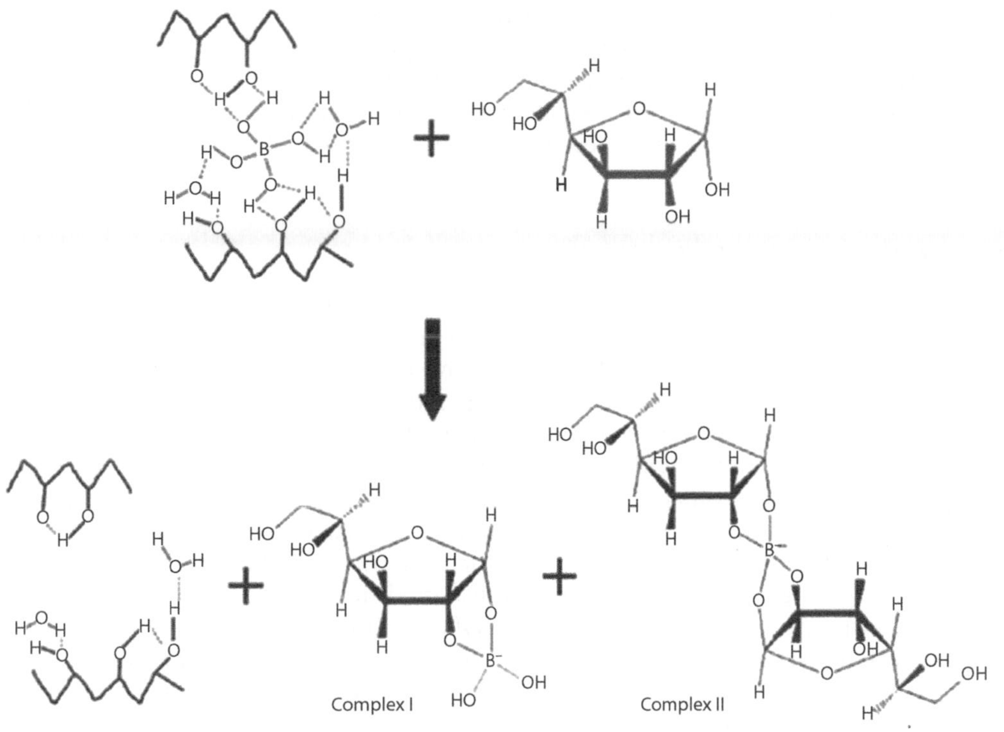

FIGURE 6.17
Disintegration of physically cross-linked PVA–borate complex by glucose. (From Manna, U. and Patil, S. 2010. *ACS Appl Mater Interfaces* 2: 1521–1527. With permission.)

Chitosan nanoparticles with anticancer drugs physically entrapped usually serve as tumor-targeting DDSs. Kim et al. [146] prepared a hydrophobically modified glycol chitosan (HGC) that can form nanosized self-aggregates in an aqueous medium. An insoluble anti-cancer drug, cisplatin (CDDP), was encapsulated into the hydrophobic cores of HGC nano-particles by a dialysis method. The drug loading efficiency was up to 80%. Chitosan-based nanoparticles released the drug in a sustained manner for a week under physiological condi-tions, controlled by the diffusion mechanism as a result of partitioning between polymer nanoparticles and surrounding aqueous phase. When the CDDP-HGC nanoparticles were injected into tumor-bearing mice, they were found to be successfully accumulated by tumor tissues because of the EPR effect. The selectively localized CDDP-HGC nanoparticles in tumor tissue showed higher antitumor efficacy and lower toxicity compared to free CDDP.

Polymer–drug conjugates composed of hydrophilic polymers to which drugs are chemi-cally conjugated via a biodegradable spacer are also used as targeted drug release systems. By EPR effects, such conjugates can be selectively accumulated at the tumor site, followed by release of the drug by cleavage of the spacer via hydrolysis or enzymatic degradation. For example, doxorubicin was conjugated to glycol–chitosan via EDC/NHS coupling chemistry and a *cis*-aconityl bond was formed between the drug and the chitosan-based carrier [138,147]. Liberation of doxorubicin was believed to be caused by cleavage of such *cis*-aconityl spacers, which are known to be pH-sensitive with a short hydrolysis half-life in acidic medium [147]. A noticeable amount of glycol–chitosan self-aggregates was found to accumulate at the tumor sites due to the EPR effect when they were systemically administered via the tail vein to tumor-bearing mice [138]. *In vivo* antitumor activity results showed that polymer–drug conjugates effectively suppressed tumor growth and reduced the toxicity against animal body when compared with commercial doxorubicin hydrochloride injection. Additionally, pH-sensitiveness of the *cis*-aconityl spacers may facilitate the targeting and release of anticancer drugs to tumor sites where the pH condition is weak acid (pH 5–6).

6.6.3.2 Active Targeting: RME

Passive targeting of drugs to tumor sites through the EPR effect does not always guarantee successful therapy if the drug does not reach the target site of the tumor cell such as the cell membrane, cytosol, or nucleus. A more effective mechanism needs to be developed so that the therapeutic medicine is able to reach the molecular targets. RME is a highly specific process happening in the human body. During the process, cells take in only certain molecules, the specificities of which are determined by receptors on the cell's membrane. This internalization of extraneous molecules can be utilized to achieve active targeting.

Compared to most normal cells, human cancer cells frequently overexpress some specific antigens or receptors on their surfaces, which can be utilized as targets in nanomedicine. Active targeting can be achieved by chemical modification of nanosized drug carriers with ligands that precisely recognize and specifically interact with receptors on the targeted tissue. For improving therapeutic effects on cancer treatment, therapeutic agents are frequently entrapped physically in the nanosized carrier where the ligands are chemically conjugated through covalent bonds. The merits of this system for delivering drugs include the following: (1) the physically entrapped drugs can preserve its activity; (2) a relatively large payload of drugs can be loaded into the hydrophobic cores of the carriers exceeding their intrinsic water solubility; (3) the targeting moieties on the carriers can be precisely tuned to increase the probability of binding to the target cells; and (4) owing to the small size of the carrier system, it can effectively infiltrate across- the inflamed leaky disease vasculature but not at the normal vasculature [144].

Folate-conjugated stearic acid-grafted chitosan (Fa-CSOSA) was synthesized by the EDC-mediated coupling reaction [148]. It can be used as an active targeting carrier, because folic acid (folate) is a low-molecular-weight vitamin whose receptor (folate receptor) is frequently overexpressed in many human cancer cells, including malignancies of the ovary, brain, kidney, breast, myeloid cells, and lungs. In the meantime, folate is always highly restricted by most normal cells [149]. The anticancer drug paclitaxel was physically encapsulated into the hydrophobic domains of nanosized Fa-CSOSA micelles by a dialysis method. The internalization of Fa-CSOSA micelles by RME was faster and greatly improved in the folate receptor overexpressing cell line, compared with the folate receptor-deficient cell line [148].

Recently, Sahu et al. [150] synthesized folate–carboxymethyl chitosan (Fa–CMCS) conjugates using 2,2'-(ethylenedioxy)-bis-ethylamine as the coupling agent. They used Fa–CMCS nanoparticles as an active targeting carrier to deliver doxorubicin, which was physically encapsulated into the nanoparticles. An *in vitro* study indicated that nanoparticles are more effectively targeting cancerous cells than normal cells because of the folate receptor overexpressing on the cancerous cell membrane. More importantly, they proposed that the basis of their research lies in the pH-sensitiveness of nanoparticles. According to them, nanoparticles can be taken up by cells via an endocytosis process. As the endocytic pathway begins near the physiological pH of 7.4, drops to a lower pH of 5.5–6.0 in endosomes, and approaches pH 4.5–5.0 in lysosomes, polymeric nanoparticles that are responsive to pH can be designed to selectively release their payload in tumor tissue or within tumor cells. In this study, a drug release test showed that the amount of doxorubicin released from nanoparticles decreased with increasing pH and the release profile exhibited a sustained pattern. Therefore, this pH-responsiveness may benefit cancer treatment via the RME mechanism.

6.6.3.3 Physical Targeting

As mentioned above, some environmental factors such as pH and temperature can be used as signals for targeting application. Here, another interesting physical targeting signal, magnetic signal, has attracted more and more attention recently. Magnetic nanoparticles, composed of a magnetic (e.g., iron oxide) core and a biocompatible polymeric shell (e.g., chitosan), are an effective DDS of this kind. The particles encapsulate drugs and can be targeted to a desired treatment location by externally localized magnetic steering [151].

For example, magnetic targeting chitosan nanoparticles were prepared through the electrostatic interaction of cationic chitosan and the negatively charged core that was composed of Fe_3O_4 nanoparticles [151]. A photodynamic therapy (PDT) agent, namely the photosensitizer, was physically entrapped in the magnetic chitosan particle by adsorption in order to develop an *in vivo* chitosan-based magnetic DDS for magnetic resonance imaging (MRI)-monitored targeting PDT. The magnetic particles were administered to tumor-bearing mice followed by exposure to an externally localized magnetic field (1 T). The results showed that the drug-loaded nanoparticles could be used in MRI-monitored targeting PDT with excellent targeting and imaging ability. Moreover, it was shown that non-toxicity and high photodynamic efficacy on SW480 carcinoma cells were achieved, and localization of nanoparticles in skin and hepatic tissue was significantly less than in tumor tissue due to the magnetic targeting effect.

The example above just shows the targeting ability of the chitosan-based magnetic DDS. Drug release from this type of DDS has also been investigated. Shen and coworkers [152] developed chitosan-coated magnetic nanoparticles containing 5-fluorouracil through a reverse microemulsion method, as a potential DDS. The resulting nanoparticles released their drugs in a sustained manner under *in vitro* conditions. After FITC labeling, the drug-loaded chitosan-based magnetic nanoparticles were found to effectively gain entry into the SPCA-1 cancer cells and induce cell apoptosis.

6.7 Application

Chitosan-based hydrogels have been used to deliver a variety of drugs, including some molecules, macromolecules, or even therapeutic cells, for treating special disease or regenerate tissues. The drugs have been loaded in chitosan gels to various sites in the human body for oral, rectal, ocular, epidermal, subcutaneous, and other applications. The literature on hydrogel formulations for pharmaceutical applications is reviewed in this section, according to the sites of administration of the drugs.

6.7.1 Drug Delivery in the Oral Cavity

Drug delivery to the oral cavity can have versatile applications in local treatment of diseases of the mouth, such as fungal and viral infections, periodontal disease, stomatitis, and oral cavity cancers. A major difficulty of achieving success in delivering drugs to these sites is the dilution and rapid elimination of topically applied medicines as a result of the flushing action of saliva that is abundant in the oral cavity. Therefore, long-term adhesion of the DDS as well as prolonging the retention of the loaded drug is required in order to achieve this local drug delivery.

Because of its excellent bioadhesive property, chitosan is widely used as carrier material for oral drug delivery. Initial studies showed that chitosan provides an extended retention time on the oral mucosa and has the ability to inhibit the adhesion of *Candida albicans* cells to human buccal cells, preventing the development of mycosis [153]. TPP-cross-linked chitosan gel and film were prepared for local delivery of chlorhexidine gluconate, an antifungal agent, to the oral cavity. An *in vitro* study indicated that a prolonged release of chlorhexidine gluconate of up to 4 h was achieved with the film. Also, an increase in antifungal activity of the drug was observed with the chitosan gel [153]. Chitosan is, moreover, an excellent candidate for the development of DDSs aiming to treat oral mucositis, which is a frequent severe complication of cancer chemotherapy and increases the risk of infection trigger by *Candida*. The hitosan gel prepared as above was also used to deliver a prophylactic agent for oral mucositis (nystatin) to the oral cavity [154]. This chitosan gel formulation significantly reduced the severity and incidence of oral mucositis, reduced weight loss and increased survival, and provided significant healing.

Chitosan microspheres were utilized for the controlled release of triclosan in oral-care formulations [155]. Triclosan was encapsulated into chitosan microspheres using a double-emulsion solvent evaporation technique, and the release profiles were established under simulated "in use" conditions. The controlled release of the drug over extended time periods was obtained, and the kinetics study showed that the release was a diffusion-controlled one.

In addition, buccal bilayered tablets composed of a drug-containing mucoadhesive layer of chitosan with polycarbophil and a backing layer of ethylcellulose were obtained by direct compression [156]. The double-layered structure provided unidirectional drug delivery toward the mucosa, and avoided a loss of drug resulting from wash-out with saliva flow. A striking feature of this device was the utilization of an *in situ* cross-linking reaction between cationic chitosan and anionic polycarbophil, which progressed upon penetration of the aqueous medium into the tablet. As a result of the cross-linking effect, the tablets showed controlled swelling and prolonged drug release, and an adequate adhesiveness could be obtained.

6.7.2 Nasal Drug Delivery

The nasal route for drug delivery has received a great deal of attention as a convenient and reliable method for the systemic administration of drugs, especially for those that are difficult to deliver via routes other than injection. The nasal route could be important for drugs that are used in crisis treatments, such as for pain and for centrally acting drugs where the putative pathway from nose to brain might provide a faster and more specific therapeutic effect [157].

In the case of patients affected by schizophrenia or other psychotic disorders, nasal delivery administration can provide more acceptable forms of medication and simultaneously enhance drugs' pharmacological profiles. Recently, Barbara Luppi et al. [158] developed freeze-dried chitosan/pectin nasal inserts for antipsychotic drug delivery. Chitosan/pectin PECs were prepared at pH 5.0 with different polycation/polyanion molar ratios and lyophilized in small inserts in the presence of chlorpromazine hydrochloride. Upon water uptake, PEC inserts became hydrogels and showed excellent mucoadhesiveness, which effectively prevented the rapid clearance of the drug formulation from the nose. For PEC with proper molar ratios, a controlled release of drugs according to hydration/diffusion mechanisms was obtained and drug permeation can be prolonged up to and over 6 h, indicating the potential for long-term treatments.

Because of the cationic characteristics of chitosan hydrogel, it is able to efficiently deliver polar drugs (including peptides and DNA) to the systemic circulation as a nasal delivery system and provide therapeutically relevant bioavailability. Chitosan–plasmid DNA complex nanoparticle, as a flu vaccine, was prepared to deliver DNA expressing nuclear protein of Influenza A virus [159]. After nasal administration of this chitosan–DNA flu vaccine, better antibody response and better protection from flu were observed in mice compared with those treated with the naked DNA system.

In order to relieve the pain and inconvenience of injections of insulin, nasal delivery of insulin to diabetic patients is preferred. Wu et al. [160] designed a new thermosensitive hydrogel for nasal delivery of insulin by simply mixing quaternized chitosan and PEG with a small amount of GP. The formulation was a solution at room temperature that transformed to a gel form when kept at 37°C. Animal experiments demonstrated that hydrogel formulation decreased the blood glucose concentration by 40–50% of the initial values for 4–5 h after administration with no apparent cytotoxicity.

6.7.3 Gastric Drug Delivery

Because the pH in the stomach is ca. 1–3 due to the strong acidity of gastric juice, drugs can be released primarily in this location when employing a proper pH-sensitive biopolymer as the drug delivery vehicle. Chitosan proves to be a good candidate owing to the protonation of amine groups when pH is low, which is favorable for the release of drugs. Targeted drug delivery to the stomach is extremely important for the treatment of local maladies, such as gastritis, gastroduodenal ulcer, and gastric cancer. *Helicobacter pylori*, which is located at the adherent mucus layer and adheres to the gastric epithelial cells *in vivo*, is responsible for most of the above disease. Anti-*H. pylori* agents include antimicrobials, such as amoxicillin, clarithromycin, and metronidazole. However, the failure of single antibiotic therapies could be attributed to the poor stability of the drug in gastric acid and the poor permeation of the antibiotic across- the mucus layer. To achieve a sustained release and a long gastric retention time of these antimicrobials, a PEC of chitosan and PAA was employed as the vehicle for amoxicillin delivery to the stomach [161]. The results indicated that antibiotics were released in a sustained way and its gastric residence time was clearly prolonged. Local gastric drug action was improved in this way. Recently, a PEC of chitosan and carboxymethylcellulose formed using a novel method "tablets-in-capsule" was utilized for gastric-specific delivery of clarithromycin. The drug release profile can be controlled more effectively [162].

6.7.4 Colonic Drug Delivery

Specific drug delivery into the colon is highly desirable for local treatment of a variety of bowel diseases such as ulcerative colitis, amebiosis, and colonic cancer, local treatment of colonic pathologies, and systemic delivery of protein and peptide drugs [163]. An oral route is usually preferred for the sake of convenience and comfort. However, the DDS employed should prevent the bioactive agent from degradation and avoid drug release and absorption in the stomach (pH 1–3) unless the system reaches the colon. The release of drug can be triggered by specific hydrolysis of the polymer matrix in the colon or the enzymatic reactions by colonic flora there. Chitosan is biodegradable by colonic bacterial flora; thus it is a commonly used polymer for colon drug delivery.

Particles of chitosan/pectin PEC particles were prepared by complex coacervation from chitosan and pectin dispersions [164]. By adding acetate phthalate into the system, the formulation presented the slowest triamcinolone release rate, of only 1.33%, in acidic medium after 2 h, which reduced the drug release in gastric juice. Therefore, particles selectively release their contents in colon sites where the crucial condition to allow drug release remain on the enzymatic degradation of polysaccharides by the specific colonic flora.

Proteins can also be delivered to the colon using a chitosan-based hydrogel carrier. Chitosan-alginate beads loaded with BSA were studied to explore the protection of protein against acidic and enzymatic degradation during gastric passage [165]. The beads showed no sign of erosion in gastric fluid, whereas they were found to erode, burst, and release the protein in intestinal fluid.

In addition, some chitosan derivatives show excellent association with insulin and improved its intestinal absorption to a great extent. Nanoparticles were prepared by the polyelectrolyte complexation method using chitosan, triethylchitosan, and dimethyl-ethylchitosan for colon delivery of insulin [166]. These nanoparticles carried positive charges and showed a size distribution in the range of 170–270 nm. Insulin loading was more than 80% for all the nanoparticles. Insulin release showed a small burst effect at the beginning and then a sustained release characteristic for 5 h. Also better insulin transport across- the colon membrane of rats was found for nanoparticles made of quaternized derivatives than for those made of chitosan. *In vivo* studies in rats have shown enhanced colon absorption of insulin by using these nanoparticles compared to free insulin in diabetic rats [166].

6.7.5 Ocular Drug Delivery

In ocular drug delivery, the major problem is to maintain an effective drug concentration at the site of action for an appropriate period of time in order to achieve the expected pharmacological response. Essential protective mechanisms of the eye, such as effective tear drainage, blinking, and low permeability of the cornea, prevent the success. Many attractive properties, such as mucoadhesive character, penetration-enhancing property, and cellular permeability, of chitosan allow it to be a very promising polymer for ocular drug delivery [167].

A novel *in situ* forming gel composed of chitosan and gellan gum was developed as an ocular DDS. The gelation was triggered by dual physiological mechanisms (pH and ion-activated gelation). Timolol maleate, the drug that is frequently used for glaucoma therapy, was used as a model drug to check the efficacy of the formulation. Clarity, gelation pH, isotonicity, sterility, viscosity, transcorneal permeation profile, and ocular irritation of the formulation have all been investigated. A significant increase in ocular retention time of this vehicle was observed. The developed system can be a viable alternative to conventional eye drops for the treatment of various ocular diseases and is suitable for clinical application [168].

Peptu et al. [169] prepared gelatin/chitosan microparticles for ocular drug delivery by a two-step cross-linking process performed in an emulsion-phase separation system.

Diameters of the particles were 0.202–4.596 µm. Adrenalin was used as the drug to be delivered. The *in vivo* adrenalin ocular delivery was tested on both animals and a voluntary human patient to determine the adrenalin action and by tears. The particles showed good adherent properties without irritation to the patient; adrenalin was released and this cleared the ocular congestion.

Nanocarriers are frequently used for ocular drug delivery, mainly because of their capacity to protect the encapsulated molecule while facilitating its transport to different compartments of the eye [167]. Chitosan nanoparticles with an average diameter of 280 nm, developed by modified ionic gelation of chitosan with TPP, were fabricated to prolong IM precorneal residence time and to improve its ocular bioavailability. Release studies showed a small initial burst release during the first hour followed by slow sustained drug release of 76% from nanoparticles during a 24 h period. According to the author, the chitosan nanocarriers developed were able to contact intimately with the cornea, providing slow gradual IM release with long-term drug level and thereby increasing delivery to both external and internal ocular tissues [170].

6.7.6 Transdermal Drug Delivery

The transdermal route is an attractive alternative to deliver therapeutic drugs. The possible benefits of transdermal drug delivery include the following: drugs can be delivered for a long duration at a constant rate, drug delivery can be easily interrupted on demand by simply removing the devices, and drugs can bypass hepatic first-pass metabolism [110]. Furthermore, drug carriers in the form of hydrogels are preferred because of their high water content, providing a comfortable feeling on the patient's skin in comparison with conventional ointments and patches.

Glimepiride, an antidiabetic sulfonylurea drug, often has adverse effects and bioavailability problems due to its poor solubility when delivered via the oral route. A transdermal delivery system for glimepiride was developed by using chitosan film as a drug vehicle. In order to optimize drug delivery and circumvent the skin barrier function, inclusion complexation of glimepiride with β-cyclodextrin was used in the formulation. Permeation studies through rat abdominal skin showed that high drug flux values were obtained from films containing glimepiride–β-cyclodextrin complex. More importantly, an evident therapeutic efficacy sustained for about 48 h was obtained on diabetic rats treated with this chitosan transdermal delivery system [171].

Recently, Lee et al. [172] prepared multifunctional core–shell polymeric nanoparticles for transdermal DNA delivery. The developed nanoparticles comprised a hydrophobic PLGA core and a positively charged glycol chitosan shell. Fluorescent quantum dots (QDs) were loaded in the core for ultrasensitive detection of Langerhans cell (LC) migration following transdermal delivery. An emulsion–diffusion–evaporation method was used to fabricate the QD-loaded nanoparticles, while a reporter gene was electrostatically adsorbed onto the glycol chitosan shell layer by mixing the nanoparticles with DNA. Chitosan-based nanoparticles can rapidly release a significant amount of their loaded DNA at pH 7.4 while being minimal at pH 6.0, indicating a pH-mediated mechanism. In addition, the mouse model study demonstrated that bombardment of nanoparticles transfected DNA directly into LCs present in the epidermis; the transfected LCs then migrated and expressed the encoded gene products in the skin draining lymph nodes, as shown in Figure 6.18 [172]. Thus, the developed nanoparticles have potential use in immunotherapy and vaccine development.

6.8 Commercial Products

Pharmaceutical companies have looked increasingly toward drug delivery companies for help in life-cycle management of drugs on the market and with promising yet hard-to-deliver drugs. The drug delivery market is valued at US$50 billion (or 12.5% of the global pharmaceutical market) by 2003 [173] and has increased remarkably during the last decade. From 2000 to 2009, about 200 FDA (Food and Drug Administration)-approved drug delivery products appeared [174].

Synthetic polymer-based DDSs, such as PLGA-based microsphere products and PEGylation drugs, have been developed by some biotech companies. For example, the PLGA-based microsphere product, known as Nutropin Depot®, provided sustained release of human growth hormone over 2–4 weeks from a single injection to treat growth hormone deficiency in pediatric patients [175]. However, this kind of product always brings about relatively severe side effects, such as erythema, bruising, and nodules. Moreover,

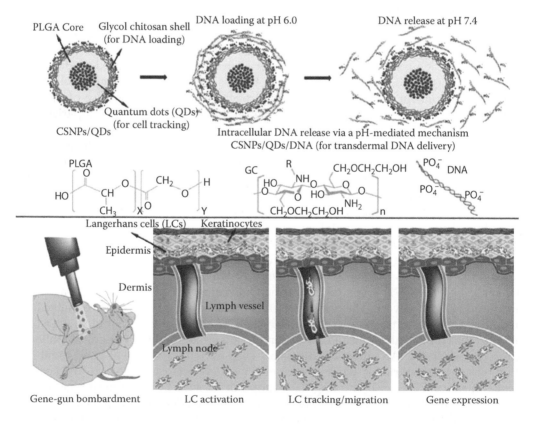

FIGURE 6.18
Schematic illustrations of the concept of multifunctional core–shell polymeric nanoparticles designed in the study: transdermal DNA delivery, tracking of LC migration, a pH-mediated DNA release mechanism, and gene expression in lymph nodes. CSNPs/QDs: core–shell nanoparticles incorporation with QDs. Abbreviation: CSNPs/QDs/DNA: CSNPs/QDs loaded with DNA. (From Lee, P. W. et al. 2010. *Biomaterials* 31: 2425–2434. With permission.)

drug (i.e., protein) loading is low and the carrier is difficult to manufacture, which have led to reduced yield and increased manufacturing costs [175].

Chitosan has been recently highlighted for its unique features in pharmaceutical formulations, especially in DDSs such as micro/nanoparticles and hydrogels for mucosal and vaccine delivery. It is particularly well suited for the formulation of drugs such as peptides, proteins, RNA, and DNA, offering unique functionalities such as mucoadhesiveness, enhanced bioavailability, enhanced cross-ing of biological barriers, bioresorbability, targeting power, and easy and robust processing into various forms [176]. Unfortunately, despite the high number of published studies, chitosan is not approved by the FDA for any product in drug delivery [177]. Some companies are conducting trials to develop chitosan-based DDS products. For example, West Pharmaceutical Services, Inc. has developed ChiSys™, a versatile transmucosal delivery system based on chitosan to deliver leuprolide for the treatment of prostate cancer [173]. Several human trials have been carried out on ChiSys™ for delivering a range of compounds from small molecules and peptides to proteins and vaccines, and a higher bioavailability of drugs and few adverse effects have been reported to date [173]. With the aim of developing chitosan-based DDS products approved by FDA in the future and enabling the provision of health benefits over current formulations, more clinical trials need to be carried out and more precautions, that is, purification of chitosan, shape/geometries/size of the vehicle, biodistribution, and degradability, should be taken [177].

6.9 Conclusions

Owing to their well-documented biocompatibility, biodegradability, low toxicity, mucoadhesivity, pH-sensitivity, and so on, as well as the merits of hydrogels, chitosan-based hydrogels in various geometries have long been used as DDSs. Additionally, because of the chemical activity of the amine groups along the macromolecules, chitosans are modified and an impressive number of chitosan derivatives have been developed to broaden the applications of chitosan-based gels as drug delivery carriers. The approach of chemical modification of chitosan or grafting chitosan with other functional materials such as stimuli-responsive polymers, cyclodextrins, and biomolecules is of potential importance in drug delivery fields since the resulting materials exhibit an improved drug loading capacity and sustained release behavior along with other unique properties such as stimuli-sensitivity, good mechanical strength, and so on. Today, the most attractive and significant drug delivery such as environment stimuli-controlled delivery, targeted or specific local delivery, as well as tough drug delivery such as delivery of macromolecules, hydrophobic drugs, bioactive molecules, DNA, gene, and vaccine are all achieved by using chitosan-based gel DDSs. These kinds of hydrogels are becoming one of the most significant and promising DDSs.

However, extensive research is still necessary to demonstrate the safety of novel chitosan derivatives. Clinical trials should be given emphasis to optimize chitosan-based formulations for DDSs with a broad range of therapeutic applications. With a better understanding of the fundamental loading and release criteria of different therapeutics as well as the mechanisms of action of novel chitosan-based hydrogel carriers, further optimizations of these systems can be made by researchers, and chitosan hydrogel DDSs could be applied clinically in the near future to relieve the suffering of patients.

References

1. Cukierman, E. and Khan, D. R. 2010. The benefits and challenges associated with the use of drug delivery systems in cancer therapy. *Biochem Pharm* 80: 762–770.
2. Balasubramanian, V., Onaca, O., Enea, R., Hughes, D. W., and Palivan, C. G. 2010. Protein delivery: From conventional drug delivery carriers to polymeric nanoreactors. *Expert Opin Drug Deliv* 7: 63–78.
3. Ravi Kumar, M. N. V. 2008. *Handbook of Particulate Drug Delivery* (2-Volume Set). Stevenson Ranch, CA: American Scientific Publishers. ISBN 1-58883-123-X.
4. Bhattarai, N., Gunn, J., and Zhang, M. Q. 2010. Chitosan-based hydrogels for controlled, localized drug delivery. *Adv Drug Deliv Rev* 62: 83–99.
5. Peter, M. G. 1995. Applications and environmental aspects of chitin and chitosan. *J Macromol Sci-Pure Appl Chem* A32: 629–640.
6. Hoffman, A. S. 2002. Hydrogels for biomedical applications. *Adv Drug Deliv Rev* 54: 3–12.
7. Jagur-Grodzinski, J. 2010. Polymeric gels and hydrogels for biomedical and pharmaceutical applications. *Polym Adv Technol* 21: 27–47.
8. Wang, C. M., Varshney, R. R., and Wang, D. A. 2010. Therapeutic cell delivery and fate control in hydrogels and hydrogel hybrids. *Adv Drug Deliv Rev* 62: 699–710.
9. Deligkaris, K., Tadele, T. S., Olthuis, W., and Berga, A. V. D. 2010. Hydrogel-based devices for biomedical applications. *Sens Actuators B Chem* 147: 765–774.
10. Hoare, T. R. and Kohane, D. S. 2008. Hydrogels in drug delivery: Progress and challenges. *Polymer* 49: 1993–2007.
11. Klouda, L. and Mikos, A. G. 2008. Thermoresponsive hydrogels in biomedical applications. *Eur J Pharm Biopharm* 68: 34–45.
12. Langer, R. 2001. Drug delivery: Drugs on target. *Science* 293: 58–59.
13. Jung, K. O., Ray, D., Daniel, J. S., and Matyjaszewski, K. 2008. The development of microgels/nanogels for drug delivery applications. *Prog Polym Sci* 33: 448–477.
14. Lapidota, S. A. and Kost, J. Hydrogels. *Encyclopedia of Materials: Science and Technology*, pp. 3878–3882. England: Elsevier Ltd.
15. Katz, J. S. and Burdick, J. A. 2009. Hydrogel mediated delivery of trophic factors for neural repair. *Wiley Interdiscip Rev Nanomed Nanobiotechnol* 1: 128–139.
16. Denkbas, E. B. and Ottenbrite, R. M. 2006. Perspectives on: Chitosan drug delivery systems based on their geometries. *J Bioact Compat Polym* 21: 351–368.
17. Belgacem, M. N. and Gandini, A. 2008. *Monomers, Polymers and Composites from Renewable Resources*. England Elsevier Ltd.
18. Agnihotri, S. A., Mallikarjuna, N. N., and Aminabhavi T. M. 2004. Recent advances on chitosan-based micro- and nanoparticles in drug delivery. *J Control Release* 100: 5–28.
19. Prabaharan, M., Borges, J. P., Godinho, M. H., and Mano, J. F. 2006. Liquid crystalline behaviour of chitosan in formic, acetic, and monochloroacetic acid solutions. *Mater Sci Forum* 514–516: 1010–1014.
20. Mani, P. 2008. Review paper: Chitosan derivatives as promising materials for controlled drug delivery. *J Biomater Appl* 23: 5–35.
21. Gupta, K. C. and Kumar, M. N. V. R. 2000. An overview on chitin and chitosan applications with an emphasis on controlled drug release formulations. *J Macromol Sci—Rev Macromol Chem Phys* C40: 273–308.
22. Berscht, P. C., Nies, B., Liebendorfer, A., and Kreuter, J. 1994. Incorporation of basic fibroblast growth factor into methylpyrrolidinone chitosan fleeces and determination of the *in vitro* release characteristics. *Biomaterials* 15: 593–600.
23. Dung, P. L., Milas, M., Rinaudo, M., and Desbrières, J. 1994. Water soluble derivatives obtained by controlled chemical modification of chitosan. *Carbohydr Polym* 24: 209–214.
24. Rinaudo, M., Auzely, R., Vallin, C., and Mullagaliev, I. 2005. Specific interactions in modified chitosan systems. *Biomacromolecules* 6: 2396–2407.

25. Tien, C. L., Lacroix, M., Szabo, P. I., and Mateescu, M. A. 2003. N-acylated chitosan: Hydrophobic matrices for controlled drug release. *J. Control Release* 93: 1–13.
26. Liu, W., Zhang, X., Sun, S. J., Sun, G. J., Yao, K. D., Liang, D. C., Guo, G., and Zhang, J. Y. 2003. N-alkylated chitosan as a potential nonviral vector for gene transfection. *Bioconjugate Chem* 14: 782–789.
27. Klotzbach, T. L., Watt, M., Ansari, Y., and Minteer, S. D. 2008. Improving the microenvironment for enzyme immobilization at electrodes by hydrophobically modifying chitosan and Nafion polymers. *J Memb Sci* 311: 81–88.
28. Li, F., Liu, W. G., and Yao, K. D. 2002. Preparation of oxidized glucose-cross linked N-alkylated chitosan membrane and *in vitro* studies of pH-sensitive drug delivery behavior. *Biomaterials* 23: 343–347.
29. Bernkop-Schnürch, A., Hornof, M., and Guggi, D. 2004. Thiolated chitosans. *Eur J Pharm Biopharm* 57: 9–17.
30. Krauland, A. H., Guggi, D., and Bernkop-Schnurch, A. 2006. Thiolated chitosan microparticles: A vehicle for nasal peptide drug delivery. *Int J Pharm* 307: 270–277.
31. Hornof, M. D., Kast, C. E., and Schnurch, A. B. 2003. *In-vitro* evaluation of the viscoelastic properties of chitosan–thioglycolic acid conjugates. *Euro J Pharm Biopharm* 55: 185–190.
32. Krauland, A. H., Hoffer, M. H., and Bernkop-Schnurch, A. 2005. Viscoelastic properties of a new *in situ* gelling thiolated chitosan conjugate. *Drug Dev Ind Pharm* 31: 885–893.
33. Teng, D. Y., Wu, Z. M., Zhang, X. G., Wang, Y. X., Zheng, C., Wang, Z., and Li, C. X. 2010. Synthesis and characterization of *in situ* cross-linked hydrogel based on self-assembly of thiol-modified chitosan with PEG diacrylate using Michael type addition. *Polymer* 51: 639–646.
34. Kim, M. S., Choi, Y. J., Noh, I., and Tae, G. 2007. Synthesis and characterization of *in situ* chitosan-based hydrogel via grafting of carboxyethyl acrylate. *J Biomed Mater Res A* 83: 674–684.
35. Chung, H. J., Bae, J. W., Park, H. D., Lee, J. W., and Park, K. D. 2005. Thermosensitive chitosans as novel injectable biomaterials. *Macromol Symp* 224: 275–286.
36. Park, K. M., Lee, S. Y., Joung, Y. K., Na, J. S., Lee, M. C., and Park K. D. 2009. Thermosensitive chitosan–pluronic hydrogel as an injectable cell delivery carrier for cartilage regeneration. *Acta Biomater* 5: 1956–1965.
37. Bhattarai, N., Matsen, F. A., and Zhang, M. Q. 2005. PEG-grafted chitosan as an injectable thermoreversible hydrogel. *Macromol Biosci* 5: 107–111.
38. Bhattarai, N., Ramaya, H. R., Gunna, J., Matsenb, F. A., and Zhang, M. Q. 2005. PEG-grafted chitosan as an injectable thermosensitive hydrogel for sustained protein release. *J Control Release* 103: 609–624.
39. Tojima, T., Katsura, H., Han, S. M., Tanida, F., Nishi, N., Tokura, S., and Sakairi, N. 1998. Preparation of an α-cyclodextrin-linked chitosan derivative via reductive amination strategy. *J Polym Sci A Polym Chem* 36: 1965–1968.
40. Prabaharan, M. and Mano, J. F. 2005. Hydroxypropyl chitosan bearing β-cyclodextrin cavities: Synthesis and slow release of its inclusion complex with a model hydrophobic drug. *Macromol Biosci* 5: 965–973.
41. Carreira, A. S., Gonçalves, F. A. M. M., Mendonça, P. V., Gila, M. H., and Coelho, J. F. J. 2010. Temperature and pH responsive polymers based on chitosan: applications and new graft copolymerization strategies based on living radical polymerization. *Carbohydr Polym* 80: 618–630.
42. Kim, S. Y., Cho, S. M., Lee, Y. M., and Kim, S. J. 2000. Thermo- and pH-responsive behaviors of graft copolymer and blend based on chitosan and N-isopropylacrylamide. *J Appl Polym Sci* 78: 1381–1391.
43. Cai, H., Zhang, Z. P., Sun, P. C., He, B. L., and Zhu, X. X. 2005. Synthesis and characterization of thermo- and pH-sensitive hydrogels based on chitosan grafted N-isopropylacrylamide via gamma-radiation. *Radiat Phys Chem* 74: 26–30.
44. dos Santos, K., Coelho, J. F. J., Ferreira, P., Pinto, I., Lorenzetti, S. G., Ferreira, E. I., Higac, O. Z., and Gilb, M. H. 2006. Synthesis and characterization of membranes obtained by graft copolymerization of 2-hydroxyethyl methacrylate and acrylic acid onto chitosan. *Int J Pharm* 310: 37–45.

45. Shantha, K. L., Bala, U., and Rao, K. P. 1995. Tailor-made chitosans for drug delivery. *Eur Polym J* 31: 377–382.
46. Kweon, D. K. and Kang, D. W. 1999. Drug-release behavior of chitosan-g-poly(vinyl alcohol) copolymer matrix. *J Appl Polym Sci* 74: 458–464.
47. Tang, J., Hua, D. B., Cheng, J. X., Jiang, J., and Zhu, X. L. 2008. Synthesis and properties of temperature-responsive chitosan by controlled free radical polymerization with chitosan-RAFT agent. *Int. J. Biol. Macromol.* 43: 383–389.
48. Hennink, W. E., De Jong, S. J., Bos, G. W., Veldhuis, T. F. J., and van Nostrum, C. F. 2004. Biodegradable dextran hydrogels cross-linked by stereocomplex formation for the controlled release of pharmaceutical proteins. *Int J Pharm* 277: 99–104.
49. Shu, X. Z. and Zhu, K. J. 2002. Controlled drug release properties of ionically cross-linked chitosan beads: The influence of anion structure. *Int J Pharm* 233: 217–225.
50. Anal, A. K., Stevens, W. F., and Remuñán-López, C. 2006. Ionotropic cross-linked chitosan microspheres for controlled release of ampicillin. *Int. J. Pharm.* 312: 166–173.
51. Yao, K. D., Yao, F. L., Li, J. J., and Yin, Y. J. 2008. Chitosan-based gels. In *Smart Materilas*, M. S. Schwartz, ed. 10-2–10-13. Boca Raton, FL: Taylor& Francis.
52. Yin, Y., Li, Z., Sun, Y., and Yao, K. 2005. A preliminary study on chitosan/gelatin polyelectrolyte complex formation. *J Mater Sci* 40: 4649–4652.
53. Chenite, A., Chaput, C., Wang, D., Combes, C., Buschmann, M. D., Hoemann, C. D., Leroux, J. C., Atkinson, B. L., Binette, F., and Selmani, A. 2000. Novel injectable neutral solutions of chitosan form biodegradable gel *in situ*. *Biomaterials* 21: 2155–2161.
54. Chenite, A., Buschmann, M., Wang, D., Chaputa, C., and Kandanic, N. 2001. Rheological characterization of thermogelling chitosan/glycerolphosphate solutions. *Carbohydr Polym* 46: 39–47.
55. Jarry, C. and Shive, M. S. Chitosan-based hydrogels in biomedical and pharmaceutical sciences. In *Smart Materilas*, M. S. Schwartz, ed. 10-13–10-20. Boca Raton, FL: Taylor & Francis.
56. Philippova, O. E., Volkov, E. V., Sitnikova, N. L., Khokhlov, A. R., Desbrieres, J., and Rinaudo, M. 2001. Two types of hydrophobic aggregates in aqueous solutions of chitosan and its hydrophobic derivative. *Biomacromolecules* 2: 483–490.
57. Nguyen, M. K. and Lee, D. S. 2010. Injectable biodegradable hydrogels. *Macromol Biosci* 10: 563–579.
58. Tang, Y. F., Du, Y., M., Hu, X. W., Shi, X. W., and Kennedy, J. F. 2007. Rheological characterisation of a novel thermosensitive chitosan/oly(vinyl alcohol) blend hydrogel. *Carbohydr Polym* 67: 491–499.
59. Xiao, C. M., Gao, F., and Gao, Y. K. 2010. Controlled preparation of physically cross-linked chitosan-g-poly(vinyl alcohol) hydrogel. *J Appl Polym Sci* 117: 2946–2950.
60. Koyano, T., Koshizaki, N., Umehara, H., Naguru, M., and Minoura, N. 2000. Surface states of PVA/chitosan blended hydrogels. *Polymer* 41: 4461–4465.
61. Tang, Y. F. and Du, Y. M. 2008. Chitosan-based injectable and thermosensitive hydrogel. *Prog Chem* 20: 239–244.
62. Muzzarelli, R. A. A. 2009. Genipin-cross-linked chitosan hydrogels as biomedical and pharmaceutical aids. *Carbohydr Polym* 77: 1–9.
63. Marguerite, R. 2010. New way to cross-link chitosan in aqueous solution. *Eur Polym J* 46: 1537–1544.
64. Weng, L., Romanov, A., Rooney, J., and Chen, W. 2008. Non-cytotoxic, *in situ* gelable hydrogels composed of N-carboxyethyl chitosan and oxidized dextran. *Biomaterial* 29: 3905–3913.
65. Simi, C. K. and Abraham, T. E. 2010. Transparent xyloglucan–chitosan complex hydrogels for different applications. *Food Hydrocolloids* 24: 72–80.
66. Hiemstra, C., van der Aa, L. J., Zhong, Z. Y., Dijkstra, P. J., and Feijen, J. 2007. Rapidly *in situ*-forming degradable hydrogels from dextran thiols through Michael addition. *Biomacromolecules* 8: 1548–1556.
67. Van de Wetering, P., Metters, A. T., Schoenmakers, R. G., and Hubbell, J. A. 2005. Poly(ethylene glycol) hydrogels formed by conjugate addition with controllable swelling, degradation, and release of pharmaceutically active proteins. *J Control Release* 102: 619–627.

68. Sakai, S., Yamada, Y., Zenke, T., and Kawakami, K. 2009. Novel chitosan derivative soluble at neutral pH and *in-situ* gellable via peroxidase-catalyzed enzymatic reaction. *J Mater Chem* 19: 230–235.

69. Jin, R., Moreira Teixeira, L. S., Dijkstra, P. J., Karperien, M., van Blitterswijk, C. A., Zhong, Z. Y., and Feijen, J. 2009. Injectable chitosan-based hydrogels for cartilage tissue engineering. *Biomaterials* 30: 2544–2551.

70. Sakai, S., Hirose, K., Taguchi, K., Ogushi, Y., and Kawakami, K. 2009. An injectable, *in situ* enzymatically gellable, gelatin derivative for drug delivery and tissue engineering. *Biomaterials* 30: 3371–3377

71. Jin, R., Moreira Teixeira, L. S., Dijkstra, P. J., van Blitterswijk, C. A., Karperien, M., and Feijen, J. 2010. Enzymatically-cross-linked injectable hydrogels based on biomimetic dextran–hyaluronic acid conjugates for cartilage tissue engineering. *Biomaterials* 31: 3103–3113.

72. Sakai, S., Matsuyama, T., Hirose, K., and Kawakami, K. 2010. *In situ* simultaneous protein-polysaccharide bioconjugation and hydrogelation using horseradish peroxidase. *Biomacromolecules* 11: 1370–1375.

73. Ono, K., Saito, Y., Yura, H., Ishikawa, K., Kurita, A., Akaike, T., and Ishihara, M. 2000. Photocross-linkable chitosan as a biological adhesive. *J. Biomed Mater Res* 49: 289–295.

74. Ishihara, M., Obara, K., Nakamura, S., Fujita, M., Masuoka, K., Kanatani, Y., Takase, B. et al. 2006. Chitosan hydrogel as a drug delivery carrier to control angiogenesis. *J Artif Organs* 9: 8–16.

75. Amsden, B. G., Sukarto, A., Knight, D. K., and Shapka, S. N. 2007. Methacrylated glycol chitosan as a photopolymerizable biomaterial. *Biomacromolecules* 8: 3758–3766.

76. Gao, X. Y., Zhou, Y. S., Ma, G. P., Shi, S. Q., Yang, D. Z., Lu, F. M., and Nie, J. 2010. A water-soluble photocross-linkable chitosan derivative prepared by Michael-addition reaction as a precursor for injectable hydrogel. *Carbohydr Polym* 79: 507–512.

77. Renbutsu, E., Hirose, M., Omura, Y., Nakatsubo, F., Okamura, Y., Okamoto, Y., Saimoto, H., Shigemasa, Y., and Minami, S. 2005. Preparation and biocompatibility of novel UV-curable chitosan derivatives. *Biomacromolecules* 6: 2385–2388.

78. Alvarez-Lorenzo, C., Concheiro, A., Dubovik, A. S., Grinberg, N. V., Burova, T. V., and Grinberg, V. Y. 2005. Temperature-sensitive chitosan-poly(*N*-isopropylacrylamide) interpenetrated networks with enhanced loading capacity and controlled release properties. *J Control Release* 102: 629–641.

79. Chow, K. S. and Khor, E. 2000. Novel fabrication of open-pore chitin matrixes. *Biomacromolecules* 1: 61–67.

80. Geng, L. Feng, W. Hutmacher, D. W., Wong, Y., Loh, H., and Fuh, J. Y. H. 2005. Direct writing of chitosan scaffolds using a robotic system. *Rapid Prototyping J* 11: 90–97.

81. Cardea, S., Pisanti, P., and Reverchon, E. 2010. Generation of chitosan nanoporous structures for tissue engineering applications using a supercritical fluid assisted process. *J Supercrit Fluids* 54: 290–295.

82. Sinha, V. R., Singla, A. K., Wadhawan, S., Kaushik, R., Kumria, R., Bansal, K., and Dhawan, S. 2004. Chitosan microspheres as a potential carrier for drugs. *Int J Pharm* 274: 1–33.

83. Sundar, S., Kundu, J., and Kundu, S. C. 2010. Biopolymeric nanoparticles. *Sci Technol Adv Mater* 11: 014104 (13pp).

84. Jung, K. O., Drumright, R., Siegwart, D. J., and Matyjaszewski, K. 2008. The development of microgels/nanogels for drug delivery applications. *Prog Polym Sci* 33: 448–477.

85. Denkbas, E. B. and Odabasl, M. 2000. Chitosan microspheres and sponges: Preparation and characterization. *J Appl Poly Sci* 76: 1637–1643.

86. Denkbas, E. B., Seyyal, M., and Piskin, E. 1998. 5-Fluorouracil loaded chitosan microspheres for chemoembolization. *J Microencapsulation* 16: 741–749.

87. Jung, K. O., Lee, D. I., and Park, J. M. 2009. Biopolymer-based microgels/nanogels for drug delivery applications. *Prog Polym Sci* 34: 1261–1282.

88. Leong, Y. S. and Candau, F. 1982. Inverse microemulsion polymerization. *J Phys Chem* 86: 2269–2271.

89. Mitra, S., Gaur, U., Ghosh, P. C., and Maitra, A. N. 2001. Tumor targeted delivery of encapsulated dextran–doxorubicin conjugate using chitosan nanoparticles as carrier. *J Control Release* 74: 317–323.

90. Berthod, A. and Kreuter, J. 1996. Chitosan microspheres-improved acid stability and change in physicochemical properties by cross-linking. *Proc Int Symp Control Release Bioact Mater* 23: 369–370.

91. Bodnar, M., Hartmann, J. F., and Borbely, J. 2006. Synthesis and study of cross-linked chitosan-N-poly(ethylene glycol) nanoparticles. *Biomacromolecules* 7: 3030–3036.

92. Csaba, N., Köping-Höggård, M., and Alonso, M. J. 2009. Ionically cross-linked chitosan/tripolyphosphate nanoparticles for oligonucleotide and plasmid DNA delivery. *Int J Pharm* 382: 205–214.

93. Cuna, M., Alonso-Sandel, M., Remunan-Lopez, C., Pivel, J. P., Alonso-Lebrero, J. L., and Alonso, M. J. 2006. Development of phosphorylated glucomannan-coated chitosan nanoparticles as nanocarriers for protein delivery. *J Nanosci Nanotechnol* 6: 2887–2895.

94. Zhou, X., Liu, B., Yu, X., Zha, X., Zhang, X., Chen, Y., Wang, X. et al. 2007. Controlled release of PEI/DNA complexes from mannose bearing chitosan microspheres as a potent delivery system to enhance immune response to HBV DNA vaccine. *J Control Release* 121: 200–207.

95. Silva, C. L., Pereira, J. C., Ramalho, A., Pais Alberto, A. C. C., and Sousa Joao, J. S. 2008. Films based on chitosan polyelectrolyte complexes for skin drug delivery: Development and characterization. *J Memb Sci* 320: 268–279.

96. Ammar, H. O., Salama, H. A., El-Nahhas, S. A., and Elmotasem, H. 2008. Design and evaluation of chitosan films for transdermal delivery of glimepiride. *Curr Drug Deliv* 5: 290–298.

97. Ganji, F. and Abdekhodaie, M. J. 2010. Chitosan–g-PLGA copolymer as a thermosensitive membrane. *Carbohydr Polym* 80: 740–746.

98. Bernabé, P., Peniche, C., and Argüelles-Monal, W. 2005. Swelling behavior of chitosan/pectin polyelectrolyte complex membranes. Effect of thermal cross-linking. *Polym Bull* 55: 367–375.

99. Bhattarai, N., Edmondson, D., Veiseh, O., Matsen, F. A., and Zhang, M. Q. 2005. Electrospun chitosan-based nanofibers and their cellular compatibility. *Biomaterials* 26: 6176–6184.

100. Lee, K. Y., Jeong, L., Kang, Y. O., Lee, S. J., and Park, W. H. 2009. Electrospinning of polysaccharides for regenerative medicine. *Adv Drug Deliv Rev* 61: 1020–1032.

101. Jiang, H., Fang, D., Hsiao, B., Chu, B., and Chen, W. 2004. Preparation and characterization of ibuprofen-loaded poly(lactide-co-glycolide)/poly(ethylene glycol)-g-chitosan electrospun membranes. *J Biomat Sci Polym Ed* 15: 279–296.

102. Kim, S. W., Bae, Y. H., and Okano, T. 1992. Hydrogels: Swelling, drug loading, and release. *Pharm Res* 9: 283–290.

103. Liu, X. D., Howard, K. A., Dong, M. D. Andersena, M. Ø., Rahbek, U. L., Johnsen, M. G., Hansenc, O. C., Besenbacher, F., and Kjems, J. 2007. The influence of polymeric properties on chitosan/sirna nanoparticle formulation and gene silencing. *Biomaterials* 28: 1280–1288.

104. Urrusuno, R. F., Calvo, P., Lopez, C. R., Vila Jato, J. L., and Alonso, M. J. 1999. Enhancement of nasal absorption of insulin using chitosan nanoparticles. *Pharm Res* 16: 1576–1581.

105. Boonsongrit, Y., Mitrevej, A., and Mueller, B. W. 2006. Chitosan drug binding by ionic interaction. *Eur J Pharm Biopharm* 62: 267–274.

106. Boonsongrit, Y., Mueller, B. W., and Mitrevej, A. 2008. Characterization of drug–chitosan interaction by ^{1}H NMR, FTIR and isothermal titration calorimetry. *Eur J Pharm Biopharm* 69: 388–395.

107. Wu, P., He, X. X., Wang, K. M., Tan, W., He, C., and Zheng, M. 2009. A novel methotrexate delivery system based on chitosan-methotrexate covalently conjugated nanoparticles. *J Biomed Nanotechnol* 5: 557–564.

108. Lee, E., Kim, H., Lee, I. H., and Jon, S. Y. 2009. *In vivo* antitumor effects of chitosan-conjugated docetaxel after oral administration. *J Control Release* 140: 79–85.

109. Cho, Y. I., Park, S. Y., Jeong, S. Y., and Yoo, H. S. 2009. *In vivo* and *in vitro* anti-cancer activity of thermo-sensitive and photo-cross-linkable doxorubicin hydrogels composed of chitosan–doxorubicin conjugates. *Eur J Pharm Biopharm* 73: 59–65.

110. Peppas, N. A., Bures, P., Leobandung, W., and Ichikawa, H. 2000. Hydrogels in pharmaceutical formulations. *Eur J Pharm Biopharm* 50: 27–46.
111. Tang, Y. F., Zhao, Y. Y. Li, Y., and Du, Y. M. 2010. A thermosensitive chitosan/poly(vinyl alcohol) hydrogel containing nanoparticles for drug delivery. *Polym Bull* 64: 791–804.
112. Lee, J. E., Kim, S. E., Kwon, I.C., Ahn, H. J., Cho, H., Lee, S. H., Kim, H. J., Seong, S. C., and Lee, M. C. 2004. Effects of a chitosan scaffold containing TGF-beta1 encapsulated chitosan microspheres on *in vitro* chondrocyte culture. *Artif Organs* 28: 829–839.
113. Cai, D. Z., Zeng, C., Quan, D. P., Bu, L. S., Wang, K., Lu, H. D., and Li, X. F. 2007. Biodegradable chitosan scaffolds containing microspheres as carriers for controlled transforming growth factor-beta1 delivery for cartilage tissue engineering. *Chin Med J* 120: 197–203.
114. Hong, Y., Gong, Y. H., Gao, C. Y., and Shen, J. C. 2008. Collagen-coated polylactide microcarriers/chitosan hydrogel composite: Injectable scaffold for cartilage regeneration. *J Biomed Mater Res A* 85: 628–637.
115. Martin, L., Wilson, C. G., Koosha, F., and Uchegbu, I. F. 2003. Sustained buccal delivery of the hydrophobic drug denbufylline Using physically cross-linked palmitoyl glycol chitosan hydrogels. *Eur J Pharm Biopharm* 55: 35–45.
116. Tojima, T., Katsura, H., Nishiki, M., Nishi, N., Tokura, S., and Sakairi, N. 1999. Chitosan beads with pendant α-cyclodextrin: Preparation and inclusion property to nitrophenolates. *Carbohydr Polym* 40: 17–22.
117. Li, C. and Metters, A. T. 2006. Hydrogels in controlled release formulations: Network design and mathematical modeling. *Adv Drug Deliv Rev* 58:1379–1408.
118. Hamid, M., Azadi, A., and Rafiei, P. 2008. Hydrogel nanoparticles in drug delivery. *Adv Drug Deliv Rev* 60: 1638–1649.
119. Peppas, N. A., Bures, P., Leobandung, W., and Ichikawa. H. 2000. Hydrogels in pharmaceutical formulations. *Eur J Pharm Biopharm* 50: 27–46.
120. Brazel, C. S. and Peppas, N. A. 2000. Modeling of drug release from swellable polymers. *Eur J Pharm Biopharm* 49: 47–58.
121. Qiu, Y. and Park, K. 2001. Environment-sensitive hydrogels for drug delivery. *Adv Drug Deliv Rev* 53: 321–339.
122. Liu, W. G., Sun, S. J., Cao, Z. Q., Zhang, X., Yao, K. D., Lu, W. W., and Luk, K. D. K. 2005. An investigation on the physicochemical properties of chitosan/DNA polyelectrolyte complexes. *Biomaterials* 26: 2705–2711.
123. Jayakumar, R., Reis, R. L., and Mano, J. F. 2007. Synthesis and characterization of pH-sensitive thiol-containing chitosan beads for controlled drug delivery applications. *Drug Delivery,* 14(1): 9–17.
124. Gong, S. Q., Tu, H. W., Zheng, H. et al. 2010. Chitosan-g-PAA hydrogels for colon-specific drug delivery: Preparation, swelling behavior and *in vitro* degradability. *Journal of Wuhan University of Technology- Mater Sci Ed* 25: 248–251.
125. AL-Kahtani Ahmed, A., Bhojya Naik, H. S., and Sherigara, B. S. 2009. Synthesis and characterization of chitosan-based pH-sensitive semi-interpenetrating network microspheres for controlled release of diclofenac sodium. *Carbohydr Res* 344: 699–706.
126. Zhou, Y. S., Yang, D. Z., Ma, G. P., Tan, H., Jin, Y., and Nie, J. 2008. A pH-sensitive water-soluble N-carboxyethyl chitosan/poly(hydroxyethyl methacrylate) hydrogel as a potential drug sustained release matrix prepared by photopolymerization technique. *Polym Adv Technol* 19: 1133–1141.
127. Guo, B. L., Yuan, J. F., and Gao, Q. Y. 2008. pH and ionic sensitive chitosan/carboxymethyl chitosan IPN complex films for the controlled release of coenzyme A. *Colloid Polym Sci* 286: 175–181.
128. Lin, W. C., Yu, D. G., and Yang, M. C. 2005. pH-sensitive polyelectrolyte complex gel microspheres composed of chitosan/sodium tripolyphosphate/dextran sulfate: Swelling kinetics and drug delivery properties. *Colloids Surf B Biointerfaces* 44: 143–151.
129. Alvarez-Lorenzo, C., Concheiro, A., Dubovik, A. S., Grinberg, N. V., Burova, T. V., and Grinberg, V. Y. 2005. Temperature-sensitive chitosan- poly(N-isopropylacrylamide) interpenetrated

networks with enhanced loading capacity and controlled release properties. *J Control Release* 102: 629–641.

130. Shi, J., Alves, N. M., and Mano, J. F. 2008. Chitosan coated alginate beads containing poly (*N*-isopropylacrylamide) for dual-stimuli-responsive drug release. *J Biomed Mater Res Part B: Appl Biomater* 84: 595–603.

131. Ma, L. W., Liu, M. Z., Liu, H. L., Chen, J., Gao, C. M., and Cui, D. P. 2010. Dual cross-linked pH- and temperature-sensitive hydrogel beads for intestine-targeted controlled release. *Polym Adv Technol* 21: 348–355.

132. Yoshizawa, T., Shin-Ya, Y., Hong, K. J., and Kajiuchi, T. 2005. pH- and temperature-sensitive release behaviors from polyelectrolyte complex films composed of chitosan and PAOMA copolymer. *Eur J Pharm Biopharm* 59: 307–313.

133. Leung, M. F., Zhu, J. M., Harris, F. W., and Li, P. 2004. New route to smart core–shell polymeric microgels: Synthesis and properties. *Macromol Rapid Commun* 25: 1819–1823.

134. Bajpai, A. K., Shukla, S. K., Bhanu, S., and Kankane, A. 2008. Responsive polymers in controlled drug delivery. *Prog Polym Sci* 33: 1088–1118.

135. Murdan, S. 2003. Electro-responsive drug delivery from hydrogels. *J Control Release* 92: 1–17.

136. Ramanathan, S. and Block, L. H. 2001. The use of chitosan gels as matrices for electrically-modulated drug delivery. *J Control Release* 70: 109–123.

137. Kaewpirom, S. and Boonsang, S. 2006. Electrical response characterisation of poly(ethylene glycol) macromer (PEGM)/chitosan hydrogels in NaCl solution. *Eur Polym J* 42: 1609–1616.

138. Park, H. J., Kwon, S., Lee, M., Chung, H., Kim, J. H., Kim, Y. S., Park, R. W., Kim, I. S., Bong, S. S., Kwon, I. C., and Jeong, Y. S. 2006. Self-assembled nanoparticles based on glycol chitosan bearing hydrophobic moieties as carriers for doxorubicin: *In vivo* biodistribution and anti-tumor activity. *Biomaterials* 27: 119–126.

139. Zhang, H., Alsarra, I. A., and Neau, S. H. 2002. An *in vitro* evaluation of a chitosan-containing multiparticulate system for macromolecule delivery to the colon. *Int J Pharm* 239: 197–205.

140. Zhao, X. L., Li, K. X., Zhao, X. F., Pang, D. H., and Chen, D. W. 2008. Study on colon-specific 5-fu pH-enzyme di-dependent chitosan microspheres. *Chem Pharm Bull* 56: 963–968.

141. Nunthanid, J., Huanbutta, K., Luangtana-Anan, M., Sriamornsak, P., Limmatvapirat, S., and Puttipipatkhachorn, S. 2008. Development of time-, pH-, and enzyme-controlled colonic drug delivery using spray-dried chitosan acetate and hydroxypropyl methylcellulose. *Eur J Pharm Biopharm* 68: 253–259.

142. Kashyap, N., Viswanad, B., Sharma, G., Bhardwaj, V., Ramarao, P., and Ravi Kumar, M. N. 2007. Design and evaluation of biodegradable, biosensitive *in situ* gelling system for pulsatile delivery of insulin. *Biomaterials* 28: 2051–2060.

143. Manna, U. and Patil, S. 2010. Glucose-triggered drug delivery from borate mediated layer-by-layer self-assembly. *ACS Appl Mater Interfaces* 2: 1521–1527.

144. Park J. H., Saravanakumar, G., Kim, K., and Kwon, I. C. 2010. Targeted delivery of low molecular drugs using chitosan and its derivatives. *Adv Drug Deliv Rev* 62: 28–41.

145. Wang, J. Q., Sui, M. H., and Fan, W. M. 2010. Nanoparticles for tumor targeted therapies and their pharmacokinetics. *Curr Drug Metab* 11: 129–141.

146. Kim, J. H., Kim, Y. S., Park, K., Lee, S., Nam, H. Y., Min, K. H., Jo, H. G., Park, J. H., Choi, K., Jeong, S. Y., Park, R. W., Kim, I. S., Kim, K., and Kwon, I. C. 2008. Antitumor efficacy of cisplatin-loaded glycol chitosan nanoparticles in tumor-bearing mice. *J Control Release* 127: 41–49.

147. Son, Y. J., Jang, J. S., Cho, Y. W., Chung, H., Park, R. W., Kwon, I. C., Kim, I. S., Park, J. Y., Seo, S. B., Park, C. R., and Jeong, S. Y. 2003. Biodistribution and anti-tumor efficacy of doxorubicin loaded glycol-chitosan nanoaggregates by EPR effect. *J Control Release* 91: 135–145.

148. You, J., Li, X., Cui, F., Du, Y. Z., Yuan, H., and Hu, F. 2008. Folate-conjugated polymer micelles for active targeting to cancer cells: Preparation, *in vitro* evaluation of targeting ability and cytotoxicity. *Nanotechnology* 19: 045102.

149. Park, E. K., Kim, S. Y., Lee, S. B., and Lee, Y. M. 2005. Folate-conjugated methoxy poly(ethylene glycol)/poly(ε-caprolactone) amphiphilic block copolymeric micelles for tumor-targeted drug delivery. *J Control Release* 109: 158–168.

150. Sahu, S. K., Mallick, S. K., Santra, S., Maiti, T. K., Ghosh, S. K., and Pramanik, P. 2010. *In vitro* evaluation of folic acid modified carboxymethyl chitosan nanoparticles loaded with doxorubicin for targeted delivery. *J Mater Sci Mater Med* 21: 1587–1597.

151. Sun, Y., Chen, Z. L., Yang, X. X., Huang, P., Zhou, X. P., and Du, X. X. 2009. Magnetic chitosan nanoparticles as a drug delivery system for targeting photodynamic therapy. *Nanotechnology* 20: 135102 (8pp).

152. Zhu, L., Ma, J., Jia, N., Zhao, Y., and Shen, H. 2009. Chitosan-coated magnetic nanoparticles as carriers of 5-fluorouracil: Preparation, characterization and cytotoxicity studies. *Colloids Surf B Biointerfaces* 68: 1–6.

153. Senel, S., Ikinci, G., Kaş, S., Yousefi-Rad, A., Sargon, M. F., and Hincal, A. A. 2000. Chitosan films and hydrogels of chlorhexidine gluconate for oral mucosal delivery. *Int J Pharm* 193: 197–203.

154. Aksungur, P., Sungur, A., Unal, S., Iskit, A. B., Squier, C. A., and Senel, S. 2004. Chitosan delivery systems for the treatment of oral mucositis: *In vitro* and *in vivo* studies. *J Control Release* 98: 269– 279.

155. Kockisch, S., Rees, G. D., Tsibouklis, J., and Smart, J. D. 2005. Mucoadhesive, triclosan-loaded polymer microspheres for application to the oral cavity: Preparation and controlled release characteristics. *Eur J Pharm Biopharm* 59: 207–216.

156. Remunan-Lopez, C., Portero, A., Vila-Jato, J. L., and Alonso, M. J. 1998. Design and evaluation of chitosan/ethylcellulose mucoadhesive bilayered devices for buccal drug delivery. *J Control Release* 55: 143–152.

157. Illum, L. 2002. Nasal drug delivery: New developments and strategies. *Drug Discov Today* 7: 1184–1189.

158. Luppi, B., Bigucci, F., Abruzzo, A., Corace, G., Cerchiara, T., and Zecchi, V. 2010. Freeze-dried chitosan/pectin nasal inserts for antipsychotic drug delivery. *Eur J Pharm Biopharm* 75: 381–387.

159. Illum, L., Jabbal-Gill, I., Hinchcliffe, M., Fisher, A. N., and Davis, S. S. 2001. Chitosan as a novel nasal delivery system for vaccines. *Adv Drug Deliv Rev* 51: 81–96.

160. Wu, J., Wei, W., Wang, L. Y., Su, Z. G., and Ma, G. 2007. A thermosensitive hydrogel based on quaternized chitosan and poly (ethylene glycol) for nasal delivery system. *Biomaterials* 28: 2220–2232.

161. Torrado, S., Prada, P., de la Torre, P. M., and Torrado, S. 2004. Chitosan-poly(acrylic) acid polyionic complex: *In vivo* study to demonstrate prolonged gastric retention. *Biomaterials* 25: 917–923.

162. Gómez-Burgaz, M. García-Ochoa, B., and Torrado-Santiago, S. 2008. Chitosan–carboxymethylcellulose interpolymer complexes for gastric-specific delivery of clarithromycin. *Int J Pharm* 359: 135–143.

163. Philip, A. K. and Philip, B. 2010. Colon targeted drug delivery systems: A review on primary and novel approaches. *Oman Med J* 25: 70–78.

164. Oliveira, G. F., Ferrari, P. C., Carvalho, L. Q., and Evangelista, R. C. 2010. Chitosan–pectin multiparticulate systems associated with enteric polymers for colonic drug delivery. *Carbohydr Polym* 82: 1004–1009.

165. Anal, A. K., Bhopatkar, D., Tokura, S., Tamura, H., and Stevens, W. F. 2003. Chitosan-alignate multilayers beads for gastric passage and controlled intestinal release of protein. *Drug Dev Ind Pharm* 29: 713–724.

166. Bayat, A., Dorkoosh, F. A., Dehpour, A. R., Moezi, L., Larijani, B., Junginger, H. E., and Rafiee-Tehrani, M. 2008. Nanoparticles of quaternized chitosan derivatives as a carrier for colon delivery of insulin: *Ex vivo* and *in vivo* studies. *Int J Pharm* 356: 259–266.

167. de la Fuente, M., Raviña, M., Paolicelli, P., Sanchez, A., Seijo, B., and Alonso, M. J. 2010. Chitosan-based nanostructures: A delivery platform for ocular therapeutics. *Adv Drug Deliv Rev* 62: 100–117.

168. Gupta, H., Velpandian, T., and Jain, S. 2010. Ion- and pH-activated novel *in-situ* gel system for sustained ocular drug delivery. *J Drug Target* 18: 499–505.

169. Peptu, C. A., Buhus, G., and Popa, M. 2010. Double cross-linked chitosan-gelatin particulate systems for ophthalmic applications. *J Bioact Compat Polym* 25: 98–116.

170. Badawi, A. A., El-Laithy, H. M., El Qidra, R. K., El Mofty, H., and El dally, M. 2008. Chitosan based nanocarriers for indomethacin ocular delivery. *Arch Pharm Res* 31: 1040–1049.

171. Ammar, H. O., Salama, H. A., El-Nahhas, S. A., and Elmotasem, H. 2008. Design and evaluation of chitosan films for transdermal delivery of glimepiride. *Curr Drug Deliv* 5: 290–298.

172. Lee, P. W., Hsu, S. H., Tsai, J. S., Chen, F. R., Huang, P. J., Ke, C. J., Liao, Z. X., Hsiao, C. W., Lin, H. J., and Sung, H. W. 2010. Multifunctional core–shell polymeric nanoparticles for transdermal DNA delivery and epidermal Langerhans cells tracking. *Biomaterials* 31: 2425–2434.

173. Koch, M. (West Pharmaceutical Services, Inc.). 2003. The growing market for nasal drug delivery. *Business Briefing: Pharmatech*.

174. Bossart, J., Sedo, K., and Kararli, T. T. 2010. Drug delivery products and technologies, a decade in review: Approved products 2000 to 2009. *Drug Deliv Technol* 5: 28–31.

175. Brown, L. R. 2005. Commercial challenges of protein drug delivery. *Expert Opin Drug Deliv* 2: 29–42.

176. Gautier, S. 2009. Ultra-pure chitosan: Insight on new non-animal sources for use in advanced drug delivery and cell therapy. *Drug Deliv Technol 10:* 20–21.

177. Kean, T. and Thanou, M. 2010. Biodegradation, biodistribution and toxicity of chitosan. *Adv Drug Deliv Rev* 62: 3–11.

7

Application of Chitosan-Based Gels in Pharmaceuticals

Yuliang Xiao, Jiangfeng Zhu, and Lianyin Zheng

CONTENTS

7.1 Introduction

The history of the studies of polysaccharide chitosan dates back to the nineteenth century. However, it is only in the last couple of decades that people have considered chitosan as a kind of biomedical and drug delivery material. Chitosan is a deacetylated form of chitin, which is the second most abundant polymer in nature after cellulose. The slight difference between the chemical structures of chitin and chitosan has, however, resulted in very different consequences in terms of their applications to drug delivery. Chitin is not soluble in water and in most of the common organic solvents used in pharmaceutical industry. Therefore, it is not useful for the development of drug delivery devices. In contrast with chitin, chitosan base can be protonized in acidic solutions and becomes soluble. The positive charges on the chitosan molecule (CM) enable it to interact with polyanions, a process that has been used to obtain micro- and nanoparticulate or nanogel drug delivery systems. In addition to its polycationic characteristics, chitosan has shown some other excellent properties (e.g., nontoxicity, biocompatibility, mucus adhesion, and biodegradation). As a result, chitosan has been used for a variety of drug delivery systems [1,2]. Some of the chitosan-based drug delivery systems are summarized in Table 7.1.

The modalities of chitosan-based drug delivery systems include tablets, capsules, microspheres/microparticles, nanoparticles, beads, films, and gels. All these modalities can be regarded as ramifications of gels. The review given below addresses the recent trends in the area of chitosan-based drug delivery systems.

7.2 Methods of Preparation of Drug Delivery Systems Based on Chitosan

Different methods have been developed to prepare chitosan drug delivery systems. The choice of the methods depends on factors such as particle size requirement, thermal and chemical stability of the active agent, reproducibility of the release kinetic profiles, stability of the final product, and residual toxicity associated with the final product. In this review we attempt to outline the different methods used in the preparation of chitosan drug delivery systems.

7.2.1 Methods of Preparation of Micro/Nanogels Based on Chitosan [1]

7.2.1.1 Emulsion Cross-Linking

This method utilizes the reactive functional amine group of chitosan to cross-link with aldehyde groups of the cross-linking agent. In this method, water-in-oil emulsion is prepared by emulsifying the chitosan aqueous solution in the oil phase. Aqueous droplets are stabilized using a suitable surfactant. The stable emulsion is cross-linked by using an appropriate cross-linking agent such as glutaraldehyde to harden the droplets. Microspheres are filtered and washed repeatedly with *n*-hexane followed by alcohol and then dried [3]. With this method, sizes of the particles can be controlled by regulating the sizes of aqueous droplets. However, the particle size of the final product depends on the amount of cross-linking agent used when hardening in addition to the speed of

TABLE 7.1

Chitosan-Based Drug Delivery Systems Prepared Using Different Methods for Various Kinds of Drugs

Type of System	Method of Preparation	Drug
Tablets	Matrix	Diclofenac sodium, pentoxyphylline, salicylic acid, theophylline
	Coating	Propranolol HCl
Capsules	Capsule	Shell insulin, 5-amino salicylic acid
Microspheres/ Microparticles	Emulsion cross-linking	Theophylline, cisplatin, pentazocine, phenobarbitone, theophylline, insulin, 5-fluorouracil, diclofenac sodium, griseofulvin, aspirin, diphtheria toxoid, pamidronate, suberoylbisphosphonate, mitoxantrone, progesterone
	Coacervation/precipitation	Prednisolone, interleukin-2, propranolol-HCl
	Spray-drying	Cimetidine, famotidine, nizatidine, vitamin D-2, diclofenac sodium, ketoprofen, metoclopramide-HCl, bovine serum albumin, ampicillin, cetylpyridinium chloride, oxytetracycline, betamethasone
	Ionic gelation	Felodipine
	Sieving method	Clozapine
Nanoparticles	Emulsion-droplet coalescence	Gadopentetic acid
	Coacervation/precipitation	DNA, doxorubicin
	Ionic gelation	Insulin, ricin, bovine serum albumin, CyA
	Reverse micellar method	Doxorubicin
Beads	Coacervation/precipitation	Adriamycin, nifedipine, bovine serum albumin, salbutamol sulfate, lidocaine-HCl, riboflavin
Films	Solution casting	Isosorbide dinitrate, chlorhexidine gluconate, trypsin, granulocyte-macrophage colony-stimulating factor, acyclovir, riboflavine, testosterone, progesterone, beta-estradiol
Gel	Cross-linking	Chlorpheniramine maleate, aspirin, theophylline, caffeine, lidocaine-HCl, hydrocortisone acetate, 5-fluorouracil

Source: Adapted from Agnihotri, S. A., Mallikarjuna, N. N., and Aminabhavi, T. M. 2004. *J Control Release* 100: 5–28.

stirring during the formation of emulsion. This method is schematically represented in Figure 7.1 [1]. The emulsion cross-linking method has a few drawbacks since it involves tedious procedures as well as uses harsh cross-linking agents, which might induce chemical reactions with the active agent. However, complete removal of the unreacted cross-linking agent may be difficult in this process.

7.2.1.2 Coacervation/Precipitation

This method utilizes the physicochemical property of chitosan since it is insoluble in an alkaline pH medium but precipitates/coacervates when it comes in contact with an alkaline solution. Particles are produced by blowing a chitosan solution into an alkali solution, such as sodium hydroxide, NaOH-methanol and ethanediamine, through a compressed air nozzle to form coacervate droplets [4]. Separation and purification of

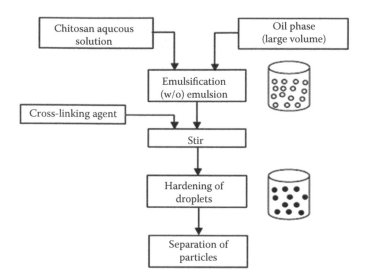

FIGURE 7.1
Schematic representation of the preparation of chitosan particulate systems by the emulsion cross-linking method.

particles are done by filtration/centrifugation followed by successive washings with hot and cold water. The method is schematically represented in Figure 7.2 [1]. Varying the compressed air pressure and spray-nozzle diameter controls the size of the particles and then hardening particles by a cross-linking agent controls the drug release. In another technique [5], a sodium sulfate solution is added dropwise to an aqueous acidic solution of chitosan containing a surfactant under stirring and ultrasonication for 30 min. Microspheres are purified by centrifugation and resuspended in demineralized water.

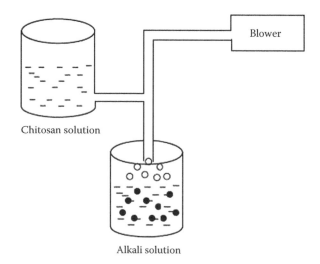

FIGURE 7.2
Schematic representation of the preparation of chitosan particulate systems by the coacervation/precipitation method.

Particles are cross-linked with glutaraldehyde. Particles produced by this method have better acid stability than those prepared by other methods.

7.2.1.3 Spray Drying

Spray drying is a well-known technique to produce powders, granules, and agglomerates from a mixture of drug and excipient solutions as well as suspensions. The method is based on drying atomized droplets in a stream of hot air. In this method, CMs are first dissolved in an aqueous acetic acid solution, and then the drug is dissolved or dispersed in the solution and, finally, a suitable cross-linking agent is added. This solution or dispersion is then atomized in a stream of hot air. Atomization leads to the formation of small droplets, from which the solvent evaporates instantaneously leading to the formation of free flowing particles [6] as depicted in Figure 7.3 [1]. Various process parameters have to be controlled to get the desired size of particles. Particle size depends on the size of the nozzle, the spray flow rate, atomization pressure, inlet air temperature, and extent of cross-linking.

7.2.1.4 Emulsion-Droplet Coalescence Method

The novel emulsion-droplet coalescence method was developed by Tokumitsu et al. [7], which utilized the principles of both emulsion cross-linking and precipitation. However, instead of cross-linking the stable droplets, this method induces precipitation by allowing coalescence of CS droplets with NaOH droplets. First, a stable emulsion containing an aqueous solution of CS along with drug is produced in liquid paraffin oil and then, another stable emulsion containing CS aqueous solution of NaOH is produced in the same manner. When both emulsions are mixed under high-speed stirring, droplets of each emulsion would collide at random and coalesce, thereby precipitating CS droplets

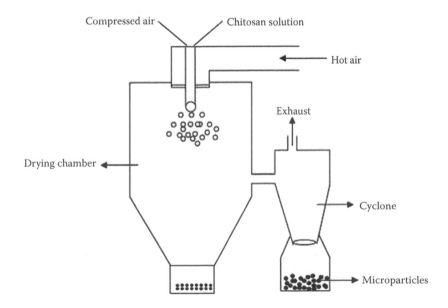

FIGURE 7.3
Schematic representation of preparation of chitosan particulate systems by means of spray drying method.

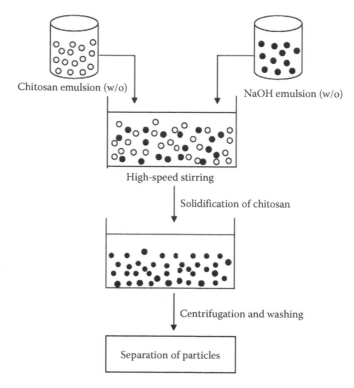

FIGURE 7.4
Schematic representation of the preparation of chitosan particulate systems by the emulsion-droplet coalescence method.

to give small-sized particles. The method is schematically shown in Figure 7.4 [1]. Gadopentetic acid-loaded CS nanoparticles have been prepared by this method for gadolinium neutron capture therapy. Particle size depends on the type of CS. When the deacetylation degree of CS decreases, the particle size increases, but the drug content decreases. Particles produced using 100% deacetylated CS had the mean particle size of 452 nm with 45% drug loading. Nanoparticles are obtained within the emulsion droplet. The size of the nanoparticle does not reflect the droplet size. Since gadopentetic acid is a bivalent anionic compound, it interacts electrostatically with the amino groups of CS, which would not have occurred if a cross-linking agent, which blocks the free amino groups of CS, is used. Thus, it is possible to achieve higher gadopentetic acid loading by using the emulsion-droplet coalescence method compared to the simple emulsion cross-linking method.

7.2.1.5 Ionic Gelation

In the ionic gelation method, CS is dissolved in an aqueous acidic solution to obtain the cation of CS. This solution is then added dropwise under constant stirring to polyanionic tripolyphosphate (TPP) solution. Due to the complexation between oppositely charged species, CS undergoes ionic gelation and precipitates to form spherical particles. The method is schematically represented in Figure 7.5 [1]. The use of complexation between oppositely charged macromolecules to prepare CS microspheres has attracted

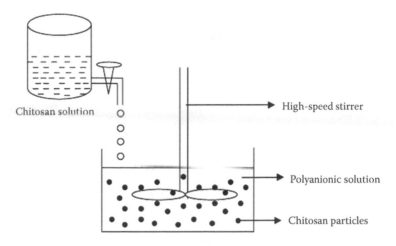

FIGURE 7.5
Schematic representation of the preparation of chitosan particulate systems by the ionic gelation method.

much attention because the process is very simple and mild [8,9]. In addition, reversible physical cross-linking by electrostatic interaction, instead of chemical cross-linking, has been applied to avoid possible toxicity of reagents and other undesirable effects. TPP is a polyanion, which can interact with the cationic CS by electrostatic forces [10,11]. However, TPP/CS microparticles have poor mechanical strength, thus limiting their usage in drug delivery.

7.2.1.6 Reverse Micellar Method

Reverse micelles are thermodynamically stable liquid mixtures of water, oil, and surfactant. Macroscopically, they are homogeneous and isotropic, structured on a microscopic scale into aqueous and oil microdomains separated by surfactant-rich films. One of the most important aspects of reverse micelle-hosted systems is their dynamic behavior. Nanoparticles prepared by conventional emulsion polymerization methods are not only large (N200 nm), but also broad in size range. The preparation of ultrafine polymeric nanoparticles with a narrow size distribution can be achieved by using a reverse micellar medium [12]. The aqueous core of the reverse micellar droplets can be used as a nanoreactor to prepare such particles. Since the size of the reverse micellar droplets usually lies between 1 and 10 nm [13] and these droplets are highly monodispersed, preparation of drug-loaded nanoparticles in reverse micelles will produce extremely fine particles with a narrow size distribution. Since micellar droplets are in Brownian motion, they undergo continuous coalescence followed by reseparation on a timescale that varies between millisecond and microsecond [14]. The size, polydispersity, and thermodynamic stability of these droplets are maintained in the system by a rapid dynamic equilibrium. In this method, the surfactant is dissolved in an organic solvent to prepare reverse micelles. To this, aqueous solutions of CS and drug are added with constant vortexing in order to avoid any turbidity. The aqueous phase is regulated in such a way as to keep the entire mixture in an optically transparent microemulsion phase. An additional amount of water may be added to obtain nanoparticles of larger size. To this transparent solution, a cross-linking agent is added with constant stirring, and cross-linking is achieved by stirring overnight. The maximum amount of drug that can be dissolved in reverse micelles varies from drug

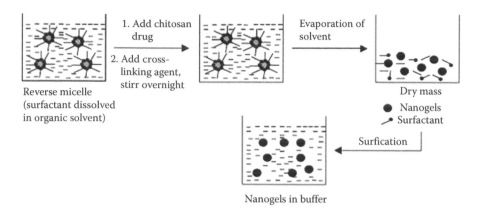

FIGURE 7.6
Schematic representation of the preparation of chitosan particulate systems by the reverse micellar method.

to drug and has to be determined by gradually increasing the amount of drug until the clear microemulsion is transformed into a translucent solution. The organic solvent is then evaporated to obtain the transparent dry mass. The material is dispersed in water and then a suitable salt is added to precipitate the surfactant. The mixture is then subjected to centrifugation. The supernatant solution is decanted, which contains the drug-loaded nanoparticles. The aqueous dispersion is immediately dialyzed through a dialysis membrane for about 1 h and the liquid is lyophilized to dry powder. The method is schematically represented in Figure 7.6 [15].

7.2.1.7 Sieving Method [15]

In this method, microparticles are prepared by cross-linking CS to obtain a nonsticky glassy hydrogel followed by passing through a sieve as shown in Figure 7.7 [1]. A suitable quantity of CS is dissolved in 4% acetic acid solution to form a thick jelly mass that is cross-linked by adding glutaraldehyde. The nonsticky cross-linked mass is passed through a

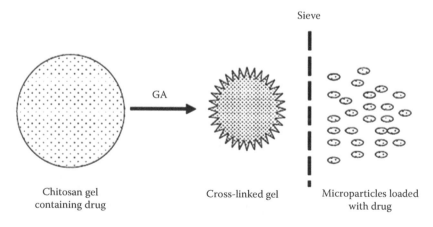

FIGURE 7.7
Schematic representation of the preparation of chitosan particulate systems by the sieving method.

sieve with a suitable mesh size to get microparticles. The microparticles are washed with a 0.1 N NaOH solution to remove the unreacted excess glutaraldehyde and dried overnight in an oven at 40°C. Clozapine is incorporated into CS before cross-linking with entrapment efficiency up to 98.9%. This method is devoid of tedious procedures, and can be scaled up easily. Microparticles are irregular in shape, with the average particle sizes in the range of 543–698 μm. The *in vitro* release is extended up to 12 h, while the *in vivo* studies indicated a slow release of clozapine.

7.2.2 Methods of Preparing Films Based on Chitosan

A chitosan solution (50 mM acetic acid), prepared allowing for the content of water and ash, was filtered through a sterile 0.22 μm filter. Then 200 μL aliquots were layered over 1 cm² dishes. The solvent was allowed to evaporate in an open plate inside a sterile laminar flow hood overnight at room temperature. Gelated films were treated with phosphate buffer (0.25 M), pH 7.0. Afterwards, the films were extensively washed with phosphate-buffered saline (PBS).

7.2.3 Methods of Preparation of Mass Gels Based on Chitosan

7.2.3.1 Cross-Linking

Chitosan was dissolved in distilled water with 50 mM acetic acid, and other additives (such as polyvinyl alcohol, polyethylene glycol, carboxymethyl cellulose, sodium alginate, etc.) solutions were added into the chitosan solution with stirring. Afterwards, the stable solution was cross-linked by using an appropriate cross-linking agent such as glutaraldehyde to harden the mass gels. The resultant mixture was dipped in distilled water for 3 days at 10°C to completely remove the unreacted cross-linking agent.

7.2.3.2 Freeze/Thawing Process

Chitosan and other additive solutions were prepared by dissolving chitosan in distilled water in an autoclave at 121°C for 1 h. Solutions were stirred till they cooled to room temperature to prevent aggregation of polymers. Air bubbles were removed by resting the solution at room temperature. The solutions were cast into Perspex molds that were 1.5 mm in thickness. Then they were physically cross-linked by five freeze/thawing cycles, which consisted of freezing at –20°C for 12 h and thawing at room temperature (21°C) for 12 h. The hydrogels were further submerged in a constantly stirred coagulation bath (7.5% KOH and 1 M Na_2SO_4) for 1 h. After removing from the coagulation bath, the resulting hydrogels were washed several times with distilled water [16].

7.2.4 Methods of Preparation of Thermosensitive *In Situ* Gels Based on Chitosan

The chitosan solution was obtained by dissolving 400 mg of chitosan (medium viscosity, 75–80% deacetylated) in 18 mL of 0.1 M acetic acid solution prepared in PBS. Then 150 mg of glycerol phosphate was dissolved in 1 mL of PBS. And then a glycerol phosphate solution was carefully added dropwise to the chitosan solution. The final liquid solution was clear and homogeneous. The solution was filtered through a 0.22 mm membrane filter. The pH value of the final solution before heating was 7.15 [17].

7.3 Drug Loading into Chitosan-Based Drug Delivery Systems

Loading drug into chitosan-based drug delivery systems can be achieved in two steps: during the preparation of carriers (incorporation) and after the formation of carriers (incubation). In these systems, drug is physically embedded into the matrix or adsorbed onto the surface. Various methods of loading have been developed to improve the efficiency of loading, which largely depends on the method of preparation, as well as physicochemical properties of the drug. Maximum drug loading can be achieved by incorporating the drug during the formation of carriers, but it may get affected by the process parameters such as the method of preparation, presence of additives, and so on.

Both water-soluble and water-insoluble drugs can be loaded into chitosan-based particulate systems. Water-soluble drugs are mixed with a chitosan solution to form a homogeneous mixture and then carriers can be produced by any of the methods discussed before. Water-insoluble drugs and drugs that can precipitate in acidic pH solutions can be loaded after the formation of carriers by soaking the preformed particles with the saturated solution of the drug.

7.4 Pharmaceutical Applications of Chitosan-Based Drug Delivery Systems

Chitosan and its derivatives have been widely studied for drug delivery. Some of the biomedical applications of chitosan-based gels discussed in the following sections include large-molecule drug delivery (protein and peptide delivery, enzyme delivery, gene delivery, and vaccines delivery), ocular, oral, mucosal, and pulmonary drug delivery.

7.4.1 Large-Molecule Drug Delivery

7.4.1.1 Protein and Peptide Delivery

Advanced research in biotechnology and genetic research has led to the discovery of a large number of proteins and peptides that are very effective in disease treatment [18,19]. Routinely, peptides and proteins are administered through the parenteral route, which has poor absorption efficiency in patients. A large amount of work has focused on protein delivery by the oral route [20–22]. However, the bioavailability of peptide after oral administration is usually low because of instability and poor absorption of proteins in the gastrointestinal (GI) tract. One possible way to improve the GI uptake of peptides is to encapsulate them in colloidal nanoparticles that can protect the peptide from being degraded in the GI tract and facilitate their transportation into systemic circulation [23].

Chitosan-based gels and their ramifications have important applications in the controlled release of protein and peptide drugs because they show excellent mucoadhesiveness [24] and a permeation-enhancing effect across the biological surfaces. Superoxide dismutase, the most potent antioxidant enzyme, has been encapsulated into chitosan microparticles to obtain suitable sustained protein delivery based on the complex coacervation process. The addition of polyethylene glycol to the protein solution or a change of pH enhanced the encapsulation efficiency for controlled release [25]. Luteinizing hormone-releasing hormone (LH-RH), a decapeptide, is a naturally occurring hormone that controls human sex hormones. Numerous LH-RH analogues (TX46) have been synthesized to manipulate the menstrual cycle and treat various steroid-dependent disorders, sex-hormone-dependent cancers and gynecological conditions [26]. A novel kind of chitosan microparticles has been prepared to prevent TX46 degradation by proteases or other enzymes [27]. Insulin-loaded chitosan microparticles have been prepared by combining a membrane emulsification technique and a stepwise cross-linking method. The chitosan microparticles showed high encapsulation efficiency (80%), high chemical stability of insulin (>95%), low burst release, and steady release behavior [28]. Chitosan gel beads prepared with chelated copper (II) ions are vehicles for the delivery of peptide and protein drugs, and have been studied for the release of insulin as well. In this study, insulin was scarcely released from the chitosan gel beads *in vitro*, which was proposed to be due to the interactions occurring among insulin, chitosan, and copper (II) ions. The efficacy of insulin released from the chitosan gel beads was confirmed by implantation into diabetic mice [29]. Human growth hormone encapsulated in chitosan microparticles has also been shown to be effective in early bone consolidation in distraction osteogenesis [30].

7.4.1.2 Enzyme Delivery

Chitosan is known as an ideal support material for enzyme immobilization because of its characteristics, such as improved mechanical strength, resistance to chemical degradation, protection of enzymes from the action of metal ions, and antibacterial properties. In D. S. Jiang's study, laccase immobilized on magnetic chitosan microcarriers improved the performance of a fiber optic biosensor of oxygen consumption in relation to analyte oxidation, and was reported to have potential applications in medical examination and diagnostics [31]. Catalase is another enzyme that has been immobilized, by a phase-inversion method [32], with sulfoxine as a chelating resin fixed to CMs acting as a support matrix [33].

7.4.1.3 Gene Delivery

Gene therapy refers to the transmission of DNA encoding a therapeutic gene of interest into the targeted cells or organs with consequent expression of the transgene. In efficient gene delivery, plasmid DNA is introduced into target cells and transcribed and the genetic information is ultimately translated into the corresponding protein. In order to achieve that goal, the gene delivery system has to overcome a number of obstacles (Figure 7.8) [34].

Transfection is hampered by (a) targeting the delivery system to the target cell, (b) transporting DNA through the cell membrane, (c) being uptaken and degraded in endolysosomes, and (d) intracellular trafficking of plasmid DNA to the nucleus. Gene delivery systems include viral vectors, cationic liposomes, polycation complexes, and microencapsulated systems [35–38]. Viral vectors are advantageous for gene delivery because they are highly efficient and have a wide range of cell targets. However, when used *in vivo*, they cause immune responses and oncogenic effects. In addition, sometimes it is difficult to reproducibly prepare viral vectors in large batches. To overcome the limitations of viral vectors, nonviral delivery systems based on chitosan are considered for gene therapy. Some of the advantages of chitosan-based delivery systems are listed below [39]:

1. Conjugation of ligands to the nanospheres, for targeting or stimulating receptor-mediated endocytosis.
2. Incorporation of lysosomolytic agents to reduce the degradation of DNA in the endosomal and lysosomal compartments.

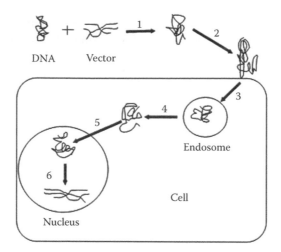

FIGURE 7.8

Gene delivery system. 1: Transfection of target cells with plasmid DNA is dependent on the condensation of the plasmid DNA by a suitable vector system; 2: the specific binding of the vector–DNA complex to the target cell; 3: the uptake of the complex into intracellular endosomes; 4: successful release from endosomes into the cytoplasm; 5: intracellular transport and nuclear localization of the DNA; 6: followed by decomplexation.

3. Coencapsulation of other bioactive agents for multiple plasmids.

4. Improvement of DNA bioavailability due to the protection from serum nuclease degradation by the polymer matrix.

5. Lyophilization of nanospheres for storage, without losing too much activity.

Chitosan was first used as a carrier of DNA for gene delivery applications in 1995 [40] by mixing a solution of the respective chitosan with plasmid DNA. Chitosan has an average amino group density of 0.837 per monosaccharide D-glucosamine unit. This amino group density depends on the degree of deacetylation. The cationically charged chitosan will form polyelectrolyte complexes with the negatively charged plasmid DNA. Chitosan–DNA complexes could be protected from DNase to improve the bioavailability of the plasmid DNA delivered into the body for gene therapy. The complex sizes yielded (150–500 nm) depends on both the molecular weight of the chitosan (108–540 kDa) used and the chitosan/DNA ratio [41,42].

Objectively speaking, few of the researchers have made efforts to correlate the transfection efficacy with the size of chitosan–DNA complexes, although there are several reports supporting the use of chitosan for gene transfection [43,44]. Typically, the particles smaller than 100 nm can be enclosed within endocytic vesicles, allowing entry into target cells via transferrin cytosis [45]. For chitosan–DNA complexes systems, Erbacher et al. [43] proposed that zeta potential was close to 0 mV (N:P 52) with a size range of 1–5 mm. In studying cationic cholesterol derivative-mediated gene transfection, Nikanishi found that moderate sizes of particles (0.4–1.4 mm) yielded the highest transfection [46], while small vesicles less than 400 nm in size showed lower transfection efficiency. The results obtained by different authors seem to be contradictory. Thus, the mechanism of cationic polymer-mediated transfection is still underappreciated.

The DNA delivered by nonviral carriers is vulnerable to degradation by DNase. A critical parameter of DNA delivery systems therefore is the ability of the carrier material to protect incorporated DNA against degradation by DNase. As physiological concentrations of the enzyme can merely be estimated, protection against DNase is routinely checked by incubation of the chitosan–DNA complexes or nanoparticles with DNase I or II as a model enzyme at different concentrations [47], followed by gel electrophoresis. Complexation of DNA with highly purified chitosan fractions (molecular weights of <5000, 5000–10,000, and >10,000 Da) at a charge ratio of 1:1 resulted in almost complete inhibition of degradation by DNase II. Leong's studies have shown that cross-linked chitosan/DNA nanoparticles stored in water remained stable for more than 3 months, whereas uncross-linked nanoparticles stored in PBS remained stable for only a few hours [39]. Lyophilized chitosan/DNA nanoparticles retained their transfection potency for more than 4 weeks [48].

In summary, chitosan and chitosan derivatives effectively condense plasmid DNA, protecting it from DNase degradation. These gene delivery systems based on chitosans can also be equipped with ligands for specific cell interaction, such as transferrin or galactose. A number of *in vitro* and *in vivo* studies showed that chitosan is a suitable material for efficient nonviral gene delivery.

7.4.1.4 Vaccine Delivery

Immunization has been the most effective way to protect individuals and the community against debilitating infectious diseases, thereby preventing economic losses and morbidity. The use of vaccines has achieved great success in the last two decades, contributing significantly to an increase in life expectancy and improving the quality of life, especially in children, both locally and globally. Today most vaccines are given by parenteral injection, which stimulates the immune system to produce antibodies in the serum but fails to generate a mucosal antibody response.

Chitosan and chitosan derivatives have been developed and studied recently for various vaccines, such as influenza, pertussis, and diphtheria antigens [49]. The immune-stimulating factor of *Bordetella bronchiseptica* dermonecrotoxin, a major virulence factor of a causative agent of atropic rhinitis, has been loaded in CMs. *In vivo* activity of immune induction was investigated by intranasal administration of the loaded CMs into mice. *Bordetella bronchiseptica* dermonecrotoxin-specific IgA titers in the nasal cavity were time- and dose-dependently increased by this administration. Similar phenomena were observed with the analysis of systemic IgA and IgG in sera that suggest that direct vaccination via the nasal cavity is effective for targeting nasal-associated lymphoid tissues, and that CMs are an efficient adjuvant in nasal mucosal immunity for atropic rhinitis vaccine [50]. CMs prepared by an ionic gelation process with TPP were also used for loading *Bordetella bronchiseptica* dermonecrotoxin. TNF-α and nitric oxide from RAW264.7 cells that were exposed to the loaded CMs were gradually secreted with time, suggesting that the antigen released from the CMs had the immune-stimulating activity [51].

A single injection of PLGA or CM containing tetanus toxoid could maintain the antibody response from days to over months at a level comparable to the booster injections of conventional aluminum hydroxide-adsorbed vaccines. Hence, CMs have potential application in replacing the expensive polymer PLGA in vaccine delivery [52].

Porous CMs suitable for the delivery of antigen have been prepared using a wet phase-inversion method, and were chemically modified with 3-chloro-2-hydroxypropyltrimethylammonium chloride. The antigen of the Newcastle disease vaccine was immobilized into the pores of CMs. Sustained release of the Newcastle disease vaccine's antigen was achieved through an adsorption–desorption release test [53].

Recombinant *Streptococcus mutans* glucan-binding protein D has also been incorporated into PLGA microspheres for intranasal administration, and was then surface coated with chitosan. The microspheres were shown to be potentially useful for antigen delivery in dental caries vaccination in rats [54].

Adenoviral vectors were encapsulated into a microparticulate system for mucosal delivery. Microencapsulation of the vectors was performed by ionotropic coacervation of chitosan, with bile salts as counteranions. Not only was the adenovirus protected from the low pH of the external medium, but also its release was delayed and dependent on cell contact, which is an advantage for mucosal vaccination purposes. The adenoviral infectivity was maintained and the onset of delivery was host-controlled [55].

For the future development of microparticles for oral vaccine delivery, a modified-cell *in vitro* model has been developed. Using this model, commercially available FluoSpheres® (Molecular Probes, Inc.) and CMs (1.7 µm) have been shown to be transported at a significantly higher amount by the human modified-cell model than when transported using a Caco-2 cell monoculture [56,57]. This *in vitro* model improves the study of targeting modified-cells of human origin.

7.4.2 Oral Drug Delivery

The oral route is the most popular and the most practical way to administer a therapeutic agent, particularly from the point of view of the patient. However, it is not always the most suitable route for some active compounds, such as nonsteroidal antiinflammatory drugs, which cause gastric mucosal damage; for drugs poorly absorbed, such as peptides; or for drugs that undergo an extensive first-past effect (e.g., nitroglycerin, alprenolol, fluorouracil, and desipramine) [58]. Furthermore, the possibility to control drug delivery after oral administration is very limited since it depends on the residence time of the dosage in the GI tract. Indeed, the drug will follow the gastric emptying rate, a physiological parameter that is subject to significant interindividual variability [59]. For these reasons, researchers have tried new excipients for manufacturing tablets or to develop drug carrier systems capable of controlling drug delivery after oral administration (e.g., microparticles). For several years, chitosan has been largely evaluated as a potential vehicle for drugs administered orally.

7.4.2.1 Gastric Delivery

The main function of the stomach is to digest food and deliver chyme to the intestine. The gastric motor activities cause the emptying process of the gastric contents. A successful gastric retention delivery system should be able to overcome the housekeeper waves and remain in the stomach during the fasted state.

Floating hollow chitosan microspheres would be an interesting gastroretentive controlled-release delivery system for drugs. The oral administration of tetracycline chitosan microspheres prepared by chemical cross-linking in fasted gerbils shows that they provide a longer residence time than either tetracycline solution or microspheres prepared by ionic precipitation [60].

The release of the drug from floating microcapsules containing melatonin prepared by the ionic interaction of chitosan and sodium dioctyl sulfosuccinate was greatly retarded in simulated gastric fluid, and the microspheres maintained their integrity for more than three days compared with nonfloating microspheres, where drug release was almost instant [61].

A stomach-specific drug delivery system using chitosan microspheres has been developed to increase the efficacy of tetracycline against *Helicobacter pylori* by ionic cross-linking

[62]. However, the high aqueous solubility of chitosan restricts the utility of CMs for gastric drug delivery. Reacetylated chitosan microspheres were prepared with suitable properties for the controlled release of amoxicillin and metronidazole in the gastric cavity and, hence, for the eradication of *H. pylori* in gastric ulcers and possibly gastric carcinoma [63].

7.4.2.2 Colon-Selective Drug Delivery

The colon is a site for the administration of protein and peptides that are degraded by digestive enzymes in the upper GI tract. The absorption of peptide and protein drugs could be enhanced in the colon because of the low activity of proteolytic enzymes there and the long residence time. In addition, it is more effective in treating colonic diseases such as ulcerative colitis, colorectal cancer, and Crohn's disease with direct delivery of drugs to the affected area [64].

Chitosan is a promising polymer for colon drug delivery since it can be biodegraded by the colonic bacterial flora and is toxicologically harmless with low cost. As a result, this compound could be promising for colon-specific drug delivery [65].

Hydroxypropyl methylcellulose phthalate, an enteric-coating material, was used to coat chitosan capsules loaded with insulin [66]. At 2 h after oral administration, the capsules were eliminated from the stomach. After 2–6 h, the capsules moved into the small intestine and were in the large intestine after 6–12 h. For *in vitro* release medium, cecal content from rats was suspended in two volumes of bicarbonate buffer and the pH was adjusted to 7.0. The release of 5(6)-carboxyfluorescein loaded in chitosan capsules, a model water-soluble compound, was increased in the rat cecal content suspension as compared to simulated gastric juice (pH 1.2) and simulated intestinal juice (pH 6.8). While the entire drug was released after 12 h in the cecal suspension, only 20% was released in the simulated intestinal juice after 6 h, and none was released in the simulated gastric juice after 2 h. Degradation of chitosan capsules in cecal contents facilitated the release of 5(6)-carboxyfluorescein.

Tominaga et al. [67] prepared a colon-targeted formulation by using a double coating system. The core, composed of acetaminophen, was coated with an inner coating layer made of chitosan and an outer coating layer made of phytin, a gastric acid-resistant material. While the outer layer protected the core from acidic conditions in the stomach and was then dissolved in the small intestine, the inner layer protected the core in the small intestine and was then biodegraded in the colon where the drug was released.

5-Aminosalicylic acid, a cyclooxygenase inhibitor and an antiinflammatory drug effective against Crohn's disease and ulcerative colitis, is rapidly absorbed from the small intestine. Eudragit-coated chitosans (200 μm) have been developed by an emulsion–solvent evaporation technique based on a multiple water/oil/water emulsion to deliver it specifically to the colon [68].

Albendazole was delivered specifically into the colon by microspheres of chitosan hydrochloride, and drug release in 24 h was 48.9% and 76.5% in colonic fluid without and with rat cecal contents, respectively [69].

Sadeghi et al. [70] synthesized the TMC- and diethylmethyl-chitosan nanoparticles loaded with insulin by the polyethylcyanoacrylate (PEC) technique and the ionic gelation technique, and the results showed that nanoparticles prepared by the PEC method had a higher insulin loading efficiency and zeta potential than those prepared by the ionotropic gelation method . The PEC method of nanoparticle preparation gave particles in the range of 170–270 nm with spherical and smooth surface morphology and the polydispersity index (PDI) below 0.3. *In vitro* release studies showed a small burst effect at the beginning and then a sustained release characteristic for 5 h. *Ex vivo* investigations revealed better insulin transport across the colon membrane of rats for nanoparticles made with quaternized derivatives than those made of chitosan. *In vivo* studies in rats have shown enhanced colonic absorption of insulin by using these nanoparticles compared to free insulin in diabetic rats [71].

A pH-sensitive multicore microparticulate system containing chitosan microcores entrapped in enteric acrylic microspheres has been reported [72]. Sodium diclofenac was efficiently entrapped within these CS microcores and then microencapsulated into Eudragit L-100 and Eudragit S-100 to form a multireservoir system. An *in vitro* release study revealed no release of the drug in gastric pH for 3 h, and after the lag time, a continuous release for 8–12 h was observed in the basic pH.

7.4.3 Mucosal Delivery

Nowadays, mucosal surfaces such as nasal, peroral, and pulmonary are receiving a great deal of attention as alternative routes of systemic administration. Chitosan has mucoadhesive properties, and, therefore, it is particularly useful in formulating bioadhesive dosage forms for mucosal administration (ocular, nasal, buccal, gastroenteric, and vaginal–uterine therapy) [73]. Nasal mucosa has high permeability and easy access of drug to the absorption site. The particulate delivery to peroral mucosa is easily taken up by Peyer's patches of the gut-associated lymphoid tissue. Chitosan has been found to enhance the drug absorption through mucosae without damaging the biological system. Here, the mechanism of action of chitosan was suggested to be a combination of bioadhesion and a transient widening of the tight junctions between epithelial cells [74].

7.4.3.1 Nasal Delivery

Nasal drug delivery represents an interesting alternative to the parenteral route for administration of drugs that show poor oral bioavailability, such as peptides and proteins. In addition, the nose has a further advantage for the absorption of drugs in that it has a large epithelial surface area available due to the presence of numerous microvilli. On the other hand, one of the major drawbacks of the nasal cavity is its rapid mucociliary clearance mechanism, which can reduce the bioavailability of drugs given intranasally. A possible strategy to circumvent this problem, without using absorption enhancers, is to prevent the clearance of the delivery system from the nasal cavity and thereby prolong contact between the drug and the mucosa. This aim can be reached by employing bioadhesive systems that form a gel-like structure at the contact of the mucus [75]. Chitosan is able to swell and form a gel-like layer in an aqueous environment (here, e.g., by absorbing water from the mucous layer in the nasal cavity), which is favorable for the interpenetration of polymer and glycoprotein chains of the mucus.

Mucoadhesive microspheres composed of hydroxypropyl methylcellulose, chitosan, carbopol 934P (and a combinations of polymers) [76], and chitosan-poly(methyl vinyl ether-*co*-maleic anhydride)-microparticles were prepared by spray drying, for the nasal delivery of propranolol HCl. These microspheres affected the integrity of tight junctions, without causing cell damage, relative to their swelling and charge of polymer. Cell viability was not affected, except with chitosan, but this was recoverable [77].

An emulsifying method used for the production of ethylcellulose–CMs suitable for the nasal delivery of loratadin was shown to result in improved drug entrapment and moderate swelling, compared with conventional CMs [78]. Chitosan-4-thiobutylamidine (TBA) microspheres have also displayed the controlled release of fluorescein isothiocyanate-labeled insulin over 6 h and have the potential to be a useful formulation for the nasal administration of peptides. Chitosan–TBA–insulin, chitosan–insulin, and mannitol–insulin microparticles led to an absolute bioavailability of $7.24 \pm 0.76\%$, $2.04 \pm 1.33\%$, and $1.04 \pm 0.27\%$, respectively, in rats [79].

The loading of carbamazepine in chitosan/glutamate microspheres, produced by spray drying, has been shown to increase the amount of the drug absorbed through the nose, when compared with the nasal administration of the pure drug as a powder ($C_{max} = 800$ and 25 ng/mL for CMs and pure drug as a powder, respectively) [80].

Nasal administration of the chitosan/antigen nasal vaccines was found to be superior to parenteral administration in the induction that the nasal formulation induced significant serum IgG responses similar to and secretory IgA levels superior to what was induced by a parenteral administration of the vaccine. Animals vaccinated via the nasal route with the various chitosan–antigen vaccines were also found to be protected against the appropriate challenge. So far the nasal chitosan vaccine delivery system has been tested for vaccination against influenza in human subjects. The nasal chitosan influenza vaccine was both effective and protective according to the CPMP requirements [49].

7.4.3.2 Pulmonary Delivery

The pulmonary tract tends to be considered as a very promising and attractive route for the administration of active substances intended for local delivery and for the treatment of systemic diseases (e.g., diabetes).

Non-cross-linked and glutaraldehyde-cross-linked chitosans have been found to be potential candidates for carriers of proteins, peptides, and pDNA to the lung via a pressurized metered-dose inhaler system [81].

Betamethasone-loaded CMs containing gelatin and Pluronic F68 have demonstrated good drug stability (1% less hydrolysis product), a high entrapment efficiency (95%), and a positive surface charge (37.5 mV). *In vitro* drug release from the CMs displayed a prolonged release pattern for 12 h that was suitable for pulmonary delivery [81–84].

Spray drying is a very valuable technique for producing dry powders adequate for the pulmonary delivery of drugs. Chitosan/TPP nanoparticles that promote peptide absorption across lung mucosal surfaces are used to microencapsulate insulin-loaded chitosan nanoparticles using typical aerosol excipients, such as mannitol and lactose [85].

Surface-modified PLGA nanospheres containing chitosan are also used for the pulmonary delivery of elcatonin. After pulmonary administration, chitosan-modified PLGA nanospheres have been shown to be more slowly eliminated from the lungs than unmodified PLGA nanospheres, and reduced blood calcium levels to 80% of the initial calcium concentration with prolonged pharmacological action to 24 h [86].

Pulmonary administration of a new pDNA, encoding eight HLA-A*0201-restricted T-cell epitopes from *Mycobacterium tuberculosis*, has been incorporated in chitosan nanoparticles to produce a pulmonary vaccine. The results showed that it induced increased levels of IFN-γ secretion compared with the pulmonary delivery of plasmid in solution or the more frequently used intramuscular immunization route [87].

7.4.3.3 Ocular Delivery

Conventional aqueous solutions topically applied to the eye have the disadvantage that most of the instilled drug is lost within the first 15–30 s after instillation due to reflex tearing and to drainage via the nasolacrimal duct [88]. One of the goals in ophthalmic research has been to increase drug absorption and the duration of contact time. The most commonly used approaches to achieve improved drug efficacy are exemplified by the use of viscosified solutions. Chitosans have superior mucoadhesives owing to their ability to develop molecular attraction forces by electrostatic interactions with the negative charges of the mucus [89,90]. In addition, the pseudoplastic and viscoelastic properties [91] of chitosan solutions make it a potential vehicle for instillation of drugs to the eye.

At present, the use of chitosan in the ophthalmic field is still in the preliminary stages of investigation. El-Samaligy et al. [92] tested three biodegradable polymers, including chitosan, to prepare ganciclovir nanoparticles for the treatment of cytomegalovirus retinitis. *In vitro* data have shown that drug release from chitosan nanoparticles was encouraging. In fact, ganciclovir was released for up to 4 days following a first-order pattern. Furthermore, the release rate was lower for chitosan devices than for the two other polymers (Bovine serum albumin (BSA) and PEC).

De Campos et al. [93] investigated the potential of chitosan nanoparticles as a new vehicle to improve the delivery of drugs to ocular mucosa. Cyclosporin A (CyA) was chosen as a model drug. A modified ionic gelation technique was used to produce CyA-loaded CS nanoparticles. These nanoparticles with a mean size of 293 nm, a zeta potential of +37 mV, high CyA association efficiency, and loading of 73% and 9%, respectively, were obtained. The *in vitro* release studies, performed under sink conditions, revealed the fast release during the first hour followed by a more gradual drug release during the 24 h period. The *in vivo* experiments showed that after topical instillation of CyA-loaded CS nanoparticles to rabbits, therapeutic concentrations were achieved in the external ocular tissues (i.e., cornea and conjunctiva) within 48 h while maintaining negligible or undetectable CyA levels in the inner ocular structures (i.e., iris/ciliary body and aqueous humor), blood, and plasma. These levels were significantly higher than those obtained following the instillation of a CS solution containing CyA and an aqueous CyA suspension. The study indicated that CS nanoparticles could be used as a vehicle to enhance the therapeutic index of the clinically challenging drugs with potential application at the extraocular level.

7.4.4 Transdermal Drug Delivery

It has been increasingly recognized that intact skin represents an interesting way to provide controlled delivery of drugs to the systemic circulation. Drugs administered via transdermal devices approach a zero-order input, which is quite equivalent to the administration of therapeutic agents after a constant intravenous infusion [94]. In addition, transdermal administration represents a reliable alternative to oral administration for substances that are subject to an extensive hepatic first-pass metabolism [95].

Because of its well-known film-forming property, a number of studies have been performed on the usefulness of chitosan membranes as transdermal devices. Thacharodi and Panduranga Rao [94–96] evaluated the efficacy of chitosan membranes as rate-controlling membranes by testing series of hydrophilic and hydrophobic drugs. They concluded that water-soluble drugs, such as propranolol, could be transported through chitosan membranes principally via a pore mechanism [94], whereas hydrophobic solutes, such as nifedipine, would be influenced by both partition and pore mechanisms operating concurrently [96]. The data of Nakatsuka and Andrady are in agreement with these results since they have suggested that the transport of the hydrosoluble vitamin < vitamin B_{12} > B-12 through cross-linked or blended chitosan films followed predominantly a pore mechanism [97].

Comparing the capacities of chitosan versus cellulose membranes, Sawayanagi et al. [98] found that the diffusion constant for acidic substances such as nonsteroidal antiinflammatory drugs was two to three times larger through the chitosan membrane.

Regarding the kinetic characteristics of several films described in the literature, it can be seen that permeability coefficients are affected by different parameters, including the degree of cross-linking [94,96], the acid or base nature of the drug [98], the molecular volume of the drug [98], the pH of the environmental medium [99], and the thickness of the membrane [97].

Until now, little information has been available concerning the influence of the site of application of such systems. Furthermore, most of the literature consists of *in vitro* release tests, which provides information on pharmacokinetic parameters affected by the biopolymeric membrane solely. It could be interesting to conduct *in vitro* skin permeation tests using excised skin mounted on a diffusion cell such as the Franz diffusion apparatus [100]. This type of test could provide useful indications of the pharmaceutical flux from the membrane to the skin sample, which in turn may provide information on *in vivo* performance of the transdermal system [101].

7.5 Conclusions

Chitosan has the desired properties for safe use as a pharmaceutical excipient. This has prompted accelerated research activities worldwide on chitosan micro- and nanoparticles as drug delivery vehicles. These systems have great utility in controlled release and targeting studies of almost all classes of bioactive molecules as discussed in this review. Recently, chitosan is also extensively explored in studies of gene delivery. However, studies on the optimization of process parameters and scale-up from the laboratory to pilot plant and then to production level are yet to be undertaken. Most of the studies carried out so far are only under *in vitro* conditions. More *in vivo* studies need to be carried out. Chemical modifications of chitosan are important for obtaining the desired physicochemical properties such as solubility, hydrophilicity, and so on. The published literature indicates that in the near future, chitosan-based particulate systems will have more commercial status in the market than in the past.

References

1. Agnihotri, S. A., Mallikarjuna, N. N., and Aminabhavi, T. M. 2004. Recent advances on chitosan-based micro- and nanoparticles in drug delivery. *J Control Release* 100: 5–28.
2. Kumar, M. N. V. R., Muzzarelli, R. A. A., Muzzarelli, C., Sashiwa, H., and Domb, A. J. 2004. Chitosan chemistry and pharmaceutical perspectives. *Chem Rev* 104: 6017–6084.
3. Akbuga, J. and Durmaz, G. 1994. Preparation and evaluation of cross-linked chitosan microspheres containing furosemide. *Int J Pharm* 111: 217–222.
4. Nishimura, K., Nishimura, S., Seo, H., Nishi, N., Tokura, S., and Azuma, I. 1986. Macrophage activation with multi-porous beads prepared from partially deacetylated chitin. *J Biomed Mater Res* 20: 1359–1372.

5. Berthold, A. and Kreuter, J. 1996. Chitosan microspheres—Improved acid stability and change in physicochemical properties by cross-linking. In *Proceedings of 23rd International Symposium on Control Release Bioactive Materials*. Tokyo, Japan. pp. 369–370.

6. He, P., Davis, S. S., and Illum, L. 1999. Chitosan microspheres prepared by spray drying. *Int J Pharm* 187: 53–65.

7. Tokumitsu, H., Ichikawa, H., and Fukumori, Y. 1999. Chitosan–gadopentetic acid complex nanoparticles for gadolinium neutron-capture therapy of cancer: Preparation by novel emulsion-droplet coalescence technique and characterization. *Pharm Res* 16: 1830–1835.

8. Liu, L. S., Liu, S. Q., Ng, S. Y., Froix, M., Ohno, T., and Heller, J. 1997. Controlled release of interleukin-2 for tumour immunotherapy using alginate/chitosan porous microspheres. *J Control Release* 43: 65–74.

9. Polk, A., Amsden, B., Yao, K. D., Peng, T., and Goosen, M. F. A., 1994. Controlled-release of albumin from chitosan–alginate microcapsules. *J Pharm Sci* 83: 178–185.

10. Kawashima, Y., Handa, T., Kasai, A. Takenaka, H., and Shan, Y. L. 1985. The effects of thickness and hardness of the coating film on the drug release rate of theophylline granules coated with chitosan sodium tripolyphosphate complex. *Chem Pharm Bull* 33: 2469–2474.

11. Kawashima, Y., Handa, T., Kasai, A., Takenaka, H., Lin, S. Y., and Ando, Y. 1985. Novel method for the preparation of controlled-release theophylline granules coated with a poly-electrolyte complex of sodium polyphosphate chitosan. *J Pharm Sci* 74: 264–268.

12. Leong, Y. S. and Candau, F. 1982. Inverse microemulsion polymerization. *J Phys Chem* 86: 2269–2271.

13. Maitra, A. 1984. Determination of size parameters of water aerosol of oil reverse micelles from their nuclear magnetic-resonance data. *J Phys Chem* 88: 5122–5125.

14. Luisi, P. L., Giomini, M., Pileni, M. P., and Robinson, B. H. 1998. Reverse micelles as hosts for proteins and small molecules. *Biochim Biophys Acta* 947: 209–246.

15. Agnihotri, S. A. and Aminabhavi, T. M. 2004. Controlled release of clozapine through chitosan microparticles prepared by a novel method. *J Control Release* 96: 245–259.

16. Liu, Y., Vrana, N. E., Cahill, P. A., and McGuinness, G. B. 2009 . Physically cross-linked composite hydrogels of PVA with natural macromolecules: Structure, mechanical properties, and endothelial cell compatibility. *J Biomed Mater Res Part B—Appl Biomater* 90B: 492–502.

17. Cho, M. H., Kim, K. S., Ahn, H. H., Kim, M. S., Kim, S. H., Khang, G., Lee, B., and Lee, H. B. 2008. Chitosan gel as an *in situ*-forming scaffold for rat bone marrow mesenchymal stem cells *in vivo*. *Tissue Eng Part A* 14: 1099–1108.

18. Castro, G. R., Kamdar, R. R., Panilaitis, B., and Kaplan, D. L. 2005. Triggered release of proteins from emulsan-alginate beads. *J Control Release* 109: 149–157.

19. Takakura, Y., Kaneko, Y., Fujita, T., Hashida, M., Maeda, H., and Sezaki, H. 1989. Control of pharmaceutical properties of soybean trypsin-inhibitor by conjugation with dextran 1. Synthesis and characterization. *J Pharm Sci* 78: 117–121.

20. Ponchel, G. and Irache, J. M. 1998. Specific and non-specific bioadhesive particulate systems for oral delivery to the gastrointestinal tract. *Adv Drug Deliv Rev* 34: 191–219.

21. Russell-Jones, G. J. 2000. Oral vaccine delivery. *J Control Release* 65: 49–54.

22. Sood, A. and Panchagnula, R. 2001. Peroral route: An opportunity for protein and peptide drug delivery. *Chem Rev* 101: 3275–3303.

23. Bodmeier, R., Chen, H., and Paeratakul, O. 1989. A novel-approach to the oral delivery of microparticles or nanoparticles. *Pharm Res* 6: 413–417.

24. He, P., Davis, S. S., and Illum, L. 1998. *In vitro* evaluation of the mucoadhesive properties of chitosan microspheres. *Int J Pharm* 166: 75–88.

25. Celik, O. and Akbuga, J. 2007. Preparation of superoxide dismutase loaded chitosan microspheres: Characterization and release studies. *Eur J Pharm Biopharm* 66: 42–47.

26. Schally, A. V. 1999. LH-RH analogues: I. Their impact on reproductive medicine. *Gynecol Endocrinol* 13: 401–409.

27. Xue, Z. X., Yang, G. P., Zhang, Z. P., and He, B. L., 2006. Application of chitosan microspheres as carriers of LH-RH analogue TX46. *Reac Func Polym* 66: 893–901.

28. Wang, L. Y., Gu, Y. H., Zhou, Q. Z., Ma, G. H., Wan, Y. H., and Su, Z. G., 2006. Preparation and characterization of uniform-sized chitosan microspheres containing insulin by membrane emulsification and a two-step solidification process. *Colloid Surface B* 50: 126–135.

29. Kofuji, K., Murata, Y., and Kawashima, S. 2005. Sustained insulin release with biodegradation of chitosan gel beads prepared by copper ions. *Int J Pharm* 303: 95–103.

30. Cho, B. C., Kim, J. Y., Lee, J. H., Chung, H. Y., Park, J. W., Roh, K. H., Kim, G. U. et al. 2004. The bone regenerative effect of chitosan microsphere-encapsulated growth hormone on bony consolidation in mandibular distraction osteogenesis in a dog model. *J Craniofac Surg* 15: 299–311.

31. Jiang, D. S., Long, S. Y., Huang, J., Xiao, H. Y., and Zhou, J.Y. 2005. Immobilization of *Pycnoporus sanguineus* laccase on magnetic chitosan microspheres. *Biochem Eng J* 25: 15–23.

32. Shentu, J. L., Wu, J. M., Song, W. H., and Jia, Z. S. 2005. Chitosan microspheres as immobilized dye affinity support for catalase adsorption. *Int J Biol Macromol* 37: 42–46.

33. Martins, A. O., Da Silva, E. L., Carasek, E., Laranjeira, M. C. M., and De Favere, V. T. 2004. Sulphoxine immobilized onto chitosan microspheres by spray drying: Application for metal ions preconcentration by flow injection analysis. *Talanta* 63: 397–403.

34. Borchard, G. 2001. Chitosans for gene delivery. *Adv Drug Deliv Rev* 52: 145–150.

35. Kim, J. S., Maruyama, A., Akaike, T., and Kim, S. W. 1997. *In vitro* gene expression on smooth muscle cells using a terplex delivery system. *J Control Release* 47: 51–59.

36. Knowles, M. R., Hohneker, K. W., Zhou, Z., Olsen, J. C., Noah, T. L, Hu, P. C., Leigh, M. W., Engelhardt, J. F., Edwards, L. J., and Jones, K. R. 1995. A controlled-study of adenoviral-vector-mediated gene-transfer in the nasal epithelium of patients with cystic-fibrosis. *New Engl J Med* 333: 823–831.

37. Lee, K. Y., Kwon, I. C., Kim, Y. H., Jo, W. H., and Jeong, S. Y. 1998. Preparation of chitosan self-aggregates as a gene delivery system. *J Control Release* 51: 213–220.

38. Xiang, Z. Q., Yang, Y., Wilson, J. M., and Ertl, H. C. 1996. A replication-defective human adenovirus recombinant serves as a highly efficacious vaccine carrier. *Virology* 219: 220–227.

39. Leong, K. W., Mao, II. Q., Truong Le, V. L., Roy, K., Walsh, S. M., and August, J. T. 1998. DNA-polycation nanospheres as non-viral gene delivery vehicles. *J Control Release* 53: 183–193.

40. Mumper, R. J., Wang, J. J., Claspell, J. M., and Rolland, A. P. 1995. Novel polymeric condensing carriers for gene delivery. *Int Symp Contro Release Bioact Mater* 22: 178–179.

41. MacLaughlin, F. C., Mumper, R. J., Wang, J. J., Tagliaferri, J. M., Gill, I., Hinchcliffe, M., and Rolland, A. P. 1998. Chitosan and depolymerized chitosan oligomers as condensing carriers for *in vivo* plasmid delivery. *J Control Release* 56: 259–272.

42. Thanou, M., Florea, B. I., Geldof, M., Junginger, H. E., and Borchard, G. 2002. Quaternized chitosan oligomers as novel gene delivery vectors in epithelial cell lines. *Biomaterials* 23: 153–159.

43. Erbacher, P., Zou, S. M., Bettinger, T., Steffan, A. M., and Remy, J. S. 1998. Chitosan-based vector/DNA complexes for gene delivery: Biophysical characteristics and transfection ability. *Pharm Res* 15: 1332–1339.

44. Sato, T., Ishii, T., and Okahata, Y. 2001. *In vitro* gene delivery mediated by chitosan. Effect of pH, serum, and molecular mass of chitosan on the transfection efficiency. *Biomaterials* 22: 2075–2080.

45. Vinogradov, S. V., Bronich, T. K., and Kabanov, A. V. 2002. Nanosized cationic hydrogels for drug delivery: Preparation, properties and interactions with cells. *Adv Drug Deliv Rev* 54: 135–147.

46. Mao, H. Q., Roy, K., Troung-Le, V. L., Janes, K. A., Lin, K. Y., Wang, Y., August, J. T., and Leong, K. W. 2001. Chitosan–DNA nanoparticles as gene carriers: Synthesis, characterization and transfection efficiency. *J Control Release* 70: 399–421.

47. Richardson, S. C. W., Kolbe, H. V, J., and Duncan, R. 1999. Potential of low molecular mass chitosan as a DNA delivery system: Biocompatibility, body distribution and ability to complex and protect DNA. *Int J Pharm* 178: 231–243.

48. Leong, K. W., Mao, H. Q., Truong-Le, V. L., Roy, K., Walsh, S. M., and August, J. T. 1997. DNA–chitosan nanospheres: Derivatization and storage stability. In *Proceedings of International Symposium on Control Release Bioactive Materials*. Stockholm, Sweden, pp. 671–672.

49. Illum, L., Jabbal-Gill, I., Hinchcliffe, M., Fisher, A. N., and Davis, S. S. 2001. Chitosan as a novel nasal delivery system for vaccines. *Adv Drug Deliv Rev* 51: 81–96.

50. Kang, M. L., Kang, S. G., Jiang, H. L., Shin, S. W., Lee, D. Y., Ahn, J. M., Rayamahji, N. et al. 2006. *In vivo* induction of mucosal immune responses by intranasal administration of chitosan microspheres containing *Bordetella bronchiseptica* DNT. *Eur J Pharm Biopharm* 63: 215–220.

51. Jiang, H. L., Park, I. K., Shin, N. R., Kang, S. G., Yoo, H. S., Kim, S. I., Suh, S. B., Akaike, T., and Cho, C. S. 2004. *In vitro* study of the immune stimulating activity of an athrophic rhinitis vaccine associated to chitosan microspheres. *Eur J Pharm Biopharm* 58: 471–476.

52. Jaganathan, K. S., Rao, Y. U. B., Singh, P., Prabakaran, D., Gupta, S., Jain, A., and Vyas, S. P. 2005. Development of a single dose tetanus toxoid formulation based on polymeric microspheres: A comparative study of poly(D, L-lactic-*co*-glycolic acid) versus chitosan microspheres. *Int J Pharm* 294: 23–32.

53. Mi, F. L., Shyu, S. S., Chen, C. T., and Schoung, J. Y. 1999. Porous chitosan microsphere for controlling the antigen release of Newcastle disease vaccine: Preparation of antigen-adsorbed microsphere and *in vitro* release. *Biomaterials* 20: 1603–1612.

54. Zhao, H. P., Wu, B., Wu, H., Su, L. Y., Pang, J. L., Yang, T. H., and Liu, Y. L. 2006. Protective immunity in rats by intranasal immunization with *Streptococcus mutans* glucan-binding protein D encapsulated into chitosan-coated poly(lactic-*co*-glycolic acid) microspheres. *Biotechnol Lett* 28: 1299–1304.

55. Lameiro, M. H., Malpique, R., Silva, A. C., Alves, P. M., and Melo, E. 2006. Encapsulation of adenoviral vectors into chitosan-bile salt microparticles for mucosal vaccination. *J Biotechnol* 126: 152–162.

56. Van der Lubben, I. M., Konings, F. A. J., Borchard, G., Verhoef, J. C., and Junginger, H. E. 2001. *In vivo* uptake of chitosan microparticles by murine Peyer's patches: Visualization studies using confocal laser scanning microscopy and immunohistochemistry. *J Drug Target* 9: 39–47.

57. Van der Lubben, I. M., Van Opdorp, F. A. C., Hengeveld, M. R., Onderwater, J. J. M., Koerten, H. K., Verhoef, J. C., Borchard, G., and Junginger, H. E. 2002. Transport of chitosan microparticles for mucosal vaccine delivery in a human intestinal M-cell model. *J Drug Target* 10: 449–456.

58. Oie, S. and Benet, L. Z. 1996. The effect of route of administration and distribution on drug action. In *Modern Pharmaceutics*, G. S. Banker and C. T. Rhodes, eds. New York, NY: Marcel Dekker, 155–178.

59. Buri, P. 1985. Voie oral. In Formes pharmaceutiques nouvelles : aspects technologique, biopharmaceutique et medical, eds. P. Buri, F. Puisieux, E. Doelker, J. P. Benoit. Paris: Technique et documentation (Lavoisier) 175–228.

60. Hejazi, R. and Amiji, M. 2004. Stomach-specific anti-*H-pylori* therapy Part III: Effect of chitosan microspheres cross-linking on the gastric residence and local tetracycline concentrations in fasted gerbils. *Int J Pharm* 272: 99–108.

61. El-Gibaly, I. 2002. Development and *in vitro* evaluation of novel floating chitosan microcapsules for oral use: Comparison with non-floating chitosan microspheres. *Int J Pharm* 249: 7–21.

62. Hejazi, R. and Amiji, M. 2002. Stomach-specific anti-*H-pylori* therapy. 1: Preparation and characterization of tetracyline-loaded chitosan microspheres. *Int J Pharm* 235: 87–94.

63. Portero, A., Remunan-Lopez, C., Criado, M. T., and Alonso, M. J. 2002. Reacetylated chitosan microspheres for controlled delivery of anti-microbial agents to the gastric mucosa. *J Microencapsul* 19: 797–809.

64. Tozaki, H., Komoike, J., Tada, C., Maruyama, T., Terabe, A., Suzuki, T., Yamamoto, A., and Muranishi, S. 1997. Chitosan capsules for colon-specific drug delivery: Improvement of insulin absorption from the rat colon. *J Pharm Sci* 86: 1016–1021.

65. Pantaleone, D. et al. 1991. Advances in chitin and chitosan. In *Fifth International Conference on Chitin and Chitosan*. Princeton, New York, NY.

66. Zhang, H., Alsarra, I. A., and Neau, S. H. 2002. An *in vitro* evaluation of a chitosan-containing multiparticulate system for macromolecule delivery to the colon. *Int J Pharm* 239: 197–205.

67. Tominaga, S. et al. 1998. Colon drug delivery system. *J Pol Appl* JP 10 324, 642 (98324,642) (C1 A61K47/36).

68. Wittaya-areekul, S., Kruenate, J., and Prahsarn, C. 2006. Preparation and *in vitro* evaluation of mucoadhesive properties of alginate/chitosan microparticles containing prednisolone. *In J Pharm* 312: 113–118.

69. Rai, G., Jain, S. K., Agrawal, S., Bhadra, S., Pancholi, S. S., and Agrawal, G. P. 2005. Chitosan hydrochloride based microspheres of albendazole for colonic drug delivery. *Pharmazie* 60: 131–134.

70. Sadeghi, A. M. M., Dorkoosh, F. A., Avadi, M. R., Saadat, P., Rafiee-Tehrani, M., and Junginger, H. E. 2008. Preparation, characterization and antibacterial activities of chitosan, *N*-trimethyl chitosan (TMC) and *N*-diethylmethyl chitosan (DEMC) nanoparticles loaded with insulin using both the ionotropic gelation and polyelectrolyte complexation methods. *Int J Pharm* 355: 299–306.

71. Bayat, A., Dorkoosh, F. A., Dehpour, A. R., Moezi, L., Larijani, B., Junginger, H. E., and Rafiee-Tehrani, M. 2008. Nanoparticles of quaternized chitosan derivatives as a carrier for colon delivery of insulin: *Ex vivo* and *in vivo* studies. *Int J Pharm* 356: 259–266.

72. Lorenzo-Lamosa, M. L., Remunan-Lopez, C., Vila-Jato, J. L., and Alonso, M. J. 1998. Design of microencapsulated chitosan microspheres for colonic drug delivery. *J Control Release* 52: 109–118.

73. Genta, I., Costantini, M., Asti, A., Conti, B., and Montanari, L. 1998. Influence of glutaraldehyde on drug release and mucoadhesive properties of chitosan microspheres. *Carbohyd Polym* 36: 81–88.

74. Artursson, P., Lindmark, T., Davis, S. D., and Illum, L., 1994. Effect of chitosan on the permeability of monolayers of intestinal epithelial-cells (Caco-2). *Pharm Res* 11: 1358–1361.

75. Felt, O., Buri, P., and Gurny, R., 1998. Chitosan: A unique polysaccharide for drug delivery. *Drug Develop Ind Pharm* 24: 979–993.

76. Harikarnpakdee, S., Lipipun, V., Sutanthavibul, N., and Ritthidej, G. C. 2006. Spray-dried mucoadhesive microspheres: Preparation and transport through nasal cell monolayer. *Aaps Pharm* 7: 12.

77. Cerchiara, T., Luppi, B., Chidichimo, G., Bigucci, F., and Zecchi, V. 2005. Chitosan and poly(methyl vinyl ether-*co*-maleic anhydride) microparticles as nasal sustained delivery systems. *Eur J Pharm Biopharm* 61: 195–200.

78. Martinac, A., Filipovic-Grcic, J., Perissutti, B., Voinovich, D., and Pavelic, Z. 2005. Spray-dried chitosan/ethylcellulose microspheres for nasal drug delivery: Swelling study and evaluation of *in vitro* drug release properties. *J Microencapsul* 22: 549–561.

79. Krauland, A. H., Guggi, D., and Bernkop-Schnurch, A. 2006. Thiolated chitosan microparticles: A vehicle for nasal peptide drug delivery. *Int J Pharm* 307: 270–277.

80. Gavini, E., Hegge, A. B., Rassu, G., Sanna, V., Testa, C., Pirisino, G., Karlsen, J., and Giunchedi, P. 2006. Nasal administration of Carbamazepine using chitosan microspheres: *In vitro/in vivo* studies. *Int J Pharm* 307: 9–15.

81. Williams, R. O., Barron, M. K., Alonso, M. J., and Remunan-Lopez, C. 1998. Investigation of a pMDI system containing chitosan microspheres and P134a. *Int J Pharm* 174: 209–222.

82. Huang, Y. C., Chiang, C. H., and Yeh, M. K. 2003. Optimizing formulation factors in preparing chitosan microparticles by spray-drying method. *J Microencapsul* 20: 247–260.

83. Huang, Y. C., Yeh, M. K., Cheng, S. N., and Chiang, C. H. 2003. The characteristics of betamethasone-loaded chitosan microparticles by spray-drying method. *J Microencapsul* 20: 459–472.

84. Huang, Y. C., Yeh, M. K., and Chiang, C. H. 2002. Formulation factors in preparing BTM–chitosan microspheres by spray drying method. *Int J Pharm* 242: 239–242.

85. Grenha, A., Seijo, B., and Remunan-Lopez, C. 2005. Microencapsulated chitosan nanoparticles for lung protein delivery. *Eur J Pharm* 25: 427–437.

86. Yamamoto, H., Kuno, Y., Sugimoto, S., Takeuchi, H., and Kawashima, Y. 2005. Surface-modified PLGA nanosphere with chitosan improved pulmonary delivery of calcitonin by mucoadhesion and opening of the intercellular tight junctions. *J Control Release* 102: 373–381.

87. Bivas-Benita, M., van Meijgaarden, K. E., Franken, K. L. M. C., Junginger, H. E, Borchard, G., Ottenhoff, T. H. M., and Geluk, A. 2004. Pulmonary delivery of chitosan–DNA nanoparticles enhances the immunogenicity of a DNA vaccine encoding HLA-A*0201-restricted T-cell epitopes of *Mycobacterium tuberculosis*. *Vaccine* 22: 1609–1615.

88. Shell, J. W. 1982. Pharmacokinetics of topically applied ophthalmic drugs. *Surv Ophthalmol* 26: 207–218.

89. Lehr, C. M., Bouwstra1, J. A., Schacht, E. H., and Junginger, H. E., 1992. *In vitro* evaluation of mucoadhesive properties of chitosan and some other natural polymers. *Int J Pharm* 78: 43–48.

90. Park, K. and Robinson, J. R. 1984. Bioadhesive polymers as platforms for oral-controlled drug delivery—Method to study bioadhesion. *Int J Pharm* 19: 107–127.

91. Wang, X. and D. Xu, D. 1994. Viscosity and flow properties of concentrated solutions of chitosan with different degrees of deacetylation. *Int J Biol Macromol* 16: 149–152.

92. El-Samaligy, M. S., Rojanasakul, Y. R., Charlton, J. F., Weinstein, G. W., and Lim, J. K. 1996. Ocular disposition of nanoencapsulated acyclovir and ganciclovir via intravitreal injection in rabbit's eye. *Drug Deliv* 3: 93–97.

93. De Campos, A. M., Sanchez, A., and Alonso, M. J. 2001. Chitosan nanoparticles: A new vehicle for the improvement of the delivery of drugs to the ocular surface. Application to cyclosporin A. *Int J Pharm* 224: 159–168.

94. Thacharodi, D. and Rao, K. P. 1993. Propranolol hydrochloride release behaviour of cross-linked chitosan membranes. *J Chem Technol Biotechnol* 58: 177–181.

95. Thacharodi, D. and Rao, K. P. 1996. Rate-controlling biopolymer membranes as transdermal delivery systems for nifedipine: Development and *in vitro* evaluations. *Biomaterials* 17: 1307–1311.

96. Thacharodi, D. and Rao, K. P. 1993. Release of nifedipine through cross-linked chitosan membranes. *Int J Pharm* 96: 33–39.

97. Nakatsuka, S. and Andarady, A. L. 1992. Permeability of vitamin B-12 in chitosan membranes. Effect of cross-linking and blending with poly(vinyl alcohol) on permeability. *J Appl Polym Sci* 44: 17–28.

98. Sawayanagi, Y., Nambu, N., and Nagai, T. 1982. The use of chitosan for sustained-release preparations of water-soluble drugs. *Chem Pharm Bull* 30: 4213–4215.

99. Kim, J. H., Kim, J. Y., Lee, Y. M., and Kim, K. Y, 1992. Controlled release of riboflavin and insulin through cross-linked poly(vinyl alcohol)/chitosan blend membrane. *J Appl Polym Sci* 44: 1823–1828.

100. Tojo, K. 1987. In *Transdermal Controlled Systemic Medications*, Y. W. Chien, ed. New York,. NY: Marcel Dekker, p. 127.

101. Shah, V. P., Lesko L. J., and Williams, R. L. 1995. *In Vitro* evaluation of transdermal drug delivery. *Eur J Pharm Biopharm* 41: 163–167.

8

Enzyme Immobilization on Chitosan-Based Supports

Kang Wang

CONTENTS

8.1 Introduction

Enzymes have been used since time immemorial in cheese manufacturing and indirectly via yeasts and bacteria in food manufacturing. Isolated enzymes were first used in the year 1914, their protein nature was proven in 1926 and their large-scale microbial production started in the 1960s. The industrial enzyme business is steadily growing due to improved production technologies, engineered enzyme properties, and new application fields. The global market for industrial enzymes is expected to increase to over $2.7 billion by 2012 [1]. In recent years, enzymes have found applications in the food, agrochemical, and pharmaceutical industries and now increasingly in organic chemical synthesis.

Biocatalysis capitalizes on the metabolic diversity of enzymes and exhibits a number of features compared with conventional chemicals. The major advantages of using enzymes in biocatalytic transformations are their chemo-, regio-, and stereospecificity. These specificities warrant that the catalyzed reaction is not perturbed by side reactions, resulting in the production of one wanted end product, whereas production of undesirable by-products is eliminated. In addition, enzymes are more suited to working with natural and renewable feedstock than those derived from petrochemicals. Also, enzymes practically do not present disposal problems since, being mostly proteins and peptides, they are biodegradable and easily removed from contaminated streams [2].

However, even when an enzyme is identified as being useful for a given reaction, its application is often hampered by its lack of long-term stability under process conditions and also by difficulties in recovery and recycling. The instability of enzyme structures was revealed once they are isolated from their natural environments. Furthermore, unlike conventional heterogeneous chemical catalysts, most enzymes operate dissolved in water in homogeneous catalysis systems, which is why they contaminate the product and as a rule cannot be recovered in the active form from reaction mixtures for reuse.

Immobilization is achieved by fixing enzymes to or within solid supports, as a result of which heterogeneous immobilized enzyme systems are obtained. Biocatalytic process economics can be enhanced by enzyme reuse and the improvement in enzyme stability afforded by immobilization. It can also improve enzyme performance under optimal process reaction conditions (e.g., acidity, alkalinity, organic solvents, and elevated temperatures), a requirement that has often retarded enzyme application in industrial chemical synthesis [3].

There is no general universally applicable method of enzyme immobilization. The main task is to select a suitable carrier. The selected method should meet both the catalytic needs (expressed in productivity, space–time yield, stability, and selectivity) and the noncatalytic needs (e.g., separation, control, and downstreaming process) that are required by a given application. Cao [4] believes that a rational combination of various immobilization methods and methodologies is a valuable method to obtain robust immobilized enzymes, which cannot be obtained by the straightforward immobilization.

Of the many carriers that have been considered and studied for immobilizing enzymes, organic or inorganic, natural or synthetic, chitin and chitosan are of interest in that they offer advantages such as high affinity to proteins, availability of reactive functional groups ($-OH$ and $-NH_2$) for direct reactions with enzymes and for chemical modifications, hydrophilicity, mechanical stability and rigidity, regenerability, and ease of preparation in different geometrical configurations that provide the system with permeability and surface area suitable for a chosen biotransformation [2].

Krajewska [2] has reviewed the application of chitin- and chitosan-based materials in enzyme immobilization and the range of uses of such complexes. Here we will mainly review the immobilization supports such as chitosan gel (see Section 8.3), chitosan modifications (see Section 8.4), and chitosan composites (see Section 8.5). Compared with tissue engineering and drug delivery application *in vivo*, chitosan supports for enzyme immobilization were more abundant due to little limitation from *in vitro*. The application of chitin is not introduced in this chapter. Methods of enzyme immobilization on a chitosan/chitin-based support are described in Section 8.2 (including the current methods and supports for enzyme immobilization).

8.2 Enzyme Immobilization and Chitosan-Based Supports

8.2.1 Current Methods of Enzyme Immobilization

Enzymes may be immobilized by a variety of methods, which may be traditionally classified as physical, where weak interactions between the support and the enzyme exist, and chemical, where covalent bonds are formed with the enzyme. Brady [5] presents enzyme immobilization strategies the can be broadly divided into four groups (Figure 8.1): entrapment, encapsulation, solid support and self-immobilization.

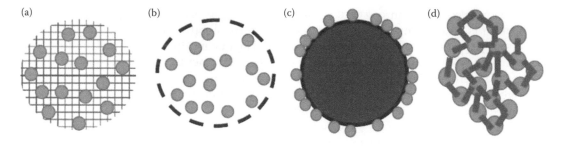

FIGURE 8.1

Enzyme immobilization strategies: (a) Entrapment, (b) encapsulation, (c) solid support, and (d) self-immobilization. Enzymes are represented by circles. (From Brady, D. and Jordaan, J. 2009. *Biotechnol Lett* 31: 1639–1650. With permission.)

Enzyme entrapment (Figure 8.1a) and encapsulation (Figure 8.1b) protects enzymes by preventing direct contact with the environment, thereby minimizing the effects of gas bubbles, mechanical shear, and hydrophobic solvents, but has the drawback of mass transfer limitations. For support-based immobilization (Figure 8.1c), adsorption is a relatively simple and inexpensive method of immobilization, and does not chemically modify the enzyme, but it has limitations as the enzyme tends to leach out, especially in aqueous solvents. This can result in difficulties in process design and downstream processing. Hence the method is best suited to immobilize lipases for use in organic solvents. Ionic binding is another simple noncovalent immobilization technique. Enzymes can be bound to polysaccharide biopolymers such as dextran, agarose, and chitosan. The most interesting recent developments are in the area of immobilization through covalent binding. Improvements in current strategies for carrier-based immobilization have been developed using heterofunctionalized supports that enhance binding efficacy and stability through multipoint attachment (MPA) [5].

Multipoint covalent attachment of enzymes on highly activated preexisting supports via short spacer arms and involving many residues placed on the enzyme surface promotes a rigidification of the enzyme structure of the immobilized enzyme (Figure 8.2). The relative distances among all residues involved in the multipoint immobilization have to be maintained unaltered during any conformational change induced by any distorting agent (heat, organic solvents, and extreme pH values). This should reduce any conformational change involved in enzyme inactivation and greatly increase the enzyme stability. The characteristics of the support, reactive groups, and immobilization conditions need to be carefully selected to be able to involve the maximum number of enzyme groups in the immobilization. A support suitable for protein multipoint immobilization requires fulfilling some characteristics, for example, large internal surface, high superficial density of reactive groups, minimal satiric hindrances of reactive groups between the protein and the support, and enough stable reactive groups placed in the enzyme surface [6].

Moreover, novel methods of enzyme self-immobilization (Figure 8.1d) have been developed (cross-linked enzyme crystals (CLECs) and cross-linked enzyme aggregates (CLEAs)). As mentioned above, the use of solid supports for enzyme immobilization can reduce the specific and volumetric activity of the biocatalyst by a factor of 10 or more. Carrier-free enzyme immobilization is possible using bifunctional cross-linkers, such as glutaraldehyde (GA), to bind enzymes to each other without resorting to a support. CLEC formation requires extensive protein purification and method development and, although broadly applicable, it only works for crystallizable enzymes. Then, a less-expensive method of

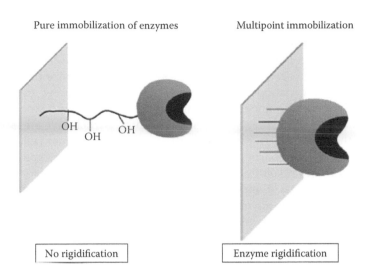

FIGURE 8.2
Effect of immobilization on enzyme stability. (From Mateo, C. et al. 2007. *Enzyme Microb Technol* 40: 1451–1463. With permission.)

enhancing enzyme proximity for cross-linking is by simply precipitating the protein and cross-linking the aggregates to form particles of about 50–100 μm diameter. These CLEAs were developed in Sheldon's laboratory and commercialized by CLEA Technologies (the Netherlands) [5].

Several enzymes have been successfully immobilized using CLEA techniques, including penicillin G acylase, lipases, and nitrilases [7–9]. Precipitants were found to have a profound influence on both specific activities and total activity recovery of CLEAs, as exemplified by *Candida antarctica* lipase B (CALB) [9]. Among the CLEAs of CALB studied, those obtained using PEG600, ammonium sulfate, PEG200, and acetone as precipitants were observed to attain over 200% total activity recovery in comparison with acetone powder directly precipitated from the liquid solution by acetone. PEG200-precipitated CLEA gave the best specific activity (139% relative to acetone powder). The results of kinetic studies showed that V_{max}/K_m does not significantly change upon CLEA formation. The diversity of enzymes able to form active CLEA, however, might be restricted by their ability to resist chemical cross-linking. Extensive enzyme aggregation in CLEAs must also be avoided to prevent mass-transfer limitations during catalysis.

8.2.2 Several Supports of Enzyme Immobilization

The results of immobilization, including the performance of immobilized enzymes, strongly depend on the properties of supports, which are usually referred to as material type, composition, structure, and so on. So far, different nanostructured materials have been used as supports, such as nanoparticles, nanofibers, nanotubes and mesoporous silica, and single enzyme nanoparticles [10,11]. They stand out from other supports because of their extremely high surface area-to-volume ratios, which can provide large specific surface areas for highly efficient immobilization as well as stabilize enzymes. Several involved materials in this chapter are briefly described below.

Nanoparticles provide an ideal remedy for the usually contradictory issues encountered in the optimization of immobilized enzymes: minimum diffusional limitation, maximum surface area per unit mass, and high enzyme loading. Moreover, the MPA of enzyme molecules to nanomaterial surfaces reduces protein unfolding, resulting in enhanced stability of the enzyme attached to the nanoparticle surface. Furthermore, for nanometals or metal oxides, their unique ability is to promote faster electron transfer between the electrode and the active site of the desired enzyme. In addition to the promising performance features, the unique solution behaviors of the nanoparticles also point to an interesting transitional region between heterogeneous and homogeneous catalysis. Theoretical and experimental studies demonstrated that particle mobility, which is governed by particle size and solution viscosity, could impact the intrinsic activity of the particle-attached enzymes [12].

As mentioned above, nanoparticles are desirable from several perspectives. However, their dispersion in reaction solutions and their subsequent recovery for reuse are often found to be a daunting task. It appears that the use of nanofibers would overcome this limitation while providing the advantageous features of nanosize materials. The collection of randomly arrayed nanofibers usually forms a nonwoven mesh (or membrane) with reusability. Thus enzyme-immobilized nanofibrous membranes have functions of biocatalysis and separation simultaneously, which is generally accepted as the fundamental requirement for the enzymatic membrane-bioreactor. Applications in biosensors and biofuel cells are also allowed for these nanofibrous membranes. Compared with other nanostructured supports, nanofibrous supports show many advantages for their high porosity and interconnectivity. Electrospun nanofibers have been proven to be excellent supports for enzyme immobilization [13]. However, studies of this issue are still limited to a small number as there are still problems in their large-scale application.

Carbon nanotubes (CNTs), discovered in 1991 by Iijima, represent an important group of nanoscale materials. CNTs can display metallic, semiconducting, and superconducting electron transport, possess a hollow core suitable for storing guest molecules, and have the largest elastic modulus of any known material. Basically, there are two groups of CNTs, multiwall carbon nanotubes (MWCNTs) and single-walled carbon nanotubes (SWCNTs). An MWCNT is a central tubule of nanometric diameter surrounded by graphitic layers separated by ca. 34 nm, and an SWCNT is only the tubule and no graphitic layers. CNT-based electrochemical transducers offer substantial improvements in the performance of amperometric enzyme electrodes, immunosensors, and nucleic acid sensing devices. The greatly enhanced electrochemical reactivity of hydrogen peroxide and NADH at CNT-modified electrodes makes these nanomaterials extremely attractive for numerous oxidase- and dehydrogenase-based amperometric biosensors [14].

Enzyme encapsulation via the sol–gel approach has been one of the most popular methods for enzyme immobilization since the first report by Avnir et al. [15]: that enzymes encapsulated into sol–gel matrices maintained their activities. In a typical synthetic protocol, tetramethoxysilane (TMOS) or tetraethoxysilane (TEOS) is hydrolyzed into "sol," and the addition of enzyme solution into "sol" initiates condensation reaction leading to "gel," where enzymes are encapsulated into silicate matrices. In this approach, various pores and channels are formed in the final silicate matrices, ranging from 0.1 to 500 nm in size. A careful optimization process is required in order to prevent the leaching of encapsulated enzymes. Once enzyme leaching is prevented, the sol–gel approach results in a fairly stable form of enzyme immobilization since the close fit of the enzyme molecule within the sol–gel pore likely prevents unfolding and denaturation of encapsulated enzymes [10]. However, due to the small pore size, the immobilized enzymes usually show lower activity than the free enzymes. Furthermore, the nonuniform pore sizes of most silica gel supports made processes less reproducible.

Each nanomaterial has unique advantages as well as disadvantages. Thus other important support composites were attracting more attention. Composites are engineered materials made from two or more constituents with significantly different physical or chemical properties from their components, which remain separate and distinct within the finished structure. A synergism results in material properties, which are unique prior to used constituents, could be presented. Among the composites, organic–inorganic hybrid nanobiocomposites have attracted much interest as a new class of materials that utilize the synergy of organic and inorganic components to obtain improved characteristics.

The benefits of using composites mainly include the following: (1) better mechanical properties: organic–inorganic hybrid materials can effectively eliminate the brittleness of pure inorganic materials and the swelling property of some pure polymers or hydrogels; (2) enhancement of the surface biocompatibility of polymer materials or inorganic supports by the addition of biomaterials; (3) the existing problem of aggregation of inorganic nanoparticles can be overcome by modifying these nanoparticles using polymers; (4) ease of chemical modification via reactive functional groups in organic materials: in hybrid nanobiocomposites, surface fuctionalization of nanoparticles allows their covalent attachment and self-assembly on surfaces that can be used for loading the desired biomolecules in a favorable microenvironment; (5) versatile enzyme immobilization methods: numerous enzymes have been stabilized by entrapment in a composite support; (6) ease of preparation in different configurations: for example, composite films for biosensors were fabricated by simple solvent evaporation.

For example, despite the many advantages of a silica sol–gel immobilization matrix, the brittleness of the silica sol–gel matrix is a major obstacle in their wide adoption as an immobilization matrix for biomolecules. In order to improve the performance of silica sol–gel hybrid materials, some polymers such as poly(ethylene oxide) (PEO), polyhydroxyl, hydrophobic poly(vinylpyridine), and poly(vinyl alcohol) (PVA) were hybridized into a silica sol–gel matrix. Miao and Tan reported on the first attempt to develop an amperometric H_2O_2 biosensor with horseradish peroxidase (HRP) immobilized by the sol–gel/chitosan–inorganic–organic hybrid film. It overcomes the shortcomings of a silica sol–gel matrix and the many amino groups present in chitosan provide a biocompatible environment for enzyme immobilization [16]. The carboxyl-containing nanofibers can be modified with chitosan or gelatin to build a dual-layer biomimetic surface. The abundant reactive groups on the backbone of chitosan or gelatin can provide sufficient bonding sites for enzyme immobilization. The tethering of chitosan or gelatin increases the activity retention of immobilized lipase, with little sacrifice of enzyme loading [17]. Immobilization of bioactive molecules onto surface-charged superparamagnetic nanoparticles (size ~25 nm) is of special interest, since the magnetic behavior of these bioconjugates may result in improved delivery and recovery of biomolecules. Besides this, the existing problem of aggregation and rapid biodegradation of Fe_3O_4 nanoparticles onto a given matrix containing biomolecules can perhaps be overcome by modifying these nanoparticles using chitosan by preparing a hybrid nanobiocomposite (see Section 8.5.3.1).

8.2.3 Methods of Enzyme Immobilization on Chitosan-Based Supports

Based on the characteristics of chitosan/chitin, methods of enzyme immobilization can be divided into six groups:

   I. Adsorption of the enzyme on the support: (I-i) physical adsorption; (I-ii) affinity by the metal ion; (I-iii) affinity by the dye; and (I-iv) affinity by the chitin-binding domain (ChBD).

   II. Chemical cross-linking by covalent binding: (II-i) in the presence of an enzyme solution; (II-ii) in the absence of an enzyme solution (the enzyme may be absorbed or entrapped); (II-iii) on the agent-activated support; (II-iv) cross-linking by covalent binding of the enzyme to an agent-activated support following cross-linking with other agents.

III. Entrapment: (III-i) entrapment of the enzyme within a polymer network; (III-ii) covering the surface of the enzyme with a film.

IV. Electrochemically conjugated protein.

V. Enzyme–chitosan conjugate.

Methods such as adsorption, entrapment, and cross-linking involve some immobilization processes described in Section 8.2.1. However, the operations in detail take on diversity due to special properties of chitosan/chitin. In addition, some peculiar enzyme immobilization methods (IV and V) are also presented here.

Immobilization of the enzyme on chitosan/chitin powder can be easily fulfilled by physical adsorption. Furthermore, chitosan has been widely used as a sorbent for transition metal ions and organic species because the amino ($-NH_2$) and hydroxyl ($-OH$) groups on chitosan chains can serve as the coordination and reaction sites. Thus chitosan particle-adsorbed metal ions or dye can be used as an affinity support for enzyme immobilization in chromatography or biosensors (see Section 8.3.4.3).

In addition, a protein engineered to carry affinity tags from heterologous sources is able to bind specifically to its unnatural cognate ligands. This approach has become widely acceptable for enzyme immobilization based on the following merits: (1) strong binding of enzymes to the support, (2) proper exposure of the enzyme active site, (3) mild conditions for immobilization, and (4) the lack of substrate diffusion barriers. Chao et al. have explored the utilization of the ChBD as an affinity tag to retain D-hydantoinase or *Z. mobilis levansucrae* (encoded by *levU*) on chitin beads. ChBD of chitinase A1 from *Bacillus circulans* WL-12 comprises 45 amino acids and exhibits remarkably high specificity to chitin. To investigate the feasibility of exploiting ChBD as affinity tags to confine enzymes of interest on chitin, ChBD fused to the C-terminus of the gene encoding enzyme was constructed. After direct absorption of the protein mixture from *Escherichia coli* onto chitin beads, the enzyme tagged with ChBD was found to specifically attach to the affinity matrix. Subsequent analysis indicated that the linkage between the enzyme and chitin beads was substantially stable. In comparison with its unbound counterpart, D-hydantoinase immobilized in this way exhibits higher tolerance to heat and can be reused 15 times to achieve conversion yields exceeding 90% [18]. With 20% sucrose, the production of levan was enhanced by 60% to reach 83 g/L using the immobilized levansucrase as compared with that by the free counterpart [19]. As illustrated in the above studies, this approach is marked by high stability as well as facile operation and provides a promising way for enzyme immobilization.

Protocols for covalent enzyme immobilization often begin with a surface modification or activation step. Chitosan has reactive amino and hydroxyl groups that, after further chemical modifications, can make covalent bonds with reactive groups of the enzyme. Mostly, immobilization of enzymes on such prepared gels does not require chemical activation, as the cross-linker, normally a bifunctional agent, fulfills two functions: cross-linking and activation. GA, as the most commonly used cross-linking agent, was applied for activating the $-NH_2$ group. Other bifunctional agents, such as carbodiimide and epoxide reactants (glycidol (Gly) and epichlorohydrin (ECO)), were used to activate $-OH$ groups.

Spagna et al. presented various enzyme immobilization trials by covalent binding. α-L-Arabinofuranosidase (Ara) from *Aspergillus niger* was immobilized on chitin or chitosan (particle sizes between 75 and 125 μm) by means of the activation of the supports with

GA before bringing them into contact with the enzyme (functionalization, the method of II-iii) or, alternatively, the adsorption of the enzyme on chitosan and its cross-linking, always with GA, which is added either in the absence (cross-linking, the method of II-i) or in the presence (conjugation, the method of II-i) of the enzyme solution. Conjugation proved to be a better method as it ensured good biocatalyst activity and stability, better than that reported for the free enzyme. It may be assumed in this case that the enzyme was at least partially cross-linked already in the solution itself before forming any bonds with the support, thus being able to benefit from the protective effects previously described for the free enzyme [20]. However, functionalization, the method of II-iii, was most used in enzyme immobilization by covalent binding (see Section 8.3.4.1).

An MPA mode would occur when the enzyme is immobilized via epoxy activation of the support. Chitosan hydroxyl groups can be activated by using epoxide reactants such as Gly and ECO, for instance, followed by oxidation with sodium periodate to produce reactive aldehyde-glyoxyl groups. These aldehyde groups are less reactive than the ones from GA. While the latter can immobilize the enzyme after linking with only one amine group, the former will only be able to keep the enzyme linked if at least two bonds are formed. Thus the higher the concentration of amine groups in the enzyme and of glyoxyl groups in the support, more bonds can occur [21]. The method of immobilization involving the amino and hydroxyl groups of chitosan is named "binary immobilization," which is also MPA [22] (see Section 8.3.4.2). In addition, changing the gel structure and immobilization conditions led to significant improvement in the covalent MPA of chymotrypsin on chitosan [23]. Adequate geometrical congruence between the enzyme and the support is very important: the greater the enzyme–support congruence, the higher the possibility of achieving an intense MPA. Therefore, the internal area of the support is one important variable to obtain active and stable enzyme derivatives. The use of sodium alginate, gelatin, or κ-carrageenan, activation with GA, Gly, or ECO, and the addition of microorganisms followed by cellular lysis allowed modification of the chitosan gel structure.

Entrapment usually refers to an immobilization enzyme within a polymer network (II-i). Covering the surface of the enzyme with a film can also be considered as a kind of entrapment. For example, Miao and Tan developed a silica sol–gel/organic hybrid material for the fabrication of an amperometric H_2O_2 biosensor by using TMOS as the silylating agent. The homogeneous stock sol–gel/chitosan solution was pipetted to cover the HRP-modified carbon paste electrode (CPE) and finally it was dried for ca. 10 min at room temperature. The developed HRP electrode exhibits high sensitivity and fast response. It also shows very good reproducibility and stability [16].

Chitosan films can be activated for protein assembly by anodic oxidation of the underlying electrode in the presence of NaCl (method IV, electrochemically conjugate protein) [24]. Although the mechanism of anodic activation of chitosan has not been definitively established, the working hypothesis is that a reactive mediator (possibly hypochlorite OCl-) is electrochemically generated at the anode, and this mediator reacts with the chitosan film to generate reactive substituents (possibly aldehydes) along chitosan's backbone. The electrodeposited and electroactivated chitosan films react with proteins to assemble them with spatial selectivity and quantitative control. The evidence presented indicates that the assembled proteins retain their native structure and biological functions. This method for on-demand biofunctionalization of individual electrode addresses should offer a generic approach to assemble proteins for multiplexed analysis.

Polymer conjugation has been reported to reduce the autolysis of proteolytic enzymes and to allow enzymes to dissolve in nonaqueous solvents. Advantages of these biocatalytic composites are that the matrix can be selected to enhance performance and the composites can be cast or formed into various shapes and sizes including foams and monoliths. Two kinds of enzyme–chitosan conjugates that can further form a smart gel or immobilize on the support were introduced in this chapter (see Section 8.4.3).

8.2.4 Preparation Methods of Chitosan-Based Supports

Preparation methods of chitosan gel, chitosan modifications and chitosan composites for enzyme immobilization are shown in Figure 8.3.

The formation of chitosan gel is mainly based on three principles:

1. Change in pH. It is easy to form an insoluble network in solution above pH 6.3 because chitosan containing abundant amino groups with pK_a 6.3 is soluble in a slightly acidic solution. This group includes the solvent evaporation method, the phase-inversion technique, the electrodeposition method, and the electrospinning technique.

2. Electrostatic interaction. Chitosan can form a gel by ionotropic gelation with certain anionic counterions, such as tripolyphosphates (TPPs) or the oppositely charged surfactant SDS.

3. Cross-linking. Freezing–thawing treatment, as a physical cross-linking, leads to a gel-like polymer system. Chemical cross-linking methods resulting in gel are often used by a mixture of an acidic chitosan solution with cross-linking agents. Mostly, the immobilization of enzymes on such prepared gels does not require chemical activation, as the cross-linker, normally a bifunctional agent, fulfills two functions: cross-linking and activation. Thus, the processes by which chitosan gels are further activated by bifunctional agents are also discussed in this group.

Chitosan-based composites, especially chitosan-inorganic nanocomposites, have been attracting extensive attention and are widely used in enzyme-membrane reactors and biosensors. The involved inorganic materials include metal and metal oxide nanoparticles, silica gels, CNTs, clay, and inorganic salt. The above methods can also be applied to fabricate chitosan composites. For instance, chitosan, as a polyelectrolyte, is able to form polyelectrolyte complexes (PECs). Two different types of complexes are considered here: the

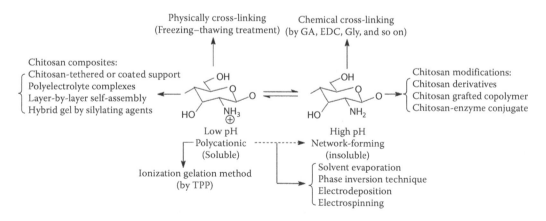

FIGURE 8.3
Preparation methods of chitosan-based supports.

complex network prepared by a mixture of polycation and polyanion and the layer-by-layer (LBL) self-assembly system formed by sequential deposition of interactive polymers from their solutions. Self-assembly of matter is of fundamental importance in different fields, including life sciences. It is widely used to describe the phenomenon of self-organization. LBL self-assembly is also used in the chitosan organic–inorganic hybrid system, such as self-assembly of chitosan and nano-Au (see Section 8.5.4.3). In addition, based on the above sol–gel approach from ref. [15], chitosan hybrid gelling is developed by the use of organosilane agents that are often regarded simply as cross-linkers.

It is an easy method to directly tether or coat natural macromolecules on the surface of the support to form a biomimetic layer for enzyme immobilization. It is considered as an effective method to increase the biocompatibility of synthesis polymers or inorganic supports, by introducing a biofriendly interface on the support surface for enzyme immobilization through surface modification technologies, which may reduce some nonbiospecific enzyme–support interactions, create a specific microenvironment for the enzyme, and benefit the enzyme activity. In comparison with the inorganic supports, the synthesis polymers are easier to entrust functional groups for chemical reactions. In fact, this method has been widely used in tissue engineering very recently.

Moreover, chemical modification methods for chitosan supports have been used to improve stability, mechanical strength, and modification of different functional groups that may be superior for enzyme immobilization. For example, hydrophobic modification of the hydrophilic chitosan backbone allows for the formation of micellar structures that have been shown to be attractive for enzyme encapsulation, often increasing thermal tolerance, chemical tolerance, and long-term stability. Furthermore, one of the ways to improve these properties is the grafting of monomers onto the matrix. The properties of the resulting graft copolymers are broadly controlled by the characteristics of the side chains, including molecular structure, length, and number. To date, a number of research works have been published that aim to study the effects of these variables on the grafting parameters and the properties of grafted chitosan polymers. In addition, two kinds of enzyme–chitosan conjugates that can further form gel or immobilize on the support were approximately considered as one of the chitosan modifications and are also described in this chapter (see Section 8.4.3).

8.3 Chitosan Gel for Enzyme Immobilization

Commonly, methods of chitosan gel preparation can be divided into four groups: the solvent evaporation method, the neutralization method, the chemical cross-linking method, and the ionotropic gelation method [2]. In this section, the phase-inversion technique is described by combining the neutralization method and solidification by a nonsolvent such as ethanol. In addition, several new methods are also briefly presented. For example, chitosan cryogels based on physical cross-linking were obtained by freezing–thawing repeated treatments. Stable chitosan films were fabricated via the electrodeposition method. Nanofibers were produced through the electrospinning technique.

8.3.1 Solvent Evaporation

The method is mainly used for the preparation of membranes and films, the latter being especially useful in preparing minute enzymatically active surfaces deposited on the tips of electrodes. For example, the chitosan-modified electrode was fabricated by casting the chitosan solution on the surface of a glassy carbon electrode (GCE) and evaporating the solvent under room temperature in air. A cross-linking agent may also be mixed with the initial chitosan solution before drying. For composites of chitosan and polymer or inorganic materials, such as PECs, metal oxide–chitosan nanocomposite, chitosan–silica hybrid material, and so on, this technique involves depositing/casting a complex fluid on a substrate by dip, spin coating, or spray drying, followed by allowing the film to evaporate and form self-assembled structures. Sometimes, repeated cross-linking is necessary. Enzymes may be immobilized on such prepared membranes by adsorption or entrapment or chemical cross-linking.

8.3.1.1 Spin Coating

Spin coating is a procedure used to apply uniform thin films to flat substrates. In short, an excess amount of a solution is placed on the substrate, which is then rotated at high speed in order to spread the fluid by centrifugal force. A machine used for spin coating is called a spin coater, or simply a spinner. Azmi et al. described an optical biosensor based on glutamate dehydrogenase (GLDH) immobilized in a chitosan film for the determination of ammonium in water samples. The GLDH–chitosan mixture was deposited onto a glass slide. Then it was spun at 2000 rpm for 3 s. The biosensor was kept at 4°C for drying. The reproducibility of the biosensor was good [25].

8.3.1.2 Spray Drying

The spray drying technique is widely used in the food and pharmaceutical industries. The method is based on drying atomized droplets in a stream of hot air. González Siso et al. prepared microbeads by spray drying of a 0.3% chitosan solution with different concentrations of an enzyme and a reticulating agent (GA). The average size of the microbeads was 2.5–4 μm. Microencapsulation on chitosan beads has been shown to be an effective immobilization method for α-amylase and invertase and the observed differences in their behavior are explained mainly by the molecular weight of their substrates [26].

8.3.2 Phase-Inversion Technique

The phase-inversion technique can produce chitosan gel via precipitation under an alkali solution or an organic medium or their mixture solution. This method is exploited to produce chitosan precipitates, membranes, and fibers, but most importantly spherical beads of different sizes and porosities. However, these supports cannot endure low pH and their intensity is low; therefore, chemical cross-linking is often used. Enzyme immobilization is similar to the solvent evaporation method. It is a simple, easy, and inexpensive method for using the deposition of chitosan as an enzyme immobilization support.

8.3.2.1 Chitosan Powders

Briante et al. described a methodology to produce in high yield hydroxytyrosol from a commercially available oleuropein by using the immobilized recombinant β-glycosidase from the hyperthermophilic archaeon *Sulfolobus solfataricus* on a chitosan support. Chitosan precipitates were prepared by adding NaOH (1.5 M final concentration) into a low-molecular-weight chitosan acetic acid solution. Neutralized chitosan suspension was lyophilized overnight. Enzyme immobilization was carried out by absorption and subsequently cross-linking by GA [27]. Zhang et al. reported that a powdery carrier of chitosan was obtained by adding chitosan solution to 2 mol/L NaOH and subsequently cross-linking with GA. Laccase is immobilized in the GA-activated powdery carrier. Immobilized laccase could be used repeatedly, and its removal efficiency for 2,4-dichlorophenol (2,4-DCP) remained above 50% for up to six usages [28].

8.3.2.2 Spherical Beads

Juang et al. prepared highly swollen beads by spraying a chitosan acetic acid 0.1 L solution into 125 mL of deionized water containing 15 g NaOH and 25 ml of 95% ethanol through a nozzle (diameter 1.2 mm). The diameter of the wet beads was approximately 2.3 mm. The activities of both acid phosphatase and β-glucosidase immobilized onto GA-activated chitosan beads remained 76% and 94% of the original ones, respectively, up to 42 days [29].

Chitosan beads were also prepared by the emulsion method and used for the immobilization of ω-transaminase of *Vibrio fluvialis*. The water-in-oil emulsion was poured into a 12% NaOH solution with stirring and was left for 3 h to allow the formation of chitosan beads. The average sizes of the prepared wet and dried chitosan beads were 1 mm and 150 μm, respectively. The specific surface area and the average pore size of the dried chitosan beads were measured to be 90 m^2/g and 15 nm, respectively. Enzyme was immobilized in GA-activated chitosan beads. The yield of enzyme immobilization (54.3%) and its residual activity (17.8%) were higher than those obtained with other commercial beads (Eupergit®C and Tentagel SCOOSu) [30].

8.3.2.3 Nanoparticles

In recent years, chitosan nanoparticles have been synthesized through different approaches, such as the chemical coprecipitation process, sol–gel self-propagation and using a water-in-oil microemulsion. The use of water-in-oil microemulsion is a potentially very useful technique for the preparation of nanoparticles. The nanosized water droplets offer a unique microenvironment for the formation of highly monodispersed nanoparticles. The growth of particles is controlled by the size of the microemulsion droplets, particularly in anionic microemulsion systems; therefore, chitosan nanoparticles could be prepared by microemulsion. Commonly, hydrochloric acid (HCl) or acetic acid (HAc) was used to dissolve chitosan in the water phase, and NaOH or organic solution was used as precipitant.

Wu et al. prepared chitosan nanoparticles in a water-in-oil microemulsion by using 2% (wt) HAc and 30% (wt) tri-*n*-octylamine (TOA) as solvent and precipitant, respectively. It was found that particle diameters were about 7 nm and the particles formed ovoid-shaped aggregates. Using 0.05% HCl and 5.0 M NaOH as solvent and precipitant resulted in nanoparticles 10 nm in size that aggregated in the form of snowflakes. Enzyme immobilization was carried out by absorption and subsequently cross-linking by GA. These particles showed good loading ability for lipase immobilization and little loss of enzyme activity was observed. The stability of the catalyst was very good; only 9% of enzyme activity was lost after five cycles [31].

8.3.2.4 Chitosan Films

Zhang et al. reported that hemoglobin (Hb) can be effectively immobilized on chitosan films as mimetic peroxidase. The dried film obtained by solvent evaporation is further neutralized by 2.0 wt% NaOH aqueous solution. Hb is immobilized in GA-activated chitosan film. The enzymatic assay indicates that immobilized Hb showed a higher thermal stability than free Hb, and catalytic activity in organic solvents was also enhanced [32].

8.3.3 Ionization Gelation Method

Chitosan can form gel by ionotropic gelation with certain anionic counterions, such as polyphosphates. Sodium TPP is a multivalent anion that can cross-link by ionic interaction between positively charged amino ($-NH_3^+$) groups of chitosan and multivalent negatively charged TPP molecules in an acid medium. The method is utilized chiefly for the preparation of gel beads or nanoparticles, within which enzymes are usually entrapped. Chitosan complexation with anionic polyelectrolytes will be described in Section 8.5.3.

8.3.3.1 Chitosan Beads

Betigeri and Neau prepared immobilized lipase by entrapment in three polysaccharides. Chitosan beads are obtained by adding a mixture of acidic chitosan solution and lipase dropwise into a TPP solution, after which the characteristics of immobilized enzyme are compared with other hydrophilic polymers, including alginate beads prepared by ionic gelation using calcium chloride and agarose beads by adding the heated solution dropwise into chilled vegetable oil. Agarose beads exhibited undesirable swelling in the leaching and activity medium and the polymer was not used further. The fact that the lipase activity in chitosan beads is higher than that in alginate beads could be attributed to an alginate–enzyme interaction [33].

8.3.3.2 Micro/Nanoparticles

Micro- or nanochitosan can be obtained by a reversed process by comparing with the formation of chitosan beads discussed in ref. [33]. Fernandes et al. developed a novel biosensor based on laccase immobilized on microspheres of chitosan cross-linked with tripolyphosphate for rutin determination in pharmaceutical formulations by square wave voltammetry. Microspheres of chitosan were obtained by adding 2% (m/v) TPP solution into 1% (m/v) chitosan solution (1% acetic acid) under stirring and subsequently spray drying this mixture solution. The microspheres had an irregular shape and were 3.0–8.9 μm in diameter. This proposed bioelectrode exhibited high sensitivity, good reproducibility, low detection, rapid response and excellent long-term stability. The determination of rutin in three pharmaceutical formulations was successfully carried out without any separation step before the electrochemical measurement [34].

In order to investigate the characterization of chitosan nanoparticles prepared by the ionization gelation method, neutral proteinase and lipase were selected as model enzymes to assess its potential applicability for enzyme immobilization. Chitosan nanoparticles of mean particle size smaller than 100 nm were obtained by adding 0.75 mg/mL TPP to chitosan solution (20 mg of chitosan was dissolved in 40 mL of 2.0% (v/v) acetic acid). Enzyme could be immobilized on the surface of chitosan nanoparticles by adsorption. The thermal, operational, and storage stabilities of immobilized enzymes were improved after they were immobilized on chitosan nanoparticles. They could improve 13.17% of neutral proteinase or lipase activity than that of free neutral one [35,36].

Biró et al. prepared macro-, micro-, and nanosized chitosan particles suitable as immobilization carriers by precipitation, emulsion cross-linking, and ionic gelation methods, respectively. The ionotropic gelation method with two different gelation agents including sulfate and TPP was used for nanoparticle preparation. The activities of β-galactosidase covalently attached to GA-activated different sized particles were evaluated and compared. The highest activity was shown by the biocatalyst immobilized on nanoparticles obtained by means of the ionotropic gelation method with sodium sulfate as a gelation agent. β-Galactosidase fixed on macro- and microspheres exhibited excellent storage stability in aqueous solution, with no more than 5% loss of activity after 3 weeks of storage at 4°C and pH 7.0 [37].

8.3.4 Chemical Cross-Linking Method

As a cross-linking and surface-activating agent, mostly GA is used. This is due to its reliability and ease of use, but more importantly, due to the availability of amino groups for the reaction with GA, not only on enzymes but also on chitosan. Other difunctional agents include carbodiimide, epoxide reactants (Gly and ECO), tris(hydroxymethyl)phosphine $P(CH_2OH)_3$, and so on.

8.3.4.1 Chemical Cross-Linking by One Agent

8.3.4.1.1 GA as a Cross-Linking Agent

Probably the mildest and most straightforward route for functionalizing primary amine containing materials is reaction with an aldehyde to form the corresponding imine. The process is very simple and superior to that of other immobilization processes on synthetic supports. Cross-linking with dialdehyde such as glyoxal and GA is a key technique in chitosan chemistry, and leads to more stable chitosan derivatives as the amine groups in different chains link together via the diimine.

Cetinus et al. reported that chemically cross-linked chitosan beads were prepared by the addition of an acidic chitosan solution to a mixture of di-ion (diphosphate) and nontoxic dialdehyde (glyoxal) and then treating GA for stability in both alkaline and acidic media. As chitosan is soluble in acidic solutions, the continuous prolonged exposure of chitosan beads, made via counterion precipitation, may result in gel softening and bead disintegration. Moreover, Schiff base formed between chitosan and glyoxal is essentially reversible; long time operation under acidic conditions may lead to gradual leakage of glyoxal. GA irreversible cross-linking via Schiff base may lead to chitosan beads exhibiting high operational stability. The catalase (CAT) and pepsin immobilized in these chitosan beads exhibit improved resistance against thermal and pH denaturation [38,39]. As a result, GA was often used.

The various enzyme immobilization trials by chemical cross-linking have been introduced in Section 8.2.4 [20]. In particular, immobilization of enzyme on support materials activated with GA has received a great deal of attention. Juang et al. reported that the equilibrium amount of cross-linking can be described by a pseudo-second-order equation. The amounts of sorption of reactive dye RR222 and Cu (II), and the activities of immobilized enzymes (phosphatase and β-glucosidase), onto cross-linked beads were greatly affected by the degree of cross-linking [29]. Thus the control of support activation with GA is very important.

The precise control of the conditions during support activation with GA has enabled the modification of the amino groups of the matrix with one or two GA molecules. It has been reported that monomers and dimers of GA have different reactivities: while the dimer is able to rapidly immobilize proteins via a direct covalent attachment, the monomer yields a very low immobilization rate. The activity/stability properties of enzymes immobilized on GA-activated supports depend on the exact immobilization protocol employed. Moreover, due to the existence of one or two ionic groups (amino groups) under GA, which provide a certain anionic exchanger nature to the support, altering the ionic strength during immobilization can modify the immobilization rate and also the region of the protein that is implied in the interaction with the support. Since in this contribution immobilization was performed in neutral medium, the reaction should have involved the most reactive amino groups in the protein [40,41].

It was possible that enzyme conformation was not changed by covalent binding to GA-pretreated chitosan beads. Desai et al. reported that the Michaelis constant (K_m) and the maximum reaction velocity (V_{max}) of the free and immobilized porcine pancreatic lipase were almost the same, indicating no conformational change taking place during immobilization [42]. Moreover, the different structures of the lipases chosen for catalysis led to very different activity levels. Lipases from *Candida rugosa*, *Pseudomonas fluorescens*, and *C. antarctica* B were immobilized onto chitosan and GA-pretreated chitosan powders, the latter derivatives being the most active [41].

8.3.4.1.2 Carbodiimide as a Cross-Linking Agent

Carbodiimide is generally utilized as a carboxyl-activating agent for amide bonding with primary amines. It has been used in peptide synthesis, in cross-linking of proteins to nucleic acids, and in the preparation of immunoconjugates, for example.

Chiou and Wu have demonstrated that 1-ethyl-3-(3-dimethylaminopropyl)carbodiimide (EDC) can be used for activating the hydroxyl groups of chitosan. Chitosan beads were produced by the deposition of chitosan solution under a mixture of ethanol and NaOH solution. Figure 8.4 shows the hypothetical illustration of lipase immobilized on chitosan beads using the activation method with EDC in the pH range of 4.0–6.0. It was assumed that the hydroxyl groups of chitosan upon activation using EDC formed an unstable

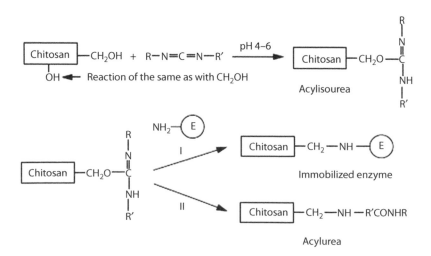

FIGURE 8.4
Scheme of lipase immobilized on chitosan by EDC activation. (From Chiou, S. H. and Wu, W. T. 2004. *Biomaterials* 25: 197–204. With permission.)

complex, acylisourea, which then complexed with the amino groups of the enzyme to form the immobilized enzyme (product I). On the other hand, it could be rearranged to form another product, acylurea (product II). The process appreciably increased the activity of lipase immobilized on wet chitosan beads [43].

8.3.4.1.3 Epoxide Reactants as a Cross-Linking Agent

Chitosan hydroxyl groups can also be activated by using epoxide reactants such as Gly and ECO. An MPA mode appeared when the enzyme was immobilized via epoxy activation of the support [21].

Spagna et al. studied the coimmobilization of two glycosidases, Ara and β-D-glucopyranosidase (βG), on chitosan or glyceryl chitosan (GCh), a derivative especially prepared by the reaction of chitosan with Gly. The glycosidases adsorbed on this latter support were then cross-linked with GA to prevent them from being released into the wine. Finally, the biocatalyst was reduced with sodium borohydride to increase its stability over time. GCh further increased the adsorption of Ara while allowing significant increases in activity. When cross-linking the enzymes adsorbed on GCh with GA, the activity of βG was not affected even though that of Ara was reduced [44].

Giordano and coworkers reported that trypsin was immobilized on chitosan gels coagulated with 0.1 or 1 M NaOH and activated with GA or Gly. Activation with Gly led to lower immobilization yields than the ones obtained with GA, but allowed obtaining the most stable derivative chitosan-glyoxyl (ChGly), which was 660-fold more stable than the soluble enzyme at 55°C and 70°C. The ChGly derivative also presented the highest stability during incubation at pH 11. Analyses of lysine residue contents in soluble and immobilized trypsin indicated the formation of multipoint bonds between the enzyme and the support for glyoxyl derivatives [45].

Supports activated with ECO displayed a higher degree of activation than the ones activated with Gly. However, chitosan-EDC was only 1.6-fold more thermally stable than the soluble enzyme CALB, which indicates that immobilization of CALB on chitosan-ECO is not the result of a multipoint covalent attachment. It was observed that chitosan activated by ECO lost a great amount of water, which may decrease the porous diameter of the support and increase its hydrophobicity. Then, despite the high aldehyde concentration, the enzyme would not reach most of these groups. Therefore, physical changes in the support surface may not favor immobilization of CALB [21].

8.3.4.1.4 Tris(Hydroxymethyl)Phosphine as Cross-Linking Agent

The most commonly used coupling reagent is GA, although its chemistry creates some inherent difficulties because of the continuing polymerization of GA upon storage and the reversibility of the Schiff base linkage. To overcome these difficulties of coupling with GA, Cochrane et al. reported that a coupling agent, $P(CH_2OH)_3$, which contains $>P-CH_2-OH$ groups, is well known to undergo Mannich-type condensation reactions at room temperature with N–H group-containing compounds. The potential advantages of using $P(CH_2OH)_3$ as a coupling agent include an increase in the number of immobilizing groups, together with an improved hydrolytic stability of the resulting $P-CH_2-N$-enzyme linkages. The use of $P(CH_2OH)_3$ as a coupling reagent for the immobilization of alcohol dehydrogenase onto chitosan films and for the attachment of the chitosan film to a glass support resulted in enzyme activities far above those obtained by adsorption of enzyme and greater than those observed when using the more conventional GA-coupling protocol [46].

8.3.4.2 Chemical Cross-Linking by Multiagents

The method of immobilization involving the amino and hydroxyl groups of chitosan is named "binary immobilization" [22]. The enzyme immobilization via chemical cross-linking of multiagents generally emerges MPA.

8.3.4.2.1 Carbodiimide and Glutaraldehyde

Hung et al. reported that lipase was immobilized on chitosan beads by a binary method in which lipase was first linked to the hydroxyl groups of chitosan activated with EDC followed by cross-linking more lipase to the amino group of chitosan using GA. The binary immobilization method yielded the highest protein loading and activity in comparison with the immobilized lipase prepared by activation with EDC and by cross-linking with GA. Broader pH tolerance and higher heat stability could be achieved by this method. Immobilized lipase retained 74% residual activity after ten hydrolysis cycles and 67% after 7 days of storage [47].

de Oliveira and Vieira describe the procedures and performance of four different methods (physical adsorption, EDC, GA, and EDC-GA) for gilo (as a source of peroxidase) crude extract immobilization on a chitosan biopolymer-CPE. The highest biosensor performance was obtained after the immobilization of peroxidase in chitosan by the activation of hydroxyl groups with EDC and cross-linking with GA, which was incorporated in a CPE. The lifetime of this biosensor was 6 months (at least 300 determinations) [48].

8.3.4.2.2 Glutaraldehyde and Epichlorohydrin

de Oliveira et al. also developed a new biosensor for gilo immobilization on a chitosan biopolymer that was chemically cross-linked with ECO and GA. Figure 8.5 shows a suggestion for the immobilization of peroxidase on (a) chitosan by cross-linking with GA and ECO.

The bifunctional GA reacts with the amine groups of chitosan to form Schiff bases, and with the addition of the ECO, through the opening of the epoxide ring links are formed with carbon atoms and the chloride group is discharged. The chemical cross-linking of chitosan with GA-ECO and peroxidase immobilization shows strong interactions, long-term stability, thermostability, and high sensitivity compared with other recently constructed biosensors. The lifetime of this biosensor was 8 months (at least 500 determinations) [49].

8.3.4.2.3 Glycidol and Glutaraldehyde

The influence of activation agents (Gly, GA, and ECO) and immobilization time (5, 24, and 72 h) on hydrolytic activity, thermal and alkaline stabilities of CALB was evaluated by Rodrigues et al. The best derivative, 58-fold more stable than the soluble enzyme, was obtained when CALB was immobilized on chitosan activated in two steps, using Gly and GA, in 72 h immobilization time. The stabilization degree of the derivative increased with the immobilization time, an indication that a multipoint covalent attachment between the enzyme and the support had really occurred. However, the longer the immobilization time, the lower the derivative activity. Therefore, the immobilization time that should be chosen to produce the derivative is a trade-off between these two parameters [21].

8.3.4.3 Cross-Linking Chitosan as Affinity Support

8.3.4.3.1 Metal Affinity Support

Immobilized metal affinity chromatography (IMAC) has been developed as a popular chromatographic tool for the purification of enzymes and proteins. Immobilized metal

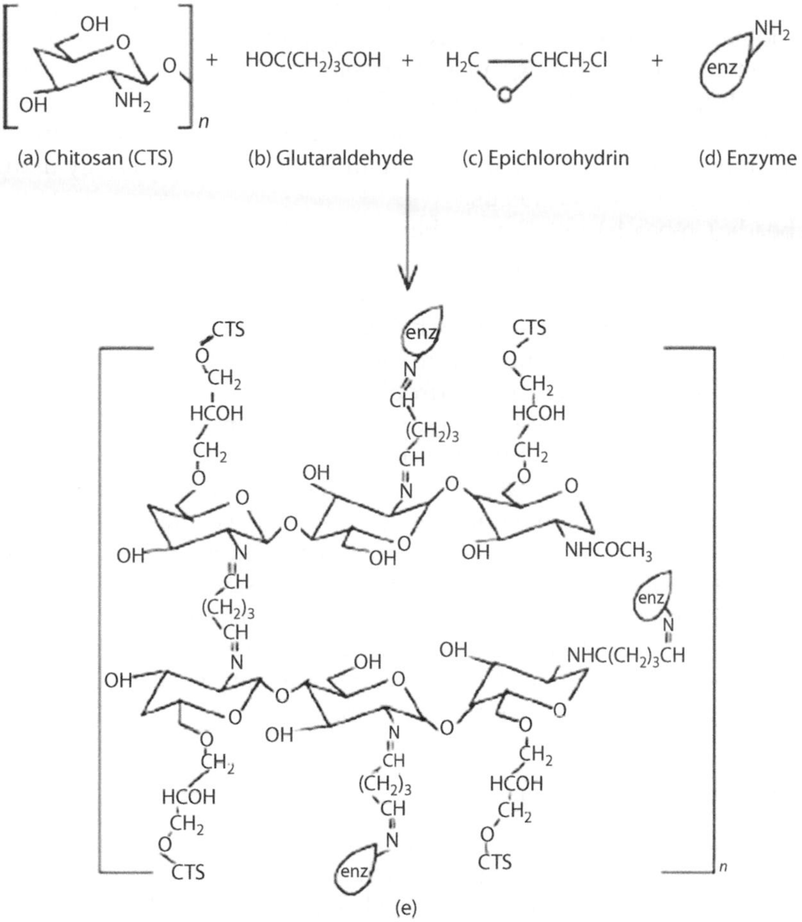

FIGURE 8.5
Reaction between chitosan, ECO, GA, and peroxidase enzyme. (From de Oliveira, I. R. W. Z., Fernandes, S. C., and Vieira, I. C. 2006. *J Pharm Biome Anal* 41: 366–372. With permission.)

affinity adsorbents provide moderate affinity to macromolecules by covalently coupling chelating compounds on solid supports to entrap metal ions. Chitosan has been described as a suitable biopolymer for the collection of metal ions since the amino groups and hydroxyl groups on the chitosan chain can act as chelation sites for metal ions.

Çetinus et al. first prepared Cu^{2+}-adsorbed GA-pretreated cross-linked chitosan beads (Cu-Ch) and then performed CAT immobilization onto this matrix. The immobilized protein amount and the maximum reaction velocity for Cu-Ch-CAT were higher than that for Ch-CAT. In both immobilization situations, although activities of immobilized CAT were lower than that of free CAT, Cu-Ch-CAT showed a high temperature stability, operational stability, and storage stability. In addition, these copper-adsorbed chitosan beads can be used as chromatographic column resin for protein purification in IMAC [50].

8.3.4.3.2 Dye Affinity Support

Dye-ligands have been considered as one of the important alternatives to natural counterparts for specific affinity chromatography. They are commercially available, inexpensive, and can easily be immobilized, especially on matrices bearing hydroxyl groups. Dye-ligands are able to bind most types of proteins, especially enzymes, in a remarkably specific manner. The interaction between the dye-ligand and proteins can be by a complex combination of electrostatic, hydrophobic, and hydrogen bonding. Selection of the supporting matrix is the first important consideration in dye-affinity systems. Chitosan's structure possesses a large number of reactive groups (hydroxyl and amino) that can be readily modified using different ligands to meet various needs.

Chitosan beads (Ch-beads) and cibacron blue F3GA(CB)-attached chitosan beads (CB-Ch-beads) were prepared by Çetinus et al. CAT was immobilized onto these beads. The CAT adsorption capacity of Ch-beads is higher than that of CB-Ch-beads, but CB-Ch-CAT showed better activity according to the Ch-CAT. Because CB molecules on the CB-Ch-beads are negatively charged, the dominant force contributing to dye and protein interactions is electrostatic rather than hydrophobic [51].

Wei et al. reported a film-forming solution for the efficient immobilization of enzymes on solid substrates. The solution consisted of a biopolymer, chitosan (CHIT), which was chemically modified with a permeability-controlling agent, Acetyl Yellow 9 (AY9), using GA as a molecular tether. A model enzyme, glucose oxidase (GOx), was mixed with the CHIT-GDI-AY9 solution and cast on the surface of platinum electrodes to form robust CHIT-GDI-AY9-GOx films for glucose biosensing. Chitosan chains were modified with anionic AY9 dye in order to introduce a perm-selectivity against anions. A relatively low sensing potential, in conjunction with the film's permeability controlling agent, allowed for interference-free determination of the enzyme's substrate, such as ascorbate and urate, which are commonly present in physiological samples [52].

8.3.5 Freezing–Thawing Treatment

When gelification is performed by freezing–thawing repeated cycles, the resultant gel-like polymer systems are called cryogels, which is a process of noncovalently physically cross-linking different from chemical hydrogels formed by covalent bonds. The porous structure of cryogels, in combination with their chemical and mechanical stability, makes them attractive matrices for immobilization of cells and enzymes. These materials were often used in porous scaffold production to immobilize cell cultures or as tissue regeneration templates. Scarce studies have reported the use of them as catalytic supports.

Knowledge of thermal and surface properties of the membrane is of importance for chitosan-based enzyme support systems. It was demonstrated by Orrego et al. that the above properties of dried cryogel chitosan membranes can be controlled by six freezing and thawing (F/T) treatments, as well as by crown ether or GA activation or cross-linking. The combined F/T and cross-linking technique increases the thermal stability of chitosan. It seems that freezing and thawing (F/T) treatment of membranes has a superior effect on the biopolymer crystallinity when compared with cross-linking [53,54]. In Table 8.1, the authors have made a comparison between the activities of *C. rugosa* lipase immobilized on chitosan membranes used in this work and the same information published for the same lipase on similar supports for use as catalysts in nonaqueous media [56].

8.3.6 Electrodeposition Method

Chitosan's pH-responsive properties allow it to be directed to assemble (i.e., to electrodeposit) in response to locally applied electrical stimuli. Chitosan can be electrodeposited

TABLE 8.1

Catalytic System Activities for *C. rugosa* Lipase on Chitosan in Nonaqueous Media

References	Supports	Activity (mM min⁻¹ g Protein⁻¹)
This work[a]	QSR	0.88
This work[a]	QGAR	2.21
This work[a]	QCER	1.78
Magnin, Dumitriu, Magny, and Chornet (2001)[b]	Chitosan/xanthan	0.0008
Chen and Lin (2003)[c]	Chitosan beads	0.0033–0.0167

Source: Orrego, C. E., et al. 2010. *Carbohydr Polym* 79: 9–16. With permission.

Note: Cryogel chitosan membranes (QS), Lipase immobilized on QS (QSR), GA cross-linked QS (QGAR), and CE cross-linked QS (QCER).

[a] This work: 40°C, *n*-butanol 0.1 M, and oleic acid 0.1 M/iso-octane.
[b] Magnin et al.: 37°C, olive oil hydrolysis/iso-octane [55].
[c] Chen and Lin: 35°C, ethanol 0.25 M, and butyric acid 0.3 M/*n*-hexane [54].

at a cathode surface by the mechanism illustrated in Figure 8.6 [57, 58]. When the applied voltage is sufficient for protons to be reduced at the cathode surface, a localized pH gradient is generated. If this localized gradient is created in the presence of chitosan (i.e., if the electrodes are immersed and biased in a slightly acidic chitosan solution), then chitosan chains that experience the high localized pH at the cathode surface can deposit as a thin film. This directed assembly can be controlled spatially and temporally. Once deposited and rinsed, the chitosan film is stable on the electrode in the absence of an applied potential provided the pH is retained above about 6.3. Until now, there are no reports of the nano- and microscale morphologies of the electrodeposited chitosan [58].

Furthermore, chitosan deposition can be used to mediate the assembly of additional components (e.g., nanoparticles and enzymes). Proteins can be enzymatically assembled onto the stimuli-responsive backbone (Section 8.2.3, IV method: electrochemically conjugate protein), whereas nucleic acids can be tethered to electrodeposited films to serve as sites for self-assembly. For example, chitosan-coated wires are an interesting platform that can be viewed as either conducting fibers or functionalized wires. As illustrated in

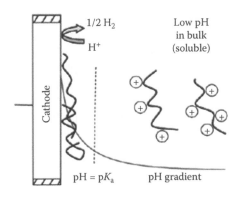

FIGURE 8.6
Mechanism for chitosan's directed assembly by electrodeposition. (From Yi, H. et al. 2005. *Biomacromolecules* 6: 2881–2894. With permission.)

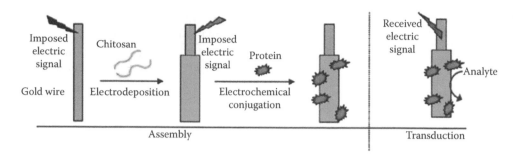

FIGURE 8.7

Gold wires are biofunctionalized using cathodic signals to electrodeposit chitosan and anodic signals to activate the chitosan for protein assembly. (From Meyer, W. et al. 2009. *Biomacromolecules* 10: 858–864. With permission.)

Figure 8.7, Meyer et al. use chitosan to serve as the interface between the protein-based recognition element and a metal wire. Importantly, chitosan allows proteins to be assembled in response to imposed electrical signals without the need for reactive reagents or harsh conditions. Thus, biofunctionalization is simple, safe, and rapid. Further, the chitosan coating is permeable to small molecules and allows the detection of electrochemically active compounds that are either present in the solution or generated during the biological recognition event. Thus, chitosan-coated electrodes can transduce chemical and biological information into convenient electrical signals [59]. Yi et al. shows a sequence of steps in which chitosan is first electrodeposited onto the patterned surface of our "chip," the deposited chitosan is next activated by GA, and then an amine-terminated single-stranded DNA probe (20 bases) is conjugated onto the activated chitosan film. This chitosan-bound probe DNA can hybridize with a fluorescently labeled target nucleic acid that has a complementary sequence [60].

8.3.7 Electrospinning Method

Electrospinning is a progressive method that produces fibers ranging from the submicron level to several nanometers in diameter in a high-voltage electrostatic field. As the electric field surpasses a threshold value where the electrostatic repulsion force of surface charges overcome surface tension, the charged fluid jet is ejected from the tip of the Taylor cone and the bending jet produces highly stretched polymeric fiber with simultaneous rapid evaporation of the solvent. Important parameters in electrospinning are not only polymer and solution properties such as molecular weight, viscosity, conductivity, and surface tension, but also electrospinning conditions such as applied electric voltage, tip-to-collector distance, feeding rate, and so on [61]. Nowadays, chitosan nanofibers can be promising materials for many biomedical applications such as tissue templates, medical prostheses, artificial organ, wound dressing, drug delivery, and pharmaceutical composition [62].

The electrospinning process was employed by Xu and coworkers to prepare a stabilized chitosan nanofibrous membrane as a support for enzyme immobilization. Figure 8.8 shows a schematic representation of lipase immobilization on chitosan nanofibers. A chitosan nanofibrous membrane was directly fabricated from a mixture solution of chitosan and PVA and then treated with an NaOH solution in order to remove PVA and stabilize the morphologies of the chitosan nanofibrous membrane in aqueous media. Lipase from *C. rugosa* was chosen as a model enzyme and immobilized on the prepared nanofibrous

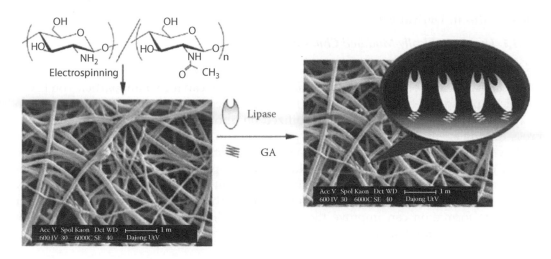

FIGURE 8.8
Schematic representation of lipase immobilization on the chitosan nanofibrous electrospun membrane. (From Huang, X. J., Ge, D., and Xu, Z. K. 2007. *Eur Polym J* 43: 3710–3718. With permission.)

membrane by GA. This chitosan nanofibrous membrane was used as a support for lipase immobilization with the advantages of high enzyme loading up to 63.6 mg/g and activity retention of 49.8%. The stabilities of the immobilized lipase toward pH, temperature, reuse, and storage were also enhanced [63,64].

8.4 Chitosan Modifications for Enzyme Immobilization

In this section, chitosan modifications for enzyme immobilization broadly include chitosan derivatives and chemical-grafted chitosan copolymer. An ideal support for enzyme immobilization should be chosen in order to achieve essential properties such as chemical stability, hydrophilicity, rigidity, mechanical stability, larger surface area, resistance to microbial attack, and so on. Without disturbing the degree of polymerizationof chitosan, one can chemically modify this acquiescent polymer since it provides functional groups such as primary amine and primary as well as secondary hydroxyl groups in its monomers. Furthermore, one way of improving these properties is by grafting monomers onto the matrix.

There are a number of reasons for coupling polymers with enzymes. Polymer conjugation has been reported to reduce the autolysis of proteolytic enzymes and to allow enzymes to dissolve in nonaqueous solvents. "Smart" biocatalysts have been prepared by conjugating enzymes to stimuli-responsive polymers that respond to changes in pH, ionic strength, temperature, redox potential, and light. Moreover, there are numerous examples in which the enzymes bound to sugars or sugar-based polymers are stabilized. Although the stabilization mechanism is not understood, it may be due to a reduction of autolysis (for proteases), MPA that may limit enzyme distortions, or microenvironmental effects.

8.4.1 Chitosan Derivatives

8.4.1.1 Hydrophobically Modified Chitosan

8.4.1.1.1 Modified by Linolenic Acid

Chitosan (CS) was modified by linolenic acid (LA), which can form nanoparticles on LACS in pH 7.4 phosphate-buffered saline buffer after sonication and can also be used as an enzyme carrier. Trypsin could be immobilized on linolenic acid chitosan using GA as a cross-linking agent. The immobilized trypsin at certain GA concentrations (from 0.03% to 0.07% v/v) can form nanoparticles after sonication, which still have catalytic activities. The kinetic constant (K_m) of trypsin immobilized on nanoparticles (71.9 mg/mL) was higher than that of pure trypsin (50.2 mg/mL), indicating that the immobilized process slightly decreased the affinity of trypsin on nanoparticles to the substrate (casein). On the other hand, this formation can improve the thermal stability and optimum temperature of trypsin, which makes it more attractive in the application aspect [65].

8.4.1.1.2 Modified by LA

Modified by aldehydes with long alkyl chain lengths. Chitosan also can be easily hydrophobically modified by reductive amination using aldehydes with long alkyl chain lengths (butanal, hexanal, octanal, or decanal). Although chitosan modified with small alkyl chains (i.e., <4 carbon chain length) is soluble in dilute aqueous acetic acid, the introduction of longer chain side groups renders the modified polymer relatively increasingly less soluble in dilute acidic aqueous solution.

Klotzbach et al. examines how hydrophobic modification of both Nafion and chitosan alters the selectivity, ion-exchange capacity, morphology, and mass transport of redox species through the membrane. It was shown that hydrophobically modified micellar polymers alter the transport properties of redox species to the electrode surface as a function of the size and charge of the redox species. GOx was immobilized within the hydrophobically modified chitosan. It was shown that the increase in hydrophobicity increases the enzyme activity, resulting in a more optimal membrane for enzyme immobilization [66].

As in the above descriptions, over the last decade, researchers have employed reductive amination to hydrophobically modify chitosan to induce a micellar structure. However, commercial sources of chitosan vary in their degree of deacetylation and there remains a paucity of information regarding how this can impact the modified polymer's functionality for enzyme immobilization. Sjoholm et al. evaluate the effect that the degree of deacetylation has on the hydrophobic modification of medium-molecular-weight chitosan via reductive amination with long-chain aldehydes (butyraldehyde) and the resulting changes in enzyme activity after the immobilization of GOx in the micellar polymeric structure. The chitosan was deacetylated to differing degrees via autoclaving in 40–45% NaOH solutions. The results suggest that a high degree of deacetylation provides optimal enzyme immobilization properties (i.e., high activity), but that the deacetylation method begins to significantly decrease the polymer molecular weight after a 20 min autoclave treatment, which negatively affects immobilized enzyme activity [67].

8.4.1.2 2-diethylaminochloroethane (DE)-Chitosan

α-L-Rhamnopyranosidase (Rha; EC 3.2.1.40) is an enzyme of considerable importance to food technology in increasing the aroma of wines, musts, fruit juices, and other beverages. Chitosan only adsorbs the Rha if activated with GA; nevertheless, the enzyme immobilized in this manner has almost no activities. The functionalization of chitosan with DE hydrochloride allows good adsorption and activity retention. Spagna et al. reported that the immobilization of Rha on supports chitin, chitosan and derivatized chitosan and DE-chitosan contained in a commercial preparation is used in the winemaking industry. In particular on DE-chitosan, the Rha was adsorbed and cross-linked with various bifunctional agents (GA, diepoxyoctane, suberimidate, and EDC), whose best results (immobilization yields and activity) were obtained with EDC that allowed a reduction in the involvement of the enzyme amine groups that are probably important in the catalytic mechanism. In addition, the use of rhamnose and a succinimide (NHS) during cross-linking enhanced the action of the EDC and so increased the immobilization yield and activity. This biocatalyst allowed an increase in the aroma in a model wine solution containing glycosidic precursors with a marked reduction in specificity toward tertiary monoterpenols as compared with the free enzyme. The results obtained seem to indicate that the amino group plays an essential role in the catalysis of Rha from *A. niger* [68].

8.4.1.3 Amino Acid-Modified Chitosan

Amino acids, the monomeric units of proteins and bio-origin materials, are chiral molecules with a relatively low molecular weight and have various properties due to their various side chains (acidic, basic, hydrophobic, etc.). They have also been used as pseudobiospecific affinity ligands for proteins. Therefore, chitosan beads with various properties could be easily prepared by introducing amino acids into their polymer backbone.

Yi et al. consider that amino acids are suitable materials for the preparation of modified chitosan beads with increased lipase-compatibility. Besides, the preparation process is simple and economical, and some amino acids are expected to improve the catalytic performances of the immobilized lipases due to the increased compatibility with the immobilized lipase. Therefore, it is considered that the development of amino acid-modified chitosan beads might be valuable for industrial applications of lipase. Various amino acids (Gly, Glu, Lys, Leu, Ala, Phe, Ser, Tyr)-modified chitosan beads (CBs) for immobilization of lipases from *C. rugosa* were prepared by activation of a chitosan backbone with ECO followed by amino acid coupling. The immobilized lipase on unmodified chitosan beads showed the highest immobilization yield (92.7%), but its activity was relatively low (10.4%). However, in spite of low immobilization yields (15–50%), the immobilized lipases on the amino acid-modified chitosan beads showed activities higher than that of unmodified chitosan beads, especially on Ala- or Leu-modified chitosan beads with 49% activity for Ala-CB and 51% for Leu-CB. Moreover, the immobilized lipases on amino acid-modified chitosan beads showed good thermal stability, storage stability, and reusability and, therefore, are suitable for industrial application [69].

Xiao et al. reported the synthesis and properties of a novel cross-linked chitosan resin modified by L-lysine (LMCCR). It is known that L-lysine is a natural alkaline amino acid and owns three reactive groups (a-carboxyl group, a-amino group, and e-amino group), making the chemical modification possible. In order to synthesize the novel resin, an acylation reaction between a-carboxyl group in L-lysine and primary amino group in chitosan has to be conducted besides a cross-linking reaction between GA and chitosan. At the same time, N, N-dicyclohexylcarbodiimide, an efficient peptide coupling reagent, is used to induce the acylation reaction. Micrographs and SEM images show that LMCCR is spherical in shape with macroporous structure. Due to its cross-linked structure and side chains, LMCCR is amorphous but more rigid and stable, and no longer dissolved in acidic media. LMCCR also exhibits considerable adsorption performances for various substances such as acetic acid, alanine, bovine serum albumin (BSA), and Zn^{2+}. LMCCR is proved to show preferable applications in enzyme immobilization, while the activity recovery and the half-life of the immobilized GOx with LMCCR as a solid support are 42.68% and 96 days [70].

8.4.1.4 Succinyl Anhydride-Modified Chitosan as pH-Sensitive Support

The drawbacks with using the insoluble chitosan in bioconversions are slow binding/catalysis due to diffusion-controlled mass transfer and steric hindrance in an already biphasic system involving water-insoluble substrates, and low geometrical congruence with protein surfaces. To overcome these problems, an attempt has been made at immobilization of the biocatalysts to reversibly soluble polymeric carriers by changing the physical conditions, such as pH, temperature, and addition of certain ions. A variety of natural and synthetic polymers with reversible solubility including alginic acid, hydroxypropyl methylcellulose acetate succinate and N-isopropylacrylamide were identified. Enzymes immobilized on such carriers could be used in biocatalysis in the soluble form and recovered by precipitation for reuse, while the substrate can easily access the active site of the immobilized enzyme, reducing the interparticle and intraparticle diffusion limitations. N-Succinyl chitosan (NSC), which was obtained by introducing succinyl groups into chitosan N-terminal of the glucosamine units, can be made soluble–insoluble by changing the pH. NSC was initially developed as wound dressing materials. Currently, it is also applied as cosmetic materials and drug carriers.

Zhou et al. prepared NSC via ring-opening reactions with succinic anhydride in the dimethyl sulfoxide system. The obtained NSC is soluble at pH above 4.8 and is insoluble at pH below 4.4. The immobilized alliinase had increased thermal stability and showed a similar dependence on pH value as NSC. Besides, the affinity of alliinase to its substrate increased when immobilized on NSC [71].

8.4.1.5 Photopolymerized Chitosan

Photopolymerized injectable chitosans have received a great deal of attention. For chitosan hydrogels by photopolymerization, their temperature and pH can be similar to body environment on the polymerization process. Additionally, control of the polymerization reaction can be accomplished through adjusting the exposure area and the time of light incidence.

Monier et al. described a versatile strategy for photopolymerized chitosan, which includes the loading of a-cyano-4-hydroxycinnamic acid onto the chitosan backbone through the amide bond formation using EDC and NSH via initial carboxyl group activation followed by reaction with chitosan-bearing amino groups. Significantly, this reaction does not require the addition of a light-sensitive initiator, which is typically required for cross-linking reactions based on photosensitive acrylate, acrylamide, or azide moieties. As a consequence, unanticipated side reactions due to the presence of free radical initiators are minimized [72].

Lipase from *C. rugosa* was entrapped in the modified photo-cross-linkable chitosan membranes and cross-linking was carried out by irradiation in the ultraviolet (UV) region. The optimum temperature for immobilized lipase was 40°C, which was identical to that of free enzyme. The optimal pH for immobilized lipase was 8.0, which was slighty higher than that of the free lipase (pH 7.5). The apparent K_m value of immobilized lipase was higher than that of free lipase. Therefore, the immobilization process slightly decreased the affinity of lipase to the substrate. On the other hand, the activity of immobilized lipase decreased slowly with time as compared with that of free lipase, and could retain 75.5% residual activity after six consecutive cycles. This immobilization remarkably improved temperature and operational stability, which made it more attractive in the application aspects [73].

8.4.2 Chemical-Grafted Chitosan Copolymer

8.4.2.1 Chitosan-Poly(Glycidyl Methacrylate) Copolymer

Chellapandian and Krishnan reported that urease (Ur) was covalently attached onto chitosan-poly(glycidyl methacrylate) by the introduction of epoxy groups to the support. The immobilized Ur retained 82% of its specific activity. The pH optimum of the free and immobilized Ur remained unchanged, but the optimum temperature of the immobilized Ur was higher than that of the free enzyme. Immobilization improved the thermal, pH, and storage stability of the enzyme [74].

8.4.2.2 Chitosan-Grafted Poly(Butyl Acrylate) by the Photochemical Technique

Compared with pure chitosan films, the chitosan-grafted poly(butyl acrylate) films have enhanced hydrophobic and impact strengths. Similar work has also been reported for grafting poly(hydroxyethyl methacrylate) (pHEMA) with chitosan in the presence of UV light. *p*-Benzoquinone has the dual functions of activating the copolymer for the immobilization of enzymes and acting as a mediator for electron shuttling in the system. That sulfite oxidase enzyme can retain its bioactivity when it is covalently bonded to the chitosan–pHEMA matrix shows that fabrication of a chitosan–pHEMA enzyme-based electrochemical biosensor can be achieved using the techniques described in [75].

8.4.2.3 Itaconic Acid-Grafted Chitosan for Reversible Enzyme Immobilization

Many protocols for enzyme immobilization involve irreversible binding between an enzyme and a functionalized support. In the reversible enzyme immobilization, the supports could be regenerated using a suitable desorption agent, and they could be recharged again with a fresh enzyme. On the other hand, when the covalently immobilized enzyme becomes inactivated upon use, both the enzyme and the support should be eliminated as wastes. In the reversible enzyme immobilization, the expensive support can be repeatedly used and the only waste produced is a solution of inactivated enzyme. For reversible enzyme immobilization, ion exchangers, hydrophobic gels, and metal-chelated supports have been used. Metal ions-chelated supports have been used extensively for separation and purification of biological macromolecules (mainly for enzyme purification) from fermentation broth or biological fluids. The low cost of metal ions and the reuse of support materials for reversible immobilization enzymes for several times without any detectable loss of metal-chelating properties can be the attractive features of metal affinity interactions with the proteins.

Among the methods of modification of polymers, grafting is one of the promising methods. For example, grafting of a functional pendant group carrying vinyl monomers such as itaconic acid onto the chitosan backbone could introduce novel oxygen-rich ligands for chelating hard Lewis metal ions. These novel comb-type polymer-grafted and metal ions-chelated matrices could be suitable for immobilization of enzyme due to their intrinsically high specific surfaces, providing the quantity and accessibility of the binding sites necessary for a high immobilization capacity and a large surface area for enzymatic reaction.

Bayramoglu et al. prepared a chitosan membrane by using the phase-inversion technique and then cross-linking with ECO under alkaline conditions. Itaconic acid was grafted on the cross-linked chitosan membrane via ammonium persulfate initiation under a nitrogen atmosphere. Poly(itaconic acid)-grafted and/or Fe(III) ions-incorporated chitosan membranes were used for reversible immobilization of CAT (from bovine liver) via adsorption. In this method, grafted poly(itaconic acid) acted as a metal-chelating ligand, and there is no need of any reaction step to activate the matrix for the chelating-ligand immobilization. In addition, grafted poly(itaconic acid) brush provides a hydrophilic microenvironment for the guest enzyme. It was observed that the same support enzyme can be repeatedly used for immobilization of CAT after regeneration without significant loss of adsorption capacity or enzyme activity [76].

8.4.2.4 Chitosan-Grafted-Polyethyl Acrylate

A method has been developed to immobilize HRP on modified chitosan beads by means of graft copolymerization of polyethyl acrylate (PEA) in the presence of potassium persulfate and Mohr's salt redox initiator. The immobilization of HRP on modified chitosan beads was carried out in three steps. The first step involves the graft copolymerization of EA onto chitosan by potassium persulfate and Mohr's salt as the combined redox initiator. In the second step, the majority of the grafted polyethylacrylate chains were converted into polyacrylic hydrazide by the reaction with hydrazine hydrate, followed by beads activation through acyl azide formation and then coupling of the enzyme by the immersion of the activated beads in the HRP enzyme solution in the third step. The activity of immobilized HRP decreased slowly with time as compared with that of free HRP and could retain 65.8% residual activity after six consecutive operations. This immobilization remarkably improved the temperature and operational stability, which made it more attractive in application aspects [77].

8.4.3 Enzyme–Chitosan Conjugate

8.4.3.1 Laccase Conjugation to Chitosan

Different from the conventional immobilization of laccase on preformed solid supports or by physically trapping in gels, conjugation of laccase and chitosan occurs in a solution by forming covalent bonds between the protein and polysaccharide molecules. Once bound, the molecules are strongly coupled and distributed uniformly in the conjugate aggregates or gels. Since the protonation of amino groups on the chitosan backbone is dependent on the solution pH, the laccase conjugate becomes a pH-sensitive biomaterial and can adjust its aggregation state in response to pH variation, as indicated in the upper part of Figure 8.9. The conjugates, therefore, can undergo repeated phase change with little loss of enzyme proteins, a useful feature for novel applications in bioremediation, organic synthesis, biosensing, and immunoenzyme assays. Additionally, chitosan's amino groups are nucelophilic and reactive at higher pH values. The reactivity of these amino groups allows chitosan to be cross-linked under mild conditions to create gel

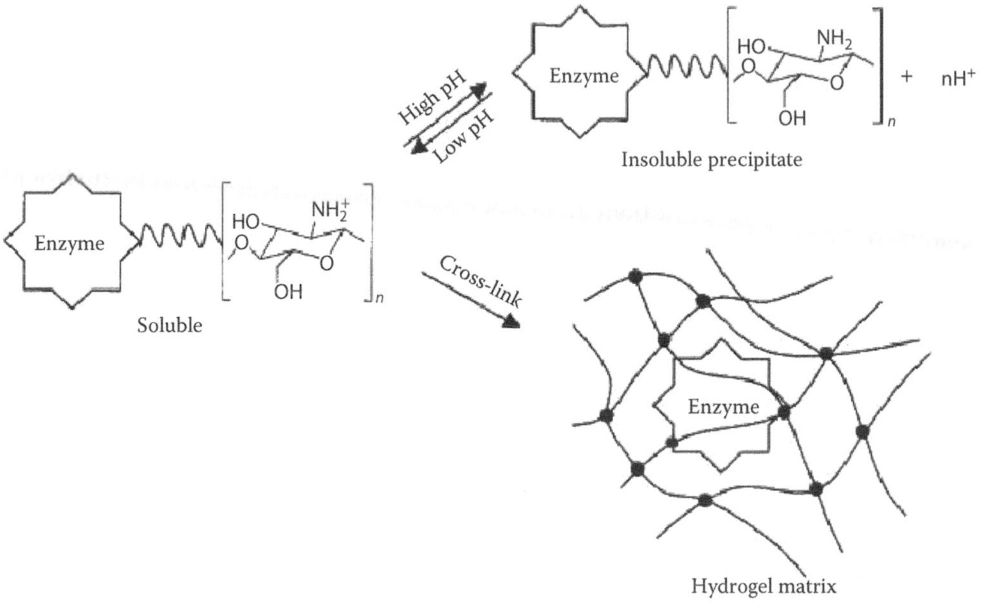

FIGURE 8.9
Enzyme–chitosan conjugate for pH-responsive solubility (upper path) and biocatalytic hydrogels (lower path). (From Vazquez-Duhalt, R. et al. 2001. *Bioconjug Chem* 12: 301–306. With permission.)

matrixes of various shapes and sizes including beads, membranes, and fibers (the lower path in Figure 8.9) [78].

One major problem of enzyme conjugation or immobilization is the loss of enzyme activity, which is attributed to many factors involving enzyme, polymer, reagents, and process conditions. Delanoy et al. investigated the effect of the molecular size of chitosan on laccase conjugation and the activity loss in the conjugation process. It was demonstrated that the chitosan molecular size has little effect on the first moderate activity loss in the conjugation reaction, but has a visible effect on the substantial activity loss associated with phase change. Small chitosan molecules gave high residual activity. The conjugated laccase exhibited a high stability in the following repeated phase changes and had the same temperature and pH profile as those of free laccase. Compared with free laccase, the conjugated laccase had a similar affinity (K_m) but reduced turnover (k_{cat}) that was adversely affected by an increase of the molecular mass of chitosan [79].

8.4.3.2 Invertase–Chitosan Conjugate

Adsorption of enzymes on charged supports through electrostatic interactions has been widely used for immobilizing enzymes because of the easiness of preparation and the possibility of reuse of the supports. However, immobilization of native enzymes on conventional ionic exchanger resins is frequently not very strong, and most proteins are fully desorbed from such matrices at moderate ionic strength or pH changes.

Gómez et al. developed a new procedure for immobilizing enzymes on charged solid supports via electrostatic interactions and it received special attention in enzyme technology. PEC formation mediated immobilization of an invertase–chitosan conjugate on sodium alginate-coated chitin supports [80]. To prepare the support for enzyme immobilization, chitin was coated with sodium alginate through amide linkages. Although different synthetic methods for conjugating polymers to enzymes have been described, in general these procedures only involve the coupling to reactive groups from the polypeptide chains of enzymes. Since the sugar residues in glycoenzymes are often not required for their activities, a novel and better approach for stabilizing these biomolecules would be the conjugation of polymers to activated carbohydrate moieties of glycoenzymes. The authors deal with the stabilization of invertase by coupling of chitosan to periodate-oxidized sugar moieties from this enzyme [81].

The yield of immobilized protein was determined as 85% and the enzyme retained 97% of the initial chitosan-invertase activity. The immobilized enzyme was stable against incubation in high-ionic-strength solutions and was fourfold more resistant to thermal treatment at 65°C than the native counterpart. The biocatalyst prepared retained 80% of the original catalytic activity after 50 h under the continuous operational regime in a packed-bed reactor [80].

8.5 Chitosan Composite for Enzyme Immobilization

Chitosan composites are divided into four groups: chitosan–biopolymer mixture prepared by mixture; chitosan-tethered membrane; chitosan-based PECs; and chitosan–inorganic composites. Inorganic materials involve magnetic particles, metal oxide (except for iron oxide), metal nanoparticles, silica, CNTs, clay, and inorganic salt.

8.5.1 Chitosan–Biopolymer Mixture Prepared by Mixture

The simplest method of preparing composites was by direct mixture of chitosan and other materials, which can change the gel structure, mechanical properties, and immobilization conditions.

Several glycosidases (βG, Ara, Rha), purified from an *A. niger* enzyme preparation, were immoblized simultaneously with a method because of their possible application in the wine-making and fruit-juice-processing industries. Immobilization of the three enzymes was carried out by inclusion using chitosan gels and subsequent cross-linking with GA. This was followed by the addition of various agents to improve the gel's physical and mechanical properties, reduce enzyme release phenomena, and increase immobilization yields and operational stability. It was shown that the best additives were gelatin and silica gel [82].

Adriano et al. reported that the use of sodium alginate, gelatin, or κ-carrageenan, activation with GA, Gly, or ECO, and addition of microorganisms followed by cellular lysis led to a modification of the gel structure. Different size distributions of pore beads may be obtained through the covalent or physical interactions of the two polymers. The biopolymers gelatin, alginate, and κ-carrageenan have groups that are negatively charged at neutral pH and can interact with the positively charged amine groups of chitosan, forming different internal nets. The hydrogen bonds formed between chitosan, alginate, or κ-carrageenan modify the porosity of the gel. They also change the chitosan molecule conformation, which becomes more resistant to drastic conditions of pH and temperature. Another way to modify the gel internal structure is its formation in the presence of a material that can be further removed. The preparation of macroporous beads and membranes in the presence of silica during gel formation, followed by the removal of the silica after dissolution at alkaline pH, has already been reported. When a similar approach is used, the gel could be formed in the presence of cells of microorganisms, followed by cell lysis. After removing the cellular material, the resulting polymer may have a higher internal surface area, favoring enzyme immobilization. It was shown that changing gel structure and immobilization conditions led to a significant improvement of the covalent MPA of chymotrypsin on chitosan. Enzyme immobilization for 72 h at pH 10.05 and 25°C and reduction with NaBH$_4$ in chitosan 2.5%–carrageenan 2.5%, with the addition of *S. cerevisiae* 5% and activation with ECO, led to the best derivative, which was 9900-fold more stable than the soluble enzyme [23].

8.5.2 Chitosan-Tethered Membrane

8.5.2.1 Chitosan-Tethered Poly(Acrylonitrile) Membrane

The chemically modified polyacrylonitrile (PAN) membrane, which possesses excellent properties, such as good thermal and mechanical stability, has been successfully applied as a membrane matrix for enzyme immobilization.

8.5.2.1.1 Chitosan-PANCMA Membrane

Ye et al. proposed a protocol to prepare a dual-layer biomimetic membrane as a support for enzyme immobilization by tethering chitosan on the surface of a poly(acrylonitrile-*co*-maleic acid) (PANCMA) ultrafiltration hollow fiber membrane in the presence of EDC and NHS. Lipase from *C. rugosa* was immobilized on this dual-layer biomimetic membrane using GA and on the nascent PANCMA membrane using EDC/NHS as a coupling agent. It was found that both the activity retention of the immobilized lipase and the amount of bound protein on the dual-layer biomimetic membrane were higher than those on the nascent PANCMA membrane. After immobilization, the pH, thermal, and reuse stabilities of the immobilized enzyme increased [83]. In order to further raise enzyme loading on the support and to reduce the diffusion resistance for the immobilized enzyme, PANCMA was fabricated into nanofibrous membranes by the electrospinning process. It was found that there is an increase of activity retention of the immobilized lipase on the chitosan-modified nanofibrous membrane ($45.6 \pm 1.8\%$) and on the gelatin-modified one ($49.7 \pm 1.8\%$) as compared with that on the nascent one ($37.6 \pm 1.8\%$). The kinetic parameter K_m of the immobilized lipase on the nanofiber membranes was lower than that of the hollow fiber membrane [17].

Immobilization of lipase on this dual-layer biomimetic support by adsorption is also investigated. The activity retention of the immobilized lipase on the chitosan-tethered membrane by adsorption (54.1%) is higher than that by chemical bonding (44.5%). Additionally, the experimental results on thermal stabilities indicate that the residual activity of the immobilized lipase at 50°C is 38% by adsorption and 65% by chemical bonding [84]. These results demonstrated that the dual-layer biomimetic membrane was a potential support in the enzyme immobilization technology for industrial applications such as the manufacture of acid by the hydrolysis of triglyceride.

8.5.2.1.2 Chitosan-Poly(Acrylonitrile–MethylMethacrylate–Sodium Vinylsulfonate) (PANMV) Membrane

Godjevargova and coworkers report the formation and characterization of ternary copolymer poly(acrylonitrile–methylmethacrylate–sodium vinylsulfonate) (PANMV)/chitosan composite membranes and their application as carriers for Ur immobilization. The chitosan layer was deposited on the surface as well as on the pore walls of the base membrane. It was found that the average size of the pore under a selective layer base PANMV membrane is 7 μm, whereas the membrane coated with 0.25% chitosan shows a reduced pore size, less than or equal to 5 μm, and that with 0.35% chitosan, about 4 μm. This resulted in a reduction of the pore size of the membrane and in an increase of their hydrophilicity. Ur was covalently immobilized onto all kinds of PANMV–chitosan composite membranes using GA. The increase of thermal stability is mainly due to MPA of Ur on the surface of the support by covalent linkage [85].

They also compared dual-layer matrices PANMV membranes coated with the physically bound chitosan PAVMVCHI-A and chemically bound chitosan PAVMVCHI-B (low-molecular-weight chitosan: 10 kDa) and PAVMVCHI-C (high-molecular-weight chitosan: 400 kDa) for immobilization of acetylcholinesterase (AChE). The chemical-modified PANMV membrane (PANMV-NaOH + ethylenediamine (EDA)) was used as a base for the prepared dual-layer membranes. For the chemical chitosan-bound membrane, chitosan was tethered onto the membrane surface to form a dual-layer biomimetic membrane in the presence of GA. The relative activities and V_{max} of the covalently immobilized enzyme on PANMVCHI-B and PANMVCHI-C membranes were higher than that on PANMVCHI-A membrane and chemical-modified membrane with NaOH + EDA. The bound enzymes on PANMVCHI-B and PANMVCHI-C have higher thermal and storage stability in comparison with AChE on PANMVCHI-A membrane and free enzyme [86].

8.5.2.2 Chitosan-Tethered Polysulfone Membrane

Edwards et al. used bench-scale, single-capillary membrane bioreactors (MRBs) to determine the influence of the chitosan coating on product removal after substrate conversion by immobilized polyphenol oxidase (PPO) during the treatment of industrial phenolic effluents. The viscous chitosan solution was circulated over the shell side of the membrane to coat the entire outer surface, and the solution was neutralized with 8% NaOH, forming the gel coating. PPO was immobilized by cross-flow circulation in pH 6.8 buffer on the shell (outer) side of the membranes. It was shown that one advantage of forming a gel-like layer of chitosan on the capillary membranes is that greater protein loading capacities can be achieved as compared with noncoated membranes. Two functions are therefore served using chitosan-coated capillary membranes and immobilized PPO: an initial highly efficient process for the removal of phenolic pollutants from water and the effective *in situ* color removal from the resultant permeate. In addition, the presence of chitosan contributes considerably to decreasing the product inhibition, which is characteristic of PPO [87].

8.5.2.3 Chitosan-Tethered Alumina Membrane

Porous membranes may exhibit pores with radii from micrometer to nanometer that determine their use in different filtration technologies. Commercial anodic alumina membranes are microfiltration membranes restricted to a very limited number of pore diameters. In general, these membranes have been employed as a template for the preparation of nanoparticles, nanotubes, nanofibrils, and nanowires of different materials including polymers, metal oxides, metals, and other nanostructured solids.

Darder prepared a set of home-made nanoporous alumina membranes of different dimensions by electrochemical oxidation of aluminum in an acidic solution, controlling

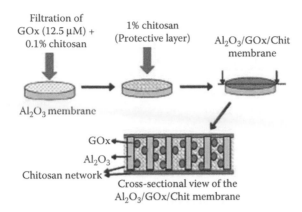

FIGURE 8.10
Immobilization of GOx in nanoporous alumina membranes. (From Darder, M. et al. 2006. *Thin Solid Films* 495: 321–326. With permission.)

the pore size and the membrane thickness by changing the anodizing voltage and the amount of transferred charge, respectively. These membranes were used to encapsulate GOx by procuring an external coverage with a thin layer of the biopolymer chitosan, which avoids enzyme leaching. The enzyme-modified membranes have been attached to the surface of a platinum electrode for the biosensor construction. GOx was immobilized on nanoporous alumina membranes by following the steps depicted in Figure 8.10.

A relatively higher amount of enzyme is retained within the pores of the membrane as the surface area of the asymmetric porous structure of the membrane increases. The thin film incorporating the enzyme is displayed on the electrode surface, without interrupting the diffusion of the product of the enzymatic reaction toward the electrode surface due to its thickness on the micrometer level and the suitable properties of the chitosan matrix. Experimental results indicate that the control of membrane dimensions, pore diameter, and thickness is a key factor in the performance of these GOx/thin film-based biosensors [88].

8.5.3 Chitosan-Based Polyelectrolyte Complexes

Many investigators have suggested ionic complexation of chitosan (having a positive charge) with polyanion to form PECs and LBL self-assembly films/microcapsules for enzyme immobilization. Gel beads/microcapsules were achieved by adding an anionic polyelectrolyte solution dropwise into an acidic chitosan solution. Enzyme immobilization is achieved here by preparing an enzyme-containing anionic polyelectrolyte solution prior to gelation. Of course, reversed chitosan polyanions, such as chitosan–alginate, a PEC for enzyme immobilization, have also been reported. Complexation network/films were obtained by precipitating a mixture of chitosan and polyanion. The technique of LBL self-assembly is based on the sequential deposition of interactive polymers from their solutions by electrostatic, van der Waals, hydrogen bonding, and charge-transfer interactions. The development of LBL self-assembly on colloidal templates has attracted considerable attention in biotechnology and promises solutions to many problems in the fields of drug delivery, biosensors, and microreactors, as well as bioseparations.

8.5.3.1 Polysaccharide–Chitosan PECs

A variety of polysaccharide–chitosan PEC gels can be obtained by changing the molecular properties of the polysaccharide and chitosan polymers, such as molecular weight, degree of acetylation of chitosan, and carboxylic acid content of polysaccharide, as well as changing the complexation conditions, such as chitosan solution pH, polymer concentration, complexation time, and mixing ratio.

8.5.3.1.1 Chitosan–Alginate Microcapsules

Alginate hydrogels, ionically cross-linked in the presence of multivalent cations, contain carboxylic acid and exhibit negative surface charge, allowing them to be used as negatively charged templates for PECs. Ehab Taqieddin and Mansoor Amiji described the development of a core–shell microcapsule technology for enzyme immobilization. The enzyme is localized and protected in the core matrix, while the shell can regulate the entry and exit of the substrate and product, respectively. A model enzyme, β-galactosidase, was immobilized in either calcium alginate or barium alginate core surrounded by a perm-selective chitosan shell. Cross-linking of chitosan with TPP resulted in the phosphate ions diffusing into the calcium alginate core and liquefying it. The enzyme loading efficiency was higher in the barium alginate core (100%) as compared with the calcium alginate core (60%). The maximum enzymatic rate (V_{max}) of calcium alginate–chitosan microcapsules was higher than that of barium alginate–chitosan microcapsules. However, the enzymatic activities of calcium alginate or barium alginate core–shell microcapsules were significantly lower than that of the free enzyme owing to the additional layer necessary for the influx of the substrate and the efflux of the product [89].

Aranaz et al. used alginate–chitosan polyelectrolyte capsules for coimmobilization of enzymes to reproduce a multistep enzymatic route for the production of D-amino acids. Encapsulation of a crude cell extract from *Agrobacterium radiobacter* containing D-hydantoinase and D-carbamoylase activities into the PECs was accomplished with negligible leakage from the formed capsules. The most suitable biocatalysts were prepared using a chitosan with a medium molecular weight (600 kDa) and a degree of deacetylation of 0.9. It was indicated that the preparation of the biocatalyst (preparation method and chitosan characteristics) play a key role in the biocatalyst's properties [90].

8.5.3.1.2 Reversed Chitosan–Alginate Beads

Sankalia et al. explored, using response surface methodology, the main and interaction effects of some process variables on the preparation of a reversed chitosan–alginate PEC with entrapped α-amylase for stability improvement [91]. The beads were prepared by dropping chitosan containing α-amylase into a sodium alginate solution without any salt. Proper selection of the reaction pH, polymer concentration and hence charge density and hardening time is important and determines the characteristics of the PECs.

8.5.3.1.3 Chitosan/Alginic Acid Complexation Network

PECs as proton-conducting biopolymer networks have potential use for biosensors. Yapar et al. reported that cholesterol oxidase was immobilized in the conducting network via complexation of chitosan with alginic acid. Chitosan was mixed with water containing cholesterol oxidase, and alginic acid was mixed with 1% glacial acetic acid. Then the two phases were put together to get the enzyme-entrapped polymer network. The complex polymer electrolyte with $x = 1$ (x is the number of moles of chitosan per mole of –COOH units in alginic acid) exhibited maximum proton conductivity. The polymer electrolyte matrix protects entrapped cholesterol oxidase; hence the enzyme shows higher stability over broader temperature and pH ranges [92].

8.5.3.1.4 Chitosan–Alginate LBL Self-Assembly Films

Deng et al. used cysteamine to form a versatile self-assembled monolayer (SAM) tightly attached to the gold surface of the piezoelectric quartz crystal, instead of directly immobilizing antibodies through GA cross-linking on the SAM, and a strong positively charged chitosan monolayer was positioned on the cysteamine SAM by using GA cross-linking. The antibodies were coupled to alginate via activation with EDC and NHS. The immobilization of the antibodies was achieved when the modified alginate was adsorbed on the chitosan monolayer by strong electrostatic interaction. The immunosensor based on the chitosan–alginate adsorption procedure shows improved performance in terms of the magnitude of the response and sensitivity compared with that observed by a similar sensor employing conventional covalent immobilization [93].

8.5.3.1.5 Chitosan/Hyaluronic Acid LBL Self-Assembly Films

A pair of biomacromolecules, positively charged chitosan and negatively charged hyaluronic acid was successfully assembled onto the surface of a poly(ethylene terephthalate) (PET) microfluidic chip using layer-by-layer deposition for the formation of a microstructured and biocompatible scaffold to immobilize trypsin. An effective multilayer assembled microchip reactor has been developed for the rapid digestion of proteins [94]. The protocol of immobilizing enzymes on the LBL-modified PET surface is depicted in Figure 8.11. Trypsin was adsorbed into the ninth layer of chitosan/hyaluronic acid assembly. A unique feature of this approach is the very short digestion time, <5 s, and the small volume of protein samples.

8.5.3.1.6 Chitosan/Xanthan Beads

Xanthan gum, a microbial exopolysaccharide consisting of a cellulosic backbone with two mannose and one glucuronic acid side chains on every second glucose residue, is considered an anionic polyelectrolyte. Magnin et al. reported that lipases were noncovalently immobilized in chitoxan, a polyionic hydrogel obtained by complexation between chitosan and xanthan. In the aqueous medium, the activity was twice as high for immobilized lipases as for free lipases. Immobilized lipases in chitoxan were able to hydrolyze triacylglycerols in three distinct organic solvent media. At the microstructural level, lipases were not distributed uniformly in the chitoxan beads. Higher concentrations of lipase were found in the outer membrane-like layer of the beads, as compared with lower concentrations in the inner part of the beads [55].

8.5.3.1.7 Chitosan/Carboxymethyl Konjac Glucomannan Nanocapsules

Konjac glucomannan (KGM), one of the high-molecular-weight water-soluble natural polysaccharides found in tubers of *Amorphophallus konjac*, is composed of β-$(1 \rightarrow 4)$-linked D-glucose and D-mannose in the molar ratio of 1:1.6 to 1:1.69. KGM has long been used as a health food to reduce the risk of developing diabetes and heart disease. Carboxymethyl konjac glucomannan (CKGM) is an anionic polymer produced by the carboxymethylation of KGM. It has good water solubility, biocompatibility, bioactivity, and excellent gelation ability when mixed with a polymer of opposite charge.

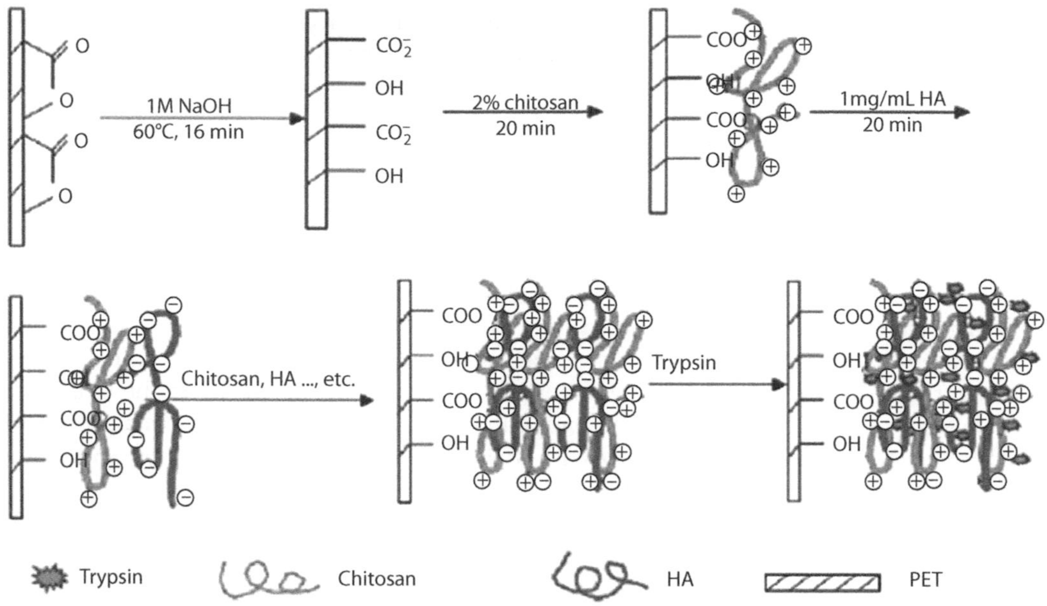

FIGURE 8.11
Process summary of the encapsulation of trypsin based on LBL self-assembly with oppositely charged polyelectrolytes on a hydrolyzed PET surface. (From Liu, Y. et al. 2006. *Anal Chem* 78: 801–808. With permission.)

Wang et al. reported a CKGM–chitosan immobilization system that entraps L-asparaginase in semipermeable CKGM–chitosan nanocapsules. The nanocapsules were prepared by dropping the CKGM solution with L-asparaginase into the chitosan solution through a needle while sonicating. The matrix has semipermeability to allow the substrate and product to pass through and to keep L-asparaginase in the matrix to prevent leaking. The immobilized enzyme has better stability and activity in contrast to the native enzyme. These studies may supply a new material for the immobilization of pH- and temperature-sensitive enzymes [95].

8.5.3.2 Enzyme or DNA–Chitosan PECs

8.5.3.2.1 Chitosan/Horseradish Peroxidase LBL Self-Assembly Films

Adsorption of material in alternated layers is now well established for immobilizing a variety of biomolecules in an equally varied range of applications. For example, antigens adsorbed on films with alternating layers for biosensing had their activity preserved for long periods of time if the layers of antigen were alternated with dendrimer layers, but not with some polyelectrolytes. It was reported by Caseli and coworkers that HRP presents negative net charge and can be immobilized in alternated layers with chitosan as the template material. The four-step procedure for the production of a single pair HRP/chitosan was repeated to yield a six-bilayer film. Although the activity in the HRP/chitosan film was lower than in a homogeneous solution or in a Langmuir–Blodgett (LB) film investigated earlier, the response was linear for a considerable length of time, which may be advantageous for sensing hydrogen peroxide [96].

8.5.3.2.2 Chitosan/Glutamate Oxidase Complexation Films

A surprisingly strong enzyme immobilization was accomplished by the precipitation of a mixture of polyanionic enzyme L-glutamate oxidase (GmOx) with polycationic chains of chitosan on the surface of the platinum electrode. The good adhesion of such composite films to the surface of platinum allowed for the construction of amperometric glutamate biosensors with an attractive analytical performance. In particular, such biosensors displayed high sensitivity, low detection limit, fast response time, and good operational and long-term stability [97].

8.5.3.2.3 Chitosan–DNA Complexation Films

Chitosan has widely been investigated for the purpose of nonviral gene delivery in the form of DNA–chitosan complexes or as nanoparticles. Tingting et al. used a DNA–chitosan polyion complex membrane as a support for the immobilization of electrocatalytic species-copper ions, which specifically bound to dsDNA and catalyzed the hydrogen peroxide reduction. The polyion complex membrane composed of the DNA–Cu(II) complex and chitosan was prepared on a GCE. The DNA–Cu(II)–chitosan/GC electrode showed excellent electrocatalytic activity for H_2O_2 reduction. Ascorbic acid and glucose have almost no interference to the measurement of H_2O_2. In addition, the sensor exhibited good reproducibility [98].

8.5.3.3 Chitosan–Polymer PECs

8.5.3.3.1 Chitosan-PTAA LBL Self-Assembly Films

Poly(thiophene-3-acetic acid) (PTAA) has many important properties such as conductivity in the doped state, thermochromism, photoluminescence, fluorescence, and absorption in the UV–VIS region. Leblanc shows a way of immobilizing organophosphorus hydrolase (OPH) using several bilayers of chitosan and negatively charged PTAA for detecting the presence of paraoxon. This polyion cushion was held together by the electrostatic attraction between chitosan and PTAA. OPH was then adsorbed on the five-bilayer chitosan–PTAA system. The fluorescence property of PTAA played a key role as the ultrathin film was monitored using emission spectroscopy. LBL adsorption allows OPH to be combined with PTAA so that in the presence of paraoxon there would be a change in the optical properties of PTAA, and hence, the presence of paraoxon could be detected. This five-bilayer macromolecular structure compared with the solid substrate rendered stability to the enzyme by giving functional integrity in addition to the ability to react with paraoxon solutions [99].

8.5.3.3.2 Polyanionic-Modified PVA-Coated Chitosan Beads

Chemically, maleic anhydride-modified PVA showed polyanionic character and was used for chitosan beads coating. The chitosan beads cross-linked by TPP can be used as a form maker. Dinçer and Azmi immobilized cellulase on the modified PVA-coated chitosan beads. ECO was selected as a convenient base catalyzed cross-linking agent. As a result of this modification, the pH optimum of enzyme shifted from pH 4.0 to 7.0 and the immobilized cellulase beads showed better pH stability than free enzyme in the neutral pH range. The activity yield of the immobilized cellulase was found to be 87%, and it was found that there was no change in the optimum temperature after immobilization [100].

8.5.4 Chitosan–Inorganic Composites

Until now, the chitosan–inorganic hybrid support presented beads, microspheres, nanoparticles, and nanofibers. Among them, nanomaterials were the most interesting. The large surface area of nanomaterials is likely to provide a better matrix for the immobilization of the desired enzyme, leading to increased enzyme loading per unit mass of particles. The enzyme-attached nanoparticles facilitate enzymes to act as free enzymes in solution that in turn provide enhanced enzyme–substrate interaction by minimizing potential aggregation of the free enzyme.

8.5.4.1 Magnetic Chitosan Support

In recent years, magnetic particles have shown great potential in protein and enzyme immobilization, bioseparation, immunoassays, and so on. Used as the support material, magnetic carriers can be quickly separated from the reaction medium and effectively controlled by applying a magnetic field, and thus the catalytic efficiency and stability properties of enzyme can be greatly improved. Moreover, magnetic nanoparticles exhibit large surface-to-volume ratio, high surface reaction activity, high catalytic efficiency, strong adsorption ability and unique fast electron transfer between the electrode and the active site of an enzyme that can be helpful for obtaining improved stability and sensitivity of a biosensor. To date, magnetic nanoparticles have been used for the immobilization of many enzymes, such as lipase, protease, glucoamylase, α-amylase, penicillin G acylase and GOx.

The preparations of magnetic chitosan were mostly prepared by two steps with the suspension cross-linking technique: the first step is the synthesis of Fe_3O_4 particles and the second one is the binding of Fe_3O_4 and chitosan; the size of the particles with this method was mostly on the micrometer scale. For biosensors, a mixture of Fe_3O_4 nanoparticles and chitosan solution could be directly dried and cast into a composite film [101]. Moreover, several methods have been developed to synthesize magnetic chitosan nanoparticles such as emulsion polymerization and *in situ* polymerization. For *in situ* polymerization, a constitution of microemulsion containing chitosan and ferrous salt was suggested as the reaction system. With the microemulsion system, the magnetic chitosan nanoparticles were *in situ* prepared by controlling the precipitation of chitosan and Fe_3O_4 with an NaOH solution as the solidification solution [102].

8.5.4.1.1 Nanobiocomposite Films by Solvent Evaporation

One very simple preparation method of magnetic chitosan supports for biosensors is the solvent evaporation/casting method. It was reported that Ur and GLDH are co-immobilized onto a superparamagnetic iron oxide (Fe_3O_4) nanoparticles–chitosan-based nanobiocomposite film deposited onto an indium-tin oxide (ITO)-coated glass plate via physical adsorption for urea detection. Fe_3O_4 nanoparticles (<22 nm) are prepared using the coprecipitation method. Chitosan–Fe_3O_4 hybrid nanobiocomposite films have been fabricated by uniformly dispersing a solution of chitosan and Fe_3O_4 nanoparticles onto an ITO surface and allowing it to dry at room temperature. It is shown that the presence of iron oxide nanoparticles results in increased active surface area of the nanobiocomposite for immobilization of enzymes, enhanced electron transfer, and increased shelf-life of the nanobiocomposite electrode [101].

Ferrites are a group of important magnetic materials for technological applications and fundamental studies. Nickel ferrite ($NiFe_2O_4$) with an inverse spinel structure shows ferrimagnetism that originates from the magnetic moment of antiparallel spins between Fe^{3+} ions at tetrahedral sites and Ni^{2+} ions at octahedral sites. The quantitative cytotoxicity test verified that both uncoated and chitosan-coated $NiFe_2O_4$ nanoparticles had noncytotoxicity. Luo et al. fabricated a glucose biosensor by integrating GOx with chitosan–$NiFe_2O_4$ nanoparticles on a GCE. Because of the excellent biocompatibility of the film with GOx, the catalytic activity of the immobilized GOx was well retained and the direct electron transfer with the underlying GCE could be realized. The resulting glucose biosensor exhibited a fast response, high sensitivity, low detection limit, and long-term stability [103].

Pure magnetic particles are likely to form a large aggregation, alter magnetic properties, and can undergo rapid biodegradation when they are directly exposed to the biological system. It has been demonstrated that the formation of a passive coating of inert materials such as silica on the surfaces of iron oxide nanoparticles could prevent their aggregation in liquid and improve their chemical stability. Qiu et al. developed a novel amperometric glucose biosensor by entrapping GOx in a chitosan composite doped with ferrocene monocarboxylic acid-modified magnetic core–shell Fe_3O_4/SiO_2 nanoparticles. It is shown that the obtained magnetic bionanoparticles attached to the surface of a CPE with the employment of a permanent magnet showed excellent electrochemical characteristics and at the same time acted as a mediator to transfer electrons between the enzyme and the electrode [104].

8.5.4.1.2 Magnetic Chitosan Beads/Microspheres by the Phase-Inversion Technique

Bayramoglu et al. prepared cross-linked magnetic chitosan beads by the phase-inversion technique in the presence of ECO under alkaline conditions, and used it for covalent immobilization of laccase. The magnetic chitosan beads were in spherical form mostly in the size range of ca. 1.0 mm and had a porous surface structure. The porous surface properties of the magnetic chitosan beads would favor a higher immobilization capacity for the enzyme due to an increase in the surface area. The laccase immobilized on magnetic chitosan beads was very effective in removal of textile dyes from aqueous solution, which creates an important environmental problem in the discharged textile dying solutions [105].

Similarly, magnetic chitosan microspheres were prepared with reversed-phase suspension methodology (combining the phase-inversion technique with the emulsification process) using GA as a cross-linking reagent for the enzyme immobilization. The microspheres have well-shaped spherical form with a smooth surface, and their mean particle size was 5.0 µm with a narrow size distribution. Laccase was immobilized on magnetic chitosan microspheres by adsorption and cross-linking with GA. The thermal, operational, and storage stabilities of the enzyme were improved greatly after they were immobilized on the surface of magnetic chitosan microspheres [106].

8.5.4.1.3 Magnetic Chitosan Nanoparticles Prepared by the Ionization Gelation Method

The preparation processes of magnetic particles in the water/oil system might impose limitations on practical applications in water systems. The problem with this method is that productivity is low; in addition, it uses a number of surfactant and cosurfactant compounds that are harmful to the environment. An efficient immobilization of β-D-galactosidase from *Aspergillus oryzae* has been developed by using magnetic chitosan nanoparticles as the support, which were prepared by electrostatic adsorption of chitosan on the surface of Fe_3O_4 nanoparticles and subsequently adding TPP. Fe_3O_4 nanoparticles could adsorb chitosan molecules on their surface due to the high surface energy. β-D-Galactosidase was covalently immobilized onto the nanocomposites using GA as an activating agent. As a result, the immobilized enzyme presented a higher storage, pH, and thermal stability than the soluble enzyme [107].

8.5.4.1.4 Combined Ionization Gelation Method with In Situ Polymerization

The order of the above preparation process, adsorption and subsequently cross-linking by TPP, can be reversed. It is well known that the NH_2 group on chitosan molecules may interact with Fe^{2+} in aqueous solution. In this study, the chitosan nanoparticles were first prepared by cross-linking with TPP in HCl solution, the chitosan nanoparticles were in the form of a gel and porous, and then Fe^{2+} was added to the solution and adsorbed by the chitosan nanoparticles. NaOH was used to adjust the pH and precipitate $Fe(OH)_2$, and a small amount of O_2 was used to oxidize the $Fe(OH)_2$ into Fe_3O_4. As the Fe_3O_4 nanoparticles were present in the pores of the chitosan gel, the monodispersion was good. The whole procedure was completed in an aqueous solution, so the method is simple and effective, and can be used for industrial production. The saturated magnetization of composite nanoparticles reached 35.54 emu/g and the nanoparticles showed the characteristics of superparamagnetism. The immobilization of lipase onto the particles showed good loading ability and little loss of enzyme activity, and the stability of the catalyst was very good; it only lost 12% of enzyme activity after five batches [108].

8.5.4.1.5 Magnetic Particles/Nanowires by LBL Self-Assembly

Lee and coworkers reported that a magnetic enzyme carrier (MEC) was prepared by immobilizing the quorum quenching enzyme (acylase) on magnetic particles to overcome the technical limitations of free enzyme. The MEC will be retained within the bioreactor because of its larger size as compared to the membrane pores and can be easily recovered and reused via magnetic capture. MIEX (ORICA, Australia), a magnetic ion-exchange resin, was adopted as a magnetic core for the follow-up enzyme immobilization. MIEX, which is made of divinyl benzene and glycidal methacrylate, has a net positive surface charge. Maghemite (γ-Fe_2O_3) makes the resin magnetic. The functionalization of MIEX was performed by LBL deposition of an anionic polyelectrolyte (polystyrene sulfonate (PSS)) and a cationic polyelectrolyte (chitosan). Porcine kidney acylase I was adsorbed physically on the MIEX–PSS–chitosan to prepare "adsorbed enzyme" or was covalently attached to the MIEX–PSS–chitosan using GA as a cross-linking agent to prepare "MEC." The MEC showed no activity decrease under both continuous shaking for 14 days and 29 iterative cycles of reuse. Furthermore, the comparison of the MEC with free enzyme in a batch-type MBR showed that the MEC efficiently alleviated the membrane biofouling and showed a great advantage over free enzyme in terms of recycled use and stability in mixed liquor. When the MEC was applied to the laboratory scale MRB in a continuous operation, it also enhanced the membrane permeability to a large extent compared with a conventional MBR with no enzyme [109].

Lei et al. reported that pectinase was immobilized on GA-activated $Fe_3O_4/SiO_2/PSS/$ chitosan microspheres by covalent attachment. In order to build more stable assembly, the polyelectrolyte brush PSS was grafted onto the surface of Fe_3O_4/SiO_2 composite particles by surface-initiated atom transfer radical polymerization using modified magnetic silica as the initiator. Subsequently, introducing an LBL self-assembly method, deposition occurs by electrostatic interactions between the adsorbed PSS and the chitosan layer with opposite charges. Biochemical studies showed an improved storage stability of the immobilized pectinase as well as enhanced performance at higher temperatures and over a wider pH range [110].

Magnin et al. have reported a facile method for the preparation of biocompatible and bioactive magnetic nanowires. The method consists of the direct deposition of polysaccharides by LBL assembly onto a brush of metallic nanowires obtained by electrodeposition of the metal within the nanopores of an alumina template supported on a silicon wafer. Carboxymethylpullulan (CMP) and chitosan multilayers were grown on brushes of Ni nanowires; subsequent grafting of an enzyme (GOx was chosen as the model system) was performed by conjugating free amine side groups of chitosan with carboxylic groups of the enzyme (EDC and NHS as chemical coupling agents). The nanowires are finally released by a gentle ultrasonic treatment. The process is very advantageous over the direct encapsulation of released nanowires because all time-consuming steps related to nanowire centrifugation, rinsing, and redispersion are eliminated. This easy and efficient route to the biochemical functionalization of magnetic nanowires can find widespread use in the preparation of a broad range of nanowires with tailored surface properties [111].

8.5.4.1.6 *Magnetic Chitosan Beads by Photochemical Polymerization*

Magnetic chitosan beads can be prepared via photochemical polymerization in Fe_3O_4 magnetite aqueous suspension under UV irradiation. Chitosan chains can be grafted from Fe_3O_4 nanoparticles via recombination of the chitosan free radicals and then the surface of Fe_3O_4 nanoparticles was coated by a cross-linked chitosan shell via further cross-linking with N,N'-methylene-bis-(acrylamide) (MBA). The magnetic chitosan beads were of regular spherical shape, had a mean diameter of 86 nm, and exhibited superparamagnetic property. Pullulanase was covalently immobilized on magnetic chitosan beads by crosslinking with GA. The K_m value of immobilized pullulanase was 3.89 mg/mL, which was three times higher than that of free pullulanase. This result indicated that the immobilized process slightly decreased the affinity of pullulanase on magnetic chitosan beads to the substrate. On the other hand, the activity of immobilized pullulanase decreased slowly with time as compared with that of free pullulanase. However, this immobilization remarkably improved the temperature and operational stability, which made it more attractive in application aspects [112].

8.5.4.2 **Metal Oxide (Except for Iron Oxide)–Chitosan Nanocomposite**

Metal oxide (except for iron oxide) semiconductors such as zinc oxide (ZnO), cerium oxide (CeO_2), tin oxide (SnO_2), titanium oxide (TiO_2) and zirconium oxide (ZrO_2) have been found to exhibit interesting properties such as large surface-to-volume ratio, high surface reaction activity, high catalytic efficiency, and strong adsorption ability. Furthermore, they have the unique ability to promote faster electron transfer between the electrode and the active site of the desired enzyme. Biosensing properties of metal oxide nanoparticles can be improved by incorporating these into chitosan in order to prepare metal oxide–chitosan hybrid nanobiocomposites.

8.5.4.2.1 *Chitosan–ZnO Nanocomposites*

Zinc oxide (ZnO) nanoparticles have been used for the fabrication of the transducer surface because of their unique ability to promote faster electron transfer between the electrode and the active site of the desired enzyme. This has been attributed to their remarkable properties such as wide band gap (3.37 eV), high surface area, high catalytic efficiency, nontoxicity, chemical stability, strong adsorption ability (high isoelectric point (IEP), ~9.5), and the immobilization of low-IEP (~5.0) proteins via electrostatic interactions. Recently, ZnO–chitosan nanobiocomposite films have been proposed for amperometric immunosensors for human IgG. Moreover, ZnO–chitosan composite films can be used for application to H_2O_2, phenol, and cholesterol biosensors, respectively. Solanki et al. reported the results of their studies on immobilization of Ur and GLDH onto ZnO–chitosan nanobiocomposite films deposited onto an ITO glass substrate for the fabrication of urea sensors.

The presence of ZnO nanoparticles in chitosan results in increased surface area and enhanced electron transfer kinetics. The low Michaelis–Menten constant (K_m) value indicates an enhanced affinity of enzyme to the nanobiocomposite [113].

8.5.4.2.2 *Chitosan–ZrO₂ Nanocomposite*

ZrO_2 has the properties of high hardness, high melting point (2700°C), and small thermal expansion coefficient. In fact, a porous ZrO_2 particle itself has been used as support for enzyme immobilization. The surface of porous zirconia has general affinity for the binding of proteins because the amine and carboxyl groups on the surface of the enzyme act as ligands to ZrO_2.

Yang et al. have used a nanoporous ZrO_2–chitosan composite matrix for fabricating the glucose biosensor. The surface of nanoporous ZrO_2 was treated with an anionic surfactant (sodium dodecylbenzene sulfonate) to improve the dispersion of ZrO_2 in chitosan solution. The results obtained from transmission electron microscopy indicated that a surface-treated ZrO_2–chitosan film is porous and highly homogeneous. GOx can be effectively entrapped in the film with a higher bioactivity compared with that of GOx cross-linked by glutaraldehyde [114].

It has also been reported that equal weights of chitosan and ZrO_2 powders were mixed in an acetic acid solution to prepare the composite beads. They were then cross-linked with GA and stored with and without freeze-drying before use. It was shown that the activity yield of enzyme immobilized on the dried chitosan–ZrO_2 beads was the highest. Acid phosphatase immobilized on wet composite beads exhibited the best storage stability and operation stability even after being reused 50 times [115].

8.5.4.2.3 *Chitosan/TiO₂ Nanocomposite*

Titanium dioxide (TiO_2) can be formed into different morphologies such as nanoparticles, nanofibers, nanotubes, and nanosheets. TiO_2 nanoparticles, as a semiconductor, showed excellent electrochemical activity toward H_2O_2, ascorbic acid, guanine, L-tyrosine, and acetaminophen, and provided direct electron transfer ability for GOx, HRP, and Hb. The catalytic activity was enhanced by taking advantage of the photovoltaic effect of TiO_2. A bioactive electrode of uniformly dispersed TiO_2 in chitosan was fabricated on an ITO substrate for the immobilization of HRP. An enhanced surface porosity and a decrease in the relative proportion of carbonyl functionality of chitosan in the chitosan–TiO_2 matrix were observed. The current–voltage characteristic of the chitosan–TiO_2 matrix was enhanced by a factor of four possibly due to covalent and hydrogen bonding of Ti atoms with hydroxyl and amino groups of chitosan. The immobilization of HRP on chitosan–TiO_2 had increased resistance for charge transfer. This is possibly due to the strong binding of HRP with the chitosan–TiO_2 matrix and controlling the transport of the ions of the supporting electrolyte [116].

TiO_2 nanotubes are very good biocompatible inorganic material, inexpensive, environmentally benign, and chemically and thermally stable. TiO_2 nanotube arrays have demonstrated a number of important applications including gas sensing, solar cells, photocatalysts, tissue engineering, and biosensors. Kafi et al. have reported on a promising H_2O_2 biosensor based on the coimmobilization of HRP and chitosan onto Au-modified titanium dioxide nanotube arrays. These titania nanotube arrays possess large surface area and good uniformity, providing an excellent matrix for the coimmobilization of HRP and chitosan. The presence of the Au thin film greatly increases the electrical activity of the formed TiO_2 nanotube arrays. Electrochemical measurements reveal that the immobilized HRP exhibits high biological activity and stability. The amperometric response of the developed biosensor to H_2O_2 concentration has long-range linearity. In addition, it was demonstrated that the presence of methylene blue further enhances the sensitivity of the designed H_2O_2 electrochemical biosensor [117].

8.5.4.2.4 Chitosan–CeO₂ Nanocomposite

CeO_2 nanoparticles as an important n-type semiconductor have attracted much interest owing to their unique properties, including high mechanical strength, oxygen ion conductivity, high IEP, biocompatibility, and high adsorption capability and oxygen storage capacity for the development of desired biosensors. NanoCeO₂–chitosan nanocomposite film was fabricated onto an ITO-coated glass plate to immobilize cholesterol oxidase (ChOx) via physiosorption for cholesterol detection. Electrochemical studies reveal that the presence of NanoCeO₂ results in an increased electroactive surface area for ChOx loading, resulting in enhanced electron transport between ChOx and the electrode [118].

Mixed ceria-based oxide systems have even higher electrocatalytic activities and oxygen storage capacity. Such examples include binary and tertiary mixtures of CeO_2/TiO_2, CeO_2/ZrO_2, and $CeO_2/ZrO_2/TiO_2$. These characteristics suggest that ceria and mixed ceria–titania oxides could potentially be used as "oxygen-rich" electrode materials for oxidase enzymes that could avoid or minimize the problems associated with variations in the oxygen level for enzymes that are using oxygen as a cosubstrate, offering the possibility of operation in "oxygen-free" environments. Andreescu and coworkers first studied the electrochemical characteristics of the CeO_2/TiO_2-modified GCE. They used a positively charged natural biopolymer, chitosan, as a binder. The ceria and titania oxides embedded within the chitosan film and the enzymatic reaction. It was demonstrated that mixed TiO_2/CeO_2 hybrid composites provide enhanced analytical characteristics to tyrosinase biosensors, including high sensitivity and the possibility of operation in "oxygen-free" conditions [119].

8.5.4.3 Metal Nanoparticles-Chitosan Nanocomposite

Metal nanoparticles, such as silver (Ag), gold (Au), platinum (Pt), and palladium nanoparticles, have attracted much interest in the construction of biosensors due to their unique chemical and physical properties. Gold nanoparticles, in particular, have been widely used to construct biosensors because of their excellent ability to immobilize biomolecules and at the same time retain the biocatalytic activities of those biomolecules. Many kinds of biosensors, such as enzyme sensors, immunosensors, and DNA sensors, with improved analytical performances have been prepared based on the application of gold nanoparticles (GNPs).

It is well known that some functional groups such as cyano (–CN), mercapto (–SH), and amino (–NH₂) groups have a high affinity for Au. Therefore, a nano-Au/chitosan composite was prepared via covalent bonds between GNPs (nano-Au) and the –NH₂ groups of the chitosan. This material combined the advantages of inorganic nanoparticles and an organic polymer. Moreover, GNPs have been shown to provide useful interfaces at which the redox processes of molecules involved in biochemical reactions of analytical significance can be electrocatalyzed.

8.5.4.3.1 Electrodeposition Method

Luo et al. have developed two kinds of biosensors based on the excellent properties of chitosan and GNPs. Gold nanoparticles, which were prepared in advance through the reduction of $HAuCl_4$ with citrate, can be self-assembled onto electrodeposited chitosan films and then immobilize enzymes effectively [120]. Also they can be mixed with chitosan and enzymes to construct biosensors through simple one-step electrodeposition [121]. However, in both of these systems, GNPs need to be prepared previously, which prolongs the duration of biosensor preparation and makes the procedure a bit complicated. Recently, the authors investigated a simple method, the coelectrochemical deposition method, for fabricating a chitosan film containing GNPs. HAuCl$_4$ solution is mixed with chitosan and electrochemically reduced to GNPs directly, and the produced GNPs were stabilized by chitosan and electrochemically deposited onto the GCE under a certain voltage along with chitosan. The characteristics of the film can be controlled by changing the deposition conditions, and the whole procedure costs only several minutes. The resulted chitosan film containing GNPs can be used to construct biosensors through assembling enzymes (GOx) on the surface of the film, and the immobilized enzymes have good bioactivity [122].

In recent years, metallic alloy nanoparticles have been of considerable interest in the field of catalysis and sensors because they often exhibit better catalytic properties than do their monometallic counterparts. Gold (Au) is relatively less reactive and more electronegative than platinum (Pt), so Au–Pt alloy nanoparticles may have unique effects on catalysis. Many studies of Au–Pt alloy nanoparticles have centered on their optical properties, selective oxidation, and dehydrogenation catalysts, electrocatalysts, and selective sensors.

By combining the advantageous features of CNTs and Au–Pt bimetallic nanoparticles, a novel glucose biosensor has been constructed by integrating CNTs with Au–Pt alloy nanoparticles. In the fabrication course, chitosan is used to disperse CNTs and to immobilize GOx. The electrodeposition method is applied to form Au–Pt alloy nanoparticles on the electrode modified with CNTs/chitosan. CNTs functionalized with carboxylic groups are well dispersed in chitosan solution with good stability owing to the presence of active amino groups of chitosan, and easily form a uniform film of CNTs/chitosan on a GCE. Because most of the amino groups of chitosan are protonated when chitosan is positively charged (pH < pK_a 6.3), it can electrostatically bind the negatively charged PtCl$_6^{2-}$ and AuCl$_4^-$. Therefore, Au–Pt alloy can cause NP size distribution by electrodeposition on the surface of GCE modified with CNTs/chitosan. The fabrication processes of the modified electrode are shown in Figure 8.12. For the immobilization of enzymes, GOx cross-link with GA-activated chitosan on the Au–PtNPs/CNTs/chitosan film. A preliminary study indicated that Au–PtNPs/CNTs had a better synergistic electrocatalytic effect on the reduction of hydrogen peroxide than did AuNPs/CNTs or PtNPs/CNTs at a low applied potential window. In addition, the biosensor was applied for the determination of glucose in human blood and urine samples, and satisfactory results were obtained [123].

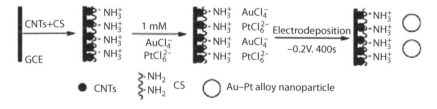

FIGURE 8.12
Preparation process of the modified electrode. (From Kang, X. H. et al. 2007. *Anal Biochem* 369: 71–79. With permission.)

8.5.4.3.2 LBL Self-Assembly Technology

Yuan reported a sensitive amperometric immunosensor for the preparation of carcinoembryonic antigen (CEA) by several steps. First, a porous nanostructure gold (NG) film was formed on GCE by electrochemical reduction of $HAuCl_4$ solution; then the nano-Au/chitosan composite was immobilized onto the electrode because of its excellent membrane-forming ability and finally the anti-CEA was adsorbed on the surface of the bilayer GNPs to construct an anti-CEA/nano-Au/chitosan/NG/GCE immunosensor [124]. They extended this methodology by using the important material nano-Pt–CHIT as the immobilization matrix and selecting Hb as a model simulation enzyme in the way of the self-assembly technology LBL to get high-sensitivity biosensor for the detection of H_2O_2 [125]. The sensor exhibited high sensitivity, selectivity, and stability.

Piezoelectric quartz crystal impedance (PQCI) analysis is a kind of piezoelectric sensing technique. A method for monitoring, in real time, the self-assembly of chitosan/GA/cysteamine (CGC) on the gold surface and the immobilization of Au colloid on a CGC membrane with PQCI was proposed by Liu et al. After the self-assembly immobilization, the electrode surface was rich in sulfur atoms, which can form covalent bonds with gold nanoparticles. The immobilization of human serum albumin (HAS) on Au colloid and the association of HAS with hesperidin were investigated by PQCI. It was shown that Au-colloid immobilization is a first-order reaction, while HSA immobilization is the sum of two exponential functions, for example, adsorption and rearrangement [126].

8.5.4.3.3 Covalent Cross-Linking Method

In recent years, electrochemical nucleic acid biosensors have received much attention due to their rapid response, high sensitivity, and inherent selectivity. A 20-mer single-stranded oligodeoxyribonucleotide (ssODN) was covalently probed onto the nanocomposite electrode, made up of an ITO glass surface coated with chitosan, which is bonded with carboxyl functionalized thiol capped GNPs (gold-mercaptopropionic acid, Au-MPA NPs). Au-MPA NPs were covalently attached onto the chitosan backbone using EDC and NHS as the condensing agents at room temperature. The resulting chitosan/Au-MPA suspension solution was uniformly spread on the ITO substrate by the spin coating technique and dried at room temperature.

The ssODN probed bioactive electrode was prepared by covalent immobilization of the ssODNs over the chitosan/Au-MPA/ITO electrode using EDC and NHS as cross-linking agents. The obtained ssODN/chitosan/Au-MPA/ITO bioelectrode was applied in the detection of the single-stranded target complementary oligodeoxyribonucleotide (cODNs) and exhibited an excellent sensitivity and reproducibility. The amperometric response of the ssODN/chitosan/Au-MPA/ITO bioelectrode to the cODNs was barely affected by the mismatched ssODNs. It was demonstrated that chitosan-based material can be used for the efficient and precise detection of cODNs associated with polygenic disease, namely cancer [127].

8.5.4.4 Chitosan–Silica Hybrid Composite Material

In 1990, Braun et al. reported on the first attempt at protein encapsulation within silica glasses. Typically, this class of silica sol–gel-based materials possesses physical rigidity, chemical inertness, high photochemical biodegradational and thermal stability, and negligible swelling in aqueous and organic solutions. Due to the inherent low-temperature process, it provides a promising means of immobilization of bioactive molecules. However, the brittleness of the silica sol–gel matrix is a major obstacle as an immobilization matrix for biomolecules. In order to overcome this problem, polymers, such as PEO, polyhydroxyl, hydrophobic poly(vinylpyridine), and PVA, were hybridized into a silica sol–gel matrix. Chitosan as a natural polymer product was also used to prepare a sol–gel/chitosan composite matrix for enzyme immobilization [16]. For the chitosan–silica hybrid system, many silylating agents such as tetraethoxysilane (TEOS), tetramethoxysilane (TMOS), tetrakis(2-hydroxy ethyl) orthosilicates (THEOS), γ-glycidoxypropyltrimethoxysilane (GPTMS), (3-aoryloxypropyl) dimethoxy methyl silane (APDMOS), and 3-amino propyl tri ethoxy silane (APTES) have been used as cross-linking agents in the formation of chitosan–silica hybrid materials.

In addition, silica gel itself had been widely used in many chromatographic adsorbents, especially when it was used as an affinity chromatographic support. Coating a high-density cross-linked chitosan layer on porous silica gel beads can be used to inhibit the nonspecific interaction. On the other hand, chitosan can be easily cross-linked by reagents such as GA to form rigid aquagels. However, severe shrinkage and deformation could not be easily avoided upon drying the chitosan carriers into the corresponding gels. This can be improved in conjunction with other solid powders to increase its density and strengthen its physical properties and thus to expand its applications.

8.5.4.4.1 Cross-Linking by Silylating Agents

Yang et al. prepared porous gels of chitosan–SiO$_2$ by coupling chitosan with TMOS through the sol–gel approach and subsequently cross-linking with formaldehyde solution. Since TMOS was water-insoluble, the mixture of chitosan acetic acid solution and TMOS initially composed of two phases was made uniform by stirring vigorously till the SiO$_2$-containing phase was distributed evenly in the aqueous solution while the hydrolysis reaction took place. GOx was selected as a model enzyme to assess its potential applicability for the enzyme immobilization purpose. The immobilized enzyme was more stable than the free one [128].

A hybrid composite material based on the cross-linking of natural polymer chitosan with APDMOS was developed for the fabrication of an amperometric H$_2$O$_2$ biosensor. The cross-linking product butyrylchitosan has the property of a hydrogel because of the interactions of hydrophilic butyrylchitosan and hydrophobic APDMOS, and the amino group has an "intelligent" pH property in the polymer. In the pH 7.4 PBS, almost all the amino are nonprotonation, and the film can exist stably. The composite film was used to immobilize HRP on a gold disc electrode. The biosensor retained approximately 75% of its original activity after about 60 days of storage in a phosphate buffer at 4°C [129].

TMOS or APDMOS as the precursor suffers from poor water solubility, which is unfavorable for the gel formation. To increase the solubility, methanol or ethanol is usually added. As a result, the resultant matrix has poor biocompatibility. Wang and Zhang developed a new amperometric H$_2$O$_2$ biosensor based on the sol–gel process of THEOS, a completely water-soluble silica precursor, in the presence of chitosan macromolecules as the nucleating centers for precipitated silica owing to the formation of hydrogen bonds between hydroxyl groups and silanols. When the silica precursor THEOS was mixed with aqueous chitosan solution, no phase separation or precipitation was observed, showing good compatibility. Moreover, it was found that such mixing was sufficient to promote the synthesis of silica hybrid material. The sol–gel process could proceed at ambient temperature without the addition of any catalysts. In the absence of chitosan, however, the sol–gel transition did not occur even at reduced temperature. It seems that chitosan has a catalytic effect on the sol–gel process of THEOS. Its gelation time and dynamic rheological properties could be modulated by the amount of added THEOS. HRP entrapped in the hybrid matrix could retain its native biocatalytic activity and provide a fast amperometric response to H$_2$O$_2$ [130].

The siloxane with an epoxide ring and trimethoxy anchor groups, GPTMS, could be used to form a dense chitosan membrane in aqueous media by the one-pot process. Because of possessing epoxy group and trimethoxy anchor groups, GPTMS acted as both an inorganic resource and a bifunctional cross-linker. On the one hand, polysiloxane network for the organic–inorganic hybrid formed resulting from self-hydrolysis and self-condensation of GPTMS. On the other hand, the reactivity between amine groups and epoxy groups offered a simple and convenient methodology for covalent incorporation of chitosan and enzyme into the inorganic framework. With GPTMS as the silylating agent, Li et al. developed a novel H_2O_2 biosensor based on *in situ* covalent immobilization of HRP into chitosan. The resultant hybrid membranes are effective in the dehydration of prevaporized isopropanol–water mixtures with satisfactory permeation selectivity, permeation flux, and long-term endurance (140 days) [131].

8.5.4.4.2 Macroporous Chitosan Layer Coated on Silica Gel

Xi and Wu prepared a new metal affinity chromatography (IMAC) adsorbent by coating chitosan–PEG solution on nonporous silica gel, followed by the steps of chitosan deposition, PEG removal, cross-linking (ECO as the cross-linking agent), and copper ion loading. The nonporous silica gel not only acted as a rigid support but also had little nonspecific interaction between its residue exposed gel surface and protein. In order to maintain the surface porous structure that was needed in affinity binding for the target protein, a macroporous structure of the coated chitosan layer was obtained by the PEG molecular imprinting and removing method. A suitable pore size could be designed in order to achieve the maximum adsorption for a given protein through changing the molecular mass and content of PEG in the coating solution. In the preparation procedure, the dried chitosan-soaked silica gel was dispersed in DMSO solution, and chitosan was deposited on the silica gel surface through the phase inversion method, which could prevent diffusion of chitosan into liquid phase. This method might acquire a relatively thick chitosan layer compared with other methods. The results proved that these kinds of ligand-free matrices had the advantage of low nonspecific interaction, ease of preparation, high adsorption capacity for metal-binding protein, and high stability. More importantly, potential selective adsorption of metal-binding protein could be achieved by designing the surface pore size using the molecular imprinting method, as well as by utilizing the difference in metal chelating ability [132].

In order to prove the latter ideas, the authors prepared the IMAC by chelating Cu^{2+}, Zn^{2+}, and Ni^{2+} ions, respectively, on chitosan–SiO_2. Trypsin could be adsorbed on the IMAC adsorbent through metal–protein interaction forces. The metal ion species had significant effects on the adsorptive capacity and the activity retention of trypsin. Zn-chitosan–SiO_2 was the best adsorbent among three kinds of M-chitosan–SiO_2 beads for trypsin immobilization since it has high enzyme loading, high stability, and activity retention [133]. In addition, the surface layer of chitosan has a porous structure and could provide a sufficient amount of amino groups, which could be easily activated with the functional group of epoxy, diazo, and aldehyde, respectively. The best results were obtained when trypsin was immobilized via direct epoxy activation, which might be ascribed to the MPA between enzyme and the support [134].

8.5.4.4.3 Chitosan Coated on Silica Gel by LBL Self-Assembly

Lei and Bi proposed a strategy for the fabrication of the silica-coated chitosan support from LBL self-assembly. The monodisperse silica particles in the range of 150 nm were prepared by a reported method [135]. The silica particles were first absorbed by dodecyl

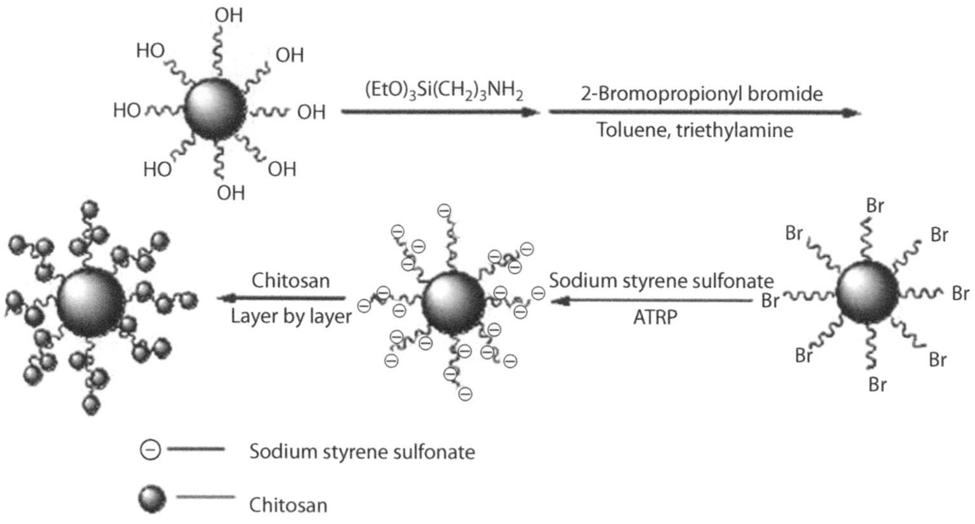

FIGURE 8.13
Schematic representation of the preparation of the silica-coated chitosan particle. (From Lei, Z. L., Bi, S. X., and Yang, H. 2007. *Food Chem* 104: 577–584. With permission.)

sulfonic acid sodium salt and then redispersed in acetate buffer of pH 3.5. A chitosan acetic acid solution was added under stirring. After 8 h, the excess polymer was removed and the particles were washed. The SiO$_2$-coated chitosan particles were cross-linked by treating with GA. The cross-linked particles were brown in color. The pectinase immobilized on the silica-coated chitosan support exhibits an improved resistance against thermal and pH denaturation. The colloidal stability is not impeded by the adsorbed proteins despite the fact that up to 247.8 mg of enzyme is adsorbed per gram of the carrier particles. The Michaelis constant K_m differs only slightly from the K_m value of the native enzyme when the amount of adsorbed enzyme is raised [136].

The authors also reported the observation of a very strong charge-controlled "spherical polyelectrolyte brush" of the core–shell structure, which was prepared by grafting poly-PSS, a negatively charged polyelectrolyte, from monodisperse SiO$_2$ nanoparticles via the surface-initiated atom transfer radical polymerization strategy. Chitosan was adsorbed on the "spherical polyelectrolyte brush" by the LBL assembly approach to fabricate a dual-layer polyelectrolyte nanoparticle support for enzyme immobilization (Figure 8.13). The silica-coated chitosan supports were treated with GA for stability in both alkaline and acidic media. The colloidal stability was not impeded by the adsorbed proteins despite the fact that up to 316.8 mg of enzyme was adsorbed per gram of the carrier particles. The activity half-lives for native and bound states of enzyme were found to be 13.5 and 30 days, respectively. Enzyme activity was found to be approximately 49.7% for immobilized enzyme after storage for 1 month [137].

8.5.4.5 Chitosan–CNT Composite Material

CNTs exhibit promising potential within the realm of bioelectrochemistry as the matrix to incorporate enzyme and construct biosensors. However, the poor solubility and chemical inertness of CNTs in aqueous solution usually limit their wide applications. Recently, chitosan has been reported to solubilize CNTs in aqueous solution for the preparation of enzyme-based nanotube sensors. The CNTs–chitosan composite provides a suitable biosensing matrix due to its good conductivity, high stability, and good biocompatibility.

8.5.4.5.1 Solvent Evaporation

The CNTs–chitosan–enzyme nanobiocomposite-modified electrode was fabricated by casting CNTs–chitosan–enzyme mixture solution on the surface of a GCE and evaporating the solvent under room temperature in air. A facilely fabricated amperometric biosensor by entrapping laccase into MWCNTs–chitosan composite film has been developed by Liu et al. The system is in favor of accessibility of the substrate to the active site of laccase, and thus the affinity to the substrate is improved greatly. On the other hand, the system can be applied in the fabrication of biofuel cells as the cathodic catalyst on the basis of its good electrocatalysis for oxygen reduction. More importantly, operation of the biosensor in pH 6.0 solution overcomes the restriction of fungi laccase exhibiting bioactivity in a solution of pH < 5.0 [138].

Tsai et al. used a composite of multiwalled CNTs–chitosan as a matrix for the entrapment of lactate dehydrogenase (LDH) onto a GCE in order to fabricate an amperometric biosensor. It was shown that the enzyme is homogeneously immobilized within MWCNT-CHIT-LDH. The inclusion of MWCNT within MWCNT-CHIT-LDH exhibits the abilities to raise the current responses, to decrease the electrooxidation potential of β-nicotinamide adenine dinucleotide, reduced form (NADH), and to prevent the electrode surface fouling [139].

The application of the composites of MWNTs and core–shell organosilica–chitosan-cross-linked nanospheres as an immobilization matrix for the construction of an amperometric hydrogen peroxide (H_2O_2) biosensor was described by Chen et al. MWNTs and positively charged organosilica–chitosan nanospheres were dispersed in acetic acid solution (0.6 wt%) to achieve organosilica–chitosan–MWNTs composites, which were cast onto a GCE surface directly. And then, HRP, as a model enzyme, was immobilized onto it through electrostatic interaction between oppositely charged organosilica–chitosan nanospheres and HRP. The direct electron transfer of HRP was achieved at HRP/organosilica–chitosan/MWNTs/GCE, which exhibited excellent electrocatalytic activity for the reduction of H_2O_2. Moreover, the proposed biosensor displayed a rapid response to H_2O_2 and possessed good stability and reproducibility. When used to detect H_2O_2 concentration in disinfector samples and sterilized milks, respectively, it showed satisfactory results [140].

8.5.4.5.2 Chemical Cross-Linking Methods

Further stabilization of the chitosan film containing SWNT (CHIT–SWNT) was performed by chemical cross-linking with GA, and free aldehyde groups produced a substrate used for covalent immobilization of galactose oxidase [141]. The use of dispersed CNTs as a transducer allows a very rapid detection of galactose with a sample throughput of 150 h^{-1} while retaining high selectivity and sensitivity. Moreover, the biosensor is mechanically robust, reliable and has been successfully used for the detection of galactose in blood plasma.

A graphite–epoxy resin composite electrode modified with functionalized MWCNTs immobilized by EDC and NHS in a chitosan matrix was prepared by Ghica et al. It was then used as a base for GOx immobilization by the simple method of cross-linking with GA using BSA as a carrier protein. The biosensor showed good reproducibility and good stability under continuous use and storage conditions. Selectivity against a number of interferences, such as wines, juices, or blood, was also good and the ascorbic acid response could be reduced using more negative potentials where the response to glucose increases [142].

Zou and coworkers describe a new type of amperometric cholesterol biosensor based on the enhancement effect of MWCNTs and sol–gel chitosan–silica hybrid composite films. The MWCNTs were treated with concentrated nitric acid and sulfuric acid to increase the solubility and dispersibility in solution. These authors chose chitosan reacting with meth-yltrimethoxysilane (MTOS) and the introduction of MWCNTs to form organic–inorganic hybrid composite films for the immobilization of cholesterol oxidase. The results show that analytical performance of the biosensor can be improved greatly after the introduction of the MWCNTs. This method has been used to determine the free cholesterol concentration in real human blood samples [143].

In order to avoid enzyme loss, cholesterol esterase and cholesterol oxidase have been immobilized using GA as a cross-linker onto sol–gel-derived silica/chitosan/MWCNT-based nanobiocomposite films deposited onto ITO glass for the estimation of esterified cholesterol [144]. It has been shown that this nanobiocomposite electrode can be used to estimate total cholesterol in serum samples.

8.5.4.6 Chitosan–Clay Composite Material

Clay is a stable aluminosilicate with a high cation-exchange capacity and different types of charges (permanent charges on the faces, pH-dependent charges at the edges), and exfoli-ated clay particles have a platelet shape with nanoscopic size. Compared with organic polyelectrolytes, clay has the advantages of high chemical stability, good adsorption prop-erty due to its appreciable surface area, special structural features, and unusual intercala-tion property.

The use of clay in making nanocomposites has recently been increased because of its cheap and easy availability. Chitosan beads or films aggregated with clay could enhance densities and mechanical strengths, thereby extending their application possibilities. Nanocomposites based on the intercalation of chitosan in clay are robust and stable three-dimensional (3D) materials by means of cationic exchange and hydrogen bonding processes.

8.5.4.6.1 Chitosan–Montmorillonite (MMT) Beads

Montmorillonite (MMT) as a natural cationic clay is the most widely used layered silicate in polymer nanocomposites. Chang and Juang prepared chitosan–clay (MMT) composite beads for immobilization of α-amylase, β-amylase, and glucoamylase by mixing an equal weight of activated clay and chitosan and cross-linked with GA. It was shown that the relative activities of immobilized enzymes are higher than free enzymes over broader pH and temperature ranges [145]. They also compared the properties of the β-glucosidase immobilized on wet (without freeze-drying) and dried (with freeze-drying) chitosan–clay composites. Although the reactivity of dried-composite enzyme was higher than that of the wet-composite enzyme, the wet-composite enzyme appeared much more reliable because a more stable behavior was observed from batch to batch. In addition, more logi-cal results and good storage stability were reported for wet-composite enzyme. Therefore, the wet-composite immobilized enzyme was more reliable if industrial applications were considered [146,147].

8.5.4.6.2 Chitosan–Synthetic Clay Composite Film

Laponite is a synthetic cationic clay of the formula of $(Mg_{5.5}Li_{0.5})Si_4O_{10}(OH)_2(Na^+_{0.73} \cdot nH_2O)$. Positively charged chitosan is expected to aggregate with negatively charged laponite nanoparticles. Different from laponite, layered double hydroxides (ldhs), $Zn_3Al(OH)_8Cl$, are anionic clays and display a layered structure built on a stacking of positive layers. The positively charged layer may be an attractive point to immobilize biomolecules depending on their IEP.

Fan et al. explore two phenol biosensors for phenol determination based on chitosan–laponite composite matrix and chitosan–ldhs composite film, respectively [148,149]. Chitosan was utilized to improve the analytical performance of the pure clay-modified bioelectrode. PPO was simply entrapped into this novel composite film. GA was avoided in making the biosensor. These biosensors exhibited good affinity to the substrate; the apparent Michaelis–Menten constant (K_m) for the chitosan–laponite sensor and the chitosan–ldh sensor was 0.16 and 0.13 mM, respectively. The enzyme electrode provided a linear response to catechol over a concentration range of 3.6×10^{-9} to 4×10^{-5} M with a sensitivity of 2750 ± 52 mA M^{-1} cm^{-2} for chitosan–laponite sensors and a concentration range of 5.3×10^{-9} to 4×10^{-5} M with a sensitivity of 674 ± 4 mA M^{-1} cm^{-2} for chitosan–ldhs sensors. It seems that substrate affinity and sensitivity of chitosan–ldhs sensors are relatively higher due to highly improved adhesive ability.

8.5.4.6.3 MMT–Chitosan–Gold Nanocomposite Film

Gold nanoparticles stabilized by chitosan (AuCS) were hybridized with exfoliated clay nanoplates through electrostatic interaction. The resulting clay (MMT)–chitosan–GNP nanocomposite (Clay–AuCS) was used to modify GCE. HRP, as a model peroxidase, was entrapped between the Clay–AuCS film and another clay layer. The results demonstrated that the quasireversible, surface-controlled electron transfer kinetics for HRP was realized on Clay–AuCS-modified GCE. The nanocomposite showed advantages over clay and AuCS alone in fabricating biosensors. Moreover, HRP retained its native secondary structure in the Clay–AuCS film and bioelectrocatalytic activity with good sensitivity and fast response toward hydrogen peroxide [150].

8.5.4.7 Chitosan–Inorganic Salt Composite Material

8.5.4.7.1 Chitosan–Nano-Calcium Carbonate Composite

A great challenge for the fabrication of biosensors comes from the effective immobilization of enzyme to the solid electrode surface. In recent years, calcium carbonate has been proved to intensify enzyme performance and has been widely used in industry, medicine, microcapsule fabrication, and many other bio-related fields. In particular, because of the large surface-to-volume ratio, the high hydrophilicity, and biocompatible characteristics, nanosized calcium carbonate (nano-$CaCO_3$) has been demonstrated to be a promising enzyme immobilization matrix.

Gong et al. present a facile approach for constructing a novel functional hybrid film composed of nano-$CaCO_3$–chitosan by a one-step coelectrodeposition method (Figure 8.14). The generated nano-$CaCO_3$-based matrix possessed a 3D porous, network-like structure, providing a favorable and biocompatible microenvironment to immobilize enzyme. By using such a composite film as an enzyme immobilization matrix, a highly sensitive and stable AChE sensor was achieved for the determination of methyl parathion as a model of organophosphate pesticide (OP) compounds. The detection limit was found to be as low as 1 ng mL^{-1} ($S/N = 3$). The designed biosensor exhibited good reproducibility and acceptable stability [151].

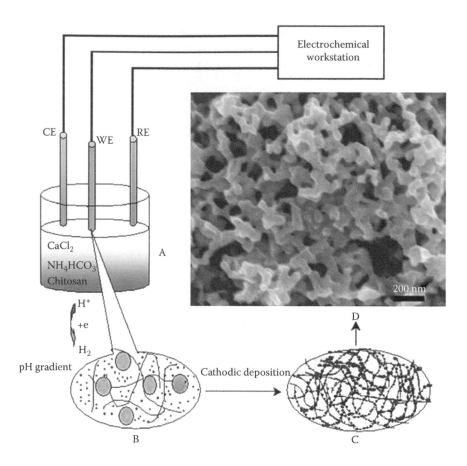

FIGURE 8.14
Illustration of the formation of the porous nano-CaCO$_3$–chitosan composite by coelectrodeposition (A–C) and SEM image of the nano-CaCO$_3$–chitosan composite film onto GCE (D). (From Gong, J. M. et al. 2009. *Electrochem Commun* 11: 1873–1876. With permission.)

8.5.4.7.2 Chitosan–Nano-Lanthanum Phosphate Composite

Monazite, especially lanthanum phosphate, has long been known as a ceramic material with high-temperature stability, chemical inertness/nonreactivity toward other ceramic oxidases, and catalytic property. Nanosized NdPO$_4$ shows greater advantages and novel characteristics than regular-sized particles, such as the much larger specific surface area. These properties may provide favorable conditions for enzyme or protein immobilization.

The direct electrochemistry of GOx immobilized on a composite matrix based on chitosan and NdPO$_4$ nanoparticles underlying on GCE was achieved [152]. The proposed biosensor can catalyze the reduction of dissolved oxygen, and glucose determination was achieved based on the decrease of peak currents due to the reduction of dissolved oxygen. The proposed composite glucose biosensor can be used for the determination of glucose in human plasma. Furthermore, an improved stability, reproducibility, and efficiency in excluding the interferences of uric acid and ascorbic acid were also obtained.

8.5.4.7.3 Chitosan–Calcium Phosphate Composite

Calcium phosphate, the main inorganic component of bone, is of superior biocompatibility, insolubility, and mechanical stability, and has been proven to be suitable for enzyme immobilization. Compared with silica, the common material in immobilized enzymes, calcium phosphate has good biocompatibility and can be prepared in mild conditions.

A novel kind of calcium phosphate-mineralized chitosan–alginate microcapsule was prepared through a bioinspired process for efficient encapsulation of yeast alcohol dehydrogenase (YADH) (Figure 8.15). In this biomimetic process, when Ca^{2+}-containing chitosan droplets were added into a phosphate-containing solution of alginate, a thin chitosan–alginate film formed immediately around the microcapsules coupled with *in situ* precipitation of calcium phosphate. The biomineralization of calcium phosphate was mimicked by the counter diffusion system in which Ca^{2+} ions and phosphate ions migrated into the chitosan–alginate film from opposite directions, respectively. YADH encapsulated in the microcapsules exhibited significantly higher activity and recycling stability in a broader temperature range than the free YADH. These hybrid materials will find promising applications in enzyme encapsulation and drug delivery systems [153].

8.5.4.7.4 Chitosan-Silica-$K_3Fe(CN)_6$ Hybrid Film

Li et al. developed a simple and effective strategy for the fabrication of hydrogen peroxide (H_2O_2) biosensors by entrapping HRP in chitosan–silica sol–gel hybrid membranes (CSHMs) doped with potassium ferricyanide ($K_3Fe(CN)_6$) and GNPs on platinum electrode surface. The hybrid membranes are prepared by cross-linking chitosan with APTES, while the presence of GNPs improved the conductivity of CSHMs, and the $Fe(CN)_6^{3-/4-}$ was used as a mediator to transfer electrons. $K_3Fe(CN)_6$, the most widely used inorganic electron mediator, has been extensively used in biosensors because of its excellent electron transferability and high degree of reversibility. Moreover, due to the possible control over pore size and hydrophobicity, the mediators could be attached specifically to the composite

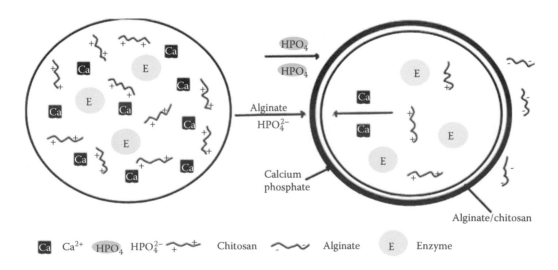

FIGURE 8.15
Schematic representation of the formation process of calcium phosphate-mineralized chitosan–alginate microcapsules. (From Jiang, Y. J. et al. 2008. *Ind Eng Chem Res* 47: 2495–2501. With permission.)

TABLE 8.2

Enzymes Immobilized on Chitin/Chitosan-Based Materials

Enzyme	Application	Support (Preparation Method—Cross-Linking Agents)	Immobilization Method (Cross-Linking Agents)	References
α-Amylase	B.	Reversed chitosan–alginate beads (i)	III-i	[91]
	F.	Chitosan microbeads (a and d-GA)	II-i	[26]
	F.	Chitosan–MMT composite beads (b and d-GA)	II-iii (GA)	[145]
β-Amylase	F.	Chitosan–MMT composite beads (b and d-GA)	II-iii (GA)	[145]
Acetylcholinesterase	E. Pesticide determination	Chitosan-tethered PANMV membrane (d-EDC and NHS)	II-iii (GA)	[86]
	E.	Nano-CaCO$_3$–chitosan composite film (f)	I-i	[151]
Acid phosphatase	F.	Chitosan beads (b and d-GA)	II-iii	[29]
	F.	Chitosan–ZrO$_2$ composite beads (b and d-GA)	II-iii	[115]
Acylase	D. Biofouling control in the membrane bioreactor	Magnetic MIEX-PSS-chitosan microspheres (j)	I-i or II-iii (GA)	[109]
Allinase	F.	Succinyl anhydride-chitosan as pH-sensitive support (h)	II-i (GA)	[71]
L-Asparaginase	B.	Carboxymethyl konjac glucomannan/chitosan nanocapsule (i)	III-i	[95]
Catalase	A. Degradation of H$_2$O$_2$	Chitosan beads (d-diphosphate and glyoxal and GA)	II-iii (GA)	[80]
	F.	Cu^{2+}-chitosan-beads (d-GA)	I-i and II-iii	[50]
	F.	CB-chitosan beads (d-diphosphate and glyoxal and GA)	I-iii and II-iii	[51]
	F.	Poly(itaconic acid) grafted and/or Fe^{3+} ions incorporated chitosan membranes (b and h)	I-i or I-ii	[76]
Anti-CEA	E. Immunosensor	Anti-CEA/nano-Au–chitosan/NG/GCE films (j)	I-i	[124]
D-Carbamoylase	B. d-Amino acids production	Alginate–chitosan capsules (i)	III-i	[90]
Cellulase	F.	Polyanionic modified PVA-coated chitosan beads (i)	II-iii (ECO)	[100]
Cholesterol esterase	E. Total cholesterol sensor	Silica–chitosan–MWCNT hybrid composite film (d-MTOS)	II-iii (GA)	[144]
Cholesterol oxidase	E. Total cholesterol sensor	Silica–chitosan–MWCNT hybrid composite film (d-MTOS)	II-iii (GA)	[144]
	E. Cholesterol biosensor	Silica–chitosan–MWCNT hybrid composite film (d-MTOS)	III-i	[143]
	E. Cholesterol biosensor	Chitosan–alginic acid complexation network (i)	III-i	[92]
	E. Cholesterol biosensor	CeO$_2$–chitosan hybrid composites (a)	I-i	[118]
Chymotrypsin	F.	Chitosan–biopolymer complexation beads (b)	II-iii (GA or Gly or ECO)	[23]
DNA	E.	Chitosan films (f)	II-iii (GA)	[60]
DNA-Cu(II)	E. Measurement of H$_2$O$_2$	DNA–Cu(II)–chitosan complexation films (i)	III-i	[98]
Anti-factor B	E. Detection of factor B	Factor B–alginate conjugate/Chitosan films (i)	V (EDC)	[93]

Enzyme	Application	Support	Immobilization method	Refs
Galactose oxidase	E. Analysis of galactose	Chitosan–SWNT (d-GA)	II-iii (GA)	[141]
β-Galactosidase	F.	Macrochitosan precipitates (b)	II-iii (GA)	[37]
	F.	Microchitosan particles (d-GA)	II-iii (GA)	[89]
	F.	Nanochitosan particles (c-TPP and d-GA)	II-iii (GA)	
	F.	Alginate–chitosan core–shell microcapsules (i)	III	
β-D-Galactosidase	A. GOS synthesis	Fe_3O_4-chitosan beads (c-TPP)	II-iii (GA)	[107]
Glucoamylase	F.	Chitosan–MMT composite beads (b and d-GA)	IV(GA)	[145]
Glucose oxidase	F.	Hydrophobically modified chitosan nanoparticles	III-i	[66–67]
	F.	L-Lysine-modified cross-linked chitosan resin (d-GA)	I-i	[70]
	F.	CMP/chitosan-magnetic nanowires (j)	V (EDC and NHS)	[111]
	E. Glucose sensor	Chitosan-AY9-GA films (a and d-GA)	I-iii	[52]
	E.	Chitosan-tethered alumina membrane (a)	III-i	[88]
	E.	FMC-AFSNPs–chitosan composite films (a)	III-i	[104]
	E.	Chitosan-$NiFe_2O_4$ nanoparticles (a)	III-i	[103]
	E.	Nano-Au–chitosan composite (f)	I-i	[120–122]
	E.	$NdPO_4$ nanoparticles/chitosan composite film (a)	III	[152]
	F.	Porous gels of chitosan–SiO_2 (d-TMOS)	II-iii (formaldehyde)	[128]
	E.	ZrO_2–Chitosan composite (a)	I-i	[114]
	E.	Functionalized MWCNT-chitosan films (d-EDC and NHS)	II-ii (GA)	[142]
	E.	Au-Pt alloy NPs/CNTs/chitosan (f)	II-iii (GA)	[123]
	E.	Chitosan-coated wires (f)	IV	[59]
β-Glucosidase	F.	Chitosan–clay composite beads (b and d-GA)	II-iii (GA)	[146,147]
	F.	Chitosan beads (b and d-GA)	II-iii	[29]
Glutamate dehydrogenase	E. Ammonium determination	Chitosan film (a)	III	[25]
L-Glutamate oxidase	E. Glutamate detection	ZnO-chitosan nanobiocomposite film (a)	I-i	[113]
		Glutamate oxidase–chitosan complexation films (i)	III	[97]
Glycosidase-Ara	A. Increase wine aroma	Chitin powders	II-iii (GA)	[68]
		Chitosan powders	II-iii (GA)	
		DE-chitosan powders	I-i and II-i (GA or DEP or SUB or EDC)	

(continued)

TABLE 8.2 (continued)

Enzymes Immobilized on Chitin/Chitosan-Based Materials

Enzyme	Application	Support (Preparation Method—Cross-Linking Agents)	Immobilization Method (Cross-Linking Agents)	References
Glycosidase-Rha	A. Oenology	Chitin or chitosan powders (b-GA)	I and II-i(GA) or II-ii (GA) or II-iii (GA)	[20]
Rha and βG	A. Increase wine aroma	Chitosan powders (d-Gly)	I-i and II-i (GA)	[44]
βG and Rha and Ara	A. Increase wine aroma	Chitosan– other biopolymer complexation (b and d-GA)	III following II-ii (GA)	[82]
Recombinant β-glycosidase	B. Hydrolysis of oleuropein	Chitosan precipitates (b)	I-i and II(GA)	[27]
Hemoglobin	E. H_2O_2 sensor	Chitosan films (b)	II-iii (GA)	[32]
	E. H_2O_2 sensor	Nano-Au/L-cysteine/nano-Au/nano-Pt–chitosan film (j)	I-i	[125]
Horseradish peroxidase	F.	Chitosan-grafted-polyethyl acrylate beads (h)	II-iii (acyl azide)	[77]
	E. Determine redox process	TiO_2–chitosan composite matrix (a)	I-i	[116]
	E. H_2O_2 sensor	Ti/TiO_2 nanotubes/Au/chitosan-HRP (a)	III-i	[117]
	E. H_2O_2 sensor	Chitosan–silica hybrid film (d-TMOS)	III-ii	[16]
	E. H_2O_2 sensor	Chitosan–silica hybrid membranes (d-THEOS)	III-i	[130]
	E. H_2O_2 sensor	Chitosan–silica porous hybrid membranes (d-GPTMS)	II-i	[131]
	E. H_2O_2 sensor	Chitosan–silica hybrid membranes (d-APDMOS)	I and III-ii	[129]
	E. H_2O_2 sensor	Chitosan–silica-$K_3Fe(CN)_6$ hybrid membranes (d-APTES)	III-i	[154]
	E. H_2O_2 sensor	Organosilica–chitosan-MWCNT composite (a)	I-i	[140]
	E. H_2O_2 sensor	Clay–chitosan–gold nanoparticle nanocomposite (a)	III-i	[150]
	E. Sensing peroxide	Horseradish peroxidase/chitosan films (j)	I-i	[96]
Human serum albumin	E. Detection of hesperidin	Chitosan/GA/cysteamine/Au-colloid film (j)	I-i	[126]
D-Hydantoinase	B. d-Amino acids production	Alginate–chitosan capsules (i)	III	[90]
ChBD-fused D-hydantoinase	F.	Chitin beads	I-iv	[18]
Invertase	F.	Invertase–chitosan conjugate on alginate-coated chitin (i)	V (Periodate)	[80]
	F.	Chitosan microbeads (a and d-GA)	II-i	[26]
Laccase	C. Dichlorophenol removal	Chitosan powder (b and d-GA)	III-i	[28]
	C. Reactive dyes degradation	$Fe3O_4$–chitosan beads (b)	II-iii (GA)	[105]

Enzyme	Application	Support	Method	References
	F.	Fe$_3$O$_4$–chitosan microspheres (d-GA and b)	II-iii (GA)	[106]
	F.	LACCASE–CHITOSAN CONJUGATE (PH RESPONSIBILITY)	V (EDC)	[78,79]
	E. Determination of rutin	Laccase–chitosan conjugate gel (a-GA)		
	E. Oxygen reduction analysis	Chitosan microspheres (c-TPP)	III-i	[34]
	E. Lactate biosensor	CNTs–chitosan composite (a)	III-i	[128]
Lactate dehydrogenase		MWCNT–chitosan composite (a)	III-i	[139]
ChBD-fused levansucrase	F.	Chitin beads	I-iv	[19]
Lipase	F.	Chitosan nanoparticles (c-TPP)	I-i	[36]
	F.	Chitosan beads	II-iii (GA and EDC), II-iv (GA and EDC), II-iv (EDC and GA)	[47]
	F.	Xanthan-chitosan beads (i)	III-i	[55]
Lipase	F.	Chitosan beads	II-iii (GA)	[42]
	A. Alcoholysis of salicornia oil	Chitosan powders	II-iii (GA)	[41]
	A. Fatty acid esterifications	Chitosan films (e)	I-i	[54]
	D. Butyl oleate synthesis	Chitosan films (e and d-GA)	II-iii	
		Chitosan films (e and d-CE)	II-iii	
	F.	Chitosan beads (b)	II-iii (EDC)	[43]
	F.	Chitosan particles (b)	II-iii (Gly, GA, ECO), II-iii (Gly and GA)	[21]
	F.	Chitosan nanofibrous membrane (f)	II-iii (GA)	[63]
	F.	Amino acid-modified chitosan beads (h)	II-iii (GA)	[69]
	F.	ACHCA–modified chitosan membranes (h and d-photo cross-link)	III	[73]
	F.	Chitosan-tethered PANCMA hollow fiber membrane (d- EDC and NHS)	II-iii (GA)	[83,84]
	F.	Chitosan-tethered nanofibrous PANCMA membranes (d- EDC and NHS)	II-iii (GA)	[17]
	F.	Fe$_3$O$_4$/chitosan nanoparticles (c-TPP and *in situ* polymerization)	I-i	[108]
	F.	Chitosan beads (c-TPP)	III-i	[33]
	F.	Chitosan nanoparticles (b)	I and II-i (GA)	[31]

(continued)

TABLE 8.2 (continued)

Enzymes Immobilized on Chitin/Chitosan-Based Materials

Enzyme	Application	Support (Preparation Method—Cross-Linking Agents)	Immobilization Method (Cross-Linking Agents)	References
Organophosphorus hydrolase	E. Detection of organophosphorus compounds	PTAA–chitosan films (j)	I-i	[99]
Pectinase	F.	Fe_3O_4/SiO_2-g-PSS/chitosan particles (j)	II-iii (GA)	[110]
	F.	SiO_2-coated chitosan particles (d-GA)	II-iii (GA)	[136]
	F.	Spherical polyelectrolyte brush-chitosan particles (j and d-GA)	II-iii (GA)	[137]
Pepsin	F.	Chitosan beads (d-diphosphate and glyoxal and d-GA)	II-iii (GA)	[39]
Peroxidase (from gilo crude extract)	E. Determination of hydroquinone	Chitosan powders	II-iii (GA and EDC)	[48]
	E. Determination of hydroquinone	Chitosan powders	II-iii (GA and ECO)	[49]
Polyphenol oxidase	C. Phenolic effluent bioremediation	Chitosan-tethered polysulfone capillary membranes (b)	I-i	[87]
	E.	Laponite clay–chitosan nanocomposite film (a)	III-i	[148]
	E.	Chitosan/layered double hydroxides composite film (a)	III-i	[149]
Proteinase	F.	Chitosan nanoparticles(c-TPP:)	I-i	[35]
Pullulanase	F.	Fe_3O_4-chitosan beads (d-MBA and UV irradiation)	II-iii (GA)	[112]
ssODN	E. Sequence-specific oligonucleotide detection	Chitosan-Au-MPA precipitates films (d-EDC and NHS)	II-iii (EDC and NHS)	[127]
Sulfite oxidase	E. Analysis of sulfite ions	Chitosan-grafted-poly(butyl acrylate) membrane (h-photo cross-link)	II-iii (p-benzoquinone)	[75]
Trypsin	E. Digestion of protein	Chitosan/hyaluronic acid films (j)	I-i	[94]
	F.	Hydrophobically modified chitosan nanoparticles (h)	II-iii (GA)	[65]
	F.	Metal ion-chelated macroporous chitosan-silica gel beads (d-EDC)	I-ii	[133,134]
	F.	Chitosan particles (b)	II-iii (Gly or GA)	[45]
Tyrosinase	E. Oxidase enzyme biosensor	TiO_2-CeO_2-chitosan hybrid composites(a)	III-i	[119]
Urease	F.	Chitosan-poly(glycidyl methacrylate) copolymer precipitate	II-iii (GA)	[74]

Enzyme	Application	Support	Immobilization	Ref.
	F.	Chitosan-tethered PANMV membrane (d-EDC and NHS)	II-iii (GA)	[85]
	E. Urea sensor	ZnO–chitosan nanobiocomposite film (a)	I-i	[113]
Urease and glutamate dehydrogenase	E. Urea sensor	Fe₃O₄–chitosan precipitations (a)	I-i	[101]
Yeast alcohol dehydrogenase	F.	Calcium phosphate-mineralized chitosan–alginate microcapsule (i)	III-i	[153]

Notes: Application of immobilization enzyme: (A) food industry; (B) pharmaceutical industries; (C) environmental industries; (D) other industries; (E) biosensors; (F) separation, purification, and recovery of enzymes; (G) immobilization study.

Support preparation methods: (a) solvent evaporation method; (b) phase-inversion technique; (c) ionotropic gelation method; (d) chemical cross-linking method; (e) freezing–thawing treatment; (f) electrodeposition method; (g) electrospinning method; (h) chemical modified; (i) PECs; (j) LBL self-assembly.

Immobilizations methods: (I) Adsorption of enzyme on support: (I-i) physical adsorption, (I-ii) affinity by dye, (I-iii) affinity by metal ion, (I-iv) affinity by ChBD; (II) chemical cross-link by covalent binding: (II-i) in the presence of enzyme solution, (II-ii) in the absence of enzyme solution (enzyme may be absorbed or entrapped), (II-iii) on agents-activated support, (II-iv) cross-linking by covalent binding of enzyme to one agent-activated support following cross-linking with the other agent; (III) entrapment: (III-i) enzyme within a polymer network, (III-ii) covering a film on the surface of enzyme; (IV) electrochemically conjugate protein; (V) Enzyme–chitosan conjugate.

Abbreviations:

Enzyme: α-L-arabinofuranosidase-Ara; Chitin-binding domain—ChBD; β-ᴅ-glucopyranosidase—βG; α-ᴅ-glucopyranosidase—Rha; carcinoembryonic antigen—CEA; A 20-mer single-stranded oligodeoxyribonucleotide—ssODN.

Application: Galactooligosaccharides—GOS.

Agents: α-cyano-4-hydroxycinnamated—ACHCA; (3-acryloxypropyl) dimethoxy methyl silane—APDMOS; 3-amino propyl tri ethoxy silane—APTES; 18-crown-6 ether—CE; 2-diethylaminochloroethane—DE; 1,2-7,8 diepoxyoctane—DEP; epichlorohydrin—ECO; 1-ethyl-3-(3-dimethylaminopropyl) carbodiimide hydrochloride—EDC; glutaraldehyde—GA; glycidol—Gly; γ-glycidoxypropyltrimethoxysilane—GPTMS; *N*,*N*-methylene-bis-(acrylamide)—MBA; methyltrimethoxysilane—MTOS; *N*-hydroxysulfosuccinimide—NHS; poly(thiophene-3-acetic acid)—PTAA; dimethylsuberimidate dihydrochloride—SUB; tetraethoxysilane—TEOS; tetrakis(2-hydroxy ethyl) orthosilicates—THEOS; tetramethoxysilane—TMOS; sodium tripolyphosphate—TPP; tetrasodium pyrophosphate—TSPP.

Supports: Acetyl Yellow 9—AY9; cibacron blue F3GA—CB; carboxymethylpullulan—CMP; carbon nanotube—CNT; ferrocene monocarboxylic acid functionalized Fe₃O₄-SiO₂ nanoparticles conjugate—FMC-AFSNPs; layer-by-layer—LBL; glassy carbon electrode—GCE; Montmorillonite—MMT; 3-mercaptopropionic acid—MPA; multiwalled carbon nanotube—MWCNT; nanostructure gold—NG; Poly(vinyl alcohol)—PVA; polyelectrolyte complexes—PECs; polystyrene sulfonate—PSS; single-walled carbon nanotube—SWCNT.

film, by which the leaching of the mediators from the composite is avoided. At the same time, negatively charged $Fe(CN)_6^{3-/4-}$ can also be tightly adsorbed within CSHMs containing robust positively charged amino groups by electrostatic interactions. CSHMs exhibit higher sensibility, wider linear range, lower detection limit, and better reproducibility and stability. In addition, this biosensor has strong antiinterference to some potential interfering substances [154].

8.6 Outlook

Chitosan/chitin, an abundant raw material, has been proved to be an excellent support for enzyme immobilization because of its hydrophilicity, biocompatibility, and biodegradability. Most of the enzymes immobilized on chitosan/chitin-based supports, reported in the literature in the last decade, are presented in Table 8.2. New methods of enzyme immobilization such as enzyme affinity by ChBD, MPA by epoxy activation of chitosan or binary immobilization, and electrochemically conjugating protein with chitosan have been used, which improved enzyme activity, stability, and selectivity. Predominantly, chitosan, pure or forming hybrids with other polymers or inorganic materials, contains a high density of primary amine and hydroxyl groups that can be cross-linked, chemically modified, or grafted. The new preparation methods of chitosan-based supports, such as freezing–thawing treatment, electrodeposition, electrospinning, LBL self-assembly and cross-linking by silylating agents, offer many opportunities for the application of immobilization enzymes, especially biosensors via chitosan–inorganic composites.

However, some supports are still difficult to fabricate in batches, and the cost is relatively high, which limits their application. In addition, few works have investigated the effect of the molecular size of chitosan and the degree of deacetylation on the new process of enzyme immobilization. These two properties influence chitosan's solubility, functionality, and reactivity and hence the properties of the immobilization enzyme. As these approaches are successfully applied to a wider range of enzymes, and production methods are developed for larger quantities, I anticipate that the resulting biocatalytic materials will enable new and expanded use of enzymes in practical applications such as biosensors and bioconversions.

Acknowledgment

The author would like to thank Professor K. D. Yao who offered the opportunity to write this chapter. The author's knowledge has certain boundaries. Therefore, there must be many mistakes in this chapter. It is hoped that the readers will kindly point out errors.

References

1. Iyer, P. V., and Ananthanarayan, L. 2008. Enzyme stability and stabilization—Aqueous and non-aqueous environment. *Process Biochem* 43: 1019–1032.

2. Krajewska, B. 2004. Application of chitin-and chitosan-based materials for enzyme immobilizations: A review. *Enzyme Microb Technol* 35: 126–139.

3. Bommarius, A. S. and Riebel, B. R. 2004. *Biocatalysis: Fundamentals and Applications*. Wiley-VCH: Germany, p. 611.

4. Cao, L. Q. 2005. Immobilised enzymes: Science or art? *Curr Opin Chem Biol* 9: 217–226.

5. Brady, D. and Jordaan, J. 2009. Advances in enzyme immobilization. *Biotechnol Lett* 31: 1639–1650.

6. Mateo, C., Palomo, J. M., Fernandez-Lorente, G., Guisan, J. M., and Fernandez-Lafuente, R. 2007. Improvement of enzyme activity, stability and selectivity via immobilization techniques. *Enzyme Microb Technol* 40: 1451–1463.

7. Langen, V., L. M., Selassa, R. P., Rantwijk, F. V., and Sheldon, R. A. 2005. Cross-linked aggregates of (R)-oxynitrilase: A stable, recyclable biocatalyst for enantioselective hydrocyanation. *Org Lett* 7: 327–329.

8. Illanes, A., Wilson, L., Caballero, E., Fernández-Lafuente, R., and Guisán, J. M. 2006. Cross-linked penicillin acylase aggregates for synthesis of beta-lactam antibiotics in organic medium. *Appl Biochem Biotechnol* 133: 189–202.

9. Prabhavathi Devi, B. L. A., Guo, Z., and Xu, X. B. 2009. Characterization of cross-linked lipase aggregates. *J Am Oil Chem Soc* 86: 637–642.

10. Kim, J., Grate, J. W., and Wang, P. 2006. Nanostructures for enzyme stabilization. *Chem Eng Sci* 61: 1017–1026.

11. Ge, J., Lu, D. N., Liu, Z. X., and Liu, Z. 2009. Recent advances in nanostructured biocatalysts. *Biochem Eng J* 44: 53–59.

12. Jia, H., Zhu, G., and Wang, P. 2003. Catalytic behaviors of enzymes attached to nanoparticles: The effect of particle mobility. *Biotechnol Bioeng* 84: 406–414.

13. Wang, Z. G., Wan, L. S., Liu, Z. M., Huang, X. J., and Xu, Z. K. 2009. Enzyme immobilization on electrospun polymer nanofibers: An overview. *J Mol Catal B: Enzyme* 56: 189–195.

14. Wang, J. 2005. Carbon-Nanotube Based Electrochemical Biosensors: A Review. *Electroanal* 17: 7–14.

15. Avnir, D., Braun, S., Lev, O., and Ottolenghi, M. 1994. Enzymes and other proteins entrapped in sol–gel materials. *Chem Mater* 6: 1605–1614.

16. Miao, Y. and Tan, S. N. 2001. Amperometric hydrogen peroxide biosensor with silica sol–gel/ chitosan film as immobilization matrix. *Analytica Chimica Acta* 437: 87–93.

17. Ye, P., Xu, Z. K., Wu, J., Innocentd, C., and Seta, P. 2006. Nanofibrous poly(acrylonitrile-*co*-maleic acid) membranes functionalized with gelatin and chitosan for lipase immobilization. *Biomaterials* 27: 4169–4176.

18. Chern, J. T. and Chao, Y. P. 2005. Chitin-binding domain based immobilization of D-hydantoinase. *J Biotechnol* 117: 267–275.

19. Chiang, C. J., Wang, J. Y., Chen, P. T., and Chao, Y. P. 2009. Enhanced levan production using chitin-binding domain fused levansucrase immobilized on chitin beads. *Appl Microbiol Biotechnol* 82: 445–451.

20. Spagna, G., Andreani, F., Salatelli, E., Romagnoli, D., and Pifferi, P. G. 1998. Immobilization of α-L-arabinofuranosidase on chitin and chitosan. *Process Biochem* 33: 57–62.

21. Rodrigues, D. S., Mendes, A. A., Adriano, W. S., Gonçalves L. R. B., and Giordano, R. L. C. 2008. Multipoint covalent immobilization of microbial lipase on chitosan and agarose activated by different methods. *J Mol Catal B: Enzyme* 51: 100–109.

22. Hung, T. C., Giridhar, R., Chiou, S. H., and Wu, W. T. 2003. Binary immobilization of *Candida rugosa* lipase on chitosan. *J Mol Catal B: Enzyme* 26: 69–78.

23. Adriano, W. S., Mendonça, D. B., Rodrigues, D. S., Mammarella, E. J., and Giordano, R. L. C. 2008. Improving the properties of chitosan as support for the covalent multipoint immobilization of chymotrypsin. *Biomacromolecules* 9: 2170–2179.

24. Shi, X. W., Yang, X., Gaskell, K. J., Liu, Y., Kobatake, E., Bentley, W. E., and Payne, G. F. 2009 Reagentless protein assembly triggered by localized electrical signals. *Adv Mater* 21: 984–988.

25. Azmi, N. E., Ahmad, M., Abdullah, J., Sidek, H., Heng, L. Y., and Karuppiah, N. 2009. Biosensor based on glutamate dehydrogenase immobilized in chitosan for the determination of ammonium in water samples. *Anal Biochem* 388: 28–32.

26. González Siso, M. I., Lang, E., Carrenö-Gómez, B., Otero Espinar, M. B. F., and Blanco Méndez, J. 1997. Enzyme encapsulation on chitosan microbeads. *Process Biochem* 32: 211–216.

27. Briante, R., Cara, F. L., Febbraio, F., Barone, R., Piccialli, G., Carolla, R., Mainolfi, P. et al. 2000. Hydrolysis of oleuropein by recombinant β-glycosidase from hyperthermophilic archaeon *Sulfolobus solfataricus* immobilised on chitosan matrix. *J Biotechnol* 77: 275–286.

28. Zhang, J. B., Xu, Z. Q., Chen, H., and Zong, Y. R. 2009. Removal of 2,4-dichlorophenol by chitosan-immobilized laccase from *Coriolus versicolor*. *Biochem Eng J* 45: 54–59.

29. Juang, R. S., Wu, F. C., and Tseng, R. L. 2002. Use of chemically modified chitosan beads for sorption and enzyme immobilization. *Adv Environ Res* 6: 171–177.

30. Yi, S. S., Lee, C. W., Kim, J., Kyung, D., Kim, B. G., and Lee, Y. S. 2007. Covalent immobilization of *v*-transaminase from *Vibrio fluvialis* JS17 on chitosan beads. *Process Biochem* 42: 895–898.

31. Wu, Y., Wang, Y. J., Luo, G. S., and Dai, Y. Y. 2010. Effect of solvents and precipitant on the properties of chitosan nanoparticles in a water-in-oil microemulsion and its lipase immobilization performance. *Bioresour Technol* 101: 841–844.

32. Zhang, Y. Y., Hu, X., Tang, K., and Zou, G. L. 2006. Immobilization of hemoglobin on chitosan films as mimetic peroxidase. *Process Biochem* 41: 2410–2416.

33. Betigeri, S. S. and Neau, S. H. 2002. Immobilization of lipase using hydrophilic polymers in the form of hydrogel beads. *Biomaterials* 23: 3627–3636.

34. Fernandes, S. C., Oliveira, I. R. W. Z., Fatibello-Filho, O., Spinelli, A., and Vieira, I. C. 2008. Biosensor based on laccase immobilized on microspheres of chitosan cross-linked with tripolyphosphate. *Sens Actuators B* 133: 202–207.

35. Tang, Z. X., Qian, J. Q., and Shi, L. E. 2006. Characterizations of immobilized neutral proteinase on chitosan nano-particles. *Process Biochem* 41: 1193–1197.

36. Tang, Z. X., Qian, J. Q., and Shi, L. E. 2007. Characterizations of immobilized neutral lipase on chitosan nano-particles. *Mater Lett* 61: 37–40.

37. Biró, E., Németh, Á. S., Sisak, C., Feczkó, T., and Gyenis, J. 2008. Preparation of chitosan particles suitable for enzyme immobilization. *J Biochem Biophys Methods* 70: 1240–1246.

38. Çetinus, Ş. A. and Öztop, H. N. 2003. Immobilization of catalase into chemically cross-linked chitosan beads. *Enzyme Microb Technol* 32: 889–894.

39. Altun, G. D. and Cetinus, S. A. 2007. Immobilization of pepsin on chitosan beads. *Food Chem* 100: 964–971.

40. Betancor, L., López-Gallego, F., Hidalgo, A., Alonso-Morales, N., Dellamora-Ortiz G., Mateo, C., Fernández-Lafuente, R., and Guisán, J. M. 2006. Different mechanisms of protein immobilization on glutaraldehyde activated supports: Effect of support activation and immobilization conditions. *Enzyme Microb Technol* 39: 877–882.

41. Foresti, M. L. and Ferreira, M. L. 2007. Chitosan-immobilized lipases for the catalysis of fatty acid esterifications. *Enzyme Microb Technol* 40: 769–777.

42. Desai, P. D., Dave, A. M., and Devi, S. 2006. Alcoholysis of salicornia oil using free and covalently bound lipase onto chitosan beads. *Food Chem* 95: 193–199.

43. Chiou, S. H. and Wu, W. T. 2004. Immobilization of *Candida rugosa* lipase on chitosan with activation of the hydroxyl groups. *Biomaterials* 25: 197–204.

44. Spagna, G., Andreani, F., Salatelli, E., Romagnoli, D., Casarini, D., and Pifferi, P. G. 1998. Immobilization of the glycosidases: α-L-Arabinofuranosidase and β-D-glucopyranosidase from *Aspergillus niger* on a chitosan derivative to increase the aroma of wine. Part II. *Enzyme Microb Technol* 23: 413–421.

45. Manrich, A., Galvão, Ć. M. A., Jesus, C. D. F., Giordano, R. C., and Giordano, R. L. C. 2008. Immobilization of trypsin on chitosan gels: Use of different activation protocols and comparison with other supports. *Int J Biol Macromol* 43: 54–61.

46. Cochrane, F. C., Petach, H. H., and Henderson, W. 1996. Application of tris(hydroxymethyl) phosphine as a coupling agent for alcohol dehydrogenase immobilization. *Enzyme Microb Technol* 18: 373–378.
47. Hung, T. C., Giridhar, R., Chiou, S. H., and Wu, W. T. 2003. Binary immobilization of *Candida rugosa* lipase on chitosan. *J Mol Catal B: Enzyme* 26: 69–78.
48. de Oliveira, I. R. W. Z. and Vieira, I. C. 2006. Immobilization procedures for the development of a biosensor for determination of hydroquinone using chitosan and gilo (*Solanum gilo*). *Enzyme Microb Technol* 38: 449–456.
49. de Oliveira, I. R. W. Z., Fernandes, S. C., and Vieira, I. C. 2006. Development of a biosensor based on gilo peroxidase immobilized on chitosan chemically cross-linked with epichlorohydrin for determination of rutin. *J Pharm Biome Anal* 41: 366–372.
50. Çetinus, Ş. A., Şahin, E., and Saraydin, D. 2009. Preparation of Cu(II) adsorbed chitosan beads for catalase immobilization. *Food Chem* 114: 962–969.
51. Çetinus, Ş. A., Öztop, H. N., and Saraydin, D. 2007. Immobilization of catalase onto chitosan and cibacron blue F3GA attached chitosan beads. *Enzyme Microb Technol* 41: 447–454.
52. Wei, X., Cruz, J., and Gorski, W. 2002. Integration of enzymes and electrodes: Spectroscopic and electrochemical studies of chitosan-enzyme films. *Anal Chem* 74: 5039–5046.
53. Orrego, C. E. and Valencia, J. S. 2009. Preparation and characterization of chitosan membranes by using a combined freeze gelation and mild cross-linking method. *Bioprocess Biosyst Eng* 32: 197–206.
54. Orrego, C. E., Salgado, N., Valencia, J. S., Giraldo, G. I., Giraldo, O. H., and Cardona, C. A. 2010. Novel chitosan membranes as support for lipases immobilization: Characterization aspects. *Carbohydr Polym* 79: 9–16.
55. Magnin, D., Dumitriu, S., Magny, P., and Chornet, E. 2001. Lipase immobilization into porous chitoxan beads: Activities in aqueous and organic media and lipase localization. *Biotechnol Prog* 17: 734–737.
56. Chen, J. P. and Lin, W. S. 2003. Sol–gel powders and supported sol–gel polymers for immobilization of lipase in ester synthesis. *Enzyme Microb Technol* 32: 801–811.
57. Fernandes, R., Wu, L. Q., Chen, T. H., Yi, H. M., Rubloff, G. W., Ghodssi, R., Bentley, W. E., and Payne, G. F. 2003. Electrochemically induced deposition of a polysaccharide hydrogel onto a patterned surface. *Langmuir* 19: 4058–4062.
58. Yi, H., Wu, L. Q., Bentley, W. E., Ghodssi, R., Rubloff, G. W., Culver, J. N., and Payne, G. F. 2005. Biofabrication with chitosan. *Biomacromolecules* 6: 2881–2894.
59. Meyer, W. L., Liu, Y., Shi, X. W., Yang, X. H., Bentley, W. E., and Payne, G. F. 2009. Chitosan-coated wires: Conferring electrical properties to chitosan fibers. *Biomacromolecules* 10: 858–864.
60. Yi, H. M., Wu, L. Q., Sumner, J. J., Gillespie, J. B., Payne, G. F., and Bentley, W. E. 2003. Chitosan scaffolds for biomolecular assembly: Coupling nucleic acid probes for detecting hybridization. *Biotechnol Bioeng* 83: 646–652.
61. Geng, X. Y., Kwon, O. H., and Jang, J. 2005. Electrospinning of chitosan dissolved in concentrated acetic acid solution. *Biomaterials* 26: 5427–5432.
62. Homayoni, H., Ravandi, S. A. H., and Valizadeh, M. 2009. Electrospinning of chitosan nanofibers: Processing optimization. *Carbohydr Polym* 77: 656–661.
63. Huang, X. J., Ge, D., and Xu, Z. K. 2007. Preparation and characterization of stable chitosan nanofibrous membrane for lipase immobilization. *Eur Polym J* 43: 3710–3718.
64. Pillai, C. K. S., Paul, W., and Sharma, C. P. 2009. Chitin and chitosan polymers: Chemistry, solubility and fiber formation. *Prog Polym Sci* 34: 641–678.
65. Liu, C. G., Desai, K. G. H., Chen, X. G., and Park, H. J. 2005. Preparation and characterization of nanoparticles containing trypsin based on hydrophobically modified chitosan. *J Agric Food Chem* 53: 1728–1733.
66. Klotzbach, T., Watt, M., Ansari, Y., and Minteer, S. D. 2006. Effects of hydrophobic modification of chitosan and Nafion on transport properties, ion-exchange capacities, and enzyme immobilization. *J Membrane Sci* 282: 276–283.

67. Sjoholm, K. H., Cooney, M., and Minteer, S. D. 2009. Effects of degree of deacetylation on enzyme immobilization in hydrophobically modified chitosan. *Carbohydr Polym* 77: 420–424.

68. Spagna, G., Barbagallo, R. N., Casarini, D., and Pifferi, P. G. 2001. A novel chitosan derivative to immobilize a-L-rhamnopyranosidase from *Aspergillus niger* for application in beverage technologies. *Enzyme Microb Technol* 28: 427–438.

69. Yi, S. S., Noh, J. M., and Lee, Y. S. 2009. Amino acid modified chitosan beads: Improved polymer supports for immobilization of lipase from *Candida rugosa*. *J Mol Catal B: Enzyme* 57: 123–129.

70. Xiao, Y. and Zhou, X. H. 2008. Synthesis and properties of a novel cross-linked chitosan resin modified by L-lysine. *React Funct Polym* 68: 1281–1289.

71. Zhou, J. Q. and Wang, J. W. 2009. Immobilization of alliinase with a water soluble–insoluble reversible N-succinyl-chitosan for allicin production. *Enzyme Microb Technol* 45: 299–304.

72. Monier, M., Wei, Y., Sarhan, A. A., and Ayad, D. M. 2010. Synthesis and characterization of photo-cross-linkable hydrogel membranes based on modified chitosan. *Polymer* 51: 1002–1009.

73. Monier, M., Wei, Y., and Sarhan, A. A. 2010. Evaluation of the potential of polymeric carriers based on photo-cross-linkable chitosan in the formulation of lipase from *Candida rugosa* immobilization. *J Mol Catal B: Enzyme* 63: 93–101.

74. Chellapandian, M. and Krishnan, M. R. V. 1998. Chitosan-poly (glycidyl methacrylate) copolymer for immobilization of urease. *Process Biochem* 33: 595–600.

75. Ng, L. T., Guthrie, J. T., Yuan, Y. J., and Zhao, H. J. 2001. UV-cured natural polymer-based membrane for biosensor application. *J Appl Polym Sci* 79: 466–472.

76. Bayramoglu, G. and Arica, M. Y. 2010. Reversible immobilization of catalase on fibrous polymer grafted and metal chelated chitosan membrane. *J Mol Catal B: Enzyme* 62: 297–304.

77. Monier, M., Wei, Y., Sarhan, A. A., and Ayad, D. M. 2010. Immobilization of horseradish peroxidase on modified chitosan beads. *Int J Biol Macromol* 46:324–330.

78. Vazquez-Duhalt, R., Tinoco, R., D'Antonio, P., Topoleski, L. D. T., and Payne, G. F. 2001. Enzyme conjugation to the polysaccharide chitosan: Smart biocatalysts and biocatalytic hydrogels. *Bioconjug Chem* 12: 301–306.

79. Delanoy, G., Li, Q., and Yu, J. 2005. Activity and stability of laccase in conjugation with chitosan. *Int J Biol Macromol* 35: 89–95.

80. Gómez, L., Ramírez, H. L., Villalonga, M. L., Hernández, J., and Villalonga, R. 2006. Immobilization of chitosan-modified invertase on alginate-coated chitin support via polyelectrolyte complex formation. *Enzyme Microb Technol* 38: 22–27.

81. Gómez, L., Ramírez, H. L, and Villalonga, R. 2000. Stabilization of invertase by modification of sugar chains with chitosan. *Biotechnol Lett* 22: 347–350.

82. Spagna, G., Barbagallo, R. N., Greco, E., Manenti, I., and Pifferi, P. G. 2002. A mixture of purified glycosidases from *Aspergillus niger* for oenological application immobilised by inclusion in chitosan gels. *Enzyme Microb Technol* 30: 80–89.

83. Ye, P., Xu, Z. K., Che, A. F., Wu, J., and Seta, P. 2005. Chitosan-tethered poly(acrylonitrile-*co*-maleic acid) hollow fiber membrane for lipase immobilization. *Biomaterials* 26: 6394–6403.

84. Ye, P., Jiang, J., and Xu, Z. K. 2007. Adsorption and activity of lipase from *Candida rugosa* on the chitosan-modified poly(acrylonitrile-*co*-maleic acid) membrane surface. *Colloid Surf B* 60: 62–67.

85. Gabrovska, K., Georgieva, A., Godjevargova, T., Stoilova, O., and Manolova, N. 2007. Poly(acrylonitrile)chitosan composite membranes for urease immobilization. *J Biotechnol* 129: 674–680.

86. Gabrovska, K., Nedelcheva, T., Godjevargova, T., Stoilova, O., Manolova, N., and Rashkov, I. 2008. Immobilization of acetylcholinesterase on new modified acrylonitrile copolymer membranes. *J Mol Catal B: Enzyme* 55: 169–176.

87. Edwards, W., Leukes, W. D., Rose, P. D., and Burton, S. G. 1999. Immobilization of polyphenol oxidase on chitosan-coated polysulphone capillary membranes for improved phenolic effluent bioremediation. *Enzyme Microb Technol* 25: 769–773.

88. Darder, M., Aranda, P., Hernáéndez-Vélez, M., Manova, E., and Ruiz-Hitzky, E. 2006. Encapsulation of enzymes in alumina membranes of controlled pore size. *Thin Solid Films* 495: 321–326.

89. Taqieddin, E. and Amiji, M. 2004. Enzyme immobilization in novel alginate–chitosan core–shell microcapsules. *Biomaterials* 25: 1937–1945.

90. Aranaz, I., Acosta, N., and Heras, A. 2009. Encapsulation of an *Agrobacterium radiobacter* extract containing D-hydantoinase and D-carbamoylase activities into alginate–chitosan polyelectrolyte complexes preparation of the biocatalyst. *J Mol Catal B: Enzyme* 58: 54–64.

91. Sankalia, M. G., Mashru, R. C., Sankalia, J. M., and Sutariya, V. B. 2007. Reversed chitosan–alginate polyelectrolyte complex for stability improvement of alpha-amylase: Optimization and physicochemical characterization. *Eur J Pharm Biopharm* 65: 215–232.

92. Yapar, E., Kayahan, S. K., Bozkurt, A., and Toppare, L. 2009. Immobilizing cholesterol oxidase in chitosan–alginic acid network. *Carbohydr Polym* 76: 430–436.

93. Deng, T., Wang, H., Li, J. S., Hu, S. Q., Shen, G. L., and Yu, R. Q. 2004. A novel immunosensor based on self-assembled chitosan/alginate multilayers for the detection of factor B. *Sens Actuators* B 99: 123–129.

94. Liu, Y., Lu, H. J., Zhong, W., Song, P. Y., Kong, J. L., Yang, P. Y., Girault, H. H., and Liu, B. H. 2006. Multilayer-assembled microchip for enzyme immobilization as reactor toward low-level protein identification. *Anal Chem* 78: 801–808.

95. Wang, R., Xia, B., Li, B. J., Peng, S. L., Ding, L. S., and Zhang, S. 2008. Semi-permeable nanocapsules of konjac glucomannan–chitosan for enzyme immobilization. *Int J Pharm* 364: 102–107.

96. Schmidt, T. F., Caseli, L., dos Santos Jr., D. S., and Oliveira Jr., O. N. 2009. Enzyme activity of horseradish peroxidase immobilized in chitosan matrices in alternated layers. *Mater Sci Eng C* 29: 1889–1892.

97. Zhang, M. G., Mullens, C., and Gorski, W. 2006. Amperometric glutamate biosensor based on chitosan enzyme film. *Electrochimica Acta* 51: 4528–4532.

98. Gu, T. T., Liu, Y., Zhang, J., and Hasebe, Y. 2009. Amperometric hydrogen peroxide biosensor based on immobilization of DNA-Cu(II) in DNA/chitosan polyion complex membrane. *J Environ Sci Suppl* : S56–S59.

99. Constantine, C. A., Mello, S. V., Dupont, A., Cao, X. H., Santos, Jr. D., Oliveira, Jr. O. N., Strixino, F. T., Pereira, E. C., Cheng, T. C., Defrank, J. J., and Leblanc, R. M. 2003. Layer-by-layer self-assembled chitosan/poly(thiophene-3-acetic acid) and organophosphorus hydrolase multilayers. *J Am Chem Soc* 125: 1805–1809.

100. Dinçer, A. and Azmi T. 2007. Improving the stability of cellulase by immobilization on modified polyvinyl alcohol coated chitosan beads. *J Mol Catal B: Enzyme* 45: 10–14.

101. Solanki, A. K. P. R., Ansari, A. A., Sumana, G., Ahmad, S., and Malhotra, B. D. 2009. Iron oxide–chitosan nanobiocomposite for urea sensor. *Sens Actuators B* 138: 572–580.

102. Jia, Z., Wang, Y. J., Lu, Y. C., Ma, J. Y., and Luo G. S. 2006. *In situ* preparation of magnetic chitosan/Fe_3O_4 composite nanoparticles in tiny pools of water-in-oil microemulsion. *React Funct Polym* 66: 1552–1558.

103. Luo, L. Q., Li, Q. X., Xu, Y. H., Ding, Y. Q., Wang, X., Deng, D. M., and Xu, Y. J. 2009. Amperometric glucose biosensor based on $NiFe_2O_4$ nanoparticles and chitosan. *Sens Actuators B* 145: 293–298.

104. Qiu, J. D., Peng, H. P., and Liang, R. P. 2007. Ferrocene-modified Fe_3O_4–SiO_2 magnetic nanoparticles as building blocks for construction of reagentless enzyme-based biosensors. *Electrochem Commun* 9: 2734–2738.

105. Bayramoglu, G., Yilmaz, M., and Arica, M. Y. 2010. Preparation and characterization of epoxy-functionalized magnetic chitosan beads: Laccase immobilized for degradation of reactive dyes. *Bioprocess Biosyst Eng* 33: 439–448.

106. Jiang, D. S., Long, S. Y., Huang, J., Xiao, H. Y., and Zhou, J. Y. 2005. Immobilization of *Pycnoporus sanguineus* laccase on magnetic chitosan microspheres. *Biochem Eng J* 25: 15–23.

107. Pan, C. L., Hu, B., Li, W., Sun, Y., Ye, H., and Zeng, X. X. 2009. Novel and efficient method for immobilization and stabilization of β-D-galactosidase by covalent attachment onto magnetic Fe_3O_4–chitosan nanoparticles. *J Mol Catal B: Enzyme* 61: 208–215.

108. Wu, Y., Wang, Y. J., Luo, G. S., and Dai, Y. Y. 2009. *In situ* preparation of magnetic Fe_3O_4-chitosan nanoparticles for lipase immobilization by cross-linking and oxidation in aqueous solution. *Bioresour Technol* 100: 3459–3464.

109. Yeon, K. M., Lee, C. H., and kim, J. 2009. Magnetic enzyme carrier for effective biofouling control in the membrane bioreactor based on enzymatic quorum quenching. *Environ Sci Technol* 43: 7403–7409.
110. Lei, Z. L., Ren, N., Li, Y. L., Li, N., and Mu, B. 2009. Fe$_3$O$_4$/SiO$_2$-g-PSStNa polymer nanocomposite microspheres (PNCMs) from a surface-initiated atom transfer radical polymerization (SI-ATRP) approach for pectinase immobilization. *J Agric Food Chem* 57: 1544–1549.
111. Magnin, D., Callegari, V., Mátéfi-Tempfli S., Mátéfi-Tempfli M., Glinel, K., Jonas, A. M., and Demoustier-Champagne S. 2008. Functionalization of magnetic nanowires by charged biopolymers. *Biomacromolecules* 9: 2517–2522.
112. Zhang, L. Y., Zhu, X. J., Zheng, S. Y., and Sun, H. 2009. Photochemical preparation of magnetic chitosan beads for immobilization of pullulanase. *Biochem Eng J* 46: 83–87.
113. Solanki, P. R., Kaushik, A., Ansari, A. A., Sumana, G., and Malhotra, B. D. 2008. Zinc oxide-chitosan nanobiocomposite for urea sensor. *Appl Phys Lett* 93: 163903.
114. Yang, Y. H., Yang, H. F., Yang, M. H., Liu, Y. L., Shen, G. L., and Yu, R. Q. 2004. Amperometric glucose biosensor based on a surface treated nanoporous ZrO$_2$/Chitosan composite film as immobilization matrix. *Anal Chim Acta* 525: 213–220.
115. Chang, M. Y. and Juang, R. S. 2007. Stability and reactivity of acid phosphatase immobilized on composite beads of chitosan and ZrO$_2$ powders. *Int J Biol Macromol* 40: 224–231.
116. Khan, R. and Dhayal, M. 2008. Electrochemical studies of novel chitosan/TiO$_2$ bioactive electrode for biosensing application. *Electrochem Commun* 10: 263–267.
117. Kafi, A. K. M., Wu, G. S., and Chen, A. C. 2008. A novel hydrogen peroxide biosensor based on the immobilization of horseradish peroxidase onto Au-modified titanium dioxide nanotube arrays. *Biosens Bioelectron* 24: 566–571.
118. Malhotra, B. D. and Kaushik, A. 2009. Metal oxide–chitosan based nanocomposite for cholesterol biosensor. *Thin Solid Films* 518: 614–620.
119. Njagi, J., Ispas, C., and Andreescu, S. 2008. Mixed ceria-based metal oxides biosensor for operation in oxygen restrictive environments. *Anal Chem* 80: 7266–7274.
120. Luo, X. L., Xu, J. J., Zhang, Q., Yang, G. J., and Chen, H. Y. 2005. Electrochemically deposited chitosan hydrogel for horseradish peroxidase immobilization through gold nanoparticles self-assembly. *Biosens Bioelectron* 21: 190–196.
121. Luo, X. L., Xu, J. J., Du, Y., and Chen, H. Y. 2004. A glucose biosensor based on chitosan–glucose oxidase–gold nanoparticles biocomposite formed by one step electrodeposition. *Anal Biochem* 334: 284–289.
122. Du, Y., Luo, X. L., Xu, J. J., and Chen, H. Y. 2007. A simple method to fabricate a chitosan–gold nanoparticles film and its application in glucose biosensor. *Bioelectrochemistry* 70: 342–347.
123. Kang, X. H., Mai, Z. B., Zou, X. Y., Cai, P. X., and Mo, J. Y. 2007. A novel glucose biosensor based on immobilization of glucose oxidase in chitosan on a glassy carbon electrode modified with gold–platinum alloy nanoparticles/multiwall carbon nanotubes. *Anal Biochem* 369: 71–79.
124. He, X. L., Yuan, R., Chai, Y. Q., and Shi, Y. T. 2008. A sensitive amperometric immunosensor for carcinoembryonic antigen detection with porous nanogold film and nano-Au/chitosan composite as immobilization matrix. *J Biochem Biophys Methods* 70: 823–829.
125. Yang, G., Yuan, R., and Chai, Y. Q. 2008. A high-sensitive amperometric hydrogen peroxide biosensor based on the immobilization of hemoglobin on gold colloid/L-cysteine/gold colloid/nanoparticles Pt–chitosan composite film-modified platinum disk electrode. *Colloid Surf B* 61: 93–100.
126. Liu, Y. J., Li, Y. L., Liu, S. C., Li, J., and Yao, S. Z. 2004. Monitoring the self-assembly of chitosan/glutaraldehyde/cysteamine/Au-colloid and the binding of human serum albumin with hesperidin. *Biomaterials* 25: 5725–5733.
127. Cao, S. S., Mishr, R., Pilla, S., Tripathi, S., Pandey, M. K., Shah, G., Mishra, A. K., Prabaharan, M., Mishra, S. B., Xin, J., Pandey, R. R., Wu, W. W., Pandey, A. C., and Tiwari, A. 2010. Novel chitosan/gold-MPA nanocomposite for sequence-specific oligonucleotide detection. *Carbohydr Polym* 82: 189–194.
128. Yang, Y. M., Wang, J. W., and Tan, R. X. 2004. Immobilization of glucose oxidase on chitosan–SiO$_2$ gel. *Enzyme Microb Technol* 34: 126–131.

129. Wang, G., Xu, J. J., Chen, H. Y., and Lu, Z. H. 2003. Amperometric hydrogen peroxide biosensor with sol/gel/chitosan network-like film as immobilization matrix. *Biosens Bioelectron* 18: 335–343.

130. Wang, G. H. and Zhang, L. M. 2006. Using novel polysaccharide–silica hybrid material to construct an amperometric biosensor for hydrogen peroxide. *J Phys Chem B* 110: 24864–24868.

131. Li, F., Chen, W., Tang, C. F., and Zhang, S. S. 2009. Development of hydrogen peroxide biosensor based on *in situ* covalent immobilization of horseradish peroxidase by one-pot polysaccharide-incorporated sol–gel process. *Talanta* 77: 1304–1308.

132. Xi, F. N. and Wu, J. M. 2004. Macroporous chitosan layer coated on non-porous silica gel as a support for metal chelate affinity chromatographic adsorbent. *J Chromatogr A* 1057: 41–47.

133. Wu, J. M., Luan, M. M., and Zhao, J. Y. 2006. Trypsin immobilization by direct adsorption on metal ion chelated macroporous chitosan–silica gel beads. *Int J Biol Macromol* 39: 185–191.

134. Xi, F. N., Wu, J. M., Jia, Z. S., and Lin, X. F. 2005. Preparation and characterization of trypsin immobilized on silica gel supported macroporous chitosan bead. *Process Biochem* 40: 2833–2840.

135. Stober, W., Fink, A., and Bohn, E. 1968. Controlled growth of monodisperse silica spheres in the micron size range. *J Colloid Interface Sci* 26: 62–69.

136. Lei, Z. L. and Bi, S. X. 2007. The silica-coated chitosan particle from a layer-by-layer approach for pectinase immobilization. *Enzyme Microb Technol* 40: 1442–1447.

137. Lei, Z. L., Bi, S. X., and Yang, H. 2007. Chitosan-tethered the silica particle from a layer-by-layer approach for pectinase immobilization. *Food Chem* 104: 577–584.

138. Liu, Y., Qu, X. H., Guo, H. W., Chen, H. J., Liu, B. F., and Dong, S. J. 2006. Facile preparation of amperometric laccase biosensor with multifunction based on the matrix of carbon nanotubes–chitosan composite. *Biosens Bioelectron* 21: 2195–2201.

139. Tsai, Y. C., Chen, S. Y., and Liaw, H. W. 2007. Immobilization of lactate dehydrogenase within multiwalled carbon nanotube–chitosan nanocomposite for application to lactate biosensors. *Sens Actuators B* 125: 474–481.

140. Chen, S. H., Yuan, R., Chai, Y. Q., Yin, B., Li, W. J., and Min, L. G. 2009. Amperometric hydrogen peroxide biosensor based on the immobilization of horseradish peroxidase on core–shell organosilica–chitosan nanospheres and multiwall carbon nanotubes composite. *Electrochim Acta* 54: 3039–3046.

141. Tkac, J., Whittaker, J. W., and Ruzgas, T. 2007. The use of single walled carbon nanotubes dispersed in a chitosan matrix for preparation of a galactose biosensor. *Biosens Bioelectron* 22: 1820–1824.

142. Ghica, M. E., Pauliukaite, R., Fatibello-Filho, O., and Brett, C. M. A. 2009. Application of functionalised carbon nanotubes immobilised into chitosan films in amperometric enzyme biosensors. *Sens Actuators B* 142: 308–315.

143. Tana, X. C., Li, M. J., Cai, P. X., Luo, L. J., and Zou, X. Y. 2005. An amperometric cholesterol biosensor based on multiwalled carbon nanotubes and organically modified sol–gel/chitosan hybrid composite film. *Ana Biochem* 337: 111–120.

144. Solanki, P. R., Kaushik, A., Ansari, A. A., Tiwari, A., and Malhotra, B. D. 2009. Multi-walled carbon nanotubes/sol–gel-derived silica/chitosan nanobiocomposite for total cholesterol sensor. *Sens Actuators B* 137: 727–735.

145. Chang, M. Y. and Juang, R. S. 2005. Activities, stabilities, and reaction kinetics of three free and chitosan–clay composite immobilized enzymes. *Enzyme Microbial Technol* 36: 75–82.

146. Chang, M. Y. and Juang, R. S. 2007. Use of chitosan–clay composite as immobilization support for improved activity and stability of β-glucosidase. *Biochem Eng J* 35: 93–98.

147. Chang, M. Y., Kao, H. C., and Juang, R. S. 2008. Thermal inactivation and reactivity of β-glucosidase immobilized on chitosan–clay composite. *Int J Bio Macromol* 43: 48–53.

148. Fan, Q., Shan, D., Xue, H. G., He, Y. Y., and Cosnier, S. 2007. Amperometric phenol biosensor based on laponite clay–chitosan nanocomposite matrix. *Biosens Bioelectron* 22: 816–821.

149. Han, E., Shan, D., Xue, H. G., and Cosnier, S. 2007. Hybrid material based on chitosan and layered double hydroxides: Characterization and application to the design of amperometric phenol biosensor. *Biomacromolecules* 8: 971–975.

150. Zhao, X. J., Mai, Z. B., Kang, X. H., and Zou, X. Y. 2008. Direct electrochemistry and electrocatalysis of horseradish peroxidase based on clay–chitosan–gold nanoparticle nanocomposite. *Biosens Bioelectron* 23: 1032–1038.

151. Gong, J. M., Liu, T., Song, D. D., Zhang, X. B., and Zhang, L. Z. 2009. One-step fabrication of three-dimensional porous calcium carbonate–chitosan composite film as the immobilization matrix of acetylcholinesterase and its biosensing on pesticide. *Electrochem Commun* 11: 1873–1876.

152. Sheng, Q. L., Luo, K., Li, L., and Zheng, J. B. 2009. Direct electrochemistry of glucose oxidase immobilized on $NdPO_4$ nanoparticles/chitosan composite film on glassy carbon electrodes and its biosensing application. *Bioelectrochemistry* 74: 246–253.

153. Jiang, Y. J., Zhang, L., Yang, D., Li, L., Zhang, Y. F., Li, J., and Jiang, Z. Y. 2008. Fabrication of polysaccharide–inorganic hybrid biocapsules with improved catalytic activity and stability. *Ind Eng Chem Res* 47: 2495–2501.

154. Li, W. J., Yuan, R., Chai, Y. Q., Zhou, L., Chen, S. H., and Li, N. 2008. Immobilization of horseradish peroxidase on chitosan/silica sol–gel hybrid membranes for the preparation of hydrogen peroxide biosensor. *J Biochem Biophys Methods* 70: 830–837.

9

Application of Chitosan-Based Biomaterials in Tissue Engineering

Changyong Wang, Junjie Li, and Fanglian Yao

CONTENTS

9.1 Introduction

Tissue engineering is an emerging interdisciplinary field that combines the knowledge and technology of cells, engineering materials, and suitable biochemical factors to create artificial organs and tissues, or to regenerate damaged tissues. The common concepts associated with tissue engineering research are based on the construction of hybrid materials obtained from the incorporation of cells into three-dimensional (3D) porous scaffolds or hydrogels. The scaffold material, which can mimic the extracellular matrix (ECM), has an essential function concerning cell anchorage, proliferation, and tissue formation in three dimensions [1]. To perform these varied functions in tissue engineering, an ideal scaffold should have the following characteristics: (1) an extensive network of interconnecting pores and spread porosity (usually exceeding 90%) so that cells can migrate, multiply, and attach deep within the scaffolds (this would allow *in vitro* cell adhesion, ingrowth, and reorganization and would provide the necessary space for neo-vascularization *in vivo*); (2) channels through which oxygen and nutrients are provided to cells deep inside the scaffold, and waste products can be easily carried away; (3) biocompatibility with a high affinity for cells to attach and proliferate; (4) the right shape, however complex as desired by the surgeon; and (5) appropriate mechanical strength and biodegradation profile. The decomposition products should be free from immunogenicity or any toxicity [2].

Recently, chitosan-based biomaterials have been reported as attractive candidates for scaffolding materials due to the inherent properties of chitosan. First, chitosans have excellent biodegradation, cytocompatibility, blood compatibility, and antimicrobial activity, and are without inflammatory reactions. Chitosan-based implants evoke minimal foreign body reaction, with little or no fibrous encapsulation. Second, they have environment–stimuli response. Third, the mechanical properties of chitosan-based biomaterials could be modulated via physical or chemical cross-linking. In addition, the degradation behaviors can also be adjusted. Fourth, chitosan can be molded in various forms with a fairly well-designed porous structure by means of different techniques, such as freeze-drying, rapid prototyping (RP), and the internal bubbling process. Seed cells may be encapsulated in gels or seeded in porous scaffolds including sponge-like or fibrous structures. Combinations of chitosan with other biocompatible materials are applied to modify biomechanical and cell–matrix interaction properties. Different adaptations of chitosan may help in optimizing cell and tissue differentiation and tailoring the transplant to different clinical cell delivery situations (*cf.* Figure 9.1) [3]. Here, the preparation of a chitosan-based scaffold and the interactions between cell/growth factor and chitosan-based biomaterial are introduced. Moreover, we focus on various types of chitosan-based biomaterials and their use in various tissue engineering applications, namely, blood vessel, skin, cartilage, bone, nerve, and liver.

9.2 Preparation of Chitosan-Based Scaffolds

9.2.1 Chitosan-Based Porous Scaffolds

The freeze-drying method is usually used to prepare chitosan-based porous scaffolds. Briefly, chitosan-based solutions or chitosan-based gels are frozen at certain temperatures for 12 h followed by lyophilization for 24 h. Chitosan scaffolds have high porosity >85%,

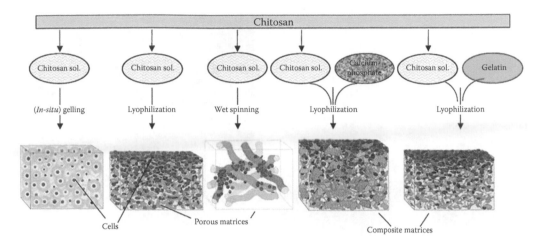

FIGURE 9.1

Illustration of selected examples of chitosan processing for use in tissue engineering. (From Martino, A. D. et al. *Biomaterials* 26: 5983–5990. With permission.)

and the porosity of chitosan scaffolds increased accordingly with decreasing chitosan concentration. The reason is obvious, since the actual volume fraction occupied by the material itself decreased as the chitosan concentration decreased [4]. Mean pore diameters could be controlled within the range 1–300 µm by varying the freezing conditions. The pore size depended on the size of ice crystals. At a lower freezing temperature, the number of nuclei of ice crystallization initially formed is more than that at a higher freezing temperature, which results in the formation of ice crystals of small size. Thus, the pore sizes become smaller and pore walls thinner, while interconnectivity increases with declining prefreezing temperature [5]. The pores of 88% and 95% degree of deacetylation (DD) chitosan scaffolds are not obviously different with variation of the pore size, whereas the pores of 70% DD scaffolds are larger [6].

In fact, these traditional chitosan-based porous scaffolds cannot achieve the requirements of complicated tissue. Bilayer chitosan-based scaffolds were prepared by quickly freezing on a stainless-steel plate, which gives direct contact with the cooling plate while being open to the air on top, as shown in Figure 9.2 [7,8]. There is a temperature gradient between the stainless-steel heat sink and the air heat sink. So a corresponding temperature gradient forms within the scaffold precursor. The pore size of the bottom layer contacting the refrigerating shutter directly is smaller than that of the air contacting top layer (*cf.* Figure 9.3). However, the microstructure of a chitosan-based scaffold prepared via freeze-drying

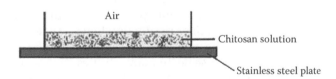

FIGURE 9.2

Formation of the bilayer chitosan scaffold model. (From Liu, H. F. et al. 2004. *J Biomater Sci Polymer Edn* 15: 25–40. With permission.)

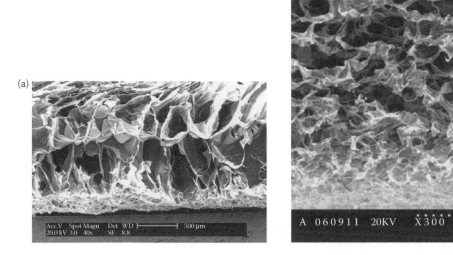

FIGURE 9.3
Scanning electron microscopy (SEM) section morphology of chitosan–gelatin (a) and chitosan–gelatin–HA scaffold (b) directed contact prefreezing methods. (From Liu, H. F. et al. 2004. *J Biomater Sci Polymer Edn* 15: 25–40; Mao, J. S. et al. 2003. *Biomaterials* 24: 1067–1074. With permission.)

technology is not easily controlled. RP makes it possible to produce tissue engineering scaffolds with predefined and reproducible internal microstructures. Moreover, the scaffold was designed to mimic the architecture of natural tissue. Li and coworkers [9] prepared chitosan–gelatin porous scaffolds with a well-defined internal morphology by RP, microreplication, and freeze-drying techniques.

9.2.2 Chitosan-Based Fiber Scaffolds

The natural ECMs in the body are mainly composed of two classes of extracellular macromolecules: proteoglycans and fibrous proteins with fiber diameters ranging from 50 to 150 nm, depending on tissue type. Nanofibrous composite scaffolds are an ideal choice for tissue engineering because of their heterogeneous nature, matching that of the ECM, large surface area-to-volume ratio, ability to facilitate diffusion (as a result of high porosity), and tunability of physical properties [10]. For chitosan, in the solid state, relatively rigid crystallites form due to the regularly arranged hydroxyl and amino groups at equatorial positions in the β(1,4)-linked D-glucosamine repeating units, while in solution, hydrogen bonding drives the formation of microfibrils, depending on chitosan concentration. Such characteristics of chitosan guide the methodology for successful electrospinning of this material [11]. Technologies for chitosan fiber production have been established during the last two decades. The electrospinning process can be used for the production of thin chitosan fibers down to the nanometer scale. In many studies, chitosan fibers are made by the wet-spinning process, which produces fibers by first dissolving the polymer in a solvent and then extruding the polymer solution via dies into a nonsolvent. Scaffolds prepared from chitosan fibers could combine adequate porous structure with sufficient degradability and mechanical properties [12].

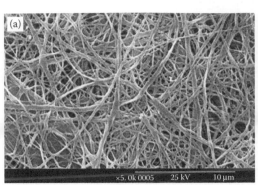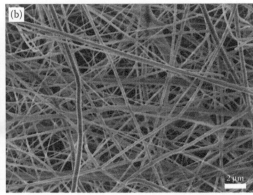

FIGURE 9.4
SEM micrographs of the chitosan nanofibrous scaffold (a) using HFIP [13] and (b) TFA as a spinning solvent. (From Schiffman, J. D. and Schauer, C. L. 2007. *Biomacromolecules* 8: 2665–2667. With permission.)

The choice of solvent is crucial to obtain the ideal chitosan-based fiber scaffold. Min et al. [13] created chitosan nanofibers by first electrospinning chitin nanofibers with 1,1,1,3,3,3-hexafluoro-2-propanol (HFIP) as the solvent, followed by deacetylation of the as-spun chitin fibers with NaOH solutions at various temperatures. The mean diameter is ca. 180 nm (*cf.* Figure 9.4a). As for the pure chitosan system, two direct spinning methods from chitosan solutions were reported. One is the concentrated acetic acid solvent system; Jang and coworkers [14] found that only chitosan with 106 kDa can be electrospun to give bead-free thin fibers with pump-feeding of the chitosan–aqueous 90% acetic acid solution. In this system, the repulsive forces between ionic groups within the chitosan backbone that arise due to the application of a high electric field during electrospinning are very strong, which restrict the formation of continuous fibers and often produce particles. The other is the trifluoroacetic acid (TFA) solvent system. Chitosan dissolved in TFA can be electrospun into randomly oriented, continuous, bead-free fibers (*cf.* Figure 9.4b) [15]. There are two possible reasons why the electrospinning of chitosan is successful when using TFA: (a) TFA forms salts with the amino groups of chitosan and this salt formation destroys the rigid interaction between chitosan molecules, making them ready to be electrospun; (b) the high volatility of TFA is advantageous for the rapid solidification of the electrified jet of chitosan–TFA solution [16,17]. The addition of dichloromethane to the chitosan–TFA solution improved the homogeneity of the electrospun chitosan fibers. The diameter of chitosan fibers is influenced by the solution concentration and molecular weight (MW) of chitosan. In general, as the solution concentration decreased, the average fiber diameter linearly decreased (*cf.* Figure 9.5) [18]. It was found that a 7% concentration produced beads on the fibers, while an 8% concentration produced an almost uniform fiber network. The average fiber diameter ranges from 74 to 108 nm and increased as the MW increased. The low MW fibers exhibited some branching, which was possibly due to the intrinsically low MW of bulk chitosan [19]. In addition, the average diameter decreased with narrower diameter distribution as the applied electric field increased.

Recently, electrospun chitosan composite nanofibrous scaffolds have been fabricated using chitosan and synthetic biodegradable protein, polysaccharide, and synthetic polymer. These composite fiber mats have advantage over the electrospinning of pure chitosan due to their intrinsic character [20]. Table 9.1 summarizes the experimental conditions adapted for the fabrication and the obtained average size of electrospun chitin nanofibers.

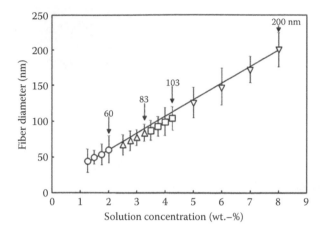

FIGURE 9.5
Relationship between the concentrations of the prespun chitosan/TFA solutions and the mean diameters of the electrospun chitosan fibers. Numbers with arrows indicate the mean fiber diameter in the optimized spinning condition, giving the relatively homogeneous fiber networks. (From Ohkawa, K. et al. 2006. *Biomacromolecules* 7:3291–3294. With permission.)

9.2.3 Chitosan-Based Microsphere Scaffolds

Recently, microspheres have also been assessed as scaffolds for tissue engineering, and new strategies, such as sintering and fusion methods, have been investigated to obtain suitable scaffolds that mimic the tissue environment for cells. Most of the concepts based on the use of such scaffolds require the implantation kind of the hybrid constructs through a surgical procedure. The process of scaffold fabrication consisted of the following steps. (1) Preparation of chitosan-based microspheres: polymer dissolving, spheres production by extrusion of the solution to the precipitating bath, pH neutralization, scaffold formation, chitosan cross-linking, rinsing, and drying. (2) Microsphere scaffold formation:

TABLE 9.1

Electrospun Chitosan Composites Nanofibers

Composites	Solvent	Average Fiber Diameter (nm)	References
Chitosan/collagen	HFP/TFA	415–810 (–)	[21,22]
Chitosan/gelatin	TFA/DCM	100–220	[23]
Chitosan/agarose	TFA/DCM	140–1500 (+)	[24]
Chitosan/PEO	aq. AA	80–180	[25]
Chitosan/PLA	TFA	40–1200 (–)	[26]
Chitosan/PCL	Formic acid/acetone	112.9–139.6	[27]
Chitosan/PVA	aq. AA	20–100	[28]
Chitosan/PLGA	Chloroform/DMF	272	[29]

Note: (+), diameter of composites increases with increasing chitosan content; (–), diameter of composites decreases with increasing chitosan content.
HFP, 1,1,1,3,3,3-hexafluoroisopropanol; TFA, trifluoroacetic acid; DMF, N,N-dimethylformamide; aq. AA, aqueous acetic acid solution; DCM, dichloromethane; PVA, poly(vinyl alcohol); PEO, poly(ethylene oxide); PLA, poly(lactic acid); PLGA, poly(lactide-co-glycolide); PCL, polycaprolactone.

scaffolds were fabricated by packing and agglomeration of the microspheres. On the one hand, chitosan-based microspheres can be packed with the use of a solvent. The acidic solvent dissolves the external surfaces of the spheres so that they get stuck together and their structure becomes tight and durable. As shown in Figure 9.6, strong union between chitosan particles was obtained through acetic acid rinsing, which partially dissolved the surface. Scaffold porous architecture is presented in the pictures. The average porosity measured was about 40% [30]. On the other hand, packing of microspheres and their aggregation can be realized at high temperature. Briefly, chitosan-based microspheres are put into a stainless-steel mold. The mold was heated to a temperature above the glass transition of polymer for a certain time period to achieve bonding between adjacent microspheres. The bonding of chitosan microspheres was achieved due to the bioadhesive character of the chitosan polymer that resulted in the union of adjacent particles at

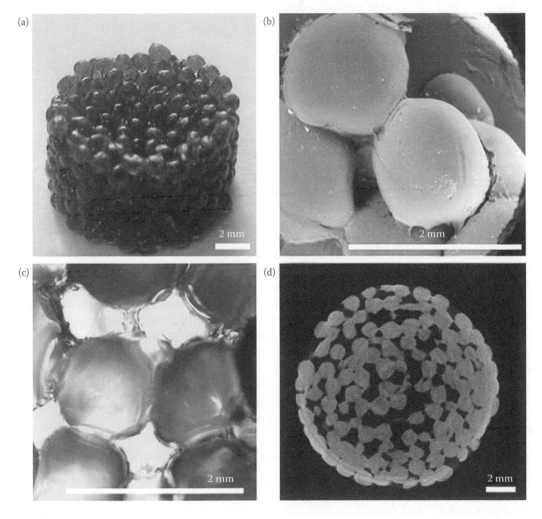

FIGURE 9.6
(a) Morphology of scaffold manufactured by the presented method. (b) SEM microphotograph of agglomerated scaffold. (c) Spheres interconnectivity observed by optical microscope. (d) One of cross-sections obtained by µCT scanning.

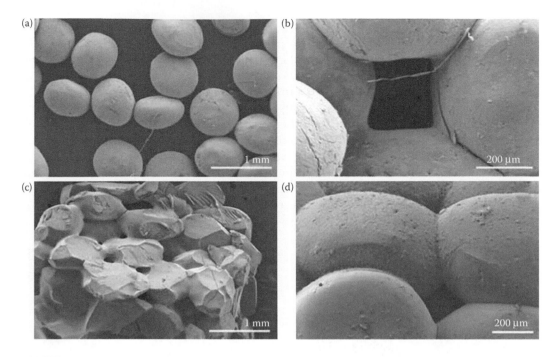

FIGURE 9.7

EM micrographs of chitosan particles obtained by the precipitation method (a); pore morphology in the chitosan scaffolds (b); cross section of chitosan scaffolds obtained by the particle aggregation method (c); and the interface between the chitosan particles after the production of the scaffolds (d). (From Malafaya, P. B. et al 2005. *J Mater Sci: Mater Med* 16: 1077–1085. With permission.)

their contact points to form the microsphere chitosan porous scaffold (*cf.* Figure 9.7) [31]. The average pore diameter was 265.46 ± 24.27 μm. Porosity and interconnectivity of the chitosan microsphere scaffold is $27.78 \pm 2.80\%$ and $94.99 \pm 1.41\%$, respectively. It is important to stress that interconnectivity was calculated with a limit in pore size of 53 μm as the minimum value for interconnected pores, meaning that interconnection diameters lower than this value were considered as closed pores [32]. A higher sintering temperature resulted in decreased porosity, because greater fusion between microspheres can occur when sintering temperature is elevated. Moreover, a higher sintering temperature and a longer sintering time have equivalent effects on the fabrication of microsphere scaffolds [7,33].

9.3 Interactions between Chitosan-Based Biomaterials and Cells

With the development of biology and genetic engineering, the design idea of chitosan-based biomaterials is gradually clear. It should be able to control the interactions between cell and materials and further control cell behaviors, such as attachment, proliferation, differentiation, and apoptosis, which is the foundation research for the application of chitosan-based biomaterials in tissue engineering. Therefore, it is necessary to understand the interactions between cells and chitosan-based biomaterials and their influencing factors. In general, molecular chain structure of chitosan, chemical composition and stiffness of chitosan-based biomaterials, and spatial architecture of scaffolds will influence these interactions. Moreover, different kinds of cells exhibit different cell responses to chitosan-based biomaterials.

9.3.1 Effect of Chitosan Chain Structure

Interactions between chitosan and cells have been attributed to nonspecific electrostatic interactions between protonated amine groups and negatively charged carboxylate and sulfate groups found in cell surface proteoglycans [34]. Therefore, structure parameters, especially the DD of chitosan, take very important roles when cells contact with chitosan-based biomaterials. Most cell behaviors, such as attachment, proliferation, migration, morphology, and differentiation, exhibit different characters due to different chain structures of chitosan.

9.3.1.1 Attachment

Cell adhesion is an important previous process for sequent cell growth, cell migration, and cell differentiation. When DD increases, the charge density of chitosan is enhanced, thus reinforcing adhesion [35]. Moreover, as little as 10% differences in the extent of DD of chitosan samples have a significant influence on the adhesion to chitosan substrates by cells in culture [36]. Chitosan with high DD has more glucosamine units and more amino groups, which results in cells getting attracted to it via electrostatic interactions. In addition, higher-DD chitosan films may also localize more growth factors in the serum near cells, therefore increasing the chances of the growth factor binding to its receptor on the cell surface [37].

9.3.1.2 Proliferation

Cell proliferation behaviors are influenced by the DD, depending on cell type. Whatever the DD of chitosan is, fibroblasts show low cell proliferation [35] owing to the extremely high adhesion of fibroblasts to chitosan-based biomaterials [38]. However, all chitosans with different DDs can support the proliferation of osteoblasts. No relationship was found between normal human bone cell proliferation and chitosan molecule structure [37]. Keratinocytes and hamster kidney cells are both reported to grow more on chitosan films than on fibroblasts and the proliferation increases considerably with increasing DD [39,40]. Buffalo embryonic stem-like cells attached and proliferated better on 88% DD and 95% DD scaffolds than on 70% DD scaffolds and there are no significant differences between 88% and 95% DD chitosan scaffolds [6,41]. The discrepancies in these results could be attributed to either the different cell types used in the experiments or the mechanism of cell adhesion to chitosan surfaces. Different DDs result in different amounts of amine groups present at the surface. Cell-specific differences in the amounts and types of negatively charged surface molecules could result in cell-specific affinities for chitosan with different DDs [42].

9.3.1.3 Migration

For fibroblasts, D-glucosamine (GlcN) is found to reduce migratory activity, while N-acetyl-D-glucosamine (GlcNAc) is not found to influence the migratory activity [43] and the content of GlcN depends on DD. For neutrophil-like HL60 cells, the migration indices for 55.8% DD chitosan elicited a significantly greater migration index than 83.3% DD chitosan. Hydrophobicity can prolong physical interactions between cells and chitosan since neutrophils demonstrate an affinity for high-DD chitosan with hydrophobic surfaces. Prolonged physical interactions between cells and chitosan may be a possibility for increased IL-8 secretion with increased N-acetylation. IL-8 will not only cause further chemotaxis toward chitosan, but migrating cells will further secrete more IL-8, resulting in a positive feedback loop that may account for the continuous migration and infiltration of neutrophils into chitosan [44]. Du and coworkers [45] reported that chitooligosaccharides can significantly offset the promotion of human hepatoma carcinoma cells–culture–fluid on the migration and tube formation of endothelial cells (ECs) in a concentration-dependent manner. Chitosan (with high DD 97.4% and MW 540 kDa) could induce inflammatory cell migration and angiogenetic activity, favoring high vascularization of the neo-tissue [46].

9.3.1.4 Differentiation

The differentiation fate of cells, especially stem cells, is influenced by transcription factor, growth factor, cell–cell interactions, mechanical stimulation, and so on. At present, there are very few reports on differentiation behaviors related to the molecular structure of chitosan. Amaral et al. [47] found that rat bone marrow stroma cells cultured on chitosan carrying a DD of 96% are able to reach a higher level of osteogenic differentiation than on other chitosans with low DD and the control. Suphasiriroj et al. [42] found that the chitosan–collagen scaffolds that contained low-DD chitosan supported greater alkaline phosphatase activity in MC3T3-E1 cells than did chitosan–collagen scaffolds that contained high-DD chitosan, irrespective of the MW. The different phenomena may be attributed to either different cell types or different materials. However, the detailed reason is unclear till now, and it is necessary to study this differentiation mechanism with the development of stem cell technology in the future.

9.3.2 Effect of Chemical Composition

Tissues of the human body contain significant extracellular space, into which ECM molecules are secreted by the cells to form a complex network (*cf.* Figure 9.8) [48]. The ECM provides mechanical support for tissues, organizes cells into specific tissues, and controls cell behavior. Chitosan exhibits cell compatibility and elicits minimal immunological responses. However, chitosan is not the main component of ECM and, to some extent, it restricts cell spreading and cytoskeleton actin distribution. The reduction in cell size is thought to be the result of strong electrostatic interactions. In order to mimic the ECM and modulate the electrostatic interactions between chitosan and cells, some polymer or inorganic minerals are incorporated into the chitosan network, and they can endow chitosan-based biomaterials with a special cell response. In general, the combination of collagen, gelatin, alginate, and hyaluronic acid (HA) into the chitosan network is mainly to modulate the cell behaviors of fibroblasts, and to also influence the behaviors of osteoblasts and chondrocytes. Adjusting the chondrocyte response to chitosan-based biomaterials is mainly by adding glycosaminoglycans (GAGs) and alginate. Introducing alginate can influence the osteoblasts and never cell behavior, while it is a more effective method to promote the proliferation of osteoblasts by introducing hydroxyapatite (HAp) into the chitosan-based network. Combining heparin can influence the character of smooth muscle cells (SMCs). In addition, the content of these materials in chitosan-based biomaterials is also

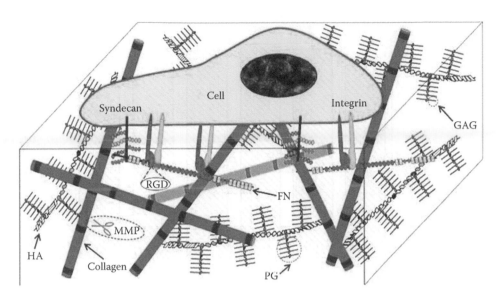

FIGURE 9.8
Model of the complex 3D structure of ECM and cell–ECM interactions. (From Zhu, J. M. 2010. *Biomaterials* 31:4639–4656. With permission.)

a very important parameter to influence cell behaviors. For example, the concentration of HA is a more important factor to affect the behavior of cells in addition to HA itself. Only the concentrations of HA in a certain range (0.01–0.1%) in chitosan–gelatin–HA composite film could enhance cell adhesion, migration, and proliferation. However, when the concentration of HA was above 0.1%, it could inhibit cell adhesion, migration, and proliferation (*cf.* Figure 9.9) [49]. The fibroblasts seeded on 0.01% HA membrane grew and proliferated with an almost extended shape and most of them were fusiform. However, fibroblasts seeded on 1% HA membrane arrayed irregularly and their shape had changed a lot. The chitosan–chondroitin sulfate (90/10 w/w) film showed excellent cytocompatibility for fibroblasts [50]. Moreover, protein adsorption is a determining step for cell adhesion and will further control cell morphology, as well as their proliferation capacity the type of adsorbed proteins and their orientation are related to the surface properties, especially to surface energy. Neither very low polar components nor very high ones were suitable for correct cell attachment/morphology. The composites of chitosan-based biomaterials are the main factor influencing surface energy. For example, plasma-treated and sulfonic acid-grafted chitosan films presented better cell viability and proliferation than untreated and acrylic acid-grafted samples [51]. Proliferation of cells seeded on more hydrophilic *N*-butyl chitosan surface was higher than that on *N*-cetyl chitosan surface [52].

9.3.3 Effect of Matrix Stiffness

Most cell types studied so far spread more, adhere better, and appear to survive better on stiffer matrices, and some cannot grow on very soft (<50 Pa) surfaces. Other cell types, such as neutrophils, appear not to respond to substrate stiffness, at least over the range of 3–50,000 Pa that can be accessed experimentally. Still other cell types, such as neurons, extend processes more avidly and appear to survive better on soft materials [53]. Matrix stiffness can regulate the degree of cell–matrix adhesion, migration, growth, and viability, as well as resistance to apoptosis [54]. Cells on stiff matrices are proliferative and fibrogenic,

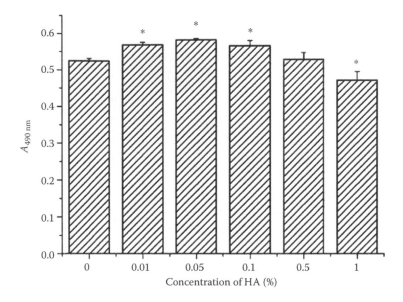

FIGURE 9.9
Adhesion of human fibroblasts on chitosan–gelatin–HA film fabricated with different concentrations of HA solutions.

with a spread phenotype, increased numbers of integrin–ECM bonds, and, in the case of fibroblasts, stress fibers. Cells migrate from soft to stiff regions of the matrix and may be most motile at intermediate stiffness [55]. For example, embryonic fibroblasts (NIH 3T3) undergo more apoptosis and less proliferation on soft as opposed to stiff substrates [56]. Moreover, the matrix also influences stem cell fate, soft matrices (elastic modulus in the range 0.1–1 kPa) favored differentiation of mesenchymal stem cells (MSCs) into neuronal-like cells, moderate elasticity (elastic modulus in the range 8–17 kPa) promoted myogenic differentiation, and a rigid matrix (elastic modulus over 34 kPa) stimulated osteogenic differentiation (*cf.* Figure 9.10) [57,58]. Different cells exhibit different cell behaviors on

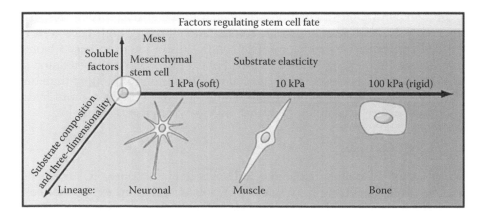

FIGURE 9.10
Multiple factors can infuence the differentiation of stem cells, including secreted soluble factors, the elasticity or compliance of the matrix substrate, and the biochemical composition and dimensionality of the matrix. (From Even-Ram, S., Vira, Artym. V., and Yamada, K. M. 2006. *Cell*; 126: 645–647. With permission.)

chitosan-based biomaterials with different stiffness. Soft chitosan-based biomaterials can provide an appropriate environment for the proliferation of neurons. An optimal stiffness of photopolymerizable methacrylamide chitosan (MAC) exists for both proliferation (3.5 kPa) and differentiation to neurons (<1 kPa). Neural stem/progenitor cell self-renewal is optimal between 1 and 7 kPa (*cf.* Figure 9.11) [59]. Proliferation and colony formation ceased on MAC surfaces when Young's elastic modulus was >10 kPa. In contrast, when elastic modulus is higher than 10 kPa, the condition is appropriate for proliferation of chondrocytes. As shown in Figure 9.12, chondrocytes showed a round morphology on chitosan film (3.8 kPa) and a flattened and spread morphology on chitosan film (15.3 and 19.9 kPa), and cell number increases with increasing stiffness [60]. A rigid chitosan-based biomaterial matrix is appropriate for the proliferation and differentiation of osteoblasts.

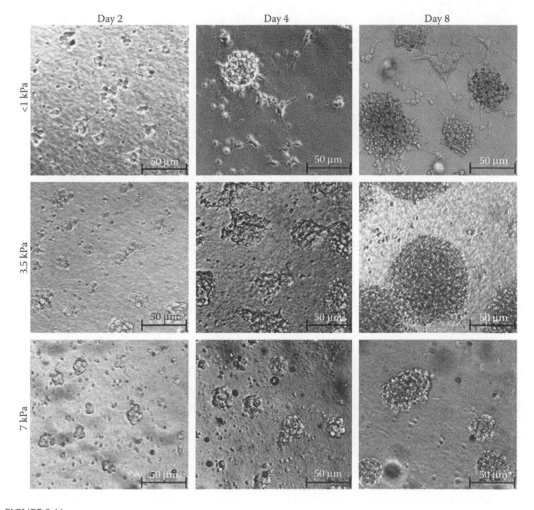

FIGURE 9.11

Representative images of neural stem/progenitor cell seeded and differentiated on MAC hydrogels of varying substrate stiffness over 8 days of culture. Cells attach as single cells and proliferate on all surfaces in the form of colonies. 3.5 kPa MAC surfaces stimulated the largest colonies by day 8. Cell process formation and migration out of colonies was only observed on <1 kPa surfaces. (From Leipzig, N. D. and Shoichet, M. S. 2010. *Biomaterials* 30: 6867–6878. With permission.)

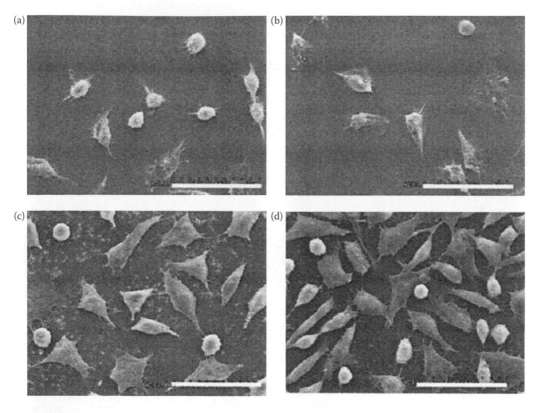

FIGURE 9.12
EM micrograph of chondrocytes seeded on uncross-linked and cross-linked films. Representative SEM images of chondrocyte cells (passage 2) on cross-linked chitosan films with (a) 3.8 kPa, (b) 7.4 kPa, (c) 15.3 kPa, and (d) 19.9 kPa. (From Subramanian, A. and Lin, H. Y. *J Biomed Mater Res* 75A: 742–753. With permission.)

For example, rigid chitosan–gelatin–pectin film can promote osteogenic differentiation of MSCs compared with the relatively soft chitosan–gelatin film [61].

9.3.4 Effect of the Spatial Architecture of Chitosan-Based Biomaterials

At present, two types of chitosan-based biomaterial scaffolds have been used in tissue engineering. One is the implanting scaffold, and the other is the injectable scaffold. The implanting chitosan-based scaffold has a special spatial architecture and can be prepared by various methods, such as thermally induced phase separation, freeze-drying, electrostatic spinning, and so on. The porosity and pore size of these scaffolds are easily controlled and have excellent mechanical properties to maintain macroscopic shape during the application. Compared with 2D film, cells seeded in these 3D scaffolds exhibit different cell behaviors. Cells seeded in chitosan-based 3D cultures showed higher cell survival relative to 2D chitosan-based substrata. On 2D substrata, cells are restricted to spreading on a flat plane and an important factor affecting cellular activity is whether the substrate contains a cell adhesion binding domain or not. On the contrary, 3D scaffolds provide spatial advantages for cell–cell and cell–matrix adhesion as well as support for cell traction (*cf.* Figure 9.13) [62,63]. In addition, the pore size of the scaffold should be greater than the size of the cell, and many cell types are unable to completely colonize scaffolds with pore sizes >300 µm

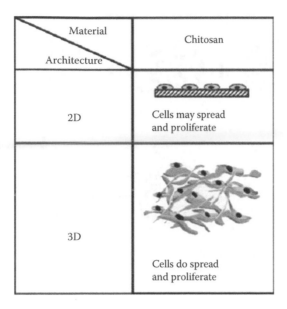

  Material Architecture	Chitosan
2D	Cells may spread and proliferate
3D	Cells do spread and proliferate

FIGURE 9.13
Schematic diagram showing the cell colonization characteristics on different architectures. (From Huang, Y., Siewe, M., and Madihally, S. V. 2006. *Biotechnol Bioeng* 93: 64–75. With permission.)

due to the difficulty in crossing large bridging distances. However, the 3D-based chitosan scaffolds cannot completely simulate the microenvironment of cell growth *in vivo*, which may dissipate some functional expression during the process of cell culture *in vitro*. And the application of the implanting chitosan-based 3D scaffold must be via surgery.

Chitosan-based injectable scaffolds for cell encapsulation or cell/hydrogels are promising substrates for tissue engineering because of *in vivo* culture environment, minimal invasion, low cost, and so on. There are several criteria that must be considered. Cells are suspended in a liquid precursor solution prior to encapsulation. The liquid precursor loaded with targeted cells can be injected into the damaged site and experiences a gel transition *in situ* due to physical or chemical stimuli. The process by which gelation occurs must be mild and cell friendly. The hydrogel's structure and chemistry composites must be suitable for cell survival and tissue formation, while its degradation must closely follow tissue growth. Finally, the degradation products must not adversely affect encapsulated cells (*cf.* Figure 9.14) [64]. Recently, layer-by-layer (LBL) encapsulation of cells has been developed. Briefly, a first layer of cells is grown on a surface to confluence, and then a hydrogel precursor solution is deposited over the confluent cells and hardened via environment stimuli. A second layer of cells is grown on top of the first layer of hardened hydrogel followed by hardening of a second hydrogel layer on the second layer of cells; the alternate deposition of cells and hydrogel is repeated several times to build a thick tissue (*cf.* Figure 9.15). The LBL cell/hydrogel buildup can potentially allow higher density, better alignment of cells, or construction of multicell-type tissues [65]. However, there are some disadvantages of chitosan-based injectable scaffolds for cell encapsulation. (1) Chitosan liquid precursor solution is not suitable for cell survival, because chitosan can dissolve in acidic medium but apparently it is less favorable for the cells. Therefore, some chemicals modified or composite with other polymers are necessary to modulate the pH value of the precursor solution. (2) The mechanical strength and shape stability of cell encapsulation or

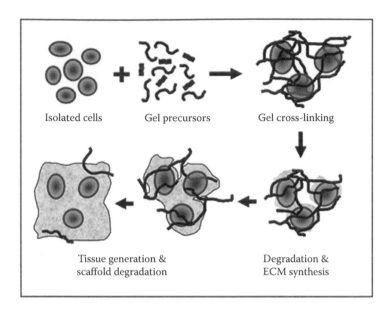

FIGURE 9.14
Cell encapsulation strategies involve mixing cells with precursors in a liquid solution followed by gelation and encapsulation of cells. (From Nicodemus, G. D. and Bryant, S. J. 2008. *Tissue Eng Part B* 14: 149–165. With permission.)

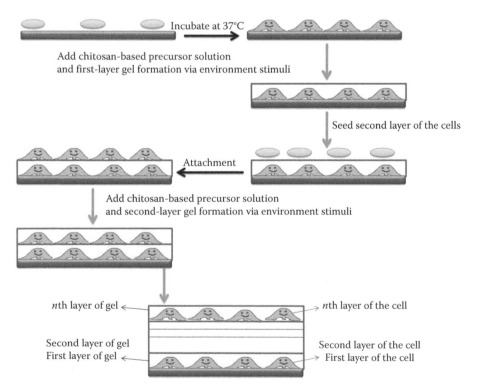

FIGURE 9.15
LBL encapsulation of cells.

hydrogels are poor. (3) Cell death usually occurs inside the hydrogel because of limited exchange of nutrition and cell metabolism products. (4) The hydrogels can be hard to handle and may be difficult to load cells. (5) The hydrogels may be difficult to sterilize.

In general, cell/hydrogels were formed by incorporating cells into thermosensitive and covalent cross-linking chitosan-based hydrogels. For example, Wang and coworkers [66] constructed cell/hydrogels by mixing sheep chondrocytes with a chitosan–glycerophosphate hydrogel. The chondrocytes remained >90% viable in the chitosan matrix after being cultured for 1 day *in vitro*. On the other hand, cell encapsulation could be prepared by combining cells in the chitosan-based polyelectrolyte complex and cross-linking the microcapsules. For example, chitosan–alginate microcapsules have been used to encapsulate mammalian cells. Some of these groups used chitosan as the main matrix entrapping the cells, while alginate was used as the coating polymer [67,68]. Other studies have used chitosan as the coating membrane of alginate microcapsules when entrapping cells [69,70]. The remarkable long-term mechanical properties provided by the chitosan outer membrane and the long-term viability achieved are of great advantage when considering this system for *in vivo* cell-based therapy [71].

9.4 Incorporation of Growth Factors in Chitosan-Based Biomaterials

Growth factors are part of a large number of polypeptides that transmit signals affecting cellular activities. They are not always promoting cell growth, but in many instances they could produce a variety of products for their composition. They have very important roles in tissue engineering. Growth factors have been introduced in many tissue-engineered systems, by various methods, for example, (1) by addition to culture, (2) by genetically engineering cells to overexpress growth factors, or (3) by constructing polymeric systems that provide for the controlled release of growth factors [72]. It is known that the half-life of growth factors is very short. Moreover, growth factors added directly to the cell culture media or injected *in vivo* may be inhibited by binding proteins or the ECM before reaching the desired target cells. The most important concern regarding the delivery of growth factors is whether or not the released protein actually retains its biological activity [73]. Therefore, the best way to enhance the efficacy of growth is by achieving sustained release and by maintaining a suitable concentration over an extended time period via the third strategy. Chitosan possesses the intrinsic advantages of being used as a carrier for loading with growth factors in order to get special bioactivity functions. Chitosan requires only mild processing conditions, and thus can avoid growth factor inactivation under harsh processing conditions [74]. Chitosan could substantially prolong the biological half-life time of fibroblast growth factor (FGF) and could protect the FGF activity from inactivation, such as heat, proteolysis, and acid. Table 9.2 summarizes chitosan and chitosan-based growth factor release systems for tissue regeneration. Growth factors can be loaded in the chitosan-based scaffold via physical adsorption, chemical immobilization, or incorporating the polymer microsphere containing growth factors.

In general, a biologically active chitosan-based scaffold for tissue engineering can be prepared by soaking a chitosan-based scaffold in growth factor solution. In this case, the growth factor can be considered only on the surface of the scaffold and so behaves as free growth factor. The binding efficiency of growth factors on the scaffold is low and is not easy to control. Moreover, the stability and release behaviors of growth factors are also

TABLE 9.2

Chitosan-Based Biological Factor or Cell Delivery Systems for Tissue Engineering

Growth Factors	Actions	Substrate Material	Applications
BMP-2	Bone morphogenesis	Chitosan	Bone regeneration
		Chitosan-poly(glutamic acid)	Osseointegration
PDGF-BB	Mitogenic	Chitosan	Bone regeneration
	Bone formation and remodeling	Chitosan-chondroitin sulfate	Periodontics
		Chitosan-poly(L-lactide)	Orthopedics
			Plastic surgery
TGF-β	Multifunctional	Chitosan	Bone and cartilage regeneration
		Chitosan-collagen	
		Chitosan-tricalcium phosphate	
		Chitosan-collagen-chondroitin sulfate	
FGF-2	Mitogenic	Chitosan-lactose hydrogel	Angiogenesis
	Angiogenic	Photocross-linkable azide-chitosan-lactose hydrogel	Wound healing
	Regulates cell differentiation		
EGF	Angiogenic	Chitosan	Wound healing
	EC proliferation		
VEGF	Angiogenic	Chitosan-dextran sulfate nanoparticles	Angiogenesis
	EC proliferation		

Source: From Jiang, T. et al. 2008. *Curr Top Med Chem* 8: 354–364. With permission.

difficult to control. That all these behaviors depended on the electrostatic interactions between growth factors and scaffolds is the main factor. One can modulate the release behaviors by adjusting the interactions between growth factors and chitosan-based scaffolds. The isoelectric points of bFGF, platelet-derived growth factor-BB (PDGF-BB), and transforming growth factor-β (TGF-β) are 9.6, 9.8, and 8.59, respectively. Under physiological conditions, ionic repulsion between chitosan and these growth factors exists, which results in low absorption and burst release. The rapid release phenomena are more obvious when some cationic polymer or protein (isoelectric point higher than 7.4) is incorporated into the chitosan scaffold. For example, the release rate of TGF-β loaded in chitosan–collagen scaffolds is higher than that in pure chitosan scaffolds [75]. It is favorable to reduce the release rate when some polyanion polymers are incorporated into chitosan due to the electrostatic attraction interaction between polyanion polymers and growth factors or chitosan. For example, a more steady release of PDGF-BB may be obtained by using the chitosan–chondroitin-4-sulfate scaffold than by using chitosan alone. And the release of PDGF-BB is efficiently sustained because the content of chondroitin-4-sulfate in the chitosan scaffold increased [76]. In order to improve the binding efficiency and decrease the burst release of bFGF, Mi and coworkers [77] conjugated heparin on the chitosan–alginate scaffold surface. The heparinized scaffolds exhibited higher affinity than the chitosan–alginate scaffold alone. The scaffolds are uniquein their ability to bind bFGF depending on the amount of conjugated heparin. The more the content of heparin, the higher the binding efficiency. Moreover, the rate of bFGF release from the scaffold decreased in a controlled manner with decreasing burst effect. For all that, the physical adsorption

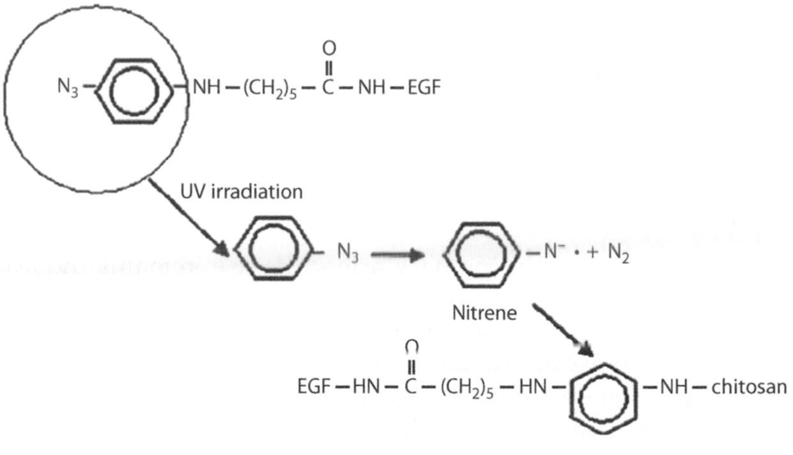

FIGURE 9.16
Production of nitrene groups in phenyl-azido derivatized EGFs by ultraviolet irradiation and immobilization on chitosan surface. (From Karakecli, A. G. et al. 2008. *Acta Biomater* 4: 989–996. With permission.)

may not be sufficient to promote long-term implantation, because of drawbacks, including protein desorption and/or exchange in contact with physiological fluid.

Growth factors or polymer microspheres containing growth factors can be directly encapsulated in the chitosan-based scaffold to construct a bioactive scaffold for tissue engineering. In this case, these growth factors are not free and the binding efficiency can be accurately controlled. The interactions between growth factors and scaffolds are still the main factors to affect the stability and release behaviors of growth factors. But growth factors are not easily released from the chitosan-based scaffolds by a diffusion mechanism. The dissolution and degradation of the scaffold itself in the biological environment are the main driving forces for the delivery of growth factors. Therefore, the release behaviors can be controlled by the swelling and degradation properties of scaffolds [78].

Growth factors are also immobilized on the surface of chitosan-based scaffolds to construct a bioactive material for tissue engineering. Chemical binding involves a covalent attachment of the target molecule to the solid surface, resulting in irreversible binding with high levels of surface coverage, which makes this approach more suitable. Gumusderelioglu and coworkers [79] bound epidermal growth factors (EGFs) on a chitosan film surface via photochemical immobilization (*cf.* Figure 9.16). The immobilized EGF activated the EGF receptor for a longer time, and a high mitogenic effect was observed. Park et al. [80] immobilized bone morphogenetic protein-2 (BMP-2) on a chitosan matrix using a bifunctional reagent succinimidyl 4-[N-maleimidomethyl]cyclohexane-1-carboxylate), which can react with chitosan on one end and BMP-2 on the other. The chemically bound BMP-2 remained bioactive and was more effective in stimulating osteoblastic cell proliferation and differentiation as compared with the BMP-2-adsorbed chitosan matrix.

9.5 Application of Chitosan-Based Biomaterials in Tissue Engineering

Tissues can be defined as an assembly of cells surrounded by an ECM. In vertebrates the main tissue types are vascular, skin, nerve, connective (bone and cartilage), and muscle tissues. The extracellular composition and physical features of tissue greatly vary based on tissue type and its physiological properties. Therefore, chitosan-based biomaterials should be constructed according to the characters of tissue. In this section, applications of chitosan-based biomaterials in blood vessel, skin, cartilage, bone, nerve, and liver tissue are introduced.

9.5.1 Blood Vessel

Cardiovascular disease, especially coronary artery disease, remains the leading cause of mortality all over the world, which has led to an increase in the economic and social burden of such diseases. When diseased arteries need to be replaced, the common clinical solution for surgeons is to use autologous grafts such as mammary artery or saphenous vein. However, these tissue sources may be inadequate or unavailable, and their harvest adds time, cost, and the potential for additional morbidity to the surgical procedure. A tissue-engineered blood vessel has been considered as an optimal alternative for a blood vessel substitute. The first tissue engineered blood vessel substitute was created by Weinberg and Bell in 1986 [81]. Current artificial vascular grafts are made of Dacron (poly(ethyleneterephthalate)) or expanded polytetrafluorethylene. These vascular grafts perform well at diameters >6 mm. However, owing to thrombus formation and compliance mismatch, none of these materials have proved suitable for generating small-diameter grafts (<6 mm) that would be required to replace the saphenous vein, internal mammary or radial artery as a vascular substitute [82].

The artery wall contains three layers. The outermost layer is the adventitia and is composed of collagen-rich connective tissue containing few elastic fibers. The middle layer consists of SMCs arranged in circumferential and more elastic fibers. The innermost layer is a monolayer of ECs. The theory of blood vessel tissue engineering can be applied by using two approaches [83]. One approach is the coculturing of SMCs with biomaterials and lining the lumen with ECs. The second approach is designed to provide a graft constructed of a material that would provide the required mechanical properties on the implant, but would also facilitate infiltration of host cells into the vessel and tissue remodeling. Based on this, a chitosan-based scaffold can be employed as a vascular substitute. The size of vascular cells is ca. 60–200 μm, which requires that the pore size of the chitosan-based scaffold is 100–300 μm. In addition, to provide appropriate microenvironments for the growth of SMCs and ECs, some proteins or polymers are usually introduced into chitosan-based networks. For example, chitosan–collagen porous and fiber scaffolds, which have the advantage of having similar components and architecture as the ECM, can improve the attachment and proliferation of vascular cells and provide a suitable cell environment for cells secreting more ECM [22,84]. Zhang et al. [85] developed a sandwich tubular chitosan–gelatin scaffold. The inner and outer surfaces were the chitosan–gelatin complex, and the middle surface was chitosan. This structure is similar to the natural blood vessel tissue. This chitosan conduit should have enough suture-retention strength to withstand *in vivo* anastomosis forces. Moreover, it is suitable for the proliferation of SMCs.

Incomplete endothelialization and SMC hyperplasia are two problems contributing to the poor performance of existing small-diameter vascular grafts. SMC hyperplasia is one of the primary causes of failure in small-diameter vascular grafts [86]. Therefore, the bioactive chitosan-based scaffold should combine some materials to both enhance the rate of endothelialization and specially inhibit the migration of smooth muscles to the graft lumen; meanwhile, the scaffold cannot decrease the bioactive functions of SMCs. Chitosan supported the proliferation of both vascular cell types, but also retarded SMC growth to a greater extent than endothelial growth. This result suggests that the scaffold material may have intrinsic biological activity, which could contribute to retardation of SMC growth relative to ECs [87]. Heparin will inhibit the proliferation of vascular SMCs, attract and protect many heparin-binding growth factors, such as bFGF, vascular endothelial growth factor (VEGF), and PDGF, and help control the release of these growth factors. Thus, chitosan–heparin composites have potential applications in small-diameter blood vessel tissue engineering [88].

9.5.2 Skin

On the surface of our body, the skin provides a protective barrier that keeps microbes out and essential body fluids in. The skin is divided into two anatomically distinct regions: the epidermis and the dermis (*cf.* Figure 9.17). The epidermis prevents moisture and heat loss from the skin and bacterial infiltration from the environment. A major component of the epidermis is the keratinocyte, which forms overlapping structures held together by desmosomes that provide cell-to-cell adhesion. The dermis is composed of various amounts of glycoproteins and GAGs. The fibroblast is the cell type that is most prevalent in the dermis and is responsible for synthesizing and depositing collagen fibers in continuous networks that form the structural scaffold [89]. It can bear daily assaults, including harmful ultraviolet radiation from the sun, and scratches and wounds [90]. Its structure can be damaged under a stronger external force and it cannot finish the self-repair. The healing of a skin wound involves complicated courses, including a wide range of cellular, molecular, physiological, and biological processes. There are millions of patients suffering from skin loss annually. The cost of skin recovery is about $36,000–117,000 per patient. Full-thickness skin defects on large scale cannot be repaired spontaneously. In past decades, many skin substitutes such as xenografts, allografts, and autografts have been employed for wound healing. However, due to the antigenicity or the limitation of donor sites, these skin substitutes cannot accomplish the purpose of skin recovery and hence are not used widely. The tissue-engineering skin strategy can

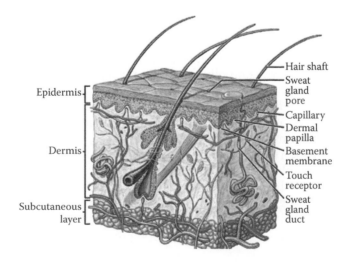

FIGURE 9.17
Structure of human skin showing the upper epidermal barrier layer and the much thicker dermal layer with hair follicles and sweat glands lined with epithelial cells. (From Shier, D., Butler, J., and Lewis, R. 1999. In *Hole's Human Anatomy and Physiology*, 8th Edn. McGraw Hill, pp. 160–183. With permission.)

overcome these disadvantages. Tissue-engineered skin needs to (a) provide a barrier layer of renewable keratinocytes (the cells that form the upper barrier layer of our skin), which is (b) securely attached to the underlying dermis, (c) well vascularized, and (d) provides an elastic structural support for skin [91], which can mimic the structure of normal skin.

Chitosan can influence the behaviors of keratinocytes and fibroblasts and can modulate human skin cell mitogenesis [41]. It has the functions of hemostasis and sterilization. Moreover, the structure of the chitosan molecule is similar to GAG and can stimulate fibroblast synthesis of collagen. These characters endow chitosan-based biomaterials with the ability to construct epidermal, dermal, or even epidermal–dermal replacement.

9.5.2.1 Epidermal Cover

Research into epidermal tissue engineering has revealed three periods: epidermal cell suspension, epidermal sheet, and epidermal cell–biomaterials composites [92]. Keratinocytes did not proliferate on the chitosan matrix. Chitosan seemed to be cytostatic toward human keratinocytes: it is not cytotoxic, but inhibits cell proliferation due to extremely high adhesion behaviors [93]. That is to say, pure chitosan is very difficult to construct the epidermal substitute. Some peptides, proteins, or polysaccharides are conjugated into the chitosan network to modulate the proliferation and migration behaviors of keratinocytes. However, it is important to note that the keratinocyte–chitosan-based biomaterials allogenic graft acts only as temporary coverage, helping to reduce inflammation and decrease the severity of hypertrophic scarring. The graft was eventually replaced by autologous keratinocytes migrating from the basement film or periphery [94].

Compared with pure chitosan, chitosan–gelatin film can improve the proliferation of keratinocytes. Moreover, increasing the contents of gelatin in chitosan–gelatin film could promote keratinocyte migration. The migration distance of cultured keratinocytes on pure chitosan film was $61.47 \pm 2.70\,\mu m$, while this value increases to $66.22 \pm 9.39\,\mu m$, $120.31 \pm 15.82\,\mu m$, and $225.38 \pm 10.48\,\mu m$ when the ratio of chitosan to gelatin is 7:3, 5:5, and 3:7, respectively [95]. That is to say, keratinocytes migrated out of the film into the wound where they aggregated to form stratified structures resembling the epidermis [96]. Human tissue-engineered epidermis can be constructed by culturing human keratinocytes onto chitosan–gelatin film (*cf.* Figure 9.18) [97]. The keratinocyte–chitosan–gelatin epidermal film can successfully promote the healing of the skin graft donor sites compared with the classic treatment method (petroleum jelly gauze). On postoperative day 7, the average healed surface area was 91% for the keratinocyte–chitosan gelatin group and 31% for the classic treatment method. At 3 months, the epidermis was well differentiated (*cf.* Figure 9.19) [98].

The development of nanotechnology provides another effective method for constructing the chitosan-based epidermal coverage. Some nanoparticles, such as silver nanocrystalline [99], nano-titanium oxide [100], and nanosized gold colloid [101], were combined into a chitosan network to modulate the behavior of keratinocytes and promote the formation of new epidermis. The viability of keratinocytes attached or proliferated on the chitosan nanofibrous scaffolds was greater than that on the chitosan film counterparts owing to the larger surface area of the fibrous scaffolds that is available for the cells to attach.

9.5.2.2 Dermal Equivalent

The dermis can increase elasticity, softness, and mechanical wear and decrease scar proliferation. The dermis is composed of various amounts of glycoproteins (e.g., collagen, elastin, fibronectin, laminin, and chondronectin) and GAGs (including HA, chondroitin

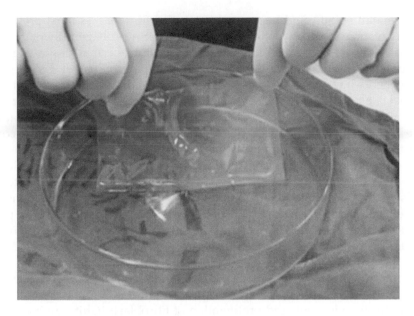

FIGURE 9.18
Human tissue-engineered epidermal membrane (keratinocyte/chitosan–gelatin film *in vitro* at 1 week). (From Yang, J. et al. 2010. *Plast Reconstr Surg* 125: 901–909. With permission.)

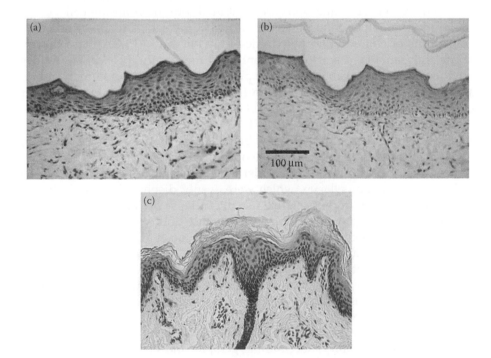

FIGURE 9.19
Immunohistochemistry testing at 3 months: (a) keratin, (b) involucrin, and (c) laminin (original magnification, ×200). (From Liu, H. F. et al. 2007. *J Biomater Appl* 21: 413–430. With permission.)

6-sulfate, dermatan sulfate, and heparan sulfate). The fibroblast is most prevalent in the dermis and is responsible for synthesizing and depositing collagen fibers in continuous networks that form the structural scaffold. Research into dermal tissue engineering is developing based on the research and application of the epidermal cover. Tissue-engineered dermal equivalents have been developed that can be used alone or in combination with epithelial sheets as for the treatment of large full-thickness skin defects. For successful dermal engineering, both selection of a suitable porous scaffold and optimization of cell seeding are important. Chitosan-based biomaterials, especially chitosan–GAG composites, can be selected for the construction of artificial dermis *in vitro*, which could be composed to mimic the mechanical characteristics of the dermis and have cytocompatibility for fibro-blasts. Moreover, fibroblast ingrowths promote the substitution of these chitosan-based biomaterials with appropriate biodegradation properties by natural components of the dermis. An ideal chitosan-based scaffold used for dermal replacement should possess the characteristics of excellent cytocompatibility for fibroblasts, suitable microstructure such as 100–200 µm mean pore size and porosity above 90%, controllable biodegradability and suitable mechanical property [102].

It has been shown that fibroblast-specific ECM components, such as type-I collagen and GAGs, play a critical role in regulating the expression of the fibroblast phenotype and in supporting both the migration and proliferation of fibroblasts. Chitosan could serve as a GAG analog component as it contains *N*-acetyl-glucosamine groups in the molecule. Therefore, collagen is usually introduced in the chitosan network to modulate the cell behavior of fibroblasts and further construct the dermal equivalent. Moreover, gelatin is the partial derivative of collagen and has been processed into composites by blending with chitosan for the construction of dermal equivalent. To better simulate the structures of the dermis, some GAGs or amino acids are combined into the chitosan–collagen scaffold [103–105]. In addition, other chitosan-based dermal equivalents are also studied. Hybrid nanofibrous films of chitosan and poly(lactic-*co*-glycolic acid) (PLGA) have been widely studied. The chitosan–PLGA scaffold has controlled mechanical properties and degrada-tion behaviors. Moreover, it can improve the proliferation capacity of human embryo skin fibroblasts. It is a potential scaffold for skin tissue engineering. However, there are few reports on the *in vivo* test of the chitosan–PLGA nanofiber scaffold. There are also many difficulties that need to be overcome [106,107].

As the dermal equivalent, chitosan-based biomaterials should have the following pro-perties: First, an appropriate microstructure of the chitosan-based porous scaffold is the basic element for obtaining an artificial dermal equivalent. The scaffold was indeed composed of chitosan and collagen, which were evenly dispersed through the scaffold. The pores of pure collagen porous scaffold usually collapse owing to the low hardness of collagen. Chitosan can improve deformation-resistance ability and reduce pore collapse because of the stiffer molecular structure of chitosan. Gao et al. [107] found that the pore size on the surface of chitosan–collagen films improved with increasing chitosan percentage. Higher chitosan (>50%) contents can yield a surface with larger pores. Of course, the micro-structure of the scaffold is also controlled by the preparation method. In addition, cross-linking is necessary in this system. The chitosan–collagen or chitosan–gelatin scaffolds quickly degraded and cannot keep the original shape if there is no cross-linking between collagen (gelatin) and chitosan. At present, glutaraldehyde, 1-ethyl-3-(3-dimethylamino-propyl)-carbodiimide/*N*-hydroxyl-succinimide, genipin, and so on are employed to prepare the chitosan–collagen scaffold. Second, the growth behaviors of fibroblasts in scaffolds are also very important for the construction of dermal replacement. Chitosan–collagen scaffolds can improve the proliferation of fibroblasts compared with pure chitosan

TABLE 9.3

The Cell Cycle of Fibroblasts on the Scaffold

Time (Days)	Cell Cycle (%)			Cell Death (%)
	G_0/G_1	S	G_2/M	
3	55.4	6.96	36.2	1.61
)	51.5	7.62	39.1	2.01
14	50.4	5.86	40.8	3.14

Source: From Sun, L. P. et al. 2009. *Biomed Mater* 4: 055008. With permission.

scaffolds. Moreover, the chitosan–collagen scaffolds with 30 wt% chitosan showed the most significant increase in relative cell viability [108]. Most fibroblasts seeded on the scaffolds come in the normal cell cycle. The cell death rate is very low (*cf.* Table 9.3). The percentages of fibroblasts cultured in the dish for 3 days in the G_0/G_1, S, and G_2/M phase cells and apoptotic cells are 57.8%, 37.8%, 4.4%, and 0.5%, respectively. The S-phase cells cultured in the chitosan–collagen scaffold decrease apparently and the G_2/M phase cells increase remarkably, which demonstrates that the collagen–chitosan scaffolds promote the S–G_2/M phase transition [109]. However, fibroblasts may locate at the peripheral area of the chitosan-based scaffold and cover some pores of the scaffold surface, which may prevent nutrition supply, limit cell growth, and result in more inhomogeneous tissues. In order to decrease these phenomena, Tan and coworkers [110] seeded human dermal fibroblasts into the chitosan–collagen scaffold using a flow perfusion system. It was found that seeding at the perfusion rate of 0.125 mL/min and 0.25 mL/min could achieve significantly higher seeding efficiencies than that at 0.5 mL/min. In comparison with the static seeding method, the perfusion seeding at 0.25 mL/min promoted a more efficient cell utilization and achieved higher initial cell densities without compromising the uniformity of initial cell distribution. The uniform distribution of cells achieved using perfusion seeding was found to be favorable to prolong cell proliferation period, increase the number of cells, and form more homogeneous morphology of constructed tissues, as shown in Figure 9.20. In addition, fibroblasts cultured under mechanical stimulation (subjected to the cyclic

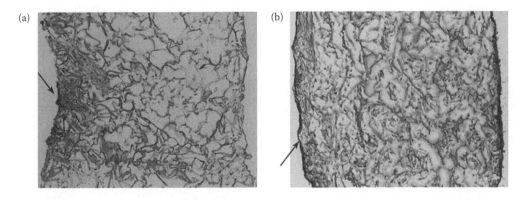

FIGURE 9.20
Cell distribution on the cross section of the 4-week chitosan–collagen constructs. Hematoxylin and eosin (H&E)-stained cross section of static cultured 4-week constructs seeded by the static (a) and perfusion (b) methods (the arrow denotes the top surface of constructs). (From Ding, C. M. et al. 2008. *Proc Biochem* 43: 287–296. With permission.)

strain, at a frequency of 1 Hz), are distributed homogeneously throughout the chitosan–collagen scaffold. Moreover, the localizations of ECM proteins, such as vimentin, fibronectin, and collagen type I, are consistent with the distribution of cellularity. The application of a cyclic strain to fibroblast–scaffold constructs may increase cell survival and integration of the artificially engineered dermis at the graft site [111]. Third, various growth factors, such as FGFs, encoding VEGFs, and EGFs, function in the process of wound healing. They can not only modulate the growth behaviors of fibroblasts but also enhance angiogenesis of the engineered constructs. Chitosan-based biomaterials-loaded FGFs can improve the attachment, proliferation, and production of the GAG capacity of fibroblasts [112]. For example, fibroblasts in chitosan–gelatin scaffolds with bFGF-loaded chitosan–gelatin microspheres achieve a relatively homogeneous distribution over time, which in turn resulted in a relatively homogeneous ECM accumulation (*cf.* Figure 9.21) [113]. More importantly, the transcript level of laminin, which is one of the most important biological noncollagenous glycoproteins that participate in angiogenesis, is markedly upregulated owing to the incorporation of FGFs or VEGFs. For example, the *N,N,N*-trimethyl chitosan chloride–pDNA-VEGF complexes-loaded chitosan–collagen scaffold could accelerate the angiogenesis in which the numbers of newly formed and matured vessels were all increased.

During the formation process of new dermis, a temporary epidermal layer on the chitosan-based scaffold is required for the dermal equivalent to be used practically, which can play a role in controlling water loss and inhibiting bacterial entry until an ultrathin epidermal autologous graft is applied [114]. The bilayer structure of chitosan-based film and scaffold has been designed to realize this function. It was processed successively via the formation of a dense chitosan film by the casting method and a porous chitosan sponge by lyophilization. The dry thickness of the film layer was 19.6 μm and that of the scaffold layer was controlled at 60–80 μm. The film layer acts as an obstacle to prevent bacterial infection and to control the loss of body fluid, while the scaffold layer of chitosan allows the ingrowth of dermal fibroblasts on a wound bed [115]. Bilayer collagen–chitosan scaffold covered with a silicone film layer is prepared by Gao and coworkers (*cf.* Figure 9.22) [116]. Comparing with the commercial product Integra® (composed of a biodegradable collagen scaffold and a silicone membrane), the bilayer chitosan-based scaffold can remain stable in shape and size during cell culture. Moreover, the chitosan-based scaffold indeed has the ability to regenerate a damaged dermis with a similar structure as the normal skin [117].

9.5.2.3 Full-Thickness Replacement

The skin, which contains the epidermis and the dermis, is the body's barrier against external harmful factors. Therefore, tissue-engineered skin should contain epidermal and dermal structures to realize the physiological function of the skin. The main objective of tissue engineering skin is to achieve permanent skin regeneration with both dermal and epidermal tissues. Keratinocytes and fibroblasts exhibit different cell behaviors on the chitosan-based scaffold. Keratinocytes prefer a more hydrophobic surface than fibroblasts. The relative viability values for both the attachment and the proliferation of keratinocytes on both chitosan scaffolds ranged between 77% and 140% (relative to those on TCPS) and that of fibroblast ranged between 35% and 62% (relative to those on TCPS) [117]. Therefore, asymmetric chitosan-based hydrogels or scaffold should be designed to obtain the epidermal–dermal replacement.

Yao and coworkers [8] prepared bilayer chitosan–gelatin and chitosan–gelatin–HA scaffolds via the freeze-drying technique. First, fibroblasts are seeded in chitosan–gelatin and

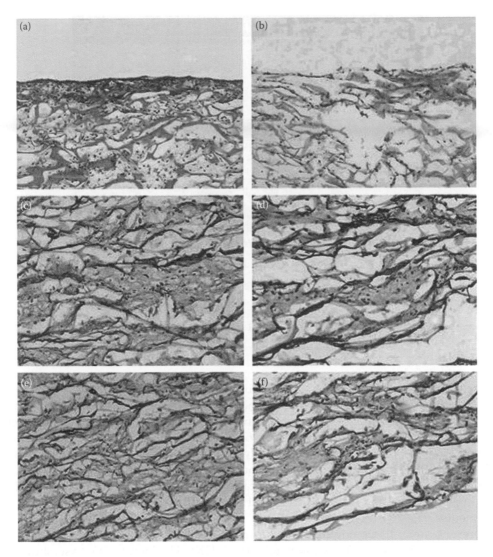

FIGURE 9.21

Histological (a, b) and immunohistochemical (c, f) observations of human fibroblasts cultured on the scaffolds with (a, c, e) and without (b, d, f) bFGF-MS for 2 weeks. Images (a) and (b) were for H&E staining (×100); images (c) and (d) were for type I collagen staining (×200); images (e) and (f) were for type III collagen staining (×200). (From Liu, H. F. et al. 2007. *Biomacromolecules* 8: 1446–1455. With permission.)

cultured for 3 weeks. During the culture process, fibroblasts can secrete ECM collagen and growth factors to form a cell–scaffold construct, which can be defined as artificial dermis. Then keratinocytes were also cocultured *in vitro* with fibroblasts in chitosan–gelatin scaffolds to construct an artificial bilayer skin to construct the artificial skin. Fibroblasts are used as the supporting layer for the primary culture of keratinocytes and they are considered to secrete some ECM molecules to provide the physiological environment needed for keratinocyte morphogenesis and differentiation. Meanwhile, keratinocytes can also affect the secretion of ECMs and growth factors of fibroblasts. After 1 week of coculture in the chitosan–gelatin–HA bilayer scaffold, a thin layer of cuboid keratinocytes is

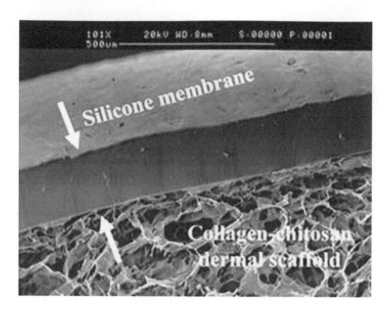

FIGURE 9.22
Microstructure of the bilayer chitosan/collagen dermal scaffold. (From Shi, Y. S. et al. 2005. *Polym Adv Technol* 16: 789–794. With permission.)

observed growing on the surface of the underlying artificial dermis (Figure 9.23a). Subsequently, after 1 week (Figure 9.23b) and 2 weeks (Figure 9.23c) of coculture at the air–liquid interface, the epithelial layer became progressively stratiform, including cubic perpendicularly oriented cells and a superficial layer of flattened cells. After 2 weeks, stratum corneum provided by longitudinally aligned cells was clearly evident [7,98,119]. Black et al. [120] also found that coculture models using keratinocytes and fibroblasts in the chitosan–collagen–chondroitin sulfate scaffold can be used to construct artificial skin including epidermal and dermal ultrastructures, the expression of major dermal ECM components.

At present, some tissue-engineering skin products that have been used in the clinic, such as OrCel (Ortec, USA), Myskin (CellTran, UK), Hyalograft 3D Laserskin (Fidia Advanced Biopolymers, Italy), and so on, can be used for the treatment of chronic skin ulcer. Integra (Integra Life Science) and Transcyte and Dermagraft (Advanced Tissue Sciences, USA) have obtained FDA approval for artificial skin. Activ Skin (Aierfu Active Tissue Engineering Co., Ltd, China) obtained State Food and Drug Administration (SFDA) approval in 2007. These tissue-engineering skin products are mostly prepared using collagen and cadaver skin. Although there are a number of research works on the chitosan-based artificial skin, there are a few chitosan-based tissue-engineering skin products. A wovenable skin substitute (Beschitin®) using chitin fiber was prepared by Morihita Resere Company of Japan in the 1980s [121]. The permeability and water absorption of Beschitin are better than that of other artificial skins prepared by collagen and pigskin. Moreover, it can significantly improve the formation of new skin. The chitosan-based biomaterial is the most potent candidate as a scaffold for skin substitutes due to its physicochemical and biological properties. Chitosan-based tissue engineered skin should have safety, can improve the "take" of cultured keratinocytes on wound beds, and promotes the rate of neo-vascularization of tissue-engineered skin.

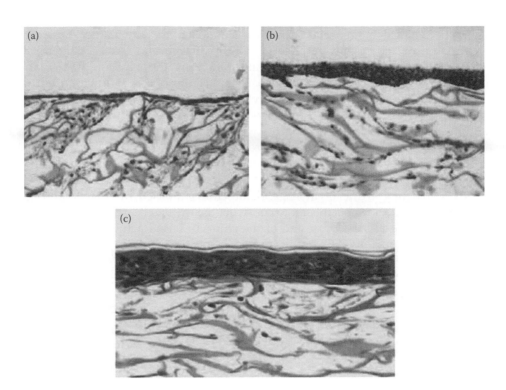

FIGURE 9.23
Histological appearance of fibroblasts and keratinocytes cocultured in chitosan–gelatin–HA scaffolds for (a) 1 week, and cocultured at an air–liquid interface for (b) 1 week and (c) 2 weeks (H&E;original magnification ×200). (From Liu, H. F., Yin, Y. J., and Yao, K. D. 2007. *J Biomater Appl* 21: 413–430. With permission.)

9.5.3 Cartilage

Articular cartilage is a unique connective tissue in the human body because blood vessels and nerves are absent in the tissue. Cartilage also contains large amounts of ECMs. Except for water, the main constituents of the ECMs in hyaline cartilage are proteoglycans and collagens [122]. Cartilage is an essential tissue for normal joint functions such as cushioning and lubrication. Articular cartilage, dense white specialized connective tissue covering the articulating surfaces of bone, contains chondrocytes and ECM. Once damaged, articular cartilage has very little capacity for spontaneous healing because of the avascular nature of the tissue. An initial surgical attempt to restore the normal articulating surface of joint cartilage was made with the introduction of Pridie's resurfacing technique [123]. Current therapies include abrasion arthroplasty, subchondral drilling, prosthetic joint replacement, and ultimately, transplantation of autologous chondrocytes or tissues. However, these treatments do not constitute a complete recovery for the patient and, in most cases, persistent problems of donor site morbidity, limitations of patient mobility and consequent disability, loss of implants, and limited durability of the prosthetics are observed. Thus, the novel cartilage tissue-engineering approach has attracted special attention. Tissue engineering of articular cartilage involves the isolation of articular chondrocytes or their precursor cells that may be expanded *in vitro* and then seeded into a biocompatible matrix, or scaffold, for cultivation and subsequent implantation into the joint. The choice of biomaterial is very critical for the success of tissue-engineering approaches. The ideal biomaterial substance should mimic the natural environment in the cartilage-specific ECM components (type II collagen and GAGs). Chitosan-based biomaterials have been extensively tested as mimicking the cartilage matrix and are considered promising candidates for the repair of articular cartilage due to the structural similarity of chitosan to various GAGs. N-acetyl-glucosamine in chitosan is an important ingredient of polysaccharide for chondrogenic expression. Chitosan has the ability to maintain the round morphology of chondrocytes, which is a normal phenotypic characteristic and preserves their capacity to synthesize cell-specific ECMs [124]. It has already been shown that chondrocytes grown on chitosan films exhibit a spherical morphology and express type II collagen and aggrecan [125]. However, the chitosan-based film is not appropriate for constructing artificial cartilage. Some chitosan-based hydrogels, porous scaffolds, or fiber scaffolds have been used to construct the artificial cartilage. There are three principles during the process of design of the chitosan-based artificial cartilage: (a) the composites should mimic the ECM of the cartilage-specific ECM; (b) the degradation rate should match with the regeneration. Chondrocytes-laden pure chitosan used to repair articular cartilage defects may proceed slower than the rate of cartilage regeneration; and (c) the fundamental structure of a scaffold should be a 3D system with adequate mechanical strength because articular cartilage is a mechanically stressed tissue. The material properties of articular cartilage are as follows: a compressive equilibrium aggregate modulus of 0.5–1.2 MPa, a tensile equilibrium modulus of 15–40 MPa, and a permeability of $(0.5–5) \times 10^{-15}$ m^4/(N s) [126].

9.5.3.1 Chitosan-Based Hydrogels–Chondrocytes Construct

Encapsulation of chondrocytes within the chitosan-based hydrogels is the main strategy to construct the artificial cartilage. Lu et al. [127] have demonstrated that a chitosan solution injected into the knee articular cavity of rats causes a significant increase in the density of chondrocytes in the corresponding articular cartilage. Recent studies have presented an initial attempt to elaborate injectable thermosensitive chitosan-based hydrogels and to assess their potency to provide a substrate for *in vitro* and *in vivo* neo-chondrogenesis. First, chondrocytes were mixed with the thermosensitive chitosan-based solution. After gentle mixing, the suspension was incubated at 37°C for several minutes to form a gel or injected quickly into the cartilage injury site. The chondrocytes are encapsulated homogeneously. The gelation process does not compromise cell viability and there is sufficient mass transport of nutrients and oxygen to the cells inside. Differentiated chondrocytes are characterized by a round morphology. Preserving this feature inside hydrogels is a prerequisite for efficient chondrogenic matrix production. Chitosan-based hydrogels can provide the constrained environment for chondrocytes that closely mimics the natural state of chondrocytes in cartilage. Chondrocytes inside chitosan hydrogels still maintained a round morphology after several weeks. Moreover, this "natural" environment may have stimulated the synthesis of the original products of collagen type II and aggrecan found in chondrocytes [128–130]. Wang and coworkers [66] found that thermosensitive chitosan–β-sodium glycerophosphate hydrogel could support matrix accumulation of chondrocytes and could repair sheep cartilage defects in 24 weeks (*cf.* Figure 9.24). On the other hand, chemical cross-linking of chitosan-based hydrogels is also used to encapsulate chondrocytes. However, some toxic cross-linking agents, such as glyoxal, glutaraldehyde, carbodiimide, and diepoxy compounds, cannot be used, because it is not impracticable to remove the residual cross-linking agents. Marra and coworkers [131] added

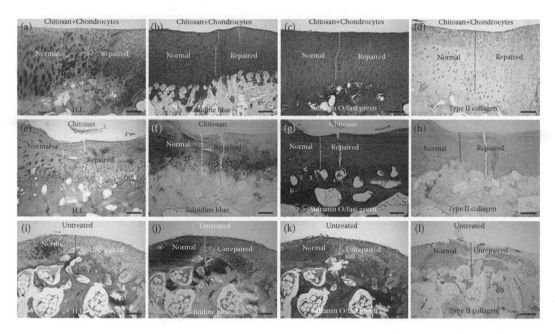

FIGURE 9.24
Histological and immunohistochemical evaluation of the articular cartilage repair at 24 weeks post operation. (a–d) In the experimental group, H&E staining showed that newly formed cartilage became more mature. The cells in the new cartilage were similar to the normal chondrocytes (a). The regenerated hyaline-like cartilage had less intensive toluidine blue staining than adjacent normal cartilage (b). A typical structure of hyaline cartilage lacunae is apparent in the regenerated area (c). The regenerated surface was demonstrated to be hyaline-like by type II collagen immunohistochemical staining (d). (e–h) In control group 1, no chitosan hydrogels were observed (e). The defects were partly filled with some renewed tissues when modestly stained with toluidine blue (f) and safranin O/fast green (g). Type II collagen immunohistochemical staining showed the cartilage to be fibrocartilage other than hyaline-like cartilage (h). (i–l) In control group 2, H&E staining indicated that the defect areas have no cell existence (i). The negative staining by toluidine blue (j) and safranin O/fast green (k) showed that the cartilage defects contain only some loose fibrous tissues. Type II collagen immunohistochemical staining contained the same (l). Dotted line indicates the boundary of the normal cartilage and the renewed cartilage. Bar 1/4 100 mm. (From Hao, T. et al. 2010. *Osteoarthritis and Cartilage* 18: 257–265. With permission.)

N-succinyl-chitosan solution into a centrifugal tube containing chondrocytes. After sufficient mixing, the cells containing *N*-succinyl-chitosan solutions were injected into a 24-well culture plate to cross-link with the aldehyde HA solutions. The formation of chondrocyte encapsulation is simple, feasible, and usually performed under mild conditions without employing any extraneous toxic cross-linking agents. And cells that were encapsulated within these hydrogels possessed normal spherical morphology (*cf.* Figure 9.25).

Reverse encapsulation of chondrocytes within the chitosan-based hydrogels is also an effective method to construct the artificial cartilage. In this system, chitosan-based hydrogels or hydrogel fragments are surrounded by chondrocytes. This situation of reverse encapsulation has the advantage of preserving the cell freedom, contrary to what happens when cells are too strongly sequestered in hydrogels. Domard and coworkers [132] mixed chondrocytes and chitosan hydrogel fragments to construct the hydrogel–chondrocytes construct. After 63 days in culture, chitosan hydrogel fragments seemed to have disappeared and be replaced by the neo-synthesized ECM (*cf.* Figure 9.26). The

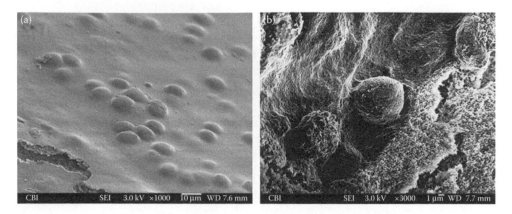

FIGURE 9.25
(a) SEM image depicting surface morphology of the *N*-succinyl-chitosan/aldehyde HA composite hydrogel encapsulated with chondrocytes after 24 h culture. (b) SEM image depicting the morphology of encapsulated chondrocytes after 24 h culture. (From Huaping Tan, H. P. et al. 2009. *Biomaterials* 30: 2499–2506. With permission.)

optimum results were obtained with chitosan hydrogel fragments of 55–70% DD and 1.5% chitosan.

9.5.3.2 Chitosan-Based Porous Hydrogels–Chondrocytes Construct

Chondrogenesis has been described on chitosan scaffolds. Since cartilage is avascular, cartilage nutrition, and metabolism are mainly influenced by local diffusion and cell–matrix

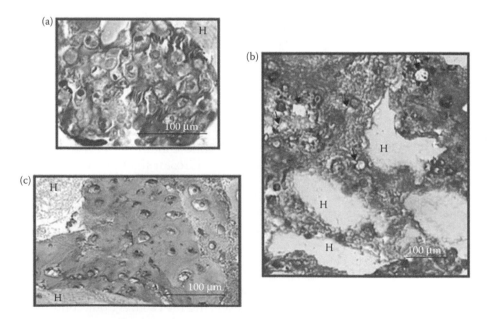

FIGURE 9.26
Histological morphology of constructs prepared with human articular chondrocytes (63-year-old female patient) and chitosan hydrogel (copolymer = 1.5%, DD of chitosan = 59.6%) and cultured for 20 days (a) or 63 days (b, c). Area: ≤50 μm² "↓", or >100 μm² "H". (From Montembault, A. et al. 2006. *Biochimie* 88: 551–564. With permission.)

interactions. The scaffold should not inhibit diffusion, which is especially relevant when culturing large amounts of cells for transplants, as is necessary for clinical applications. Therefore, the pores of the chitosan-based scaffold have a very important role in the formation process of new cartilages. On the basis of a chondrocytes diameter of approximately 10 µm, it is believed that a truly interconnecting porous structure with an average pore diameter of 70 µm would have allowed a substantial number of cells to migrate to the interior region of the scaffold. Chondrocytes cultured on chitosan scaffolds with pores <10 µm in diameter formed a film covering the surface of the scaffolds and produced small amounts of matrix (*cf.* Figure 9.27a) [133]. In this system, chondrocytes migration and tissue ingrowth within chitosan scaffolds are very difficult. Chitosan scaffolds containing larger pores appeared to contain more cells surrounded by the ECM. Cells penetrated the pores of chitosan scaffolds, especially in the group presenting the largest pores. The distribution of cells appeared more uniform throughout scaffolds as pores increased in size. Macroporous

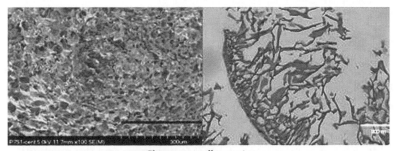

Chitosan, small pore size

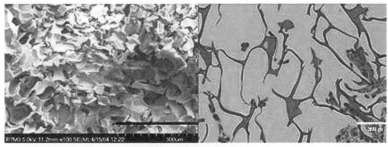

Chitosan, medium pore size

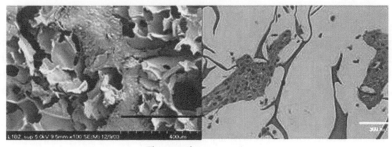

Chitosan, large pore size

FIGURE 9.27
Histology (H&E, ×40) and SEM of chitosan/chondrocytes constructs after 4 weeks of dynamic culture. (From GriVon, D. J. et al. 2006. *Acta Biomater* 2: 313–320. With permission.)

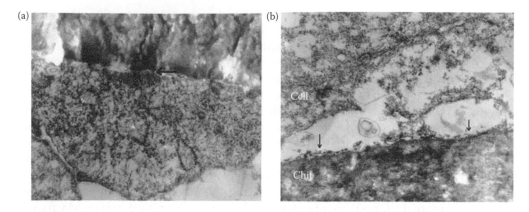

FIGURE 9.28
Representative micrographs of chondrocytes and chitosan scaffold interactions: (a) the large arrow indicates the junctional complex between the chitosan scaffold and the cell. TEM micrograph (×20,000); and (b) the thin arrows indicate the cell membrane in interaction with the chitosan scaffold. TEM micrograph (×12,000).

chitosan scaffolds can enhance the diffusion of cells and nutrients into the center of scaffolds. And chitosan allowed cell surfaces to gain resistance and attach to neighboring structures tightly. Chondrocyte membranes were strongly attached on the chitosan surface. Chondrocytes have junctional complexes that consist of plaques and filaments (*cf.* Figure 9.28) [134]. Moreover, when a concentration of 12–25 million cells/cm^2 is seeded in chitosan porous scaffolds, a lot of cartilage-specific ECMs can form and the mechanical strength of this scaffold–chondrocytes increased over time from 9.6 kPa at 14 days of 3D culture to 14.6 kPa at 28 days [135]. However, chondrocytes-laden porous chitosan scaffolds used to repair articular cartilage defects may proceed slower than the rate of cartilage regeneration [136]. And the ability of chitosan to maintain a round cellular morphology has been previously demonstrated for short periods of cell culture times (e.g., from 48 h to 2 weeks), but not for the prolonged cell culture time [137]. Therefore, pure chitosan scaffolds are not appropriate for producing artificial cartilage. Collagen, CAGs, polysaccharide, and synthetic polymer are introduced into the chitosan network to modulate the physicochemical properties, degradation behavior and mechanical properties, and bioactivities.

9.5.3.2.1 Chitosan–Collagen Scaffolds

In order to further produce the biomimetic environment for chondrocytes, chitosan scaffolds blended with collagen (or gelatin) or other GAGs were synthesized. The 3D porous chitosan–type II collagen scaffold can mimic the cartilage-specific ECM. It can improve the proliferation and differentiation of chondrocytes and synthesize type II collagen [138]. Recently, collagen is replaced by gelatin to prepare the 3D porous scaffold. The degraded products of chitosan–gelatin are involved in the synthesis of articular cartilage, such as chondroitin sulfate, dermatan sulfate, HA, keratin sulfate, and type II collagen [139]. The chitosan–gelatin scaffolds gradually experienced degradation, and cartilage tissues were developed, matured, and formed relatively homogenous cartilage [140].

9.5.3.2.2 Chitosan–CAG Scaffolds

GAGs are the main components of cartilage-specific ECM, and chitosan has a protective effect against GAG hydrolysis by their specific enzymes. Therefore, chitosan–GAG scaffolds have attracted much attention in cartilage tissue engineering. The addition of GAGs does not obviously alter the physical properties of chitosan scaffolds. Conjugating a single GAG species to chitosan is beneficial to chondrocyte culture and ECM production. The inclusion of GAG in the scaffold may promote the adhesion, migration, proliferation, and differentiation of chondrocytes. In addition, GAG can increase the water-binding capacity of scaffolds. The rich water-binding capacity may have therefore influenced the cell distribution and cluster formation, and the preservation of chondrocytes. For example, chondrocytes attached to chitosan–chondroitin sulfate scaffold had largely maintained a rounded or polygonal morphology and undergone only a modest degree of mitosis, maintaining the synthesis of cartilage-specific collagens [141]. A homogeneous cartilaginous tissue, which was similar to those of natural cartilage, formed when chondrocytes were seeded in the ternary chitosan–collagen–chondroitin sulfate porous scaffold at 12 weeks after implantation [142]. Similarly, ternary chitosan–collagen–hyaluronan scaffolds show an improvement in the mechanical strength, degradation rate, and water-binding capacity. And the chitosan–collagen–hyaluronan scaffolds reveal an increase in the total amount of GAGs and contain significantly more newly synthesized GAGs than the chitosan–collagen scaffolds alone [143]. Dermatan sulfate plays a very important role in cartilage engineering, and a low concentration of dermatan sulfate is beneficial for ECM production. However, higher concentration could enhance the activities of metalloproteases [144] which degrade ECM molecules and lead to lower GAGs and collagen production levels. Hu and coworkers [145] found that a combination of 2.8 mg chondroitin 6-sulfate and 0.01 mg dermatan sulfate in the chitosan scaffold (ca. 2.5 mg) is the optimal composite to modulate the behaviors of chondrocytes.

9.5.3.2.3 *Chitosan–Polysaccharide Scaffolds*

Some polyanion polysaccharides, whose structures are similar to GAGs, are also introduced into the chitosan network to construct the artificial cartilages. Alginate, a family of polyanionic copolymers, represents naturally occurring polysaccharides composed of (1–4)-linked β-D-mannuronic acid (M units) and α-L-guluronic acid (G units) monomers. The use of alginate may facilitate a uniform distribution of chondrocytes in the relatively wide pores of the scaffold and prevent cells from floating out. Moreover, *in vitro* experiments showed that alginate can stimulate the expression of the chondrogenic phenotype [146]. Chitosan–alginate porous scaffolds have a highly porous structure with a fairly even pore distribution and the surface of the scaffold is relatively rough and embedded with small grooves. The chondrocyte on chitosan, alginate, and chitosan–alginate scaffolds continued to increase with time. Moreover, the cell number on the chitosan–alginate scaffold became notably higher than on the pure chitosan scaffold and alginate scaffold. And the proliferation capacity of chondrocytes on chitosan–alginate (50/50 wt%) is higher than that on the chitosan–alginate (30/70 wt%) scaffold [37,147–149]. Moreover, the chitosan–alginate scaffold showed prolonged support for collagen type II production compared with the chitosan scaffold. Compared with chitosan, chitosan–alginate showed better support of maintaining the phenotype of chondrocytes, presumably resulting from special characteristics of alginate material in promoting chondrocyte recovery. At day 14, chondrocyte cells on chitosan and chitosan–alginate exhibited a spherical morphology. At day 21, however, the cells on the chitosan scaffold became more flattened and started to assume a fibroblast-like morphology, while the cells on the chitosan–alginate scaffold remained their initial spherical morphology (Figure 9.29) [137]. When the chondrocyte–chitosan–alginate–hyaluronate constructs are implanted into rabbit knee cartilage defects, partial repair is observed after 1 month [150].

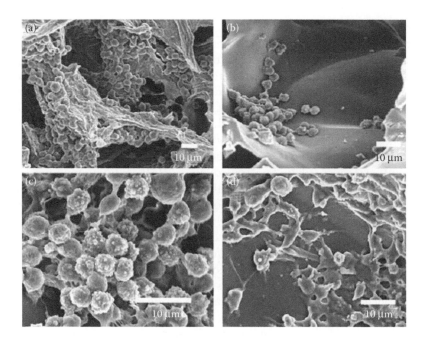

FIGURE 9.29
SEM images of chondrocyte cells grown on (a) chitosan–alginate and (b) chitosan scaffolds after 14 days cell culture, and on (c) chitosan–alginate and (d) chitosan scaffolds after 21 days of cell culture. (From Li, Z. S. and Zhang, M. Q. 2005. *J Biomed Mater Res* 75A: 485–493. With permission.)

9.5.3.2.4 Chitosan–Synthetic Polymers Scaffold

Synthetic polymers, such as polyethylene oxide (PEO), polyester, poly(DL-lactide), and so on, are also used to construct artificial skin with chitosan. These polymers can modulate the structure, degradation behaviors, and mechanical properties of the chitosan scaffold. Moreover, it can help seeded chondrocytes spread through the scaffolds and distribute homogeneously inside, can preserve the phenotype of chondrocytes, and effectively support the production of type II collagen. For example, chitosan–PEO scaffolds were employed for the cultivation of chondrocytes for the generation of cartilage tissue. The incorporation of PEO could amend porosity, mechanical brittleness, and ameliorate the biological compatibility of a chitosan scaffold. Porosity and moisture content increased as the weight percentage of PEO in chitosan–PEO scaffolds increased. The porosity can achieve the requirement for cartilage tissue engineering when the weight percentage of PEO is higher than 25%. PEO was a linear elastomeric polymer; thus an increase in the weight percentage of PEO reduced Young's modulus and improved the extensibility of the scaffolds. PEO with ether oxygen is highly hydrophilic. PEO could absorb a large amount of water. Thus an increase in the weight percentage of PEO promoted the percentage of biodegradation. The chondrocyte behaviors on the chitosan–PEO scaffold depended on the composites of the scaffold. In the chitosan–chitin–PEO scaffold, the range of the composition for a better culture of BKCs was 25% < PEO < 40%, 12.5% < chitin < 37.5%, and 30% < chitosan < 50% [26,151,152].

9.5.3.2.5 Chitosan Scaffolds Conjugated with Growth Factors

Many studies have suggested that a porous scaffold in itself is insufficient to induce rapid cartilage regeneration at the initial stages of cartilage healing. Growth factors, affecting the unique development of cartilage, are crucial for chondrogenesis. For example, TGF-β1 is one of the active growth factors regulating mitosis of chondrocytes and accelerates the synthesis of collagen, fibronectin, and proteoglycan in articular cartilage [153]. Therefore, a combination of the use of growth factors and a porous scaffold might substantially improve the cartilage-forming efficacy. A porous freeze-dried chitosan-based scaffold incorporating TGF-β1-loaded microspheres was used for the treatment of cartilage defects. Lee et al. [154] found that porous chitosan–collagen–GAG scaffolds loaded with TGF-β1 exhibited controlled release of TGF-β1 and promoted cartilage regeneration. Moreover, the proliferation capacity of chitosan-based scaffold loaded with TGF-β1 is much higher than that without TGF-β1. Long-term use of TGF-β1 can bring side effects, such as destroying the cartilage and partial ossification *in vivo*, and disturbance of proteoglycan homeostasis. TGF-β1 incorporated into the chitosan-based porous scaffold showed a burst release at the initial stage; this release kinetics is advantageous in the promotion of cartilage regeneration when the body needs high protein concentration in the initial stage and avoids the side effects of long-term use. In addition, other growth factors, such as FGFs, PDGFs, EGFs, and so on, play an important role in the proliferation of chondrocytes and production of ECM. Recently, tissue engineering and local therapeutic gene delivery systems have been paid much attention in the cartilage natural healing process. Guo et al. [155] designed a gene-activated matrix consisting of plasmid DNA and biodegradable chitosan–gelatin as scaffolds for cartilage regeneration. The plasmid DNA in the scaffolds can be partly protected from degradation by human serum and transfected to the primary chondrocytes. The combination of chitosan-based cartilage scaffolds with gene therapy and the use of growth factors will hopefully improve the long-term outcomes of cartilage repair in clinical settings.

9.5.4 Bone

Bone is a dynamic and highly vascularized tissue that continuously rebuilds its structure. Bone tissue has a hierarchical organization over length scales that span several orders of magnitude from the macro-(centimeter) scale to the nanostructured (ECM or ECM) components (*cf.* Figure 9.30) [156]. It is actually an inorganic–organic composite mainly made up of nano-HAp (nHAp) $(Ca_{10}(PO_4)_6(OH)_2$; and collagen fibers. The nanocomposite structure is integral to the requisite compressive strength and high fracture toughness of bone. Bone tissue itself is arranged either in a compact pattern (cortical bone) or in a trabecular pattern (cancellous bone). Every year, millions of patients, particularly among the aged, are suffering from bone defects arising from trauma, tumor, or bone diseases and of course several are dying due to insufficient ideal bone substitute. Bone defects represent a challenge for orthopedic and reconstructive surgeons. Surgical treatments of large bone defects include the Ilizarov method, or bone transport, and bone graft transplant. Currently, the gold standard treatment is the use of a procedure called autografting. The traditional biological methods of bone-defect management include autografting and allografting bone. Since bone grafts are avascular and dependent on diffusion, the size of the defect and the viability of the host bed can limit their application. Nevertheless, its use is severely hampered by its short supply and the considerable donor site morbidity associated with the harvest [157]. Bone tissue engineering techniques based on autogenous cell–tissue transplantation would eliminate these problems. In this regard, 3D scaffolds, osteoblasts or cells that can become osteoblasts, and regulating factors that promote cell recruitment, growth, differentiation, are very important factors to improve the formation of new bone (*cf.* Figure 9.31) [139].

Bone tissue undergoes constant remodeling in order to ensure that its structural integrity is maintained. The formation of new bone is a complicated process that involves

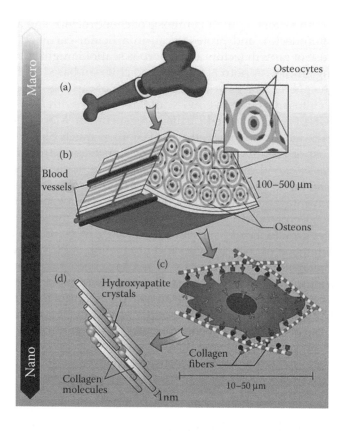

FIGURE 9.30
Hierarchical organization of bone over different length scales. Bone has a strong calcified outer compact layer (a), which comprises many cylindrical Haversian systems, or osteons (b). The resident cells are coated in a forest of cell membrane receptors that respond to specific binding sites (c) and the well-defined nanoarchitecture of the surrounding ECM (d). (From Stevens, M. M. and George, J. H. 2005. *Science* 310: 1135–1138. With permission.)

osteoblasts (improve bone forming) and osteoclasts (improve bone resorbing) [158,159]. Most research pay attention to the osteoblast response to chitosan films or scaffolds. Chitosan was shown to be an effective substrate that supports the initial attachment and the spreading of osteoblasts. The viability of the attached osteoblasts on chitosan substrates generally increased significantly with an increase in the cell seeding time. Osteoblast cells are not fully attached on the surfaces of the chitosan substrates at 2 h after cell seeding and they are round. At 8 h after cell seeding, osteoblasts on the chitosan film counterparts assumed a spindle shape [160]. Osteoblasts displayed phenotypes that were well spread with a developed cytoskeleton [161]. Moreover, chitosan supports osteoblasts to produce mineralized tissues [162]. Takakuda and coworkers [163] found that chitin–chitosan can be used as a bone formation accelerator. After the 2-week implantation of chitin–chitosan coating on PLA fiber into holes drilled into the distal metaphyses of rat femora, the mean area of bone tissue in the experimental group was 0.532 ± 0.145 mm^2, while that in the control group was 0.113 ± 0.049 mm^2. The success of an implant not only depends on the interaction with osteoblasts. Osteoclasts also play a very important role in the formation process of new bone. Cartmell SH and coworkers [164] found that chitosan supported osteoclast culture, but the proliferation capacity of osteoclasts is lower than that of osteoblasts on chitosan film. Chitosan recorded significantly higher amounts of DNA in the

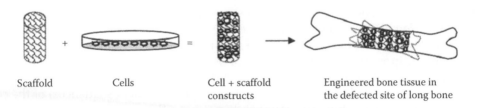

Scaffold   Cells   Cell + scaffold   Engineered bone tissue in
                     constructs   the defected site of long bone

FIGURE 9.31

Schematic diagram of the bone tissue engineering approach using scaffolds and cells. (From Thein-Han, W. W. et al. 2008. *Mater Sci Technol* 24: 1062–1075. With permission.)

osteoblast–osteoclast coculture system compared to osteoclasts. In this coculture system, osteoblasts are responsible for the generation of bone ECM but also regulate the differentiation and activity of osteoclasts.

Chitosan-based scaffold is an attractive candidate for bone because it can modulate osteoblast and osteoclast growth and differentiation, and matrix mineralization. But, as a temporary template introduced at the defective site or lost bone for tissue regeneration, which over a period of time gradually degrades and is replaced by newly formed bone tissue, the chitosan-based scaffold should also have other characters as follows: (1) An ideal bone tissue-engineering chitosan-based scaffold should have an appropriate microstructure for the growth of osteoblasts. On the basis of an osteoblast length of approximately 10–30 μm, the pore diameter of the chitosan-based scaffold should be higher than this value. In general, the pore size should range from 100 to 400 μm. When pore diameter is too small, cells may provoke pore occlusion and prevent cellular penetration within the scaffold: pore size ranging from 75 to 100 μm resulted in ingrowth of unmineralized osteoid tissue and smaller pores (down to 10 μm) were penetrated only by fibrous tissue [165]. (2) The chitosan-based scaffolds should have sufficient mechanical strength during *in vitro* culturing to maintain the spaces required for osteoblast ingrowth and matrix formation. Moreover, it can bear certain loading after *in vivo* implantation. The optimal mechanical strength of the chitosan-based scaffold should be close to the mechanical strength of natural bone. For example, the compressive strength of cortical bone is 130–180 MPa and the compressive strength of cancellous bone ranges from 4 to 12 MPa. At present, the compressive strength of some chitosan-based scaffolds mimics cancellous bone, but to obtain a compressive strength similar to cortical bone is very difficult. (3) The degradation of the chitosan-based scaffold should match with the formation of new bone. In general, it needs ca. 1–6 months according to the age and constitution of the patient. (4) Moreover, the scaffold should load and release various growth factors (BMPs and TGF-β1) to improve the formation of new bone. In short, mimicking the composites and structure of natural bone is an effective method to obtain ideal chitosan-based bone engineering. At present, some proteins, polysaccharides, synthetic polymers and inorganic minerals (HAp, calcium phosphate, etc.) have been incorporated into the chitosan network to construct artificial bone.

9.5.4.1 Chitosan-Based Polymeric Porous Scaffolds

Collagen and chitosan have intrinsic properties that support growth and differentiation of osteoblasts. Osteoblasts have a specific affinity for collagen fibers. The incorporation of collagen into a collagen–chitosan scaffold can increase the biological stability and adjust the degradation behaviors. Chitosan–collagen composite sponges promoted growth of osteoblasts into the mature stage. Moreover, osteocalcin and calcium were clearly demonstrated in chitosan–collagen sponges but not chitosan scaffold. The collagen matrix promoted osteoblastic differentiation and enhanced the osteoconductivity of chitosan–collagen scaffold. Thus a combination of collagen and chitosan matrices should create an appropriate environment for growth and differentiation of osteoblasts [166]. Moreover, combined chitosan–collagen scaffold promoted osteogenic differentiation of MSCs due to the specific cell-binding sites (particularly the RGD (Arg-Gly-Asp) amino acid sequences) of the collagen matrix. But the pure chitosan scaffolds do not have this effect [167]. The defect sites exhibited marked bone formation at the defect margin, and dense, fibrous connective tissues were observed in the center of the defect at 8 weeks after implanting chitosan–collagen in a rat calvarial defect [168]. However, the pore size and interconnected pore structure of the chitosan–collagen scaffold need to be improved through the fabrication process. Chitosan–alginate porous scaffolds are highly porous with a pore size around 100–300 µm, a structure favorable for cell attachment and new bone tissue ingrowth. Compared with pure chitosan scaffolds, chitosan–alginate scaffolds can improve the proliferation and mineral deposition of osteoblasts. A layer of small particles (calcium-rich minerals) covered the cells grown on the chitosan–alginate scaffold. Moreover, chitosan–alginate scaffolds promoted rapid vascularization and deposited connective tissue and calcified matrix within the entire scaffold structure [169]. For a porous chitosan polymeric scaffold, although they have excellent bioactivity for osteoblasts, the compressive moduli of these scaffolds were in the lower range of the trabecular bone, making them unsuitable for load-bearing bone tissue-engineering applications.

Chitosan-based polymeric microsphere scaffolds have excellent mechanical properties. Chitosan–poly(lactic acid–glycolic acid) (chitosan–PLAGA) sintered microsphere scaffolds had compressive moduli (340.96–412.37 MPa) and compressive strengths (9.68–13.32 MPa) in the range of the trabecular bone and compressive strength, and it can support well the proliferation of osteoblasts [33]. Heparinized chitosan–PLAGA microsphere scaffolds with low heparin loading are capable of stimulating MC3T3-E1 cell proliferation differentiation. *In vivo* study using the rabbit ulnar critical-sized defect mode demonstrated that scaffolds supported normal bone formation via intramembranous formation (*cf.* Figure 9.32) [170]. However, the porosity of these chitosan-based microsphere scaffolds is only ca. 30%, which may restrict the ingrowth of cells and exchange of nutrition. Therefore, enhancing porosity is a crucial factor for the application of chitosan-based microsphere scaffolds in bone tissue engineering.

9.5.4.2 Chitosan–Ceramic Composite Scaffolds

The components of bone possess a nanocomposite structure interwoven in a 3D matrix. In recent years, nanomaterials have been developed for bone tissue engineering applications. From the biomimetic point of view, chitosan–ceramic composites could potentially improve both biocompatibility and mechanical properties of bone grafting materials. Chitosan–HAp composite scaffolds have received great attention because they can mimic the composites and structure of nature. In this system, HAp cannot be absorbed but it may be inserted into new bone following the absorption of the chitosan. Chitosan–HAp composite scaffolds were characterized by a highly porous structure and the pore size (50–120 µm) was in a similar range for the scaffolds with different contents of nHAp. The compressive strength of the chitosan–HAp scaffold increases with increasing HAp content in composites. Osteoblasts on the chitosan–HAp scaffold exhibited significantly higher proliferation capacity than that on pure chitosan scaffolds [171]. Chitosan–HAp scaffolds significantly enhanced osteoblast matrices *in vitro*, as evidenced by increased osteocalcin production

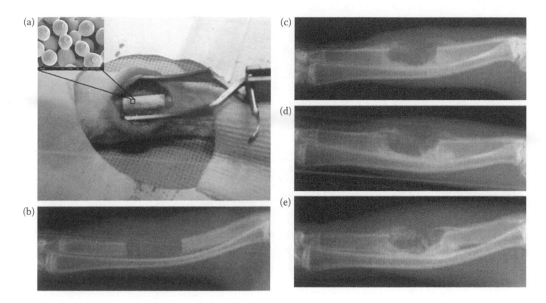

FIGURE 9.32
(a) The surgical procedure showing that a 15 mm segment of ulna was removed and a sintered microsphere scaffold was implanted into the defect site; (b) a radiograph of the defect immediately after surgery showing the removal of the segment of ulna and the creation of a segmental defect in the ulna; (c–e) typical radiographs of the defect site at 4 weeks (c), 8 weeks (d), and 12 weeks (e) post operation in the heparinized chitosan/PLAGA microsphere scaffolds. The inset in (a) shows the porous structure of the sintered microsphere scaffold used in the *in vivo* study.

when compared with pure chitosan scaffolds. Chesnutt et al. [172] found that chitosan–HAp scaffolds were also shown to be biocompatible and osteoconductive in a preliminary critical-sized rat calvarial defect study. After 12 weeks, composite scaffolds were enclosed by a thin layer of new bone and some small scaffold particles were observed to have become completely incorporated into the new bone. Moreover, the combination of the chitosan–HAp scaffolds and osteoblasts can achieve a better repair of bone defect [173].

In order to further mimic the composites and structure of nature, collagen or gelatin also be combined into chitosan–HAp scaffold. Chitosan–gelatin–HA composite scaffolds were prepared via blending chitosan–gelatin solution and HA particles. Osteoblasts adhered to the surface of the composites, performed their functions, and exhibited a good proliferation in the composite scaffolds, while interlaced ECM networks formed around the cells (*cf.* Figure 9.33) [174]. The osteoblast–scaffold constructs had good biomineralization effect after 3 weeks in culture. Hu and coworkers [175] found that chitosan–collagen–HA scaffolds have a capability for bone repair. When the composites scaffolds were implanted in the bone defect site of rabbits, the bone defect was still there at the fourth week, and there was no new bone formed in the bone defect site. At the eighth week, defect could still be found in the bone defect location. At the 12th week, the bone defect was repaired completely (*cf.* Figure 9.34). However, the HAp particles in this case did not disperse well or were easily to agglomerate, and even settle, which made it difficult to form a controlled structure. Meanwhile, the HAp crystal may migrate from the composite because of the weak interactions between HAp and the chitosan matrix. When cells interact with the composites, the interfaces between HAp crystals and polymer were destroyed and the nHA crystals were easily released from the chitosan-based matrix. The composite scaffold obtained via deposition *in situ* can avoid these disadvantages, because there are strong

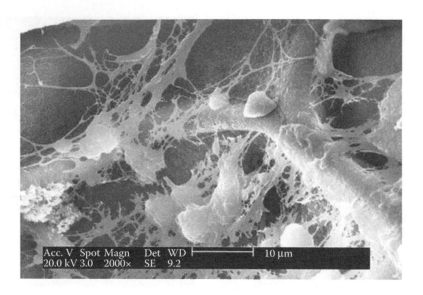

FIGURE 9.33
SEM micrographs of the osteoblasts/scaffold construct. The osteoblasts were well attached to the pore wall, and surrounded by an excreted interlaced fibrous network. (From Zhao, F. et al. 2002. *Biomaterials* 23: 3227–3234. With permission.)

interactions between HA and COO^- groups of collagen or gelatin. Moreover, the size of HAp particles could be modulated via adjusting the polymer matrix. More gelatin or collagen may result in the formation of small HAp particles [176]. This stable structure endows the composite scaffold with excellent bioactivity.

9.5.5 Nerve

Nerve injuries are common in trauma surgery. Today, even under excellent conditions, nerve regeneration can never achieve complete histological and clinical recovery. In the peripheral nervous system, the proximal segment may be able to regenerate and reestablish nerve function. However, the gap between the nerve stumps is too large (>2 mm), a device is needed to bridge the gap in order to guide outgrowing nerve fibers and to prevent the formation of neuroma. For the central nervous system, axons do not regenerate appreciably in their native environment. The autologous nerve graft, although the gold

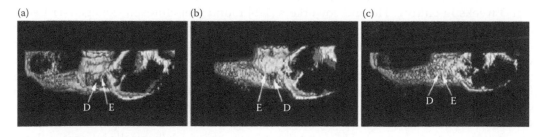

FIGURE 9.34
CT 3D reconstruction of repairing bone defect by chitosan–collagen–HA for 4 (a), 8 (b), and 12 (c) weeks. (d) The bone defect site; (e) the newly formed bone in the bone defect site. (From Wang, Y. et al. 2008. *J Biomed Mater Res* 86A: 244–252. With permission.)

standard for nerve reconstruction, is associated with some major disadvantages. The nerve graft cannot be harvested from amputated extremities in the same operation and it can result in new nerve injures. One the other hand, although allograft can overcome these major drawbacks, as soon as cellular components are transferred, immunosuppression becomes mandatory [177].

Tissue-engineered conduits have been developed as a promising option for nerve regeneration, due to their mechanical support and chemical stimulation for axonal elongation. The conduit allows for neurotropic and neurotrophic communication between the nerve stumps and provides physical guidance to regenerating axons. The topographical cues induce cabling of cells within the conduit [178]. Chitosan has been studied as a candidate conduit material for nerve regeneration due to its natural features. It can support the adhesion, migration, and proliferation of nerve cells (e.g., Schwann cells, cerebral cortex cells, and PC12). Some polymers are added into the chitosan network to modulate the nervous cell behaviors.

Besides, a chitosan-based biomaterial, in order to be an ideal nerve conduit, should have the following characteristics. (a) It must have enough internal surface area for the nerve fibers and Schwann cells to cohere. It must allow diffusion transport of nutrients while preventing external cells from entering the conduit. The optimal porosity of the nerve conduit is 70–98% [179]. (b) The chitosan-based biomaterial must have appropriate matrix stiffness. A soft biomaterial with low Young's modulus, which can better mimic the mechanical properties of soft nerve tissue, is a more favorable scaffold for nerve regeneration. But chitosan is considerably more rigid and brittle than nerve tissues. Nerve conduits made from chitosan may compress the regenerating nerve cells and may rupture *in vivo* before wounds are completely healed. Therefore, chitosan must be modified to improve its mechanical properties before it can be used in nerve repair. Some flexible molecules are introduced into the chitosan network to improve the proliferation and differentiation capacity of nerve cells. For example, the P12 cells cultured on the composite film with 60 wt% gelatin differentiated more rapidly and extended longer neurites than on the pure chitosan film [180]. (c) The chitosan-based biomaterial must have sufficient mechanical stability during nerve regeneration. It is demonstrated that the chitosan mesh tubes with a DD of 93% have sufficient mechanical properties to preserve tube space, provide a better scaffold for cell migration and attachment, and facilitate humoral permeation to enhance nerve regeneration. (d) The chitosan-based biomaterial must become revascularized fast enough to overcome nutrient transport limitations into the graft. (e) It must have appropriate degradation rate to maintain a stable support structure for the entire regeneration process, but should not remain in the body much longer than needed to prevent later compression of the nerve. (f) It must have an appropriate degree of inflammatory response after implanted *in vivo*. The potency of the chitosan-based conduits for promoting nerve regeneration will eventually depend on its interaction with the relevant tissues. Some degree of inflammatory response may therefore play a positive role; however, a high number of inflammatory cells blocked the way for the sprouting axons, and nerve regeneration was delayed. Pure chitosan conduits showed high infiltration of inflammatory cells such as macrophages during the first 2 weeks, which will limit the application of chitosan conduits in nerve regeneration. Thus, some proteins or polymers should be incorporated into the chitosan network to decrease the inflammatory response [181,182].

Typical materials for nerve guide coatings are adhesion proteins, such as laminin, fibronectin, or poly(L-lysine), which have been found to be specific for nerve regeneration, thus allowing more rapid recovery of nerve functionality. Chitosan modified by blending with proteins or poly(L-lysine) had significantly improved nerve cell affinity as indicated by increasing the attachment, differentiation, and growth of the nerve cells. The improved nerve cell affinity for the chitosan–poly(L-lysine) composite materials had been attributed to the increased hydrophilicity by the abundant hydroxyl group and the positive surface charge of chitosan [183]. The inner surface of artificial nerve conduits is expected to serve for regenerating nerves. However, recent research found that the nerve tissue regenerates not directly attached to the conduits surface but rather in a fibrin matrix scaffold inside the conduits. While laminin (an 800 kDa glycoprotein from the basement membrane) can aid nerve growth, synthetic laminin peptides were preferred in studies intended to facilitate nerve regeneration *in vivo* with the aid of chitosan conduits covalently coated with the said peptides. Laminin associating with the inner surface of the conduits may be favorable for the attachment and migration of Schwann cells and growth cones [184]. Itoh and coworkers [185] coupled laminin on the inner surface of chitosan conduits to support nerve regeneration on the inner surface of chitosan conduits. In particular, glial cell line-derived nerve growth factor and laminin were blended with chitosan to fabricate factor + laminin + chitosan guides, which can enhance both functional and sensory recovery [186].

The main drawback of using poly(L-lysine), fibronectin, and laminin is their high cost. Therefore, nerve guides are currently being fabricated by adding certain proteins that support nerve repair and regeneration, and by optimizing the biological properties of a nerve guide. The addition of collagen to the chitosan network has an effect on the quality of nerve repair compared with using the chitosan material alone. The chitosan–collagen nerve conduits have a smooth inner and outer surface texture. The chitosan–collagen conduits scaffold exhibits better physical and chemical properties at the quantity ratio of chitosan to collagen of 3:1 [187]. Chitosan–collagen composites provide a better environment to support the survival, migration, proliferation, and differentiation of neural stem cells and their differentiating cells. And the differentiating percentage from neural stem cells into neurons was significantly increased compared with pure chitosan [188]. Compared with pure chitosan, collagen–chitosan conduits improved the axonal maturation measured by a significant increase in axon diameter and axon area [189]. Moreover, the chitosan–collagen conduits enhanced motor and sensory nerve recovery [190]. Wei et al. [191] evaluated a chitosan–collagen film as a nerve wrap conduit to repair completely resected sciatic nerve. Histological analysis revealed nerve regeneration at 8 weeks post surgery using the 10 mm conduits. Ciardelli and Chiono [192] found that chitosan–gelatin can also promote nerve regeneration.

Collapse of an unfilled circular conduit is a major block to nerve regeneration in tubulization. Chitosan conduits can be molded into various configurations, which make them effective in enhancing nerve regeneration. Itoh et al. [193] prepared circular and triangular chitosan tubes via melting molding for nerve regeneration (*cf.* Figure 9.35). After implanting in a nerve defect of rat, some of the circular tubes somewhat narrowed with time, and nerve regeneration occurred toward one side. However, the volume for regenerating nerves in a triangular tube was rather preserved, and the nerve tissue equally distributed in the tube. This may be ascribed to its (a) superior mechanical property, (b) preservation of the space for nerve regeneration, and (c) contact phase enlargement between the tube surface and penetrating cells from the nerve ends.

However, the application of chitosan-based conduits prepared using melting molding is subject to certain restrictions owing to the low porosity and low permeability, which hinders the inflow of nutrients through the conduit walls. Porous and fiber chitosan-based conduits can overcome these disadvantages. Gander and coworkers [182] prepared porous chitosan–alginate conduits (*cf.* Figure 9.36). These have a good permeability for solutes and adequate mechanical strength. Recently, bilayered fiber chitosan conduits comprising an

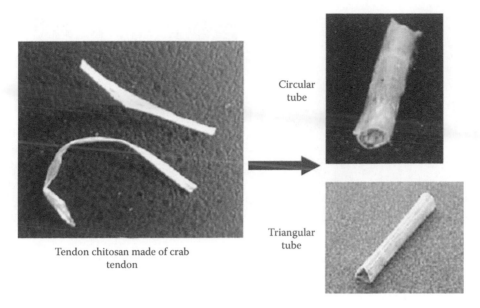

Circular tube

Triangular tube

Tendon chitosan made of crab tendon

FIGURE 9.35
Circular and triangular conduits of chitosan. (From Itoh, S. et al. 2003. *Artif Organs* 27: 1079–1088. With permission.)

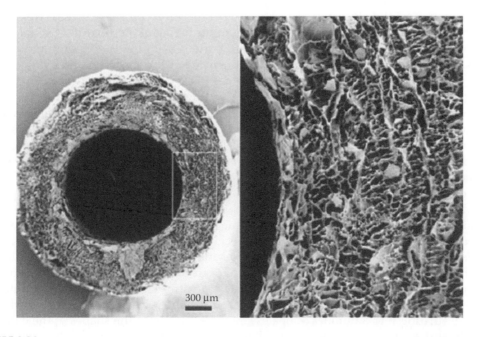

300 μm

FIGURE 9.36
SEM micrograph of the cross section through a freeze-dried alginate/chitosan nerve conduit (magnification ×70 (left) and ×350 (right)). (From Pfister, L. A. 2007. *J Biomed Mater Res* 80A: 932–937. With permission.)

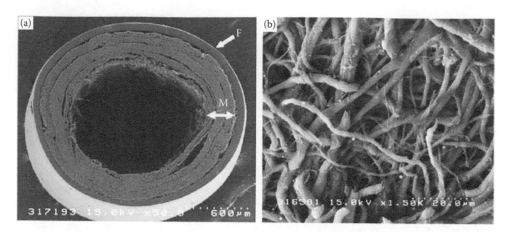

FIGURE 9.37
(a) SEM micrographs of the bilayered chitosan tube. F, chitosan film; and M, electrospun nano/microfiber mesh. (b) Enlargement of the electrospun nano/microfiber mesh. The nano/microfiber structure comprises randomly oriented fibers. 3D pores formed among fibers are interconnected and distributed throughout the structure. (From Wang, W. et al. 2008. *J Biomed Mater Res* 84A: 557–566; Wang, W. et al. 2008. *J Biomed Mater Res* 85A: 919–928. With permission.)

outer layer of chitosan film and an inner layer of electrospun chitosan nonwoven have been developed (*cf.* Figure 9.37) [194,195]. 3D pores formed between fibers were interconnected and distributed throughout the structure. The porosity improves the exchange of nutrients and metabolic waste between the scaffold and surrounding tissue. The compressive strength of the bilayered chitosan conduits was significantly greater than that of the chitosan fiber mesh conduits. The bilayer chitosan-based conduits can improve nerve regeneration, and the efficiency of nerve regeneration into bilayer chitosan tubes with immobilized CGGGGGGYIGSR peptide was similar to that of the isograft. Axonal regeneration parallel to aligned Schwann cells is reported in injured peripheral and central nerves *in vivo*. Inducing Schwann cell alignment resulting in oriented axonal growth while preventing neuroma formation in the peripheral nerve injury is very important during the process of nerve regeneration. Itoh and coworkers [196] constructed bilayered chitosan fiber conduits with an inner layer of oriented nanofibers and an outer layer of randomized nanofibers. Schwann cells aligned in the same direction as a result of secure adhesion to the oriented fibers, but had no specific orientation on randomized nanofibers. The oriented chitosan nanofiber mesh tube may be a promising substitute for an autogenous nerve graft.

The degradation of chitosan used to date in nerve regeneration is very slow and poorly controlled. As a source material of chitosan, chitin has attracted much less research interest mainly because of the difficulty in processing it into the desired shape and also because of uncertainty of its biological properties, especially nerve cell affinity. Gu and coworkers [197] developed a two-step procedure to prepare tailored chitin products indirectly starting from chitosan counterparts. This "chitin" and chitosan materials were equally biocompatible to cultured Schwann cells. The degradation rate of "chitin" is higher than that of chitosan. Moreover, the shapes of implanted chitin conduits in nerve defects were completely changed, turning into a number of opalescent pieces, whereas the shapes of the chitosan conduits still showed no conspicuous alterations and there was little inflammation at the implantation spots (*cf.* Figure 9.38). Carboxymethyl chitosan, a dissolvable chitosan derivative, also possesses many desirable physiochemical and biological features that are

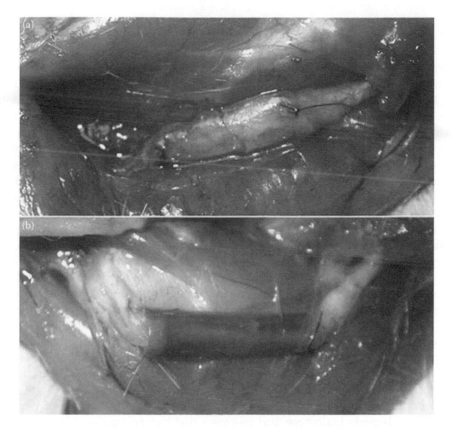

FIGURE 9.38
The reexposed sites of nerve implantation following transfusion of animals at 20 weeks after implantation for the "chitin" nerve guidance conduits (a) and the chitosan nerve guidance conduits (b). Degradation of chitin- and chitosan-based nerve guidance conduits (NGCs) was observed. (From Yang, Y. M. et al. 2009. 11: B209–B218. With permission.)

similar to chitosan. It can be degraded quickly by lysozyme due to its solubility at physiological pH. Compared with chitosan conduit, easier supply of nutrients and oxygen into the partially decomposed tube wall can occur, which results in better nerve regeneration of the carboxymethyl chitosan conduits [198]. Apart from these, incorporating other materials with a high degradation rate, such as collagen, gelatin, PDLLA, and so on, is an effective method to modulate the degradation rate of chitosan-based conduits.

9.5.6 Liver

Each year, end-stage liver disease claims thousands of lives in the world. Currently, there is very little effective treatment for the most severe liver diseases. Orthotopic liver transplant is currently the only treatment for end-stage liver disease; there are 65,000 people in China and 27,000 people in the Unite States who need to receive liver transplants. Unfortunately, the demand for liver transplantation far exceeds the limited supply; only 2000–3000 people can receive the transplantation surgery. In addition, liver transplantation is far from the ideal treatment owing to its high cost, the adverse effects associated with surgery, and immune suppression. Liver tissue engineering, where one seeks to augment liver function by implanting functional hepatocytes, offers an attractive alternative. The difficulty of liver regeneration lies in the vast complexity of tissue [199]. It is a highly organized structure and the 3D arrangement of hepatic cells is integral to its functions. Primary hepatocytes rapidly lose tissue-specific functions once they are removed from the living organism. In contrast to other simple structural tissues, such as bone and cartilage, the liver must carry out complex metabolic functions, such as biosynthesis, biotransformation, and excretion. Unlike the bone and cartilage, liver tissue has no inherent mechanical function. That is to say, it is very difficult to mimic the structure of nature. The field of liver regeneration remains one of the biggest challenges for tissue engineering. The chitosan-based biomaterials can be considered as a potential scaffold to support liver regeneration. At present, however, research on liver tissue engineering is at the initial stage.

In the human liver, hepatic cells are arranged in an intricate manner, enabling optimal communication and attachment among cells. Hepatocytes *in vivo* survive in a 3D system that is formed by various kinds of ECMs such as collagen, proteoglycan, fibronectin, and laminin. Chitosan-based biomaterials can provide an appropriate microenvironment for the growth of hepatocyte due to its various properties. It is evident that several liver-specific functions, such as albumin secretion and urea synthesis, could be enhanced when culturing hepatocytes in porous chitosan scaffolds *in vitro* [200]. In order to provide a better microenvironment, collagen or gelatin was introduced into the chitosan-based network. Hepatocytes maintain viability and perform biological functions in chitosan–gelatin, and the chitosan–gelatin is more efficient in inducing fibrin formation and vascularization at the implant–host interface [201,202].

Asialoglycoprotein receptors (ASGPRs) are expressed on the surface of hepatocytes. Therefore, some ligands (galactose and fructose) that can recognize ASGPR are usually combined into the chitosan scaffold. The scaffold with ligands can provide a new synthetic ECM for hepatocyte attachment through the specific interactions between ASGPR on hepatocytes and ligands. Moreover, they can improve hepatocyte attachment and maintain viability via the specific interactions between ASGPR on hepatocytes and galactose ligands. For example, alginate–galactosylated chitosan scaffolds have the potential ability to improve hepatocyte attachment for short-term culture. Galactose ligands facilitate hepatocyte aggregation in alginate–galactosylated chitosan scaffolds, resulting in the maintenance of high cell activity by the intercellular adhesion molecules in the 3D coculture system [203,204]. Meanwhile, fructose-modified chitosan porous scaffolds induced the formation of cellular aggregates with enhancing the liver-specific metabolic activities and cell density to a satisfactory level [205].

Pore size plays important roles in liver regeneration. Microspores (1–100 μm) significantly improve hepatocyte attachment and albumin secretion [206]. This character can be realized via freeze-drying technology. However, artificial liver manufacture requires a careful interplay of many design parameters owing to the complexity of liver tissue. Precise control of internal pore architecture parameters as well as the ECM components is essential to maintain the liver functions. Li and coworkers [9,207] prepared 3D chitosan–gelatin scaffold using RP technology. The scaffold possesses multilevel organized internal morphologies including vascular systems (portal vein, artery, and hepatic vein) and parenchymal component (hepatocyte chamber) (*cf.* Figure 9.39). The smallest channels are approximately 150 μm in width and the smallest distance between channels and chambers is about 170 μm. The scales for the hepatocyte chambers are 200 μm in width and 580 μm in length. Moreover, the volume between the blood vessels and the hepatic chambers is a

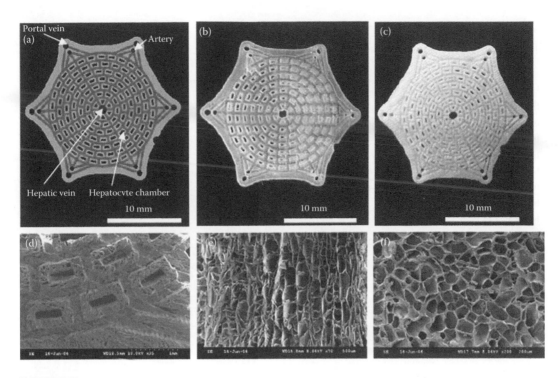

FIGURE 9.39
Porous chitosan/gelatin scaffold with specific external shape and predefined internal morphology. (a) CAD model, (b) resin mould fabricated using the SL technique, (c) porous chitosan/gelatin scaffold, (d) SEM of the predefined internal morphology, (e) microstructures when segmented longitudinally, and (f) microstructures when segmented transversely. (From He, J. K. et al. 2007. *Polymer* 48: 4578–4588. With permission.)

fully interconnected porous structure (Figures 9.39e and f). These organized architectures have the potential to allow the orderly arrangement and coculture of various liver cells, such as hepatocytes and ECs. Hepatocytes could form large colonies in the predefined hepatic chambers, and these cavities could be completely filled with hepatocytes during 7 day culture. Albumin secretion and urea synthesis further indicated that the well-organized scaffolds were more suitable for hepatocyte culture.

9.6 Summary and Outlook

In summary, chitosan is an attractive candidate biomaterial that shows a great potential in tissue engineering due to its biocompatibility, controlled biodegradability, and functionality. It can be used as a substitute for blood vessel, skin, cartilage, bone, nerve, liver, and so on. Table 9.4 summarizes the applications of chitosan-based biomaterials in tissue engineering. However, currently there are few chitosan-based tissue-engineering products. Although much progress has been made to apply chitosan-based biomaterials in tissue engineering, many limitations need to be overcome to develop more clinically meaningful chitosan scaffolds for various kinds of tissue regeneration. There are still many challenges in improving their properties.

TABLE 9.4

Application of Chitosan-Based Biomaterials in Tissue Engineering

	Blood Vessel	Skin	Cartilage	Bone	Nerve	Liver
Chitosan/collagen	+	+++	+++	+	++	++
Chitosan/gelatin	+	+++	+++	+	++	+++
Chitosan/heparin	+++					
Chitosan/GAG	++	++	+++	+	++	++
Chitosan/alginate		+	+++	++	++	++
Chitosan/pectin				+		
Chitosan/PVA	++		+			
Chitosan/PLA		++		++		
Chitosan/PEO		+	++			
Chitosan/PLGA		++		++		
Chitosan/PLAGA						
Galactosylated chitosan						+++
Fructose chitosan						+++
Chitosan/HAp				+++	+	
Chitosan/TCP				+++	+	

Note: +++, optimal; ++, excellent; +, appropriate; blank, no data.

9.6.1 Design of Complicated Scaffolds

Tissues in nature exhibit gradients across a spatial volume, in which each identifiable layer has specific functions to perform so that the whole tissue–organ can behave normally. Such a gradient is termed a functional gradient. In the process of tissue regeneration, more than one cell type is necessary. These different cell types have obviously different environments *in vivo*. The chitosan-based scaffold should have gradient chemical constitution and matrix stiffness to construct a special ECM matrix for different cells. The tissues consist of layers having different microstructures, which can vary in terms of porosity, density, and pore size. They have different scaffold requirements, such as different pore sizes, porosities, and mechanical properties [208]. Table 9.5 summarizes the optimal properties for different cells types. A chitosan-based scaffold should be designed to fit these characteristics. At present, some bilayer or multiple layer chitosan-based porous scaffolds have been developed via freeze-drying [8] or the LBL assembly technique combined with choosing salt as the porogen [209]. These multilayer structures have distinctive interfaces between

TABLE 9.5

Optimal Microstructures of Chitosan-Based Scaffolds for Different Tissues

Tissue	Pore Size (μm)	Matrix Stiffness
Blood vessel	60–150	
Nerve		Soft
Skin	20–125	↓
Liver	45–150	
Cartilage	70–120	↓
Bone	100–400	Rigid

the layers. However, the optimal scaffold should have continuous pore gradients. However, it is usually difficult to fabricate well-constructed scaffolds with continuous gradient pore sizes and porosities using common processing techniques, such as particulate leaching and freeze-drying technology. RP can accurately control the microstructure of chitosan-based scaffolds. But the porosity is low; for example, the porosities of 3D scaffolds prepared via 3D printing technology and fused deposition modeling technology are ca. 40–60% and 21–68%, respectively. Therefore, a suitable and meaningful design and preparation technology to represent the continuous gradient that can fulfill the biological and mechanical requirements of the regenerated tissue is needed.

9.6.2 Stem Cell Technology and Chitosan-Based Biomaterials

Recently, seed cells have become the main bottlenecks in the development of tissue engineering. For example, the application of chondrocytes is restricted due to its limited sources and weak capacity to maintain the chondrocyte phenotype and biological activity. Adult stem cell types are pluripotent, meaning that they can differentiate into cells derived from three germ layers. For example, hematopoietic stem cells may differentiate into brain cells, skeletal, cardiac muscle cells, and liver cells. MSCs may differentiate into skeletal muscle cells, may also differentiate into osteoblasts, chondrocytes, adipocytes, and other myocytes such as cardiac muscle cells, and so on. The plasticity provides the basic possibility for multiple-tissue engineering using a certain type of stem cells. In previous research, some bioactive molecules were incorporated into the stem cell–scaffold system to stimulate the differentiation of stem cells along the specific lineage (*cf.* Table 9.6) [210]. Even without differentiating into specific cells or tissues, the self-renewal aspect of MSCs can still provide a trophic effect in structure reparative environments. However, the applications of these bioactive molecules are limited due to their high cost and side effects to some extent. Therefore, it is a challenge to build an appropriate microenvironment for the proliferation and differentiation of stem cells. Many researchers have employed biomaterial scaffolds with different chemical signals, mechanical signals, and topographical signals to adjust the differentiation behaviors of stem cells.

Chemical functional groups of biomaterials could influence the differentiation behaviors of MSCs, such as methyl ($-CH_3$), hydroxyl ($-OH$), carboxyl ($-COOH$), and amino ($-NH_2$) groups that have been presented in biomaterials. Curran et al. [211,212] reported that the $-NH_2$ and $-SH$ modified surfaces of clean glass promoted and maintained osteogenesis both in the presence and absence of biological stimuli, but these surfaces did not support long-term chondrogenesis under any test conditions. Incorporating

TABLE 9.6

Differentiation Supplements in the Medium for MSCs

Differentiation Type	Supplements
Osteogenic differentiation	Dexamethasone (Dex), L-ascorbic acid-2-phosphate (AsAP) or ascorbic acid, β-glycerophosphate
Chondrogenic differentiation	Dex, AsAP, TGF-β or BMP-2, BMP-6
Adipogenic	1-Methyl-3-isobutylxanthine, Dex, insulin, and indomethacin
Neuronal differentiation	Transferring, putrescine, insulin, progesterone, selenium, retinoic and brain-derived neurotrophic factor
Epidermal differentiation	EGF, FGF, insulin, retinoic acid $CalCl_2$ or insulin, transferrin, and selenite (ITS), Dex

pectin, which is rich in –COOH, into the chitosan network can improve the osteogenic differentiation of MSCs [61]. Moreover, the differentiation of stem cells is also affected by the scaffold structure. A decreased fiber diameter was found to enhance the chondrogenic differentiation of MSCs [213]. And MSCs have a higher osteogenic differentiation capacity on the nano-chitosan–gelatin–HAp surface than on the micro-chitosan–gelatin–HAp surface [214]. Chondrogenic differentiation of MSCs on chitosan was improved in fibrous scaffolds compared with porous scaffolds [215]. Above all, chitosan-based biomaterials can provide a simulated natural environment with chemical, topographical signals for stem cell differentiation. Developing 3D chitosan-based biomimetic scaffolds seems to be a shortcut to modulate stem cells under the natural repair and remodeling process.

In general, the chitosan-based biomaterial system must only partly mimic living tissues and must remain sufficiently far from the strict area of native ECMs. This concept is defined according to two criteria: one is related to the chemical structure and the other to the physical organization of the material. The ultimate objective of chitosan biomaterials is to construct appropriate chemical microenvironment, physical microenvironment, mechanical microenvironment, and bioactive microenvironment for cell growth and tissue regeneration. In order to achieve this goal, the marriage between materials science and biology needs to grow stronger.

References

1. Langer, R. and Vacanti, J. P. 1993. Tissue engineering. *Science* 260: 920–927.
2. Liu, C., Xia, Z., and Czernuszka, J. T. 2007. Design and development of three-dimensional scaffolds for tissue engineering. *Chem Eng Res Design* 85: 1051–1064.
3. Martino, A. D., Sittinger, M., and Risbud, M. V. 2005. Chitosan: A versatile biopolymer for orthopaedic tissue-engineering. *Biomaterials* 26: 5983–5990.
4. Yang, B., Li, X. Y., Shi, S., Kong, X. Y., Guo, G., Huang, M. J., Luo, F. L., Wei, Y. Q., Zhao, X., and Qian, Z. Y. 2010. Preparation and characterization of a novel chitosan scaffold. *Carbohydr Polym* 80: 860–865.
5. Sundararajan, V., Madihally, S. V., and Matthew, H. W. T. 1999. Porous chitosan scaffolds for tissue engineering. *Biomaterials* 20: 1133–1142.
6. Thein-Han, W. W. and Kitiyanant, Y. 2007. Chitosan scaffolds for *in vitro* buffalo embryonic stem-like cell culture: An approach to tissue engineering. *J Biomed Mater Res Part B: Appl Biomater* 80B: 92–101.
7. Liu, H. F., Mao, J. S., Yao, K. D., Yang, G. H., Cui, L., and Cao, Y. L. 2004. A study on a chitosan-gelatin-hyaluronic acid scaffold as artificial skin *in vitro* and its tissue engineering applications. *J Biomater Sci Polymer Edn* 15: 25–40.
8. Mao, J. S., Zhao, L. G., Yin, Y. J., and Yao, K. D. 2003. Structure and properties of bilayer chitosan-gelatin scaffolds. *Biomaterials* 24: 1067–1074.
9. He, J. K., Li, D. C., Liu, Y. X., Yao, B., Lu, B. H., and Lian Q. 2007. Fabrication and characterization of chitosan/gelatin porous scaffolds with predefined internal microstructures. *Polymer* 48: 4578–4588.
10. Toh, Y. C., Ng, S., Khong, Y. M., Zhang, X., Zhu, Y., Lin, P. C., Te, C. M., Wanxin Sun, W. S., and Yu, H. 2006. Cellular responses to a nanofibrous environment. *Nano Today* 1: 34–43.
11. Ohkawa, K., Dongil Cha, D., Kim, H., Nishida, A., and Yamamoto, H. 2004. Electrospinning of chitosan. *Macromol Rapid Commun* 25: 1600–1605.

12. Heinemann, C., Heinemann, S., Bernhardt, A., Worch, H., and Hanke, T. 2008. Novel textile chitosan scaffolds promote spreading, proliferation, and differentiation of osteoblasts. *Biomacromolecules* 9: 2913–2920.
13. Min, B. M., Lee, S. W., Lim, J. N., You, Y., Lee, T. S., Pil Hyun Kang, P. H., and Park, W. H. 2004. Chitin and chitosan nanofibers: Electrospinning of chitin and deacetylation of chitin nanofibers. *Polymer* 45: 7137–7142.
14. Geng, X. Y., Kwon, O. H., and Jang, J. 2005. Electrospinning of chitosan dissolved in concentrated acetic acid solution. *Biomaterials* 26: 5427–5432.
15. Schiffman, J. D. and Schauer, C. L. 2007. One-step electrospinning of cross-linked chitosan fibers. *Biomacromolecules* 8: 2665–2667.
16. Hasegawa, M., Isogai, A., Onabe, F., Usuda, M., and Atalla, R. H. 1992. Characterization of cellulose-chitosan blend films. *J Appl Polym Sci* 45: 1873–1979.
17. Ohkawa, K., Cha, D., Kim, H., Nishida, A., and Yamamoto, H. 2004. Electrospinning of chitosan. *Macromol Rapid Commun* 25: 1600–1605.
18. Ohkawa, K., Minato, K. I., Kumagai, G., Hayashi, S., and Yamamoto, H. 2006. Chitosan nanofiber. *Biomacromolecules* 7: 3291–3294.
19. Schiffman, J. D. and Schauer, C. L. 2007. Cross-linking chitosan nanofibers. *Biomacromolecules* 8: 594–601.
20. Jayakumar, R., Prabaharan, M., Nair, S. V., and Tamura, H. 2010. Novel chitin and chitosan nanofibers in biomedical applications. *Biotechnol Adv* 28: 142–150.
21. Chen, Z. G., BoWei, B., Xiumei Mo, X. M., Lim, C. T., Ramakrishna, S., and Cui, F. Z. 2009. Mechanical properties of electrospun collagen–chitosan complex single fibers and membrane. Electrospun collagen–chitosan nanofiber: A biomimetic extracellular matrix for endothelial cell and smooth muscle cell. *Mater Sci Eng C* 29: 2428–2435.
22. Chen, Z. G., Wang, P. W., Wei, B., Mo, X. M., and Cui, F. Z. 2010. Electrospun collagen–chitosan nanofiber: A biomimetic extracellular matrix for endothelial cell and smooth muscle cell. *Acta Biomater* 6: 372–382.
23. Dhandayuthapani, B., Krishnan, U. M., and Sethuraman, S. 2010. Fabrication and characterization of chitosan-gelatin blend nanofibers for skin tissue engineering. *J Biomed Mater Res Part B: Appl Biomater* 94B: 264–272.
24. Teng, S. H., Wang, P., and Kim, H. E. 2009. Blend fibers of chitosan–agarose by electrospinning. *Mater Lett* 63: 2510–2512.
25. Duan, B., Dong, C. H., Yuan, X. Y., and Yao, K. D. 2004. Electrospinning of chitosan solutions in acetic acid with poly (ethylene oxide). *J Biomater Sci Polymer Edn* 6: 797–811.
26. Xu, J., Zhang, J. H., Gao, W. Q., Liang, H. L., Wang, H. Y., and Li, J. F. 2009. Preparation of chitosan/PLA blend micro/nanofibers by electrospinning. *Mater Lett* 63: 658–660.
27. Malheiro, V. N., Caridade, S. G., Alves, N. M., and Mano, J. F. 2010. New poly(e-caprolactone)/chitosan blend fibers for tissue engineering applications. *Acta Biomater* 6: 418–428.
28. Li, L. and Hsieh, Y. L. 2006. Chitosan bicomponent nanofibers and nanoporous fibers. *Carbohydr Res* 341: 374–381.
29. Wu, L. L., Li, H., Li, S., Li, X. R., Yuan, X. Y., Li, X. L., and Zhang, Y. 2010. Composite fibrous membranes of PLGA and chitosan prepared by coelectrospinning and coaxial electrospinning. *J Biomed Mater Res* 92A: 563–574.
30. Kucharska, M., Walenko, K., Butruk, B., Brynk, T., Heljak, M., and Ciach, T. 2010. Fabrication and characterization of chitosan microspheres agglomerated scaffolds for bone tissue engineering. *Mater Lett* 64: 1059–1062.
31. Malafaya, P. B., Pedro, A. J., Peterbauer, A., Gabriel, C., Redl, H., and Reis, R. L. 2005. Chitosan particles agglomerated scaffolds for cartilage and osteochondral tissue engineering approaches with adipose tissue derived stem cells. *J Mater Sci: Mater Med* 16: 1077–1085.
32. Malafaya, P. B., Santos, T. C., van Griensven, M., and Reis, R. L. 2008. Morphology, mechanical characterization and *in vivo* neo-vascularization of chitosan particle aggregated scaffolds architectures. *Biomaterials* 29: 3914–3926.

33. Jiang, T., Abdel-Fattah, W. I., and Laurencin, C. T. 2006. *In vitro* evaluation of chitosan/poly (lactic acid-glycolic acid) sintered microsphere scaffolds for bone tissue engineering. *Biomaterials* 27: 4894–4903.

34. Henriksen, I., Green, K. L., Smart, J. D., Smistad, G., and Karlsen, J. 1995. Bioadhesion of hydrated chitosans: An *in vitro* and *in vivo* study. *Int J Pharm* 145: 231–240.

35. Mao, J. S., Cui, Y. L., Wang, X. H., Sun, Y., Yin, Y. J., Zhao, H. M., and Yao, K. D. 2004. A preliminary study on chitosan and gelatin polyelectrolyte complex cytocompatibility by cell cycle and apoptosis analysis. *Biomaterials* 25: 3973–3981.

36. Prasitsilp, M., Jenwithisuk, R., Kongsuwan, K., Damrongchai, N., and Watts, P. 2000. Cellular responses to chitosan *in vitro*: The importance of deacetylation. *J Mater Sci Mater Med* 11: 773–778.

37. Cao, W. L., Jing, D. H., Li, J. M., Gong, Y. D., Zhao, N. M., and Zhang, X. F. 2005. Effects of the degree of deacetylation on the physicochemical properties and Schwann cell affinity of chitosan films. *J Biomater Appl* 20: 157–177.

38. Izume, M., Taira, T., Kimura, T., and Miyata, T. 1989. *Chitin and Chitosan*. Amsterdam: Elsevier Applied Science.

39. Hamilton, V., Yuan, Y. L., Rigney, D. A., Chesnutt, B. M., Puckett, A. D., Ong, J. L., Yang, Y. Z. Haggard, W. O., Elder, S. H., and Bumgardner, J. D. 2007. Bone cell attachment and growth on well-characterized chitosan films. *Polym Int* 56: 641–647.

40. Chatelet, C., Damour, O., and Domard, A. 2001. Influence of the degree of acetylation on some biological properties of chitosan films. *Biomaterials* 22: 261–268.

41. Howling, G. I., Dettmar, P. W., Goddard, P. A., Hampson, F. C., Dornish, M., and Wood, E. J. 2001. The effect of chitin and chitosan on the proliferation of human skin fibroblasts and keratinocytes *in vitro*. *Biomaterials* 22: 2959–2966.

42. Suphasiriroj, W., Yotnuengnit, P., Surarit, R., and Pichyangkura, R. 2009. The fundamental parameters of chitosan in polymer scaffolds affecting osteoblasts (MC3T3-E1). *J Mater Sci Mater Med* 20: 309–320.

43. Okamoto, Y., Watanabe, M., Miyatake, K., Morimoto, M., Shigemasa, Y., and Minami, S. 2002. Effects of chitin/chitosan and their oligomers/monomers on migrations of fibroblasts and vascular endothelium. *Biomaterials* 23: 1975–1979.

44. Park, C. J., Gabrielson, N. P., Pack, D. W., Jamison, R. D., and Johnson, A. J. W. 2009. The effect of chitosan on the migration of neutrophil-like HL60 cells, mediated by IL-8. *Biomaterials* 30: 436–444.

45. Wu, H. G., Yao, Z., Bal, X. F., Du, Y. G., and Lin, B. C. 2008. Anti-angiogenic activities of chitooligosaccharides. *Carbohydr Polym* 73: 105–110.

46. Boucard, N., Viton, C., Agay, D., Mari, E., Roger, T., Chancerelle, Y., and Domard, A. 2007. The use of physical hydrogels of chitosan for skin regeneration following third-degree burns. *Biomaterials* 28: 3478–3488.

47. Amaral, I. F., Lamghari, M., Sousa, S. R., Sampaio, P., and Barbosa, M. A. 2005. Rat bone marrow stromal cell osteogenic differentiation and fibronectin adsorption on chitosan membranes: The effect of the degree of acetylation. *J Biomed Mater Res* 75A: 387–397.

48. Zhu, J. M. 2010. Bioactive modification of poly(ethylene glycol) hydrogels for tissue engineering. *Biomaterials* 31: 4639–4656.

49. Liu, H. F., Yin, Y. J., Yao, K. D., Ma, D. R., Cui, L., and Cao, Y. L. 2004. Influence of the concentrations of hyaluronic acid on the properties and biocompatibility of Cs–Gel–HA membranes. *Biomaterials* 25: 3523–3530.

50. Yuan, N. Y., Tsai, R. Y., Ming-Hwa Ho, M. H., Wang, D. M., Lai, J. Y., and Hsieh, H. J. 2008. Fabrication and characterization of chondroitin sulfate-modified chitosan membranes for biomedical applications. *Desalination* 234: 166–174.

51. Lopez-Perez, P. M., Marques, A. P., da Silva, R. M. P., Pashkuleva, I., and Reis, R. L. 2007. Effect of chitosan membrane surface modification via plasma induced polymerization on the adhesion of osteoblast-like cells. *J Mater Chem* 17: 4064–4071.

52. Cai, K. Y., Liu, W. G., Li, F., Yao, K. D., Yang, Z. M., Li, X. Q., and Xie, H. Q. 2002. Modulation of osteoblast function using poly(D,L-lactic acid) surfaces modified with alkylation derivative of chitosan. *J Biomater Sci Polym Edn* 13: 53–66.

53. Georges, P. C. and Janmey, P. A. 2005. Cell type-specific response to growth on soft materials. *J Appl Physiol* 98: 1547–1553.

54. McDaniel, D. P., Shaw, G. A., Elliott J. T., Bhadriraju, K., Meuse, C., Chung, K. H., et al. 2007. The stiffness of collagen fibrils influences vascular smooth muscle cell phenotype. *Biophys J* 92: 1759–1769.

55. Wells, R. G. 2008. The role of matrix stiffness in regulating cell behavior. *Hepatology* 47: 1394–1400.

56. Wang, H. B., Dembo, M., and Wang, Y. L. 2000. Substrate flexibility regulates growth and apoptosis of normal but not transformed cells. *Am J Physiol Cell Physiol* 279: C1345–C1350.

57. Engler, A. J., Sen, S., Sweeney, H. L., and Discher, D. E. 2006. Matrix elasticity directs stem cell lineage specification. *Cell* 126: 677–689.

58. Even-Ram, S., Vira, Artym. V., and Yamada, K. M. 2006. Matrix control of stem cell fate. *Cell* 126: 645–647.

59. Leipzig, N. D. and Shoichet, M. S. 2010. The effect of substrate stiffness on adult neural stem cell behavior. *Biomaterials* 30: 6867–6878.

60. Subramanian, A. and Lin, H. Y. 2005. Cross-linked chitosan: Its physical properties and the effects of matrix stiffness on chondrocyte cell morphology and proliferation. *J Biomed Mater Res* 75A: 742–753.

61. Li, J. J., Sun, H., Zhang, R., Li, R. Y., Yin, Y. J., Wang, H., Liu, Y. X., Yao, F. L., and Yao, K. D. 2010. Modulation of mesenchymal stem cells behaviors by chitosan/gelatin/pectin network films. *J Biomed Mater Res Part* 95B: 308–319.

62. Huang, Y., Siewe, M., and Madihally, S. V. 2006. Effect of spatial architecture on cellular colonization. *Biotechnol Bioeng* 93: 64–75.

63. Huang, Y., Onyeri, S., Siewe, M., Moshfeghian, A., and Madihally, S. V. 2005. *In vitro* characterization of chitosan–gelatin scaffolds for tissue engineering. *Biomaterials* 26: 7616–7627.

64. Nicodemus, G. D. and Bryant, S. J. 2008. Cell encapsulation in biodegradable hydrogels for tissue engineering applications. *Tissue Eng Part B* 14: 149–165.

65. Poon, Y. F., Ye Cao, Y., Liu, Y. X., Chan, V., and Chan-Park, M. B. 2010. Hydrogels based on dual curable chitosan-graft-polyethylene glycol-graft-methacrylate: Application to layer-by-layer cell encapsulation. *ACS Appl Mater Interf* 2: 2012–2025.

66. Hao, T., Wen, N., Cao, J. K., Wang, H. B., Lv, S. H., Liuy, T., Lin, Q. X., Duan, C. M., and Wang, C. Y. 2010. The support of matrix accumulation and the promotion of sheep articular cartilage defects repair *in vivo* by chitosan hydrogels. *Osteoarthritis and Cartilage* 18: 257–265.

67. Zielinski, B. A. and Aebischer, P. 1994. Chitosan as a matrix for mammalian cell encapsulation. *Biomaterials* 15: 1049–1056.

68. Yu, S. H., Buchholz, R., and Kim, S. K. 1999. Encapsulation of rat hepatocyte spheroids for the development of artificial liver. *Biotechnol Tech* 13: 609–614.

69. Hardikar, A. A., Risbud, M. V., and Bhonde, R. R. 2000. Improved post-cryopreservation recovery following encapsulation of islets in chitosan-alginate microcapsules. *Transplant Proc* 32: 824–825.

70. Haque, T., Chen, H., Ouyang, W., Martoni, C., Lawuyi, B., Urbanska, A. M., and Prakash, S. 2005. *In vitro* study of alginate–chitosan microcapsules: An alternative to liver cell transplants for the treatment of liver failure. *Biotechnol Lett* 27: 317–322.

71. Baruch, L. and Machluf, M. 2006. Alginate–chitosan complex coacervation for cell encapsulation: Effect on mechanical properties and on long-term viability. *Biopolymers* 82: 570–579.

72. Elisseeff, J., McIntosh, W., Fu, K., Blunk, B. T., and Langer, R. 2001. Controlled- release of IGF-I and TGF-beta1 in a photopolymerizing hydrogel for cartilage tissue engineering. *J Orthop Res* 19: 1098–1104.

73. Edelman, E., Mathiowitz, E., Langer, R., and Klagsbrun, M. 1991. Controlled and modulated release of basic fibroblast growth factor. *Biomaterials* 12: 619–626.

74. Jiang, T., Kumbar, S. G., Nair, L. S., and Laurencin, C. T. 2008. Biologically active chitosan systems for tissue engineering and regenerative medicine. *Curr Top Med Chem* 8: 354–364.

75. Lee, J. Y., Kim, K. H., Shin, S. Y., Rhyu, I. C., Lee, Y. M., Park, Y. J., Chung, C. P., and Lee, S. J. 2006. Enhanced bone formation by transforming growth factor-β1-releasing collagen/chitosan microgranules. *J Biomed Mater Res* 76A: 530–539.

76. Park, Y. J., Lee, Y. M., Lee, J. Y., Seol, Y. J., Chung, C. P., and Lee, S. J. 2000. Controlled release of platelet-derived growth factor-BB from chondroitin sulfate-chitosan sponge for guided bone regeneration. *J Control Release* 67: 385–394.

77. Ho, Y. C., Mi, F. L., Hsing-Wen Sung, H. W., and Kuo, P. L. 2009. Heparin-functionalized chitosan–alginate scaffolds for controlled release of growth factor. *Int J Pharm* 376: 69–75.

78. Abarrategi, A., Civantos, A., Ramos, V., Sanz Casado, J. V. S., and Lopez-Lacomba, J. L. 2008. Chitosan film as rhBMP2 carrier: Delivery properties for bone tissue application. *Biomacromolecules* 9: 711–718.

79. Karakecli, A. G., Satriano, C., Gumusderelioglu, M., and Marletta, G. 2008. Enhancement of fibroblastic proliferation on chitosan surfaces by immobilized epidermal growth factor. *Acta Biomater* 4: 989–996.

80. Park, Y. J., Kim, K. H., Lee, J. Y., Ku, Y., Lee, S. J., Min, B. M., and Chung, C. P. 2006. Immobilization of bone morphogenetic protein-2 on a nanofibrous chitosan membrane for enhanced guided bone regeneration. *Biotechnol Appl Biochem* 43: 17–24.

81. Weinberg, C. B. and Bell, E. 1986. A blood vessel model constructed from collagen and cultured vascular cells. *Science* 231: 397–400.

82. Swathi Ravi, S. and Chaiko, E. L. 2010. Biomaterials for vascular tissue engineering. *Regen Med* 5: 107–120.

83. Lanza, R., Langer, R., and Vacanti, J. P. 2000. *Principles of Tissue Engineering*, 2nd edn. San Diego: Academic Press, pp. 427–454.

84. Zhu, C. H., Fan, D. D., Duan, Z. G., Xue, W. J., Shang, L. G., Chen, F. L., and Luo, Y. N. 2009. Initial investigation of novel human-like collagen/chitosan scaffold for vascular tissue engineering. *Biomed Mater Res* 89A: 829–840.

85. Zhang, L., Ao, Q., Wang, A. J., Lu, G. Y., Kong, L. J., Gong, Y. D., Zhao, N. M., and Zhang X. F. 2006. A sandwich tubular scaffold derived from chitosan for blood vessel tissue engineering. *J Biomed Mater Res* 77A: 277–284.

86. Couet, F., Rajan, N., and Mantovani, D. Macromolecular biomaterials for scaffold-based vascular tissue engineering. *Macromol Biosci* 7: 701–718.

87. Chupa, J. M., Foster, A. M., Sumner, S. R., Madihally, S. V., and Matthew, H. W. T. 2000. Vascular cell responses to polysaccharide materials: *In vitro* and *in vivo* evaluations. *Biomaterials* 21: 2315–2322.

88. Madihally, S. V., Flake, A. W., and Matthew, H. W. 1999. Maintenance of CD34 expression during proliferation of CD34+ cord blood cells on glycosaminoglycan surfaces. *Stem Cells* 17: 295–305.

89. Shier, D., Butler, J., and Lewis, R. 1999. In *Hole's Human Anatomy and Physiology*, 8th edn. Boston, MA: McGraw Hill, pp. 160–183.

90. Fuchs, E. 2007. Scratching the surface of skin development. *Nature* 445: 834–842.

91. MacNeil, S. 2008. Biomaterials for tissue engineering of skin. *Mater Today* 11: 26–35.

92. Horch, R. E., Debus, M., Wagner, G., and Stark, G. B. 2000. Cultured human keratinocytes on type I collagen membranes to reconstitute the epidermis. *Tissue Eng* 6: 53–67.

93. Mao, J. S., Wang, X. H., and Yao, K. D. 2003. Studied on a novel human keratinocyte membrane delivery system *in vitro*. *J Mater Sci* 38: 2283–2290.

94. Schaum, D. K. 2008. Should it be coded as a dressing or as a dermal/epidermal (substitute) tissue? *Adv Skin Wound Care* 21: 317–321.

95. Yang, G. H., Yang, J., Wang, J. M., Cui, L., Liu, W., and Cao, Y. L. 2005. Biological behaviors of keratinocytes cultured on chitosan-gelatin membrane. ASBM6: *Adv Biomater* VI 288–289: 401–404.

96. Ikemoto, S., Mochizuki, M., Yamada, M., Takeda, A., Uchinuma, E., Yamashina, S., Nomizu, M., and Kadoya, Y. 2006. Laminin peptide-conjugated chitosan membrane: Application for keratinocyte delivery in wounded skin. *J Biomed Mater Res* 79A: 716–722.

97. Yang, J., Woo, S. L., Yang, G. H., Wang, J. M., Cui, L., Liu, W., and Cao, Y. L. 2010. Construction and clinical application of a human tissue-engineered epidermal membrane. *Plast Reconstr Surg* 125: 901–909.

98. Liu, H. F., Yin, Y. J., and Yao, K. D. 2007. Construction of chitosan-gelatin-hyaluronic acid artificial skin. *J Biomater Appl* 21: 413–430.

99. Lu, S. Y., Gao, W. J., and Gu, H. Y. 2008. Construction, application and biosafety of silver nanocrystalline chitosan wound dressing. *Burns* 34: 623–628.

100. Zhang, Y., He, H., Gao, W. G., Lu, S. Y., Liu, Y., and Gu, H. Y. 2009. Rapid adhesion and proliferation of keratinocytes on the gold colloid/chitosan film scaffold. *Mater Sci Eng C* 29: 908–912.

101. Peng, C. C., Yang, M. H., Chiu, W. T., Chiu, C. H., Yang, C. S., Chen, Y. W., Chen, K. C., and Peng, R. Y. 2008. Composite nano-titanium oxide–chitosan artificial skin exhibits strong wound-healing effect-an approach with anti-inflammatory and bactericidal kinetics. *Macromol Biosci* 8: 316–327.

102. Ma, L., Gao, C. Y., Mao, Z. W., Zhou, J., Shen, J. C., and Hu, X. Q., and Han, C. M. 2003. Collagen/chitosan porous scaffolds with improved biostability for skin tissue engineering. *Biomaterials* 24: 4833–4841.

103. Tsai, S. T., Hsieh, C. Y., Wang, D. M., Huang, L. L. H., Juin-Yih Lai, J. Y., and Jen Hsieh, H. J. 2007. Preparation and cell compatibility evaluation of chitosan/collagen composite scaffolds using amino acids as cross-linking bridges. *J Appl Polym Sci* 105: 1774–1785.

104. Kellouche, S., Martin, C., Korb, G., Rezzonico, R., Bouard, D., Benbunan, M., Dubertret, L., Soler, C., Legrand, C., and Dosquet, C. 2007. Tissue engineering for full-thickness burns: A dermal substitute from bench to bedside. *Biochem Biophy Res Comm* 363: 472–478.

105. Vaissiere, G., Chevallay, B., Herbage, D., and Damour, O. 2000. Comparative analysis of different collagen-based biomaterials as scaffolds for long-term culture of human fibroblasts. *Med Biol Eng Comput* 38: 205–210.

106. Duan, B., Wu, L. L., Yuan, X. Y., Hu, Z., Li, X. L., Yang Zhang, Y., Yao, K. D., and Wang, M. 2007. Hybrid nanofibrous membranes of PLGA/chitosan fabricated via an electrospinning array. *J Biomed Mater Res* 83A: 868–878.

107. Gao, C. Y., Wang, D. Y., and Shen, J. C. 2003. Fabrication of porous collagen/chitosan scaffolds with controlling microstructure for dermal equivalent. *Polym Adv Technol* 14: 373–379.

108. Tangsadthakun, C., Kanokpanot, S., Sanchavankit, N., Pichyangkura, R., Banaprasert, T., Tabata, Y., and Damrongskkul, S. 2007. The influence of molecular weight of chitosan on the physical and biological properties of collagen/chitosan scaffolds. *J Biomater Sci Polymer Edn* 18: 147–163.

109. Sun, L. P., Wang, S., Zhang, Z. W., Wang, X. Y., and Zhang, Q. Q. 2009. Biological evaluation of collagen–chitosan scaffolds for dermis tissue engineering. *Biomed Mater* 4: 055008.

110. Ding, C. M., Zhou, Y., He, Y. N., and Tan, W. S. 2008. Perfusion seeding of collagen-chitosan sponges for dermal tissue engineering. *Proc Biochem* 43: 287–296.

111. Lim, S. H., Son, Y. S., and Kim, C. H. 2007. The effect of a long-term cyclic strain on human dermal fibroblasts cultured in a bioreactor on chitosan-based scaffolds for the development of tissue engineered artificial dermis. *Macromol Res* 5: 370–378.

112. Lefler, A. and Ghanem, A. 2009. Development of bFGF-chitosan matrices and their interactions with human dermal fibroblast cells. *J Biomater Sci* 20: 1335–1351.

113. Liu, H. F., Fan, H. B., Cui. Y. L., Chen, Y. P., Yao, K. D., and Goh, J. C. H. 2007. Effects of the controlled-released basic fibroblast growth factor from chitosan-gelatin microspheres on human fibroblasts cultured on a chitosan-gelatin scaffold. *Biomacromolecules* 8: 1446–1455.

114. Hutmacher, D. W., Goh, J. C. H., and Teoh, S. H. 2001. An introduction to biodegradable materials for tissue engineering applications. *Ann Acad Med Singapore* 30: 183–191.

115. Ma, J. B., Wang, H. J., He, B. L., and Chen, J. T. 2001. A preliminary *in vitro* study on the fabrication and tissue engineering applications of a novel chitosan bilayer material as a scaffold of human neofetal dermal fibroblasts. *Biomaterials* 22: 331–336.

116. Shi, Y. S., Ma, L., Zhou, J., Mao, Z. W., and Gao, C. Y. 2005. Collagen/chitosan-silicone membrane bilayer scaffold as a dermal equivalent. *Polym Adv Technol* 16: 789–794.

117. Ma, L., Shi, Y. C., Chen, Y. X., Haiguang Zhao, H. G., Gao, C. Y., and Han, C. M. 2007. *In vitro* and *in vivo* biological performance of collagen-chitosan/silicone membrane bilayer dermal equivalent. *J Mater Sci: Mater Med* 18: 2185–2191.

118. Neamnark, A., Sanchavanakit, N., Pavasant, P., Ratana Rujiravanit, R., and Supaphol, P. 2008. *In vitro* biocompatibility of electrospun hexanoyl chitosan fibrous scaffolds towards human keratinocytes and fibroblasts. *Eur Polym J* 44: 2060–2067.

119. Mao, J. S., Zhao, L. G., Yao, K. D., Shang, Q. X., Yang, G. H., and Cao, Y. L. 2003. Study of novel chitosan-gelatin artificial skin *in vitro*. *J Biomed Mater Res* 64A: 301–308.

120. Black, N. F., Bouez, C., Perrier, E., Schlotmann, K., Chapuis, F., and Damour, O. 2005. Optimization and characterization of an engineered human skin equivalent. *Tissue Eng* 11: 723–733.

121. Su, C. H., Sun, C. S., Wei Juan, S. W., Hu, C. H., Ket, W. T., and Sheut, M. T. 1997. Fungal mycelia as the source of chitin and polysaccharides and their applications as skin substitutes. *Biomaterials* 16: 1169–1174.

122. Mobasheri, A., Carter, S. D., Martin-Vasallo, P., and Shakibaei, M. 2002. Integrins and stretch activated ion channels; putative components of functional cell surface mechanoreceptors in articular chondrocytes. *Cell Biol Int* 26: 1–18.

123. Insall, J. 1974. The Pridie debridement operation for osteoarthritis of the knee. *Clin Orthop Relat Res* 101: 61–67.

124. Muzzarelli, R. A. A. 2009. Chitins and chitosans for the repair of wounded skin, nerve, cartilage and bone. *Carbohydr Polym* 76: 167–182.

125. Lahiji, A., Sohrabi, A., Hungerford, D. S., and Frondoza, C. G. 2000. Chitosan supports the expression of extracellular matrix proteins in human osteoblasts and chondrocytes. *J Biomed Mater Res* 51: 586–595.

126. Subramanian, A., Vu, D., Larsen, G. F., and Lin, H. Y. 2005. Preparation and evaluation of the electrospun chitosan/PEO fibers for potential applications in cartilage tissue engineering. *J Biomater Sci Polym Edn* 16: 861–873.

127. Lu, J. X., Prudhommeaux, F., Meunier, A., Sedel, L., and Guillemin, G. 1999. Effects of chitosan on rat knee cartilages. *Biomaterials* 20: 1937–1944.

128. Park, K. M., Lee, S. Y., Joung, Y. K., Na, J. S., Lee, M. C., and Park, K. D. 2009. Thermosensitive chitosan–Pluronic hydrogel as an injectable cell delivery carrier for cartilage regeneration. *Acta Biomater* 5: 1956–1965.

129. Jin, R., Moreira, L. S., Dijkstra, P. J., Karperien, M., van Blitterswijk, C. A., Zhong, Z. Y., and Feijen, J. 2009. Injectable chitosan-based hydrogels for cartilage tissue engineering. *Biomaterials* 30: 2544–2551.

130. Au, A., Ha, J., Polotsky, A., Krzyminski, K., Anna Gutowska, A., Hungerford, D. S., and Frondoza, C. G. 2003. Thermally reversible polymer gel for chondrocyte culture. *J Biomed Mater Res* 67A: 1310–1319.

131. Huaping Tan, H. P., Chu, C. R., Payne, K. A., and Marra, K. G. 2009. Injectable *in situ* forming biodegradable chitosan–hyaluronic acid based hydrogels for cartilage tissue engineering. *Biomaterials* 30: 2499–2506.

132. Montembault, A., Tahiri, K., Korwin-Zmijowska, C., Chevalier, X., Corvol, M. T., and Domard A. 2006. A material decoy of biological media based on chitosan physical hydrogels: Application to cartilage tissue engineering. *Biochimie* 88: 551–564.

133. GriVon, D. J., Sedighi, M. R., SchaeVer, D. V., Eurell, J. A., and Johnson, A. L. 2006. Chitosan scaffolds: Interconnective pore size and cartilage engineering. *Acta Biomater* 2: 313–320.

134. Senkoylu, A., Simsek, A., Sahin, F. I., Menevse, S., Ozogul, C., Denkbas, E. B., and Piskin, E. Interaction of cultured chondrocytes with chitosan scaffold. *J Bioact Compat Polym* 16: 136–144.

135. Concaro, S., Nicklasson, E., Ellowsson, L., Lindahl, A., Brittberg, M., and Gatenholm, P. 2008. Effect of cell seeding concentration on the quality of tissue engineered constructs loaded with adult human articular chondrocytes. *J Tissue Eng Regen Med* 2: 14–21.

136. Nettles, D. L., Elder, S. H., and Gilbert, J. A. 2002. Potential use of chitosan as a cell scaffold material for cartilage tissue engineering. *Tissue Eng* 8: 1009–1016.

137. Li, Z. S. and Zhang, M. Q. 2005. Chitosan–alginate as scaffolding material for cartilage tissue engineering. *J Biomed Mater Res* 75A: 485–493.
138. Shi, D. H., Cai, D. Z., Zhou, C. R., Rong, L. M., Wang, K., and Xu, Y. C. 2005. Development and potential of a biomimetic chitosan/type II collagen scaffold for cartilage tissue engineering. *Chinese Med J* 118: 1436–1443.
139. Thein-Han, W. W., Kitiyanant, Y., and Misra, R. D. K. 2008. Chitosan as scaffold matrix for tissue engineering. *Mater Sci Technol* 24: 1062–1075.
140. Xia, W. Y., Liu, W., Cui, L., Liu, Y. C., Zhong, W., Liu, D., Wu, J. J., Chua K., and Cao, Y. L. 2004. Tissue engineering of cartilage with the use of chitosan-gelatin complex scaffolds. *J Biomed Mater Res B* 71B: 373–380.
141. Francis Suh, J. K. and Matthew, H. W. T. 2000. Application of chitosan-based polysaccharide biomaterials in cartilage tissue engineering: A review. *Biomaterials* 21: 2589–2598.
142. Yan, J. H., Qi, N. M., and Zhang, Q. Q. 2007. Rabbit articular chondrocytes seeded on collagen-chitosan-GAG scaffold for cartilage tissue engineering *in vivo*. *Artif Cells Blood Substit Biotechnol* 35: 333–344.
143. Yan, J. H., Li, X. M., Liu, L. G., Wang, F. J., Zhu, T. W., and Zhang, Q. Q. 2006. Potential use of collagen-chitosan-hyaluronan tri-copolymer scaffold for cartilage tissue engineering. *Artif Cells Blood Substit Biotechnol* 34: 27–39.
144. Isnard, N., Robert, L., and Renard, G. 2003. Effect of sulfated GAGs on the expression and activation of MMP-2 and MMP-9 in corneal and dermal explant cultures. *Cell Biol Int* 27: 779–784.
145. Chen, Y. L., Lee, H. P., Chan, H. Y., Sung, L. Y., Chen, H. C., and Hu, Y. C. 2007. Composite chondroitin-6-sulfate/dermatan sulfate/chitosan scaffolds for cartilage tissue engineering. *Biomaterials* 28: 2294–2305.
146. Marijnissen, W. J. C. M., van Osch, G. J. V. M., Joachim Aigner, J., van der Veen, S. W., Hollander, A. P., Verwoerd-Verhoef, H. L., and Verhaar, J. A. N. 2002. Alginate as a chondrocyte-delivery substance in combination with a non-woven scaffold for cartilage tissue engineering. *Biomaterials* 23: 1511–1517.
147. Tigli, R. S. and Gumusderelioglu, M. 2009. Evaluation of alginate–chitosan semi IPNs as cartilage scaffolds. *J Mater Sci: Mater Med* 20: 699–709.
148. Li, Z. S., Gunn, J., Chen, M. H., Cooper, A., and Zhang, M. 2008. On-site alginate gelation for enhanced cell proliferation and uniform distribution in porous scaffolds. *J Biomed Mater Res* 86A: 552–559.
149. Iwasaki, N., Yamane, S. T., Majima, T., Kasahara, Y., Minami, A., Harada, K., Nonaka, S. et al. 2004. Feasibility of polysaccharide hybrid materials for scaffolds in cartilage tissue engineering: Evaluation of chondrocyte adhesion to polyion complex fibers prepared from alginate and chitosan. *Biomacromolecules* 5: 828–833.
150. Hsu, S. H., Whu, S. W., Hsieh, S. C., Tsai, C. L., Chen, D. C., and Tan, T. S. 2004. Evaluation of chitosan-alginate-hyaluronate complexes modified by an RGD-containing protein as tissue-engineering scaffolds for cartilage regeneration. *Artifi Organ* 28: 693–703.
151. Kuo, Y. C. and Ku, I. K. 2008. Cartilage regeneration by novel polyethylene oxide/chitin/chitosan scaffolds. *Biomacromolecules* 9: 2662–2669.
152. Kuo, Y. C. and Hsu, Y. R. 2009. Tissue-engineered polyethylene oxide/chitosan scaffolds as potential substitutes for articular cartilage. *J Biomed Mater Res* 91A: 277–287.
153. Mukai, S., Ito, H., Nakagawa, Y., Akiyama, H., Miyamoto, M., and Nakamura, T. 2005. Transforming growth factor-β1 mediates the effects of low-intensity pulsed ultrasound in chondrocytes. *Ultrasound Med Biol* 31: 1713–1721.
154. Lee, J. E., Kim, K. E., Kwon, I. C., Ahn, H. J., Lee, S. H., Cho, H., Kim, H. J., Seong, S. C., and Lee, M. C. 2004. Effects of the controlled-released TGF-beta 1 from chitosan microspheres on chondrocytes cultured in a collagen/chitosan/glycosaminoglycan scaffold. *Biomaterials* 25: 4163–4173.
155. Guo, T., Zhao, J. N., Chang, J. B., Ding, Z., Hong, H., Chen, J. N., and Zhang, J. F. 2006. Porous chitosan-gelatin scaffold containing plasmid DNA encoding transforming growth factor-b1 for chondrocytes proliferation. *Biomaterials* 27: 1095–1103.

156. Stevens, M. M., and George, J. H. 2005. Exploring and engineering the cell surface interface. *Science* 310: 1135–1138.

157. Stevens, M. M. 2008. Biomaterials for bone tissue engineering. *Mater Today* 11: 18–25.

158. Ducy, P., Schinke, T., and Gerard Karsenty, G. 2000.The osteoblast: A sophisticated fibroblast under central surveillance. *Science* 289: 1501–1504.

159. Teitelbaum, S. L. 2000. Bone resorption by osteoclasts. *Science* 289: 1504–1508.

160. Sangsanoh, P., Orawan Suwantong, O., Neamnark, A., Cheepsunthorn, P., Pavasant, P., and Supaphol, P. 2010. *In vitro* biocompatibility of electrospun and solvent-cast chitosan substrata towards Schwann, osteoblast, keratinocyte and fibroblast cells. *Eur Polym J* 46: 428–440.

161. Fakhrya, A., Schneider, G. B., Zaharias, R., and Senel, S. 2004. Chitosan supports the initial attachment and spreading of osteoblasts preferentially over fibroblasts. *Biomaterials* 25: 2075–2079.

162. Seol, Y. J., Lee, J. Y., Park, Y. J., Lee, Y. M., Young-Ku, R. I. C., Lee, S. J., Han, S. B., and Chung, C. P. 2004. Chitosan sponges as tissue engineering scaffolds for bone formation. *Biotechnol Lett* 26: 1037–1041.

163. Kawai, T., Yamada, T., Yasukawa, A., Koyama, Y., Muneta, T., and Takakuda, K. 2009. Biological fixation of fibrous materials to bone using chitin/chitosan as a bone formation accelerator. *J Biomed Mater Res Part B: Appl Biomater* 88B: 264–270.

164. Jones, G. L., Motta, A., Marshall, M. J., El Haj, A. J., and Cartmell, S. H. 2009. Osteoblast: Osteoclast co-cultures on silk fibroin, chitosan and PLLA films. *Biomaterials* 30: 5376–5384.

165. Puppi, D., Chiellini, F., Piras, A. M., and Chiellini, E. 2010. Polymeric materials for bone and cartilage repair. *Prog Polym Sci* 35: 403–440.

166. Arpornmaeklong, P., Suwatwirote, N., Pripatnanont, P., and Oungbho, K. 2007. Growth and differentiation of mouse osteoblasts on chitosan-collagen sponges. *Int J Oral Maxillofac Surg* 36: 328–337.

167. Arpornmaeklong, P., Pripatnanont, P., and Suwatwirote, N. 2008. Properties of chitosan/collagen sponges and osteogenic differentiation of rat-bone-marrow stromal cells. *Int J Oral Maxillofac Surg* 37: 357–366.

168. Jung, U. W., Kim, S. K., Kim, C. S., Cho, K. S., Kim, C. K., and Choi, S. H. 2007. Effect of chitosan with absorbable collagen sponge carrier on bone regeneration in rat calvarial defect model. *Current Appl Phys* 7S1: e68–e70.

169. Li, Z. S., Ramay, H. R., Hauch, K. D., Xiao, D. M., and Zhang, M. Q. 2005. Chitosan–alginate hybrid scaffolds for bone tissue engineering. *Biomaterials* 26: 3919–3928.

170. Jiang, T., Nukavarapu, S. P., Deng, M., Jabbarzadeh, E., Kofron, M. D., Doty, S. B., Abdel-Fattah, W. I., and Laurencin, C. T. 2010. Chitosan-poly(lactide-*co*-glycolide) microsphere-based scaffolds for bone tissue engineering: *In vitro* degradation and *in vivo* bone regeneration studies. *Acta Biomater* 6: 3457–3470.

171. Thein-Han, W. W. and Misra, R. D. K. 2009. Biomimetic chitosan–nanohydroxyapatite composite scaffolds for bone tissue engineering. *Acta Biomater* 5: 1182–1197.

172. Chesnutt, B. M., Yuan, Y. L., Buddington, K., Haggard, W. O., and Bumgardner, J. D. 2009. Composite chitosan/nano-hydroxyapatite scaffolds induce osteocalcin production by osteoblasts *in vitro* and support bone formation *in vivo*. *Tissue Eng Part A* 15: 2571–2579.

173. Mukherjee, D. P., Tunkle, A. S., Roberts, R. A., Clavenna, A., Rogers, S., and Smith, D. 2003. An animal evaluation of a paste of chitosan glutamate and hydroxyapatite as a synthetic bone graft material. *J Biomed Mater Res B* 67: 603–609.

174. Zhao, F., Yin, Y. J., Lu, W. W., Leong, J. C., Zhang, W. J., Zhang, J. Y., Zhang, M. F., and Yao, K. D. 2002. Preparation and histological evaluation of biomimetic three-dimensional hydroxyapatite/chitosan-gelatin network composite scaffolds. *Biomaterials* 23: 3227–3234.

175. Wang, Y., Zhang, L. H., Hu, M., Liu, H. C., Wen, W. S., Xiao, H. X., and Niu, Y. 2008. Synthesis and characterization of collagen-chitosan-hydroxyapatite artificial bone matrix. *J Biomed Mater Res* 86A: 244–252.

176. Li, J. J., Chen, Y. P., Yin, Y. J., Yao, F. L., and Yao, K. D. 2007. Modulation of nano-hydroxyapatite size via formation on chitosan-gelatin network film *in situ*. *Biomaterials* 28: 781–790.

177. Lohmeyer, J. A. and Machens, H. G. 2009. Basics and current approaches to tissue engineering in peripheral nerve reconstruction. *Neurosurg Quart* 19: 101–109.

178. Pearson, R. G., Molino, Y., Williams, P. M., Tendler, S. J., Davies, M. C., Roberts, C. J., and Shakesheff, K. M. 2003. Spatial confinement of neurite regrowth from dorsal root ganglia within nonporous microconduits. *Tissue Eng* 9: 201–208.

179. Li, S. T. and Qakland, N. J. 1990. U.S. Patent 4,963,146.

180. Cheng, M. Y., Deng, J. G., Yang, F., Gong, Y. D., Zhao, N. M., and Zhang, X. F. 2003. Study on physical properties and nerve cell affinity of composite films from chitosan and gelatin solutions. *Biomaterials* 24: 2871–2880.

181. Yang, Y., Gu, X., Tan, R., Hu, W., Wang, X., Zhang, P., and Zhang, T. 2004. Fabrication and properties of a porous chitin/chitosan conduit for nerve regeneration. *Biotechnol Lett* 26: 1793–1797.

182. Pfister, L. A., Papaloizos, M., Merkle, H. P., and Gander, B. 2007. Hydrogel nerve conduits produced from alginate/chitosan complexes. *J Biomed Mater Res* 80A: 932–937.

183. Gong, H. P., Zhong, Y. H., Li, J. C., Gong, Y. D., Zhao, N. M., and Zhang, X. F. 2000. Studies on nerve cell affinity of chitosan-derived materials. *J Biomed Mater Res* 52: 285–295.

184. Cheng, H., Huang, Y. C., Chang, P. T., and Huang, Y. Y. 2007. Laminin-incorporated nerve conduits made by plasma treatment for repairing spinal cord injury. *Biochem Biophys Res Commun* 357: 938–944.

185. Suzuki, M., Itoh, S., Yamaguchi, I., Takakuda, K., Kobayashi, H., Shinomiya, K., and Tanaka, J. 2003. Tendon chitosan tubes covalently coupled with synthesized laminin peptides facilitate nerve regeneration *in vivo*. *J Neurosci Res* 72: 646–659.

186. Patel, M., Mao, L., Wu, B., and VandeVord, P. J. 2007. GDNF–chitosan blended nerve guides: A functional study. *J Tissue Eng Regen Med* 1: 360–367.

187. Wang, X. M., Zhang, J., Chen, H., and Wang, Q. R. 2009. Preparation and characterization of collagen-based composite conduit for peripheral nerve regeneration. *J Appl Polym Sci* 112: 3652–3662.

188. Yang, Z. Y., Mo, L. H., Duan, H. M., and Li, X. G. 2010. Effects of chitosan/collagen substrates on the behavior of rat neural stem cells. *Sci China Life Sci* 53: 215–222.

189. Patel, M., VandeVord, P. J., Matthew, H. W., De Silva, S., Wu, B., and Wooley, P. H. 2008. Collagen–chitosan nerve guides for peripheral nerve repair: A histomorphometric study. *J Biomater Appl* 23: 101–121.

190. Patel, M., VandeVord, P. J., Matthew, H. W., DeSilva, S., Wu, B., and Wooley, P. H. 2008. Functional gait evaluation of collagen chitosan nerve guides for sciatic nerve repair. *Tissue Eng Part C* 14: 365–370.

191. Wei, X., Lao, J., and Gu, Y. D. 2003. Bridging peripheral nerve defect with chitosan-collagen film, chin. *J Traumatol* 6: 131–134.

192. Ciardelli, G. and Chiono, V. 2006. Materials for peripheral nerve regeneration found the chitosan/gelatin also can promote the nerve regeneration. *Macromol Biosci* 6: 13–26.

193. Itoh, S., Suzuki, M., Yamaguchi, I., Takakuda, K., Kobayashi, H., Shinomiya, K., and Tanaka, J. 2003. Development of a nerve scaffold using a tendon chitosan tube. *Artif Organs* 27: 1079–1088.

194. Wang, W., Itoh, S., Matsuda, A., Ichinose, S., Shinomiya, K., Hata, Y., and Tanaka, J. 2008. Influences of mechanical properties and permeability on chitosan nano/microfiber mesh tubes as a scaffold for nerve regeneration. *J Biomed Mater Res* 84A: 557–566.

195. Wang, W., Itoh, S., Matsuda, A., Aizawa, T., Demura, M., Ichinose, S., Shinomiya, K., and Tanaka, J. 2008. Enhanced nerve regeneration through a bilayered chitosan tube: The effect of introduction of glycine spacer into the CYIGSK sequence. *J Biomed Mater Res* 85A: 919–928.

196. Wang, W., Itoh, S., Konno, K., Kikkawa, K., Ichinose, S., Sakai, K., Ohkuma, T., and Watabe, K. 2009. Effects of Schwann cell alignment along the oriented electrospun chitosan nanofibers on nerve regeneration. *J Biomed Mater Res* 91A: 994–1005.

197. Yang, Y. M., Wu, J., Wang, X. D., Liu, J., Ding, F., and Gu, X. S. 2009. Fabrication and evaluation of chitin-based nerve guidance conduits used to promote peripheral nerve regeneration. *Adv Eng Mater* 11: B209–B218.

198. Wang, G., Lu, G. Y., Ao, Q., Gong, Y. D., and Zhang, X. F. 2010. Preparation of cross-linked carboxymethyl chitosan for repairing sciatic nerve injury in rats. *Biotechnol Lett* 32: 59–66.

199. Seal, B. L., Otero, T. C., and Panitch, A. 2001. Polymeric biomaterials for tissue and organ regeneration. *Mater Sci Eng R* 34: 147–230.

200. Elcin, Y. M., Dixit, V., and Gitnick, G. 1998. Hepatocyte attachment on biodegradable modified chitosan membranes: *In vitro* evaluation for the development of liver organoids. *Artif Organs* 22: 837–846.

201. Yan, Y. N., Wang, X. H., Pan, Y. Q., Liu, H. X., Cheng, J. C., Xiong, Z., Lin, F., Wu, R. D., Zhang, R. J., and Lu, Q. P. 2005. Fabrication of viable tissue-engineered constructs with 3D cell-assembly technique. *Biomaterials* 26: 5864–5871.

202. Wang, X. H., Yu, X., Yan, X. N., and Zhang, R. J. 2008. Liver tissue responses to gelatin and gelatin/chitosan gels. *J Biomed Mater Res* 87A: 62–68.

203. Yang, J., Chung, T. W., Nagaoka, M., Goto, M., Cho, C. S., and Akaike, T. 2001. Hepatocyte-specific porous polymer-scaffolds of alginate/galactosylated chitosan sponge for liver-tissue engineering. *Biotechnol Lett* 23: 1385–1389.

204. Seo, S. J., Kim, I. Y., Choi, Y. J., Akaike, T., and Cho, C. S. 2006. Enhanced liver functions of hepatocytes cocultured with NIH 3T3 in the alginate/galactosylated chitosan scaffold. *Biomaterials* 27: 1487–1495.

205. Li, J. L., Pan, J. L., Zhang, L. G., and Yu, Y. T. 2003. Culture of hepatocytes on fructose-modified chitosan scaffolds. *Biomaterials* 24: 2317–2322.

206. Ranucci, C. S. and Moghe, P. V. 1999. Polymer substrate topography actively regulates the multicellular organization and liver-specific functions of cultured hepatocytes. *Tissue Eng* 5: 407–430.

207. He, J. K., Li, D. C., Liu, Y. X., Yao, B., Zhan, H. X., Lian, Q., Lu, B. H., and Lv, Y. 2009. Preparation of chitosan–gelatin hybrid scaffolds with well-organized microstructures for hepatic tissue engineering. *Acta Biomater* 5: 453–461.

208. Leonga, K. F., Chua, C. K., Sudarmadji, N., and Yeong, W. Y. 2008. Engineering functionally graded tissue engineering scaffolds. *J Mechanical Behavior Biomed Mater* 1: 140–152.

209. Wu, H., Wan, Y., Cao, X. Y., Dalai, S., Wang, S. W., and Zhang, S. M. 2008. Fabrication of chitosan-g-polycaprolactone copolymer scaffolds with gradient porous microstructures. *Mater Lett* 62: 2733–2736.

210. Liao, S., Casey K., Chan, C. K., and Ramakrishna, R. 2008. Stem cells and biomimetic materials strategies for tissue engineering. *Mater Sci Eng C* 28: 1189–1202.

211. Curran, J. M., Chen, R., and Hunt, J. A. 2006. The guidance of human mesenchymal stem cell differentiation *in vitro* by controlled modifications to the cell substrate. *Biomaterials* 27: 4783–9473.

212. Curran, J. M., Chen, R., and Hunt, J. A. 2005. Controlling the phenotype and function of mesenchymal stem cells *in vitro* by adhesion to silane modified clean glass surfaces. *Biomaterials* 26: 7057–7067.

213. Wise, J. K., Yarin, A. L., and Megaridis, C. M. 2009. Chondrogenic differentiation of human mesenchymal stem cells on oriented nanofibrous scaffolds: Engineering the superficial zone of articular cartilage. *Tissue Eng Part A* 15: 913–921.

214. Li, J. J., Dou, Y., Yang, J., Yin, Y. J., Zhang, H., Yao, F. L., Wang, H. B., and Yao, K. D. 2009. Surface characterization and biocompatibility of micro- and nano-hydroxyapatite/chitosan-gelatin network films. *Mater Sci Eng C* 29: 1207–1215.

215. Ragetly, G. R., Griffon, D. J., Lee, H. B., Page Fredericks, L., Gordon-Evans, W., and Chung, Y. S. 2010. Effect of chitosan scaffold microstructure on mesenchymal stem cell chondrogenesis. *Acta Biomater* 6: 1430–1436.

10

Future

Dunwan Zhu, Xigang Leng, and Kangde Yao

CONTENTS

10.1 Complexity of a Live System

10.1.1 Architectures of a Live System

Cells are the basic structural and functional units of organisms. The human body is composed of numerous cells. Humans may have hundreds of types of cells, the amount of which may be up to several trillions. These cells are well orderly assembled and perform various functions. A group of similar cells formed a tissue, organs with special functions were formed by tissues, systems were constructed with related organs, and a human being was constructed with several systems.

The protoplasm is the living content of a cell that is surrounded by a plasma membrane (cell membrane), which is composed of a mixture of small molecules such as ions, amino acids, monosaccharides, and water, and macromolecules such as nucleic acids, proteins, lipids, and polysaccharides. Due to their high molecular weight and complicated structure, these macromolecules are also referred to as biomacromolecules, which play a very important role in major life events of the organism. From the viewpoint of materials science, biomacromolecules can be regarded as the basic units of an assembled organism, and tissue is regarded as a composite material that is composed of cells and their extracellular matrices (ECMs).

10.1.2 Cells and Their ECMs

The ECM is the extracellular part of animal tissue that usually provides structural support to the animal cells in addition to performing various other important functions. The ECM, cells, and capillaries are physically integrated in functional tissues. ECM is not only a physical support for cells, but also provides a natural environment for cell proliferation and differentiation or morphogenesis, which contributes to cell-based tissue regeneration and organogenesis.

Components of the ECM are produced intracellularly by resident cells, and secreted into the ECM via exocytosis. Once secreted, they then aggregate with the existing matrix. ECM is composed of (1) fibers (collagen and elastin) and (2) a largely amorphous interfibrillary matrix (mainly proteoglycans, noncollagenous cell-binding adhesive glycoproteins, solutes, and water).

Collagen comprises a family of closely related but genetically, biochemically, and functionally distinct molecules, which are responsible for tissue tensile strength. The most common protein in the animal world, collagen provides the extracellular framework for all multicellular organisms. The collagens are composed of a triple helix of three polypeptide α-chains; about 30 different α-chains form at nearly 20 distinct collagen types. Types I, II, and III are the interstitial or fibrillar collagens and are the most abundant. Types IV, V, and VI are nonfibrillar (or amorphous) and are present in interstitial tissue and basement membranes.

Glycosaminoglycans (GAGs) are highly charged (usually sulfated) polysaccharide chains up to 200 sugars long, composed of repeating unbranched disaccharide units. GAGs are divided into four major groups on the basis of their sugar residues: (1) hyaluronic acid: a component of loose connective tissue and of joint fluid, where it acts as a lubricant; (2) chondroitin sulfate and dermatan sulfate; (3) heparan sulfate and heparin; and (4) keratin sulfate.

Elastins, in contrast to collagens, give elasticity to tissues, allowing them to stretch when needed and then return to their original state. This is useful in blood vessels, lungs, skin, and ligamentum nuchae, and these tissues contain high amounts of elastins. Elastins are synthesized by fibroblasts and smooth muscle cells. Elastins are highly insoluble, and tropoelastins are secreted inside a chaperone molecule, which releases the precursor molecule upon contact with a fiber of mature elastin. Tropoelastins are then deaminated to become incorporated into the elastin strand. Diseases such as cutis laxa and Williams syndrome are associated with deficient or absent elastin fibers in the ECM.

Fibronectins are proteins that connect cells with collagen fibers in the ECM, allowing cells to move through the ECM. Fibronectins bind collagen and cell surface integrins, causing a reorganization of the cell's cytoskeleton and facilitating cell movement. Fibronectins are secreted by cells in an unfolded, inactive form. Binding to integrins unfolds fibronectin molecules, allowing them to form dimers so that they can function properly. Fibronectins also help at the site of tissue injury by binding to platelets during blood clotting and facilitating cell movement to the affected area during wound healing.

Laminins are proteins found in the basal laminae of virtually all animals. Rather than forming collagen-like fibers, laminins form networks of web-like structures that resist tensile forces in the basal lamina. They also assist in cell adhesion. Laminins bind other ECM components such as collagens, nidogens, and entactins.

10.1.3 Cell Events

Like cell–cell interactions, cell–matrix interactions have a high degree of specificity, requiring initial recognition, physical adhesion, electrical and chemical communication, cytoskeletal reorganization, and/or cell migration. Moreover, adhesion receptors may also act as transmembrane signaling molecules that transmit information about the environment to the inside of cells and mediate the effects of signals initiated by growth factors or compounds controlling tissue differentiation. Moreover, the components of the ECM (ligands) with which cells interact are immobilized and not in solution. However, soluble (secreted) factors also modulate cell–cell communication in the normal and pathological regulation of tissue growth and maturation. Cell surface adhesion molecules that interact with the ECM include the integrin adhesion receptors and the vascular selectins.

The integrins comprise a family of cell receptors with diverse specificity that bind ECM proteins, other cell surface proteins, and plasma proteins and control cell growth, differentiation, gene expression, and motility. Some integrins bind only a single component of the ECM, for example, fibronectin, collagen, or laminin. Other integrins can interact with several of these polypeptides. In contrast to hormone receptors, which have high affinity and low abundance, the integrins exhibit low affinity and high abundance, so that they can bind weakly to several different but related matrix molecules. This property allows the integrins to promote cell–cell interactions as well as cell–matrix binding.

Cell binding to the ECM through specific cell–substratum contacts is critical to cell-growth control through mechanical forces mediated through associated changes in cell shape and cytoskeletal tension. Focal adhesions are considered to represent the strongest such interactions. They comprise a complex assembly of intra- and extracellular proteins, coupled to each other through transmembrane integrins. Cell-surface integrin receptors promote cell attachment to substrates, especially those covered with the extracellular proteins fibronectin and vibronectin. These receptors transduce biochemical signals to the nucleus by activating the same intracellular signaling pathways that are used by growth factor receptors. The more the cells spread, the higher their rate of proliferation. The importance of cell spreading to their proliferation has been emphasized by experiments that used endothelial cells cultured on microfabricated substrates containing fibronectin-coated islands of various defined shapes and sizes on micrometer scale.

10.1.4 Interaction of Cell and Chitosan-Based Biomaterials

Chitosan is widely used as a drug delivery system and tissue engineering scaffold material due to its excellent properties including nontoxicity, biocompatibility, and biodegradability. Recently, many studies on chitosan material have reported that chitosan can facilitate the attachment, spreading, and proliferation of many mammalian cells, including Schwann cells, chondrocytes, and vascular smooth muscle cells.

Hwang et al. investigated the effect of chitin and its derivatives on nitrogen oxide (NO) production by activated RAW 264.7 macrophages [1]. Chitin and chitosan had a significant inhibitory effect on the production of NO by activated macrophages. Hexa-N-acetyl-chitohexaose and penta-N-acetylchitopentaose also inhibited NO production but with less potency. However, N-acetylchitotetraose, -triose, -biose, and monomer of chitin, N-acetylglucosamine, and glucosamine had little effect on the production of NO by activated cells. These results suggest that the promotional effect of chitinous material on wound healing may be related, at least partly, to inhibition of activated macrophage-mediated NO production.

Chitosan has been attracting increasing research efforts as a potential carrier owing to its excellent biocompatibility and biodegradability. Our previous study investigated the impact of arginine-modified chitosan/DNA nanoparticles on the function of the murine macrophage through observation of phagocytic activity and production of proinflammatory cytokines [2]. The results showed that both chitosan/DNA nanoparticles and arginine-modified chitosan/DNA nanoparticles, containing 20 μg/mL DNA, were internalized by almost all the macrophages in contact. This led to no significant changes, compared to the nonexposure group, in production of cytokines and phagocytic activity of the macrophages 24 h post coincubation, whereas exposure to lipopolysaccharides (LPS) induced obviously elevated cytokine production and phagocytic activity, suggesting that incorporation of arginine moieties into chitosan does not have a negative impact on the function of the macrophages.

10.1.5 Interaction of Stem Cell and Chitosan-Based Biomaterials

Stem cells with a self-renewal potential and a multilineage differentiation capacity have been considered as the best choice for the seeding cells in tissue engineering.

Bone marrow-derived mesenchymal stem cells (MSCs) have been extensively studied and have shown promising potential for applications [3]. Recent studies further show that chitosan has good characteristics for the attachment, proliferation, and viability of MSCs [4,5].

Shi et al. created a skin equivalent with characteristic dermal and epidermal architecture by combining dermal stem cells and hair follicle epidermal stem cells on a chitosan/collagen-based scaffold. The results showed that the chitosan/collagen matrix provide a suitable substrate for the tridimensional growth of skin stem cells [6].

10.2 Design of Smart Chitosan-Based Biomaterials

10.2.1 Scaffolds for Tissue Engineering

As one of the hot fields in present-day and future life sciences, tissue engineering finally aims at the restoration or replacement of a lost or damaged organ or body part with transplantation of new tissues in combination with supportive scaffolds and biomolecules.

Chitosan and its derivatives are considered as good candidates for scaffolds due to their polyelectrolyte properties, including the presence of reactive functional groups, gel-forming ability, high adsorption capacity, complete biodegradability, bacteriostatic, and fungistatic, and even antitumor influence [7]. Many chitosan derivatives are also biocompatible and nontoxic with living tissues [8,9].

The cationic nature of chitosan also allows for pH-dependent electrostatic interactions with anionic GAG and proteoglycans distributed widely throughout the body and other negatively charged species. This property is one of the important elements for tissue engineering applications because the numbers of cytokines/growth factors are known to be bound and modulated by GAG including heparin and heparan sulfate. A scaffold incorporating a chitosan–GAG complex may serve as a means of retaining and concentrating desirable factors secreted by colonizing cells. Moreover, Nishikawa et al. [10] reported that chitosan, structurally resembling GAG consisting of long-chain, unbranched, repeating disaccharide units, is considered to play a key role in modulating cell morphology, differentiation, and function.

10.2.2 Extracellular Carriers

Chitosan is a linear polysaccharide composed of randomly distributed N-acetyl-D-glucosamine and β-(1,4)-linked D-glucosamine. Compared with polyethyleneimine (PEI) (another well-studied polymer with generally high transfection efficiency but significant cytotoxicity), chitosan has lower transfectability. This is believed to be related to its comparatively weak endolysosomalytic proton sponge effect.

Park et al. [11] have used galactosylated chitosan-graft-poly(ethylene glycol) (GCP) as a DNA vector. The particle size of GCP–DNA complexes is small, with a minimal value of about 27 nm. DNA complexed with GCP is stable and protected against enzyme degradation with DNase. However, the transfection efficiency when using GCP–DNA complexes is very low, mainly because of interaction with plasma leading to dissociation of GCP–DNA complexes.

Our previous studies have proposed a DNA–N-dodecylated chitosan complex and salt-induced gene delivery (CS-12) from dodecyl bromide and chitosan (average molecular weight 700 kDa), assembled with DNA (salmon testes, average molecular weight 2 kbp) to form DNA-CS-12 polyelectrolyte complex [12]. Incorporating dodecylated chitosan can enhance the thermal stability of DNA. Pure DNA in the absence of dodecylated chitosan is hydrolyzed by DNase and can be broken into fragments. On the other hand, DNA dissociated from the complex is well protected and remains intact due to the protection from DNase offered by alkylated chitosan.

10.2.3 Intelligent Carriers

Chitosan-based environmentally sensitive hydrogels have enormous potential for various applications. Some environmental variables, such as low pH and elevated temperatures, are found in the body. For this reason, either pH-sensitive and/or temperature-sensitive hydrogels can be used for site-specific controlled drug delivery. Hydrogels that are responsive to specific molecules, such as glucose or antigens, can be used as biosensors as well as drug delivery systems.

If bonding between the therapeutic and hydrogel polymer is established by an enzyme-sensitive tether and broken by the specific enzyme produced during normal cell activity in or around the hydrogel, a "smart" drug delivery system (DDS) is created and its drug release is more specific to the target tissue. For example, a vascular endothelial growth factor (VEGF) can be covalently immobilized within a hydrogel network by enzyme-sensitive oligopeptides [13]. The release of VEGF is mediated by proteases (e.g., matrix metalloproteinases) secreted by migrating cells. The cell-demanded VEGF release matches the release profiles with the cellular activity that is critical during tissue regeneration.

A thermosensitive chitosan-Pluronic hydrogel was also produced by ultraviolet (UV) photo-cross-linking [14]. The chitosan and Pluronic groups were functionalized with photosensitive acrylate groups that were cross-linked by UV exposure. The resultant polymers could then form a physical network at temperatures above the low critical solution temperature (LCST). The hydrogel showed the sustained release of encapsulated human growth hormone and plasmid DNA, demonstrating its potential usefulness for preparing different types of drugs [14,15].

Numerous studies on DNA delivery with chitosan as a carrier biomaterial have shown effective expression of reporter genes *in vitro* and *in vivo* [16–18], promoting chitosan as an attractive candidate for siRNA delivery.

Chitosan can not only transfer plasmid DNA, but can also deliver RNA. Because of this, chitosan is useful for alleviating poor cellular uptake and rapid degradation of naked siRNA or miRNA both *in vitro* and *in vivo*. Such feasibility has been shown by Howard et al., who significantly reduced the number of enhanced green fluorescence protein-expressing epithelial cells in the bronchiole (43% and 37% reduction compared to the untreated and mismatch control, respectively) of mice via daily nasal administration of interpolyelectrolyte siRNA–chitosan complexes.

Interpolyelectrolyte complexes between chitosan and siRNA were used to form nano-particles for siRNA delivery and gene silencing applications. Physicochemical properties such as size, zeta potential, and complex stability of the nanoparticles were shown to be highly dependent on the structural parameters M_w and the degree of deacetylation (DD) of the chitosan polymer. It was found that chitosan/siRNA nanoparticles formed using high M_w (114 and 170 kDa) and DD (84%) chitosan formed at N:P 150 were the most stable and exhibited the highest (about 80%) *in vitro* gene knockdown, which was comparable to the best we have observed using other commercial reagents. This work demonstrates the application of chitosan as a nonviral carrier for siRNA and the pivotal role of polymeric properties in the optimization of gene silencing protocols.

10.2.4 Extension of Application Potential

Chitosan and its derivatives have great potential to be used in other biomedical applications. As a result of the biocompatible properties such as good blood compatibility and cell growth efficiency, grafted chitosan materials have potential to be used in cardiovascular applications [19]. It has been demonstrated that the permeability of chitosan membranes grafted with hydroxyethyl methacrylate (HEMA) may be controlled through plasma treatment that has the potential to be used in dialysis [20].

Stimuli-responsive hydrogels have shown an improved drug-loading capacity and a sustained release behavior [21]. In particular, systems that combine chitosan and poly(*N*-isopropylacrylamide) (PNIPAAm) have shown drug release profiles that can be controlled by both pH and temperature, constituting very promising materials [22,23]. This kind of smart system has also been proposed for gene delivery. Our previous research [24] coupled a carboxyl-terminated NIPAAm–vinyl laurate (VL) copolymer with chitosan (PNVLCS) and examined the gene expression of PNVLCS–DNA complexes in C_2C_{12} cells against temperature change. The results indicated that the transfection efficiency of PNVLCS–DNA complexes was improved by dissociation of the gene from the carrier by temporarily reducing the culture temperature to 20°C. By contrast, naked DNA and Lipofectamine did not demonstrate thermoresponsive gene transfection.

In addition to applications in controlled drug release, PNIPAAm-grafted chitosan-based materials have been exploited for controlling cell adhesion/detachment by changing the incubation temperature above or below its LCST [5,25]. Temperature-responsive chitosan-graft-PNIPAAm [5] were applied for culturing MSCs. Chitosan-g-PNIPAAm copolymers with chondrogenic MSCs showed promising potential for clinical applications, particularly as cell therapy technologies for treating vesicoureteral reflux [25].

10.3 Challenges Due to Interactions of Chitosan-Based Gels

Hydrogels are comprised of cross-linked polymer networks that have a high number of hydrophilic groups or domains. These networks have a high affinity for water, but are prevented from dissolving due to the chemical or physical bonds formed between the polymer chains. Water penetrates these networks causing swelling, giving the hydrogel its form.

Fully swollen hydrogels have some physical properties common to living tissues, including a soft and rubbery consistency, and low interfacial tension with water or biological fluids. The elastic nature of fully swollen or hydrated hydrogels has been found to minimize irritation to the surrounding tissues after implantation. The low interfacial tension between the hydrogel surface and body fluid minimizes protein adsorption and cell adhesion, which reduces the chances of a negative immune reaction [26].

Despite these many advantageous properties, hydrogels also have several limitations. The low tensile strength of many hydrogels limits their use in load-bearing applications and can result in the premature dissolution or flowing away of the hydrogel from a targeted local site. This limitation may not be important in many typical drug delivery applications (e.g., subcutaneous injection). More important, perhaps, are problems relating to the drug delivery properties of hydrogels. The quantity and homogeneity of drug loading into hydrogels may be limited, particularly in the case of hydrophobic drugs. The high water content and large pore sizes of most hydrogels often result in relatively rapid drug release, over a few hours to a few days. Ease of application can also be problematic; although some hydrogels are sufficiently deformable to be injectable, many are not, necessitating surgical implantation. Each of these issues significantly restricts the practical use of hydrogel-based drug delivery therapies in the clinic.

Recently, researchers have developed other hydrogels using chitosan copolymers in combination with poly(N-isopropyl acrylamide) and poloxamers whose hydrophobic group interactions dominate at elevated temperatures. These polymers have been recognized as good candidates for *in situ*, reversible hydrogel formation [27].

10.4 Challenge and Adaptability for Chitosan-Based Gels

10.4.1 Multiple Layers for Soft-Tissue Regeneration

Soft-tissue implant attempts to replace or augment most of the soft tissues in the body, such as artificial skin, ligament, tendon, cartilage, blood vessels, heart valves, and so on. Rives et al. [28] proposed a layering approach to fabricate plasmid-releasing scaffolds that provide localized transgene expression following implantation into intraperitoneal fat, a model site for cell transplantation. In our previous research, a novel absorbable scaffold composed of chitosan and gelatin was fabricated by freezing and lyophilizing methods, resulting in an asymmetric structure [29]. This bilaminar texture is suitable for preparing a bilayer skin substitute. The chitosan–gelatin scaffolds were more wettable and adsorbed more water than did chitosan alone. Keratinocytes were cocultured with fibroblasts in chitosan–gelatin scaffolds to construct an artificial bilayer skin *in vitro*. The artificial skin obtained was flexible and had good mechanical properties. Moreover, there was no contraction observed in the *in vitro* cell culture tests. The results suggested that chitosan–gelatin scaffolds were suitable for skin tissue engineering goals.

10.4.2 Vascularization and Structure for Hard Tissue Regeneration

Although tissue engineering has made significant progress in culturing large amounts of cells *in vitro* and in the design and usage of support materials to deliver the cells *in vivo*, the number of clinical applications in the field of tissue engineering is still limited. One of the current limitations of tissue engineering is its inability to provide sufficient blood supply in the initial phase after implantation. Insufficient vascularization can lead to improper cell integration or cell death in tissue-engineered constructs. It is necessary to discuss the advantages and limitations of some recent strategies aimed at enhancing the vascularization of tissue-engineered constructs.

A critical obstacle in tissue engineering is the inability to maintain large masses of living cells, upon transfer from the *in vitro* culture conditions into the host, *in vivo* [29]. To achieve the goals of engineering large complex tissues, and possibly internal organs, vascularization of the regenerating tissue is essential. A tissue more than a few millimeters in volume cannot survive by diffusion and requires the formation of new blood capillaries to supply essential nutrients and oxygen [30].

After implantation of tissue constructs, the supply of oxygen and nutrients to the implant is often limited by diffusion processes that can only supply cells in the proximity of 100–200 mm from the next capillary. In order for implanted tissues of greater size to survive, the tissue has to be vascularized, which means that a capillary network capable of delivering nutrients to the cells is formed within the tissue. After implantation, blood vessels from the host generally invade the tissue to form such a network, in part in response to signals that are secreted by the implanted cells as a reaction to hypoxia.

10.4.3 Functionalization for Organ Regeneration

The majority of current reconstructive techniques rely on donor tissue for replacement; however, a shortage of donor tissue may limit these types of reconstructions, and usually significant morbidity is associated with the harvest procedure. Furthermore, the functional aspects of the damaged organ are rarely replaced by these reconstructive procedures, and they may even lead to complications because of the inherently different functional parameters of reconstructed tissue.

Because the speed of vascularization after implantation is a major problem in tissue engineering, the successful use of tissue-engineered constructs is currently limited to thin or avascular tissues, such as skin or cartilage, for which postimplantation neovascularization from the host is sufficient to meet the demand for oxygen and nutrients [31]. To succeed in the application of tissue engineering for bigger tissues, such as bones and muscles, the problem of vascularization has to be solved [32].

10.5 Disease Information for Drug Delivery Systems

Chitosan and chitosan derivatives, because of their excellent mucoadhesive and absorption-enhancing properties, have been extensively studied for the delivery of therapeutic proteins and antigens, particularly via mucosal routes.

Diabetes mellitus is an endocrine disease that is related to disorders of carbohydrate metabolism brought about by a deficiency in insulin secretion, insulin resistance, or both [33,34]. Chitosan displays mucoadhesive property and robust physicochemical stability that have been shown to be potentially useful for the delivery of insulin via the transmucosal pathway [35,36]. The positive effect of chitosan on transmucosal delivery of insulin has been explained by its capacity to open the tight junction between epithelial cells, thus facilitating the transport of macromolecular drug through well-organized epithelia via redistribution of F-actin, a protein of the cytoskeleton which regulates paracellular flow [37,38].

The addition of poly(ethylene glycol) significantly decreased both the burst release and the encapsulation efficiency, whereas the addition of alginate reduced the burst release, while protein loading remained high [39].

In recent years, it has been demonstrated that chitosan derivatives such as thiolated or quaternized chitosan have superior mucoadhesive and absorption-enhancing properties. These chitosan derivatives might be efficient in both soluble and particulate forms. It can be concluded that so far chitosan-based particles do not fulfill all the criteria needed for the delivery of therapeutic proteins. Factors such as poor efficacy and avoidance of possible immunogenicity of therapeutic proteins as well as possible long-term toxicity of chitosan-based polymers need further investigation.

Chitosan-based systems offer great opportunities for the delivery of protein therapeutics and antigens. To achieve clinical exploitation of chitosan-based formulations of therapeutic proteins, some important hurdles need to be cleared. Chitosan-based vaccines have shown excellent potential in preclinical models and promising results in clinical trials; however, also for these systems, further optimizations are necessary for obtaining clinical approval.

References

1. Hwang, S. M., Chen, C. Y., Chen, S. S., and Chen, J. C. 2000. Chitinous materials inhibit nitric oxide production by activated RAW 264.7 macrophages. *Biochem Biophys Res Commun* 271: 229–233.
2. Liu, L. X., Bai, Y. Y., Song, C. N., Zhu, D. W., Song, L. P., Zhang, H. L., Dong, X., and Leng, X. G. 2010. The impact of arginine-modified chitosan–DNA nanoparticles on the function of macrophages. *J Nanopart Res* 12: 1637–1644.
3. Short, B., Brouard, N., Occhiodoro-Scott, T., Ramakrishnan, A., and Simmons, P. J. 2003. Mesenchymal stem cells. *Arch Med Res* 34: 565–571.
4. Dang, J. M., Sun, D. D., Shin-Ya, Y., Sieberb, A. N., Kostuik, J. P., and Leong, K. W. 2006. Temperature-responsive hydroxybutyl chitosan for the culture of mesenchymal stem cells and intervertebral disk cells. *Biomaterials* 27: 406–418.
5. Cho, J. H., Kim, S. H., Park, K. D., Jung, M. Y., Yang, W. I., Han, S. W., Noh, J. Y., and Lee, J. W. 2004. Chondrogenic differentiation of human mesenchymal stem cells using a thermosensitive poly(N-isopropylacrylamide) and water-soluble chitosan copolymer[J]. *Biomaterials* 25: 5743–5751.
6. Shi, C., Cheng, T., Su, Y., and Mai, Y. 2004. Significance of dermis-derived multipotent stem cells in wound healing and skin equivalent construction. 2004. *Joint International Tissue Engineering Society (TESI) and European Tissue Engineering Society (ETES) Meeting*, Lausanne, October 10–13, Switzerland.
7. Shahidi, F. and Abuzaytoun, R. 2005. Chitin, chitosan, and co-products: Chemistry, production, applications, and health effects. *Adv Food Nutr Res* 49: 93–135.
8. Hejazi, R. and Amiji, M. 2003. Chitosan-based gastrointestinal delivery systems. *J Control Release* 89: 151–165.
9. Khor, E. and Lim, L. Y. 2003. Implantable applications of chitin and chitosan. *Biomaterials* 24: 2339–2349.

10. Nishikawa, H., Ueno, A., Nishikawa, S., Kido, J., Ohishi, M., Inoue, H., and Nagata, T. 2000. Sulfated glycosaminoglycan synthesis and its regulation by transforming growth factor-beta in rat clonal dental pulp cells. *J Endod* 26: 169–171.

11. Park, I. K., Kim, T. H., Park YH, Shin, B. A., Choi, E. S., Chowdhury, E. H., Akaike, T., and Cho, C. S. 2001. Galactosylated chitosan-graft-poly(ethylene glycol) as hepatocyte-targeting DNA carrier. *J Control Release* 76: 349–362.

12. Liu, W. G., Yao, K. D., and Liu, Q. G. 2001. Formation of a DNA–N-dodecylated chitosan complex and salt-induced gene delivery. *J Appl Polym Sci* 82: 3391–3395.

13. Zisch, A. H., Lutolf, M. P., Ehrbar, M., Raeber, G. P., Rizzi, S. C., Davies, N., Schmokel, H. et al. 2003. Cell-demanded release of VEGF from synthetic, biointeractive cell ingrowth matrices for vascularized tissue growth. *FASEB J* 17: 2260–2262.

14. Yoo, H. S. 2007. Photo-cross-linkable and thermo-responsive hydrogels containing chitosan and Pluronic for sustained release of human growth hormone (hGH). *J Biomater Sci Polym Ed* 18: 1429–1441.

15. Lee, J. I., Kim, H. S., and Yoo, H. S. 2009. DNA nanogels composed of chitosan and Pluronic with thermo-sensitive and photo-cross-linking properties. *Int J Pharm* 373: 93–99.

16. Liu, W. G., Sun, S. J., Cao, Z. Q., Xin, Z., Yao, K. D., Lu, W. W., and Luk, K. D. K. 2005. An investigation on the physicochemical properties of chitosan/DNA polyelectrolyte complexes. *Biomaterials* 26: 2705–2711.

17. Li, X. W., Lee, D. K., Chan, A. S., and Alpar, H. O. 2003. Sustained expression in mammalian cells with DNA complexed with chitosan nanoparticles. *Biochim Biophys Acta* 1630: 7–18.

18. Kiang, T., Wen, J., Lim, H. W., and Leong, K. W. 2004. The effect of the degree of chitosan deacetylation on the efficiency of gene transfection. *Biomaterials* 25: 5293–5301.

19. Chung, T. W., Lu, Y. F., Wang, S. S., Lin, Y. S., and Chu, S. H. 2002. Growth of human endothelial cells on photochemically grafted Gly-Arg-Gly-Asp (GRGD) chitosans. *Biomaterials* 23: 4803–4809.

20. Li, Y., Liu, L., and Fang, Y. 2003. Plasma-induced grafting of hydroxyethyl methacrylate (HEMA) onto chitosan membranes by a swelling method. *Polym Int* 52: 285–290.

21. Prabaharan, M. and Mano, J. F. 2006. Stimuli-responsive hydrogels based on polysaccharides incorporated with thermo-responsive polymers as novel biomaterials. *Macromol Biosci* 6: 991–1008.

22. Alvarez-Lorenzo, C., Concheiro, A., Dubovik, A. S., Grinberg NV, Burova, T. V., and Grinberg, V. Y. 2005. Temperature-sensitive chitosan-poly(N-isopropylacrylamide) interpenetrated networks with enhanced loading capacity and controlled release properties. *J Control Release* 102: 629–641.

23. Bhattarai, N., Ramay, H. R., Gunn, J., Matsen, F. A., and Zhang, M. Q. 2005. PEG-grafted chitosan as an injectable thermosensitive hydrogel for sustained protein release. *J Control Release* 103: 609–624.

24. Sun, S. J., Liu, W. G., Cheng, N., Zhang, B. Q., Cao, Z. Q., Yao, K. D., Liang, D. C., Zuo, A. J., Guo, G., and Zhang, J. Y. 2005. A thermoresponsive chitosan-NIPAAm/vinyl laurate copolymer vector for gene transfection. *Bioconjug Chem* 16: 972–980.

25. Gil, E. and Hudson, S. 2004. Stimuli-responsive polymers and their bioconjugates[J]. *Prog Polym Sci* 29: 1173–1222.

26. Bhattarai, N., Gunn, J., and Zhang, M. 2010. Chitosan-based hydrogels for controlled, localized drug delivery. *Adv Drug Deliv Rev* 62: 83–99.

27. Hoffman, A. S. 2002. Hydrogels for biomedical applications. *Adv Drug Deliv Rev* 54: 3–12.

28. Rives, C. B., des Rieux, A., Zelivyanskaya, M., Stock, S. R., Lowe, W. L. Jr., and Shea, L. D. 2009. Layered PLG scaffolds for in vivo plasmid delivery. *Biomaterials* 30: 394–401.

29. Mao, J. S., Zhao, L. G., Yao, K. D., Shang, Q. X., Yang, G. H., and Cao, Y. L. 2003. Study of novel chitosan–gelatin artificial skin *in vitro*. *J Biomed Mater Res A* 64: 301–308.

30. Mooney, D. J. and Mikos, A. G. 1999. Growing new organs. *Sci Am* 280: 60–65.

31. Jain, R. K., Au, P., Tam, J., and Fukumura, D. 2005. Engineering vascularized tissue. *Nat Biotechnol* 23: 821–823.
32. Johnson, P. C., Mikos, A. G., Fisher, J. P., and Jansen, J. A. 2007. Strategic directions in tissue engineering. *Tissue Eng* 13: 2827–2837.
33. Carino, G. P. and Mathiowitz, E. 1999. Oral insulin delivery. *Adv Drug Deliv Rev* 35: 249–257.
34. Graves, P. M. and Eisenbarth, G. S. 1999. Pathogenesis, prediction and trials for the prevention of insulin-dependent (type 1) diabetes mellitus. *Adv Drug Deliv Rev* 35: 143–156.
35. Krauland, A. H., Guggi, D., and Bernkop-Schnurch, A. Oral insulin delivery: The potential of thiolated chitosan–insulin tablets on non-diabetic rats. *J Control Release* 95: 547–555.
36. Pan, Y, Li, Y. J., Zhao, H. Y., Zheng, J. M., Xu, H., Wei, G., Hao, J. S., and Cui, F. D. 2002. Bioadhesive polysaccharide in protein delivery system: Chitosan nanoparticles improve the intestinal absorption of insulin *in vivo*. *Int J Pharm* 249: 139–147.
37. Cano-Cebrian, M. J., Zornoza, T., Granero, L., and Polache, A. 2005. Intestinal absorption enhancement via the paracellular route by fatty acids, chitosans and others: A target for drug delivery. *Curr Drug Deliv* 2: 9–22.
38. Avadi, M. R., Jalali, A., Sadeghi, A. M. M., Shamimi, K., Bayati, K. H., Nahid, E., Dehpour, A. R., and Rafiee-Tehrani, M. 2005. Diethyl methyl chitosan as an intestinal paracellular enhancer: *Ex vivo* and *in vivo* studies. *Int J Pharm* 293: 83–89.
39. Xu, Y., Du, Y., Huang, R., and Gao, L. P. 2003. Preparation and modification of N-(2-hydroxyl) propyl-3-trimethyl ammonium chitosan chloride nanoparticle as a protein carrier. *Biomaterials* 24: 5015–5022.

Index